TOXICITY AND DRUG TESTING

Edited by **William Acree**

Toxicity and Drug Testing
Edited by William Acree

Published by InTech

Janeza Trdine 9, 51000 Rijeka, Croatia

Publishing Process Manager Molly Kaliman

Technical Editor Teodora Smiljanic

Cover Designer InTech Design Team

Additional hard copies can be obtained from orders@intechopen.com

Toxicity and Drug Testing, Edited by William Acree
p. cm.
ISBN 978-953-51-0004-1

For EU product safety concerns:
IN TECH d.o.o., Prolaz Marije Krucifikse Kozulić 3, 51000 Rijeka, Croatia,
info@intechopen.com or visit our website at intechopen.com.

Meet the editor

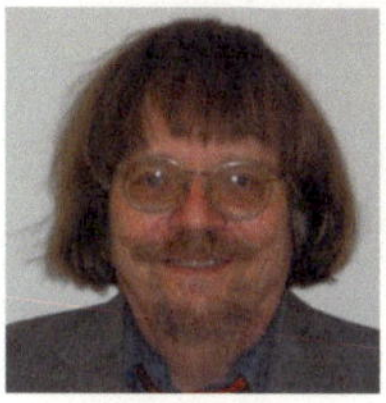

Dr William Acree is currently Professor of Chemistry at the University of North Texas. He has published more than 560 scientific research articles, plus five books, six book chapters and four encyclopedia articles. He serves as a member on the Editorial Advisory Boards of eight journals and has been a manuscript reviewer for over 60 leading international journals. Professor Acree's research interests involve developing quantitative structure-property relationships and linear free energy relationships to describe partitioning processes of chemical, environmental and pharmaceutical importance. To date he has derived expressions for predicting the solubility of drug molecules in water and in more than 70 organic solvents of varying polarity, for predicting the distribution of organic compounds and drugs between select rat (and human) tissue samples and blood, for predicting the toxicity of organic compounds to several aquatic organisms, and for predicting the solute partitioning between water and numerous organic solvents.

Contents

Preface

Book focuses on experimental in vivo and in vitro methods used to measure the ADMET properties (absorption, distribution, metabolism, excretion and toxicity) of potential drug candidates. Modern drug design also includes in silico computation methods to estimate ADMET properties, and several predictive methods are presented for drug solubility, blood-to-tissue partition coefficients, toxicity, nasal pungency and several other biological and sensory responses. One chapter is devoted to measurement uncertainty, bias and statistical treatment of experimental data. Analytical methods employed to identify and quantify genotoxic pharmaceutical impurities and drug metabolites are also described. Toxicity data from clinical studies are reported. Authors from several countries have contributed chapters detailing regulatory policies, pharmaceutical concerns and clinical practices in their respective countries. The open exchange of scientific results and ideas will hopefully lead to improved pharmaceutical products and a greater awareness of the vast toxicological issues that we all experience.

Dr. William Acree
University of North Texas,
United States

Part 1

Drug Design

1

Blood Brain Barrier Permeation

Abolghasem Jouyban[1] and Somaieh Soltani[2]
[1]Drug Applied Research Center and Faculty of Pharmacy,
[2]Liver and Gastrointestinal Diseases Research Center,
Tabriz University of Medical Sciences, Tabriz,
Iran

1. Introduction

The large surface area and the short diffusion distance from capillaries of the blood brain barrier (BBB) to the neurons facilitate the drugs and nutrients access to the brain. Penetration of chemicals to the BBB occurs using a combination of intra and intercellular passages. Tight junctions regulate the intracellular passage of molecules according to their physico- chemical properties (e.g. lipophilicity, ionisation and polarity), where inter cellular penetration is regulated by influx and efflux transporters, endocytosis and passive diffusion. Poor pharmacokinetic properties (absorption, distribution, metabolism and excretion) and toxicity are responsible for most of the failures in drug discovery projects. This problem is more evident for CNS drugs because of the restrict barrier function of blood brain barrier. The CNS drug discovery attracted more attentions since the diseases pattern has been changed during recent decades and aging disorders are one of the major health problems. Drug exposure is controlled by plasma pharmacokinetic properties of drug which are different from brain pharmacokinetic and can be studied using common pharmacokinetic studies, where BBB permeability depends on physicochemical properties of drug compound and physiologic function of the BBB (physical barrier, transport, metabolic, ...) and need special study techniques. In this chapter, fundamentals of BBB, permeation mechanisms, penetration measurement methods and penetration prediction methods are discussed.

2. Fundamentals of BBB

2.1 Cellular properties of Blood Brain Barrier

BBB consisted of a monolayer of brain micro vascular endothelial cells (BMVEC) joined together by much tighter junctions than peripheral vessels and formed a cellular membrane which known as the main physical barrier of BBB (Abbott, 2005; Cardoso et.al., 2010). The main characteristics of this cellular membrane are, uniform thickness, no fenestrae, low pinocytotic activity, continues basement membrane and negative surface charge. In addition to the BMVECs, the neurovascular unit consisted of the capillary basement membrane, pericytes, astrocytes and microglia. The BMVECs are surrounded by a basement membrane which composed of structural proteins (collagen and elastin), specialized proteins (fibronectin and laminin) and proteoglycans. This structural specificity gives the basement membrane a cell establishment role. Pericytes are cellular constituents of microvessels including capillaries and post capillary venules that covered about 22-32% of the capillaries and shared the same basement membrane. Pericytes are responsible for a wide variety of structural and non-structural tasks in BBB. In summary they synthesis some of structural and signalling proteins and they are involved in the BMVECs proliferation, migration and differentiation. More details and references about pericytes role in BBB can be found in the literature (Cardoso et al., 2010). Fine lamellae closely opposed to the outer surface of the capillary endothelium and respective basement membrane formed by astrocytes end feet. Like pericytes, astrocytes involve in various functional and structural properties of neurovascular unit.

Microglia is immunocompetent cells of the brain that continuously survey local micro environment with highly motile extensions and change the phenotype in response to the homeostatic disturbance of the CNS (Prinz & Mildner, 2011). The interactions of brain micro vascular endothelial cells with basement membrane, neighbouring glial cells (microglia and astrocytes), neurons and perivascular pericytes leads to specific brain micro vascular biology. Presence of matrix adhesion receptors and signalling proteins form an extensive and complex matrix which is essential for maintenance of the BBB (Cardoso et al., 2010). Figure 1 shows a schematic illustration of neurovascular unit and BBB cellular components.

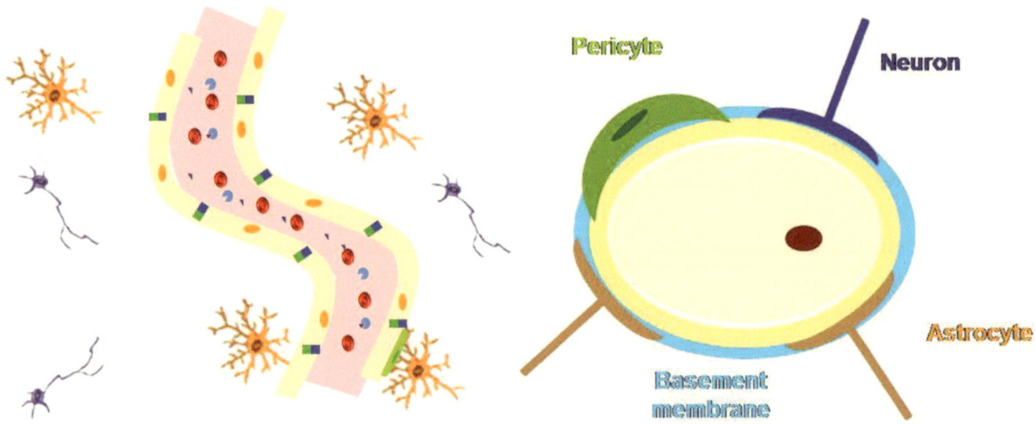

Fig. 1. Schematic illustration of the neurovascular unit and BBB cellular components adopted from (Cardoso et al., 2010).

2.2 Molecular properties of BBB

The BMVECs assembly are regulated by molecular constituents of tight junctions, adherence junctions and signalling pathways. Tight junctions are highly dynamic structures which are responsible for the barrier properties of BBB. Apical region of the endothelial cells sealed together by tight junctions and paracellular permeability of BMVECs are limited by them. Structurally tight junctions formed by interaction of integral transmembrane proteins with neighbouring plasma membrane. Among these proteins junction adhesion molecules, claudins and occludins (inter membrane) which bind to the cytoplasmic proteins (e.g. zonula occludens, cinguline, ...) are well studied and their role in tight junctions and BBB have been evaluated (Figure 2). Beyond the main role in physical restriction of BBB, other functions such as control of gene expression, cell proliferation and differentiation have been suggested for tight junctions. Below the tight junctions, actin filaments (including cadherins and catenins) linked together and form a belt of adherence junctions. In addition to the contribution in the barrier function some other events such as adhesion of BMVECs to each other, the contact inhibition during vascular growth, the initiation of cell polarity and the regulation of paracellular permeability have been suggested for adherence junctions. A dynamic interaction between tight junctions and adherence junctions through signalling pathways regulate the permeability of BBB. These signalling routes mainly involve protein kinases, members of mitogen - activated protein kinases, endothelial nitric oxide synthase and G-proteins. Dynamic interactions between these pathways control the opening and closing of the paracellular route for fluids, proteins and cells to move across the endothelial cells through two main types of signal transduction procedures (e.g. signals from cell interior to tight junctions to guide their assembly and regulate their permeability, signals transmitted from tight junctions to cell interior to modulate gene expression, proliferation and differentiation). The molecular mechanisms of these interactions can be found in the literature (Ballab et al., 2004; Abbott et al., 2006). In addition to the proteins with enzymatic activities, there are other specific proteins (drug efflux transporters, multi drug resistance proteins, organic anion transporting polypeptides) work as BBB transporters which are responsible for rapid efflux of xenobiotics from the CNS (Losscher & Potschka, 2005) and delivery of the essential nutrients and transmitters to the brain.

The combined effect of the special cellular and molecular properties of central nervous system result in the specific barrier functions of BBB which is important for preventing CNS from harmful xenobiotics. Because of these properties drug delivery to the CNS is among the most challenging drug development areas. In order to develop successful drug candidates for CNS disorders drug uptake mechanisms should be studied. In the next section, these mechanisms are briefly reviewed.

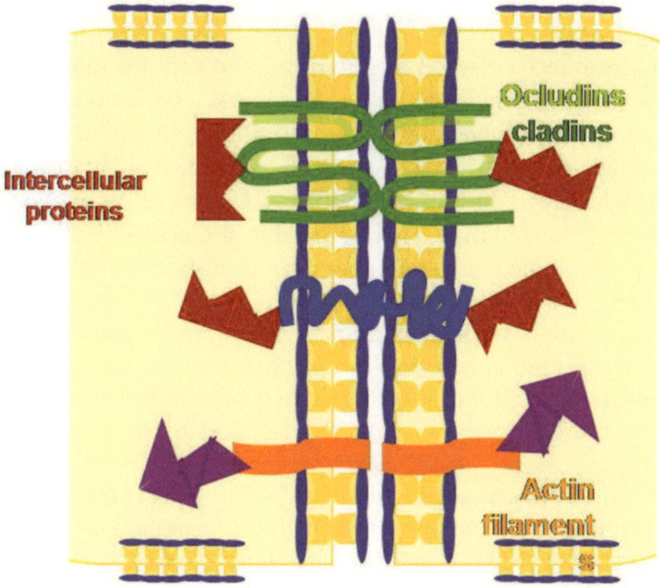

Fig. 2. Tight junctions and adherent junctions.

3. BBB permeation mechanisms

Like other cellular membranes in the body, permeation through BBB can occur by passive diffusion, endocytosis and active transport (Diagram 1). Combined effects of the mentioned mechanisms modulate the compound (e.g. Drugs) penetration to the brain.

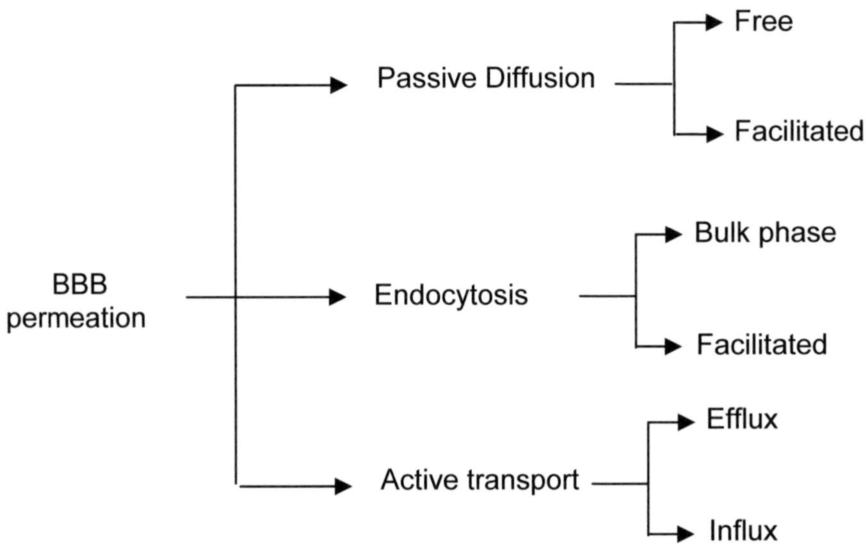

Diagram 1. Main permeation mechanisms in the brain.

3.1 Passive diffusion

A limited number of drugs and drug like compounds with high lipophilicity and low molecular size can penetrate to the brain mainly by passive diffusion. In order to overcome the surface tension difference between a compound and cellular membrane, physical work is needed and the smaller molecules will need less work. The uncharged forms of the weak acidic and basic compounds have higher permeability rate in comparison with charged molecules in physiologic pH of brain. The charged forms possess hydrophilic characteristics and hydrophilic drugs distribute within blood and cannot cross the endothelial cells and excreted from brain parenchyma. Therefore, the molecules with higher fraction of uncharged form in physiologic pH have higher permeability rate (Fischer et al., 1998).

Passive diffusion occurs via two mechanisms (Figure 3):

- Free diffusion in which some compounds move freely paracellularly (e.g. sucrose) between cells to a limited extent due to tight junctions or transcellularly (transcytosis) across the cells for lipophilic substances (e.g. ethanol) (Alam et al., 2010). These mechanisms are non-competitive, nonsaturable and occur in downhill concentration direction.
- Facilitated diffusion in which target compounds bind to a specific membrane protein and carry to the other side of the membrane through conformation change of the protein. This mechanism is a form of carrier mediated endocytosis which occurs from high to low concentration like free diffusion and contributes for transport of some amino acids, nucleosides, small peptides, mono-carboxylates and glutathione (Alam et al., 2010).

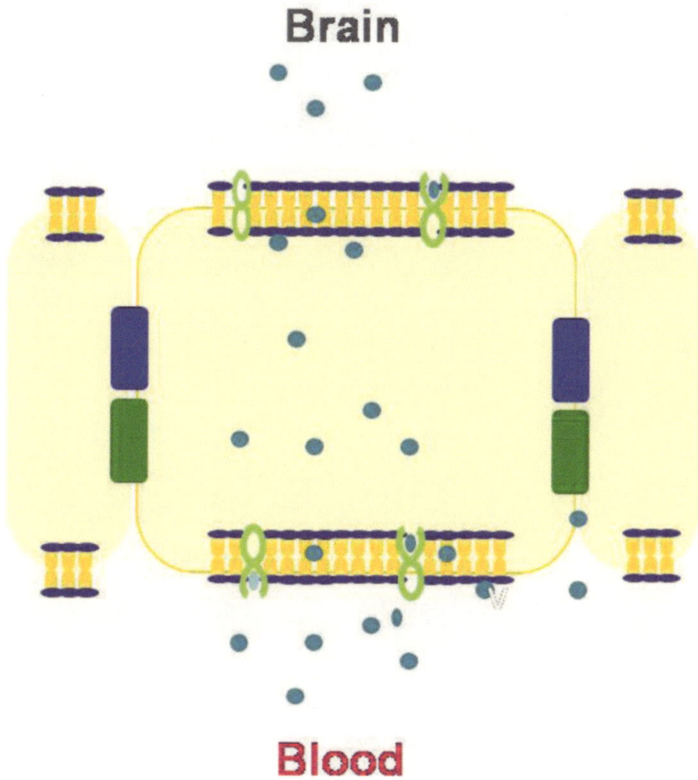

Fig. 3. Free and facilitated passive diffusion.

3.2 Endocytosis

In this method, substances (e.g. macromolecules) are engulfed by membrane and pass through the cell by vesicles and release in the other side (Kerns & Di, 2008). Endocytosis occurs via two main methods: bulk phase endocytosis (fluid phase or pinocytosis) and mediated or facilitated endocytosis (receptor and absorptive mediated). Fluid phase endocytosis is a nonsaturable, non-competitive and non-specific method for uptake of extra cellular fluids which is temperature and energy dependent.

Receptor mediated endocytosis facilitates the larger essential molecules uptake selectively using specific receptors present in luminal membrane. Hormones, growth factors, enzymes and plasma proteins are targets for specific receptors (Pardridge, 2007).

Absorptive mediated endocytosis is based on an electrostatic interaction between negatively charged plasma membrane luminal surfaces (glycocalyx which is a negatively charged proteoglycan or glycosaminoglycan) with cationic substances (e.g. peptides) and uptake it in a vesicle into the endothelial cell and release it on the other side (Figure 4) (Ueno, 2009).

This has lower affinity and higher capacity than receptor mediated endocytosis (Alam et al., 2010). Mechanism of vesicle formation (caveolin dependent, dynamin dependent and caveolin- dynamin independent) is not discussed in this chapter and more details could be found in the literature (Lajoie et al., 2010).

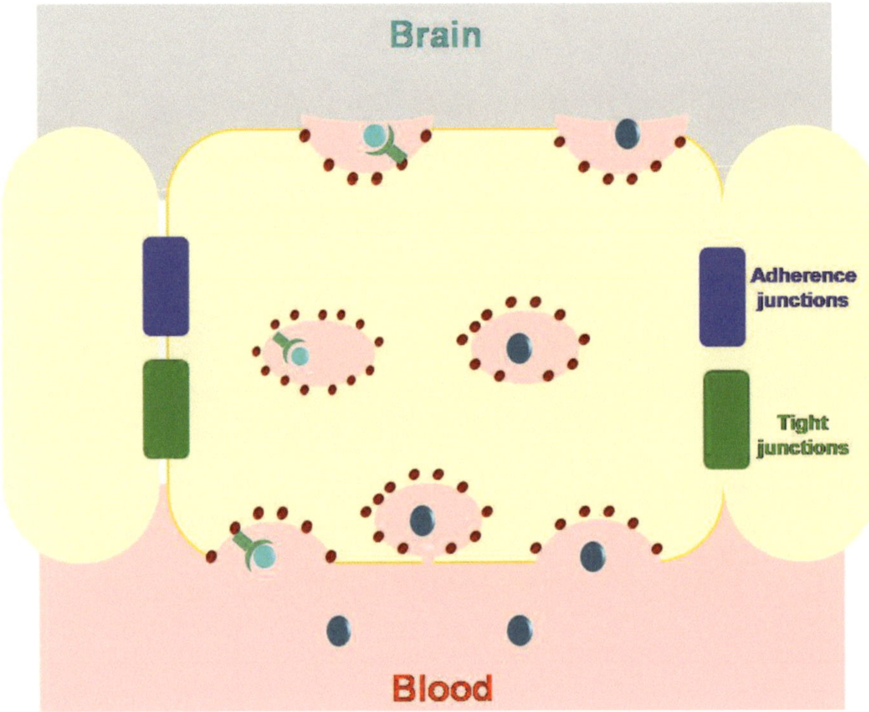

Fig. 4. Bulk phase and facilitated endocytosis.

3.3 Active transport

Hydrophilic drugs which cannot penetrate the brain through passive diffusion and lipophilic drugs which cannot penetrate the brain, in contrast of their suitable characteristics for BBB permeation are substrate for drug transporters of the BBB. Also some compounds are substrates for transporters and at the same time they are delivered by passive diffusion or endocytosis. Drug transporters are integral membrane proteins which is able to carry the drug usually against the concentration gradient into and out of the cell.

The overall exposure of xenobiotics to brain through these transporters depends on their location and expression level according to the normal and pathophysiologic conditions. Two types of drug transporters according to their driving forces (ATP dependent and ATP independent) are known. Active transporters broadly categorized as primary (ATP dependent), secondary or tertiary (ATP independent) (Murk et al., 2010).

There are two types of transporters:

1. Carrier mediated transporters which express on both the luminal and abluminal membranes and operates in both blood to brain and brain to blood directions.
2. Active efflux transporters which mediate extruding drugs and other compounds from brain (Alam et al., 2010). Although the main role of the drug transporters is carrying the drugs and other xenobiotics into and out of the brain but they are responsible for other cell processes such as inflammation, differentiation of immune cells, cell detoxification, lipid trafficking, hormone secretion and development of stem cells (Murk et al., 2010).

3.3.1 Influx transporters

Essential hydrophilic nutrients (e.g. glucose, amino acids, fatty acids, organic and inorganic ions) reach to brain through influx transporters and receptors. According to the structural similarity of the target drug to the biologic molecules; it can be delivered to the brain using appropriate transporter. Solute carrier family encodes most of the influx transporters which include facilitated, ion coupled and ion exchange transporters that do not need ATP (Eyal et al., 2009). These transporters are responsible for uptake of a broad range of substrates including glucose, amino acids, nucleosides, fatty acids, minerals and vitamins (Alam et al., 2010). The most well studied groups of these bidirectional transporters along with their properties and activities are summarized in Table 1.

3.3.2 Efflux transporters

Efflux occurs in BBB through both passive and active routes in order to detoxify the brain and prevent from drugs and xenobiotics exposures. There are several kinds of efflux transporters such as ATP binding cassette transporters (ABC), organic anion transport systems, amino acid transport systems and so on (Ueno, 2009). ABC transporters are primary active systems which are responsible for different efflux activities including P-glycoprotein (P-gp), multi-drug resistance proteins (MRPs), and breast cancer related protein (BCRP). P-gp (the most studied ABC transporter), located in luminal side of BBB, immediately pump most of the drugs and xenobiotics back to the blood and decrease the net penetration to the brain. A broad range of drugs, generally including un-conjugated and cationic substances (Table 1) are substrates for P-gp, where some of them are able to inhibit P-gp and lead to increased permeability of co-administered drugs. This fact can be used as a drug delivery strategy to the brain. Along with P-gp, MRPs and BCRP are responsible for main part of drug efflux in BBB and their effect are dependent to their localization and expression level in normal and pathologic conditions. Over expression of these transporters considered as one of the major reasons of pharmacoresistance of brain diseases and their inhibition, bypassing and regulating methods are important for CNS drug development (Loscher & Potschka, 2005).

3.4 Metabolism in BBB (Enzymatic barrier)

Existing enzymes in BBB can be regarded as second barrier after negative surface charge. These enzymes involve in disposition of drugs and xenobiotics before entering the endothelial cells of capillaries. Alkaline phosphatase, acid phosphatase, 5′-nucleotidase, adenosine tri-phosphatase and nucleoside di-phosphatase are among well studied enzymes distributed within BBB (Ueno, 2009).

4. BBB permeation measurement methods

The rate and the extent of drug transport to the brain are needed for drug discovery studies (both peripheral and CNS drugs) and different methods developed in order to study the pharmacokinetic profile of drug candidates. BBB permeability depends on physicochemical properties of drug compound and physiologic functions of the BBB (physical barrier, transport, metabolic pathways) and need special study techniques. These techniques include *in vivo, in vitro,* and *in silico* methods (Diagram 2) which are complement in most cases and researchers are able to define different aspects of drug passage to the brain using these methods.

Transporter name	Substrates	Sample drugs and nutrients	Influx/ Efflux
Organic anion transporting polypeptides	Anionic amphipathic molecules with molecular weight greater than 450 Daltons and a high degree of albumin binding	Fexofenadine, Digoxin, Methotrexate	Influx
Organic anion transporters	Anionic drugs and nucleotides	Benzylpenicillin, Valacyclovir, Zidovudine, Mercaptopurine, Methotrexate, Valproic acid	Influx
Organic cation transporters	Bidirectional transport of small hydrophilic positively charged compounds	Cimetidine , Desipramine, Metformin, Amantadine, Memantine, Cisplatine, Quinin	Influx / Efflux
System L.	Bidirectional transport of large neutral amino acids with branched or aromatic side chains	L-phenylalanine, L-tyrosine, L-tryptophan, L-lucine, Levodopa, α-Methyldopa, Baclofen, Melphalan, Gabapentin, Pregabalin	Influx / Efflux
Monocarboxylate transporters	HMG-CoA reductase inhibitors that contain a carboxylic acid moiety	Simvastatin, γ- Hydroxybutyrate	Influx
Nucleoside transporters	Purine and pyrimidine nucleosides	Adenosine	Influx
Hexose transporters	Hexose nucleosides	Glucose	Influx
Ion transporters	Bidirectional transport of small ions	Cl^-, Na^+, K^+, H^+, $HCO3^-$	Influx / Efflux
P-glycoproteins	A broad range of drugs and xenobiotics (normally un-conjugated, cationic substances)	Anti cancer drugs, corticoids	Efflux
Multi-drug resistance proteins	Drugs and xenobiotics (normally conjugated, anionic substances)	Anti cancer and anti HIV Drugs	Efflux
Breast cancer resistant proteins	Drugs and xenobiotics (overlap with P-glycoproteins and multi-drug resistance proteins)	Some anti cancer Drugs	Efflux

Table 1. Some of the well studied influx and efflux transporters of brain.

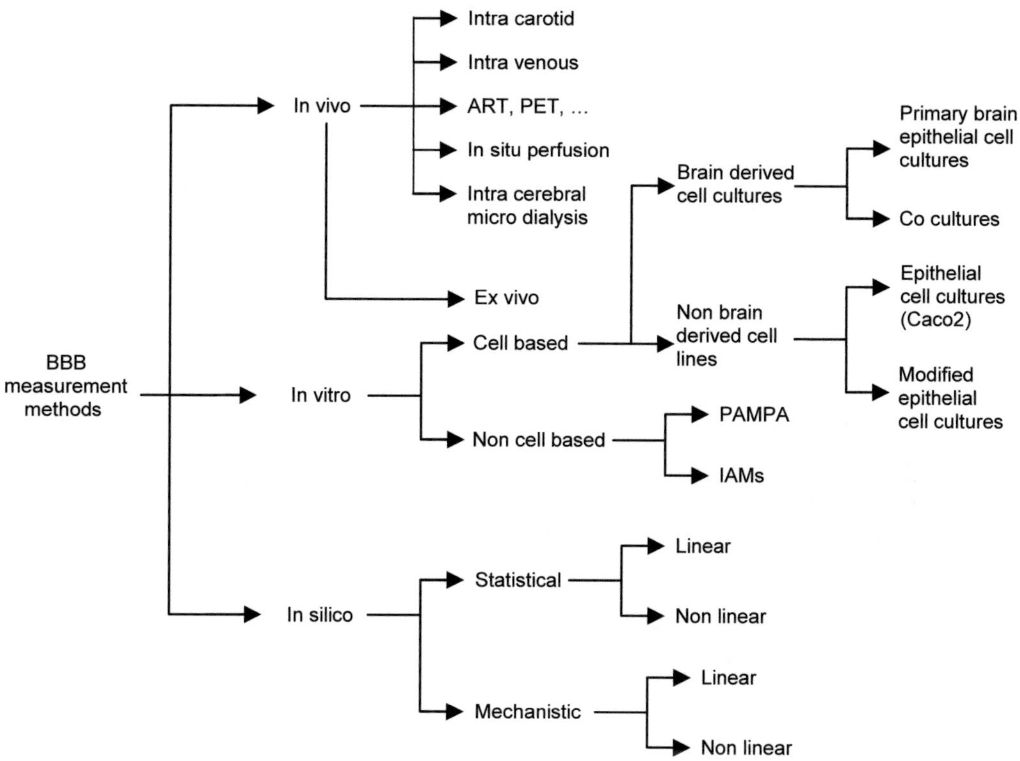

Diagram 2. Brain drug testing methods.

4.1 BBB permeation data

4.1.1 Bound and unbound drug concepts

The drug is available in blood in the free (unbound) and bounded (protein bounded, erythrocyte bounded, tissue bounded) forms. The unbound drug molecules equilibrate across the BBB and brain. The spaces that these equilibria occur are: blood, interstitial fluid, intercellular and intracellular fluids. Figure 5 shows these equilibria schematically. The speed of the equilibria to reach the steady state define the rate of drug distribution within brain, and the slowest one would be the rate limiting step. For poor CNS penetrantes, the BBB permeation or the diffusion of drug molecules within the brain tissue is the rate limiting step. Total brain concentration which allow us just to rank drug candidates according to their CNS total levels and general CNS penetrability can be measured using most of the *in vivo* methods, while there is just a few methods which are able to provide free fractions directly.

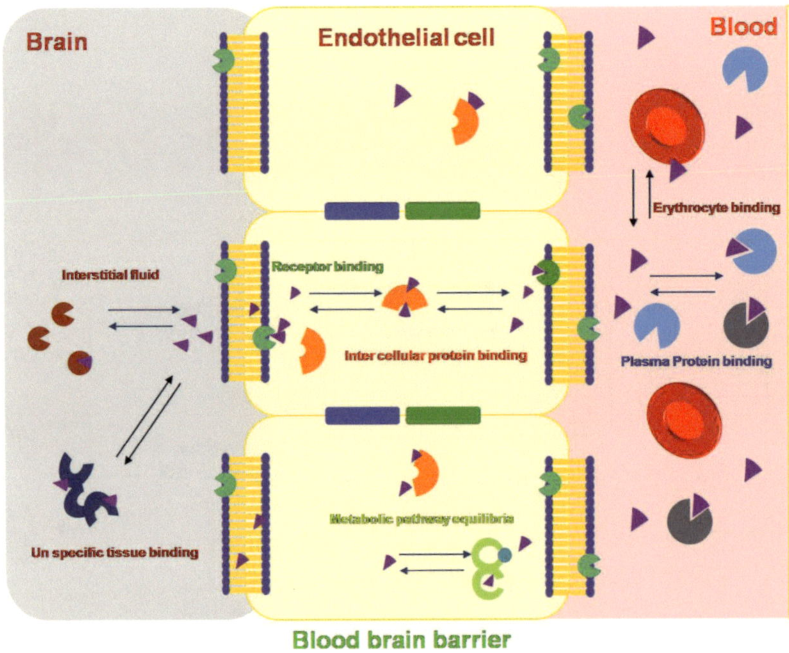

Fig. 5. Different equilibria in brain.

4.1.2 The importance of free drug measurement

The free drug is responsible for pharmacokinetic and pharmacodynamic properties of drugs and relation between dose and response is correct when free drug supplies in target tissue get into account. In this regard interstitial fluid and intra cellular fluid drug levels in brain are important data for drug discovery.

The traditional methods of brain homogenization destroy all compartments of brain (including brain tissue binding and plasma protein binding) and drug levels in specific compartments cannot be measured (Reichel, 2009). The plasma free fractions data cannot be used in CNS drug discovery studies, because of the different physiological properties, blood brain interstitial fluid free fractions. Some researchers used cerebrospinal drug levels (CSF sampling) as an estimate of the unbound drug levels in brain which is not so reliable because of lower tightness of cerebra-spinal blood barrier which leads to higher diffusion and overestimation of free drug concentration in brain (Read & Braggio, 2010). The microdialysis is the only *in vivo* method to provide such data directly, which is limited by its practicability.

4.1.3 The rate and extent of drug penetration to the brain

Neuropharmaceuticals should be able to permeate the BBB and enter the brain parenchyma in order to treat desired disorders whereas peripheral drugs should have limited entrance to the brain in order to decrease their neurological side effects. The drug entrance to the brain was evaluated and quantified using different methods, among them BUI, logBB, $K_{p,uu}$ etc, are well studied and frequently used to measure the rate and the extent of brain drug penetration (Jeffrey & Summerfield, 2010).

Brain uptake index (BUI%) is one of the earliest indicators of BBB permeability of compounds and is calculated by:

$$BUI\% = 100\frac{E}{E_{ref}} \tag{1}$$

where E denotes the first pass extraction and the E_{ref} referred to freely diffusible internal standard. This indicator provides information about the total concentration of the drug in the brain at early time point after administration (Lanevskij et al., 2010).
The logBB which describes the ratio between brain and blood (or plasma) concentrations and provide a measure of the extent of drug permeation is calculated using (Kerns & Di, 2008):

$$\log BB \; or \; K_p = \frac{AUC_{\ tot.brain}}{AUC_{\ tot.blood}} \tag{2}$$

The only information provided by K_p is passive lipid partitioning of the drug which is affected by metabolism, relative binding affinity to proteins and lipid content of brain and blood or plasma and it is not a net measure of BBB permeability (Abbott, 2004; Mehdipour & Hamidi, 2009). It is highly time dependent and in order to get an overall estimation, usually is measured under steady-state conditions.
Another approach based on unbound drug fraction, for quantifying the extent of brain penetration is recommended, which is calculated by:

$$K_{p,uu} = \frac{AUC_{\ \mathrm{u,\,brain}}}{AUC_{\ \mathrm{u,\,blood}}} \tag{3}$$

$K_{p,uu}$ affected by both passive diffusion and active influx/efflux and can give information about the permeation mechanism, beyond these, it is not affected by plasma protein and brain tissue binding which interfere in logBB values (Mehdipour & Hamidi, 2009). For drugs delivered by passive diffusion, this index will be close to unity while for efflux and influx substrates it will be less than and more than unity respectively (Hammarlund- Udenaes et al., 2008).
To assess the brain drug permeability rate, the unidirectional influx constant from blood to the brain (K_{in}) and the product of the BBB permeability surface area (PS) which is a measure of the unidirectional clearance from blood to brain have been developed. Both parameters expressed as ml/min/g of brain (Rooy et al., 2010). PS is able to reflect the BBB permeation step more accurately (Abbott, 2004) and is valuable parameter for follow up permeation ability of drug candidates in the pharmaceutical industry and although in pathologic conditions. PS gives an estimation of unbound drug in brain but it is affected by the possible association of the drug with active influx or efflux transporters (Hammarlund- Udenaes et al., 2008).
According to the measurement method K_{in} and PS can be calculated from Crone-Renkin equation:

$$K_{in} = F\left(1 - e^{\frac{-PS}{F}}\right) \tag{4}$$

where F could be considered as perfusion flow rate, or cerebral blood flow rate and PS is computed using:

$$PS = -F \times \ln\left(1 - \frac{K_{in}}{F}\right) \quad (5)$$

Methods for measuring efflux of the drugs out of the brain (brain efflux index (BEI)) have been developed which represent the elimination rate constant of the drugs in brain. Using these parameters, scientists can provide information about the mechanism of BBB permeation in which for passive diffusion the efflux and influx constants will be similar.
To measure all of these data, the remained drug in brain microvascular should be calculated and subtracted from total brain concentration.

4.2 *In vivo*

The resulted data from *in vivo* experiments are valuable and regarded as gold standard in CNS drug discoveries. This value comprises from the experiment which uses anesthetized or cautious animals which represent full physiologic condition for study and the obtained data reflect different aspects of BBB permeation. Demanding skilled scientists and equipped laboratories are the main disadvantage of these techniques.

4.2.1 Intra venous injection

Intra venous injection methods have been developed during primary CNS studies in order to assess the BBB permeability and brain distribution of the CNS drug candidates. The radio-labelled compounds are injected intravenously and blood samples are obtained in different time intervals and a single brain tissue can be obtained at the designated time point. The measured compound concentrations in plasma and brain plotted against the time and after calculating AUC values the logBB computed using equation 2. For each time interval three animals are needed and in order to get a plot using 7 data points, 21 animals are required which is the main limitation of the method (Rooy et al., 2010). The logBB are interesting for pharmaceutical companies, because they can be easily used to rank the goals and other pharmacokinetic parameters such as C_{max} and time length that the compound remains above *in vitro* determined effective concentration can be calculated. Recently these data are questioned about their ability to reflect the permeability properties of studied compounds mainly because: 1) The obtained concentrations are total, while the free fraction of the compounds are responsible for most of their pharmacokinetic properties and 2) It is a brain distribution value and the permeation rate of compounds cannot be obtained (Kerns & Di, 2008). The other parameters which can be calculated using the obtained data are rate parameters (i.e. K_{in} and PS).

4.2.2 Single carotid injection

Single intra carotid injection is one of the earliest BBB permeation study methods and can be done by injection of a given concentration of a labelled compound through common carotid artery of an animal along with a reference standard and experiment stopped after 5 - 15 seconds. Then the brain sampling is done and the brain uptake index (BUI%) can be calculated using the concentration of the compound and the reference standard (Pardridge, 2007). Because of the low sensitivity of the method (limited sampling time), this method has been replaced by *in situ* brain perfusion which provide higher control on experimental condition (Kerns & Di, 2008).

4.2.3 *In situ* brain perfusion

The desired concentration of the studied drug was prepared using the perfusion fluid and the resulted solution is perfused directly to the brain through common artery of an anesthetized animal (commonly rat) for the suitable time and the brain sampling carry out on the predefined time intervals after stopping the perfusion (Amith & Allen, 2003). Similar to the intravenous injection method the remained intravascular perfusion fluid should be removed by brain flashing or calculated using an impermeable compound injection (Rooy et al., 2010). Direct perfusion enables scientists to study the BBB drug permeation in the absence of the first pass metabolism or drug elimination methods. Using this method, the mechanism of drug permeation can be studied using co-administered transporter inhibitors. But such as intravenous injection high resource demanding is a limitation for this method. The K_{in} and PS can be calculated using the obtained data from this method.

4.2.4 Quantitative auto radiography

Another method for CNS drug partitioning study is quantitative auto radiography which can be used for regional study of total drug exposure. Using this method, the amount of radio labelled compound is measured in desired regions (e.g. stroke affected areas, brain tumours) following oral, intravenous or subcutaneous administrations to animals. Similar to previous methods after blood sampling in various time intervals, the brain is taking out and after sectioning the frozen brain to suitable sections the radioactivity is measured. Intra vascular correction is needed here too. Obtaining the regional PS values is possible using this method and the resolution of obtained data is high because of the micrometer dimensioned studied sections (Bickel, 2005; Rooy et al., 2010).

4.2.5 Positron emission tomography

Positron emission tomography is a non-invasive method which is applicable in human. The suitable tracers are administered to the body and the emission is monitored using positron emission tomography scanners. The blood sampling is done in designed intervals and the brain and plasma distribution is measured using a curve fitting method. Similar to quantitative auto radiography the regional information about drug distribution is achievable using this method (Dash & Elmquist, 2003).

4.2.6 Intra cerebral microdialysis

Microdialysis is the only technique which is able to provide the concentration of CNS drug candidates in the interstitial fluid directly. A stereotaxic probe equipped with a semi permeable membrane implanted under anesthesia. The interior of the probe perfused with a physiological solution and samples are taken from freely moving animals and analyze using suitable separation techniques (commonly chromatographic systems) (Bickel, 2005; Alivajeh & Palmer, 2010). The studied compound can be administered orally, intravenously, subcutaneously or from other routes. This method is applicable for human and by implanting the probe in different regions of brain; specific data from different parts of brain (which have different properties) could be collected. The recovery of the probe is an important point in this method to get the absolute concentration data. Pharmacokinetic

parameters of CNS drug candidates including half-life, C_{max}, T_{max}, total exposure, volume of distribution, clearance, BBB influx and efflux rates for different brain regions and most importantly the $K_{p,uu}$ at steady state can be obtained and calculated using microdialysis driven data. These data can be used for pharmacodynamic studies and dosing regimens (Alivajeh & Palmer, 2010).
The methods reviewed in sections 4.2.1 to 4.2.6 give information about the overall exposure resulted from different passive or active influx and efflux systems.

4.2.7 Permeation mechanism study *in vivo*

During drug development the detailed information about the mechanism of permeation and possible efflux or metabolic instability are needed to design the structure of the desired drug and its delivery system. To get detailed information researchers have been used different methods such as: knockout or gene deficient animals for studying the effect of a specific transporter, special enzyme or transporter inhibitors (e.g. efflux inhibitors) or receptor antagonists to eliminate the desired transport effect from the study.
In order to study passive diffusion of drug candidates without interfering of other permeation mechanisms, a number of methods have been developed. For example, it is possible to use excess molar of unlabelled compound in order to saturate the transporters, enzymes or facilitated mechanisms. Also it is possible to use efflux transporters' inhibitors (e.g verapamil for P-gp). Beside these, by studying the Michaelis-Menten behaviour of drugs, it is possible to ensure that the permeation mechanism is passive diffusion (unsaturable) or not.

4.2.8 *Ex vivo*

E*x vivo* experiments are developed to study drug candidates more reliably out of the body in the simulated physiologic condition (pH, temperature, buffer, nutrients, oxygen) which have the advantage of being applicable in post mortem human samples obtained by autopsy. The resulted data from these experiments have been shown acceptable correlation with *in vivo* experiments. Although in this method impossible experiments and studies in living organism can be conducted, but the differences between the living organism and the slices obtained by autopsy according to the degradation of some proteins should be take into account (Cardoso et al., 2010).

4.3 *In vitro*

In order to do more rigorous investigations on the complex mechanisms occurred in endothelial cell membranes and in intracellular compartments (e.g. active and passive efflux and influx) in the BBB of a living organism, *in vitro* methods can be used. *In vitro* models of BBB should be simple, reproducible and mimic the *in vivo* conditions (both normal and pathologic). Most of the *in vitro* models of BBB are based on endothelial cells as the foundation of BBB and different animals are used to prepare cell cultures. The results should be interpret carefully because of the differentiations (the lower tightness of the developed cell lines, the phenotype modification and the absence of intercellular contact and in vivo signallings occur during the cell isolation). But it is a reliable method for high throughput screening experiments, in order to compare the penetration ability of a set of compounds (Cardoso et al., 2010). The main categories of *in vitro* models include cell based and non cell based methods. Cell based models are simplification of *in vivo* system in which the brain and non brain derived cell cultures are used to study the permeation and transport of drug candidates. The brain derived cell cultures (primary endothelial cultures) show closest phenotype to the *in vivo* brain while their preparation and handling are more difficult than non-brain derived cell lines. Primary endothelial cultures prepared by isolating animal brain micro vessels and *seeding* in culture medium where the endothelial cells grow out and make suitable mono layers for experiments. In order to mimic the *in vivo* system more closely co-cultures included astrocytes have been developed which provide more physical and physiological features in comparison with primary cell cultures (Cardoso et al., 2010). Non brain derived models use the epithelial cell cultures (e.g. Caco 2) and modified epithelial cell cultures which are used for drug absorption studies in order to rank the permeability of CNS drug candidates. Non cell based *in vitro* models include the parallel artificial membrane permeability assay (PAMPA) and immobilized artificial membranes (IAMs) which used as HPLC columns and mimic the properties of biological membrane (Abbott, 2004). PAMPA models initially developed for study passive oral absorption and successfully applied in the pharmaceutical industry. Recently, it has been modified for using in BBB permeation studies and showed good correlation with *in vivo* findings (Mensch et al., 2010).

4.4 BBB permeation prediction methods (*in silico* methods)

In vivo, ex vivo and *in vitro* methods of assessing brain drug penetration leads to high quality data resemble most of the permeation mechanisms in BBB, but they are highly cost and time demanding and are not suitable for screening of large compound libraries. As soon as BBB studies have begun, attempts to predict the BBB permeation properties of drug candidates lead to primary structure activity relationships which later accepted as essential rules of CNS drug development. These structural features later used to develop quantitative relationships to predict the pharmacokinetic properties of CNS drugs. During years and improving the knowledge about the effect of different passive and active mechanisms of brain drug penetration, the prediction models improved and specific models to predict different aspects of BBB permeation have been developed. In order to develop a model first the prediction endpoint (dependent variable or experimental value) should be measured or obtained from the literature. The quality of these data is deterministic for developed model certainty. After selection of the data set, the inclusion of each point in data set should be evaluated and possible outliers should be determined. The next step is to split data set in training and test sets and measure or calculate the desired independent descriptors. The significant descriptors should be selected and the relationship between the dependent and independent variables should be developed using appropriate modelling method. While the model has been developed, its predictive ability along with other validation parameters should be calculated and the effect of selected descriptors on the experimental value should be defined. The details of each step are provided in following sections. Some commercial software have been developed to predict the brain drug penetration which can be used to get primary estimations about the CNS activity of a compound.

4.5 Prediction endpoints (Experimental data)

In order to get initial information about the BBB permeation of new drug entities, studying the existing information using different methods is more interesting than experimental measurement. There are different (*in vivo* or *in vitro*) indicators which are able to evaluate the rate or extent of drug permeation to the BBB (see section 4.1.3). Among them logBB values have been used extensively for *in silico* methods in order to predict the extent of drug penetration to the brain and the related data sets can be found in the literature. Unbound drug fraction, logPS and BUI% have been used to develop the prediction methods, while some researchers used *in vitro* data (e.g. PAMPA derived P-gp binding affinity) for their studies (Dagenais et al., 2009). Beside these BBB+/- and CNS+/- data which have been extracted from logBB experiments and implications of brain disorders or targets about primary site of action of compounds respectively, were utilized for classification purposes (Klon, 2009). It seems that using the combined information derived from different indicators will be more useful than individual ones. The quality of selected data set should be considered according to the experimental method which used to obtain it (data set homogenesity). The homogenesity of logBB data sets have been questioned, but the studies showed that these combined data sets are applicable. Also the outliers should be determined using statistical methods or according to the experimental method. One of the most common statistical methods is to compute deviations of a single data point from mean dependent or independent variables or both of them and exclude highly deviated datum. In fact an applicability domain for each prediction method should be defined and the compounds out of this domain should be excluded from analyses. For experimental procedures it should be kept in mind that if special efflux inhibitors are used or not. In some methods, scientists are used unlabeled substrate to saturate the desired enzyme or transporter or receptor and the resulted data from these experiments should not be combined with others (Lavnevskij et al., 2010). The third point which should be kept in mind is that the number of the data points should be enough for developing statistical properties (e.g. regression coefficients) of the developed model and also for excluding a part of data as test set. If it is not possible the prediction capability of developed model cannot be evaluated and it will be applicable for the entire data set.

4.6 Descriptors

The structural features and physicochemical properties (Table 2) of the studied compounds should be extracted using the available experimental and computational methods (commercial software, fragment based methods, ...). The most studied and evaluated descriptors to define the BBB permeation are those related with passive diffusion. Table 3 contains the details of most frequently used descriptors as well as their effects on BBB permeation. As can be seen from the table, the overall findings about the structural features (also known as the rule of five) of the CNS drug candidates are:

- High lipophilicity
- Low hydrogen binding
- Small molecular weight.

It should be noted that these rules should be used cautiously during drug design procedure. For example, although high lipophilicity increase the permeation rate but it causes the poor solubility, metabolic instability and higher membrane bounding which are not suitable properties for a drug candidate.

Descriptor	Topological descriptors Constitutional, Molecular properties, Quantum chemical, ACDLabs, free aqueous solubility energy
Software	Absolve, Dragon, Hyperchem, Volsurf, MOE, Cerius package

Table 2. Frequently used descriptors and software.

Property	The cutoff for BBB permeation
Molecular weight	< 400-500 Da
H bond donor	<3
H bond acceptor	<7
ClogP*	<7
logD7.4	1-3
Polar surface area	< 60-70 A°2
Rotatable bonds	<8
Flexibility	1.27
pKa	7.5-10.5
N+O	<6

* The studies showed that logPoct/water have poorer correlation with permeation data in comparision with ΔlogP or logD7.4. Recent studies showed that the ionization state of drug candidates in physiologic condition should be defined and the models should be developed accordingly (Lavenskij et al., 2009, 2010; Shayanfar et al., 2011).

Table 3. Descriptors used in rules of five methods and their cut off points (Di, 2008; Palmer, 2010)

4.7 Model development

After preparing a number of descriptors, the best descriptor or a combination of descriptors which are able to describe the desired dependent variable (prediction end point) should be selected. There are two approaches for descriptor selection:

4.7.1 Mechanistic approach

In this method, the studied property (e.g. BBB permeation) affecting parameters should be extracted from theoretical findings (several processes include in the overall result) and convert to mathematical representations. The provided descriptors depend on their effects (positive or negative, direct or inverse) on desired property should be correlated to the prediction end point and the resulted equation could be used for prediction purposes (Lavenskij et al., 2010).

4.7.2 Statistical approach

It is so important to exclude insignificant descriptors to prevent over fitting and biased results using a descriptor selection method. The number of descriptors depends on the modelling method. For simple multivariate regression methods, the number of descriptors depends on the number of data points, while for partial least square and principal component analyses methods it is not limited. In addition to the number of the descriptors and their significances, the inter correlation between them should be checked and just one of the highly correlated descriptors should be kept in multiple linear regression methods, while this is not a problem for partial least square or principal component analyses. There are different methods for descriptor selection and more information can be found in the literature. It is better to keep the penetration mechanisms and approved relationships in mind in this step and avoids complete statistical methods.

4.8 Method development

As soon as the descriptors selected or provided in mechanistic approach, the model should be developed according to the purpose of the modelling. The *in silico* methods developed for following purposes in CNS drug studies:

4.8.1 Classification

It is important to know that if the desired compound is CNS active or not. To do this a border value should be defined for the scaled dependent variable. Different data sets have been used for these models:

- logBB data (BBB+/-),
- CNS active or inactive compounds (CNS+/-)
- P-gp substrate or non-substrate (Pgp+/-).

These models are applicable for screening studies (primary steps of CNS drug development) where the goal is to select the possible CNS active compounds from large compound libraries and in advanced steps of CNS drug studies where the possible reasons of efficacy failure are investigated. Different classification methods have been developed until now using different algorithms and descriptors. The review of these studies showed that the methods were more successful for CNS+ and BBB+ compounds than CNS- and BBB- ones. One reason for this approach is raised from efflux pumps which efflux some structurally suitable compounds from brain. Considering the efflux system substrates during method development will improve the prediction accuracy for these compounds. It should be noted that there is a difference between BBB+ and CNS+, since a drug could be penetrated into brain without measurable biological effect. However in some modelling studies these data were mixed up. It seems that in order to develop more accurate classifiers, some physiological properties of brain such as the extent of non-specific protein and tissue binding, the concentration of the target protein and specific receptors in the brain should be considered.

4.8.2 Permeability prediction (The rate and extent of penetration)

The log*BB*, $K_{p,uu}$ (for exposure extent studies) and log*PS* (for rate studies) have been frequently used to develop prediction models. The multiple linear regression and least square methods are among the most studied models providing simple and interpretable equations.

Detailed review of these equations could be found in the literature (Garg et al., 2008; Klon, 2009; Mehdipour & Hamidi, 2009; Shayanfar et al., 2011). The descriptors used for rules of five (Table 3) studies originally comprised from these equations and at least one of these descriptors or similar descriptors which provide relevant information can be found in these equations. In this regard, most of the time, medicinal chemists use the same descriptors to check the new data set or new methods. Lipophilicity descriptors, size and shape descriptors, ionization states of compounds, and polar surface area descriptors proved to have effect on BBB permeation. The complexity of BBB permeation encouraged scientists to check non linear methods applicability in this field and some exponential linear equations and neural networks have been successfully developed. Although neural networks provided more accurate predictions in comparison with linear ones, their interpretation and reproducibility are in question and their usefulness for developing universal models which can be applicable for chemists have not been approved yet. In fact the best model for a chemist is a model which is able to answer him/her what is the possible modification for desired property improvement and the un-interpretable models are not able to answer this question. Because of this, using less accurate but well defined models are preferred to complicate but accurate ones.

The studies of unbound fraction of the drug in brain ($K_{p,uu}$) showed that the previously accepted trend of permeation (higher permeation for more lipophilic compounds) which was raised from log*BB* and log*PS* studies are not the same for unbound fraction, and lipophilicity have inverse relation with it. These findings showed that the absolute values for the effective descriptors are not suitable and a balanced range of descriptors should be defined for them (Lavenskij et al., 2010).

4.9 Validation

In order to check the sensitivity, specificity, prediction capability, reproducibility, error margins and chance correlations for the developed models, some validation statistics should be provided and using these parameters researchers will be able to make decision on selecting or rejecting a model in comparison with others. The details of these parameters and their usefulness for evaluating the model have been reviewed. For classification methods the lower failure in localization of compounds (both positive and negative) is better and for predictive models the higher correlation coefficients (both for training and test sets and cross validation sets), lower prediction errors (less than about 1 log unit deviation and relative mean squared errors less than 0.3)and lower correlation coefficients (e.g. <0.2) for Y randomized data sets are acceptable. These parameters are not absolute and it would be possible to accept a low quality model in the absence of the better one.

4.10 Prediction using commercial software

Using the developed models, some software has been developed in order to calculate the BBB permeation or P-gp binding affinity which can be used for estimation of compound permeation. These predictions are included in the most of the ADME prediction software which could be found on internet.

5. Conclusion

The importance of BBB for reaching CNS drugs to their targets and also undesired penetration of non CNS drugs to avoid their CNS side effects are briefly discussed. Short review of measurement methods of drug's penetration to CNS is presented along with a summary of computational aspects used for modelling purposes.

The molecular and cellular properties of BBB have been reviewed and the role of its compartments in the regulating of drugs and xenobiotics penetration to the brain has been discussed. Working as a regulatory interface BBB is able to work as a physical and physiological barrier which prevents peripheral drugs to penetrate the brain and reduce their CNS side effects. This barrier activity causes some difficulties in CNS drug delivery and different measurement methods have been developed to study the rate and extent of drug delivery to the brain and the mechanism of delivery methods have studied using these methods. Beyond the experimental methods, prediction of these properties are studied in order to provide cheaper, simpler and more rapid methods for medicinal chemists who work in brain drug development field.

6. Acknowledgment

This work is dedicated to Professor Morteza Samini, Tehran University of Medical Sciences, Tehran, Iran, for his long life efforts in training pharmacy students in Iran.

7. References

Abbott, N. J. (2004). Prediction of blood-brain barrier permeation in drug discovery from in vivo, in vitro and in silico models. *Drug Discovery Today: Technologies*. Vol. 1, pp. 407-416.

Abbott, N. J. (2005). Physiology of the blood-brain barrier and its consequences for drug transport to the brain. *International Congress Series*. Vol. 1277, 3-18.

Abbott, N. J.; Rinnback, L. & Hansson, E. (2006). Astrocyte-endothelial interactions at the blood-brain barrier. *Nature Reviews Neuroscience*. Vol.7, pp. 41-53.

Alam, M. I.; Beg, S.; Samad, A.; Baboota, S.; Kohli, K.; Ali, J.; Ahuja, A. & Akbar, M. (2010). Strategy for effective brain drug delivery. *European Journal of Pharmaceutical Sciences*. Vol. 40, pp. 385-403.

Alavijeh, M. S. & Palmer, A. M. (2010). Measurement of the pharmacokinetics and pharmacodynamics of neuroactive compounds. *Neurobiology of Disease*. Vol. 37, pp. 38-47.

Ballabh, P.; Braun, A. & Nedergaard, M. (2004). The blood-brain barrier: An overview: Structure, regulation, and clinical implications. *Neurobiology of Disease*. Vol. 16. pp. 1-13.

Bickel, U. (2005). How to measure drug transport across the blood-brain barrier. *NeuroRx* Vol. 2, pp. 15-26.

Cardoso, F. L.; Brites, D. & Brito, M. A. (2010). Looking at the blood-brain barrier: Molecular anatomy and possible investigation approaches. *Brain Research Reviews*. Vol. 64, pp. 328-363.

Dagenais, C.; Avdeef, A.; Tsinman, O.; Dudley, A. & Beliveau, R. (2009). P-glycoprotein deficient mouse In situ blood-brain barrier permeability and its prediction using an incombo PAMPA model. *European Journal of Pharmaceutical Sciences*. Vol. 38, pp. 121-137.

Dash, A. K. & Elmquist, W. F. (2003). Separation methods that are capable of revealing blood-brain barrier permeability. *Journal of Chromatography B*. Vol. 797, pp. 241-254.

Eyal, S.; Hsiao, P. & Unadkat, J. D. (2009). Drug interactions at the blood-brain barrier: Fact or fantasy?. *Pharmacology & Therapeutics*. Vol. 123, pp. 80-104.

Fischer, H.; Gottschlich, R. & Seelig, A. (1998). Blood-brain barrier permeation: Molecular parameters governing passive diffusion. *Journal of Membrane Biology*. Vol. 165, pp. 201-211.

Hammarlund-Udenaes, M.; Friden, M.; Syvonen, S. & Gupta, A. (2008). On the rate and extent of drug delivery to the brain. *Pharmaceutical Research*. Vol. 25, 1737-1750.

Jeffrey, P. & Summerfield, S. (2010). Assessment of the blood-brain barrier in CNS drug discovery. *Neurobiology of Disease*. Vol. 37, pp. 33-37.

Kerns, E. H. & Di, L. (2008). Drug-like Properties: Concepts, Structure Design and Methods: from ADME to Toxicity Optimizati. *Academic Press*, 978-0-12-369520-8,

Klon, A. E. (2009). Computational models for central nervous system penetration. *Current Computer-Aided Drug Design*. Vol. 5, pp. 71-89.

Lajoie, P.; Nabi, I. R. & Kwang, W. J. (2010). Lipid Rafts, Caveolae, and Their Endocytosis. International Review of Cell and Molecular Biology, *Academic Press*. Vol. 282, pp. 135-163.

Lanevskij, K.; Japertas, P.; Didziapetris, R. & Petrauskas, A. (2009). Ionization-specific QSAR models of blood-brain penetration of drugs. *Chemistry and Biodiversity*. Vol. 6, pp. 2050-2054.

Lanevskij, K.; Japertas, P.; Didziapetris, R. & Petrauskas, A. (2010). Prediction of blood–brain barrier penetration by drugs. *Delivery to the Central Nervous System Drug*. Vol. 45, pp. 63-83.

Loscher, W. & Potschka, H. (2005). Role of drug efflux transporters in the brain for drug disposition and treatment of brain diseases. *Progress in Neurobiology*. Vol. 76, pp. 22-76.

Mehdipour, A. R. & Hamidi, M. (2009). Brain drug targeting: a computational approach for overcoming blood-brain barrier. *Drug Discovery Today*. Vol. 14, pp. 1030-1036.

Mensch, J.; Melis, A.; Mackie, C.; Verreck, G.; Brewster, M. E. & Augustijns, P. (2010). Evaluation of various PAMPA models to identify the most discriminating method for the prediction of BBB permeability. *European Journal of Pharmaceutics and Biopharmaceutics*. Vol. 74, pp. 495-502.

Mruk, D. D.; Su, L. & Cheng, C.Y. (2010). Emerging role for drug transporters at the blood testis barrier. *Trends in pharmacological sciences*. Vol. 32, pp. 99-106.

Palmer, A. M. (2010). The role of the blood-CNS barrier in CNS disorders and their treatment. *Neurobiology of Disease*. Vol. 37, pp. 3-12.

Pardridge, W. M. (1998). *Introduction to the blood-brain barrier: methodology, biology, and pathology*. Cambridge University PRESS. 0 521 58124 9 (hb).

Pardridge, W. M. (2007). Blood-brain barrier delivery. *Drug Discovery Today*. Vol. 12, pp. 54-61.

Prabha, G.; Jitender, V. & Nilanjan, R. (2008). *Drug Absorption Studies*, Springer. 978-0-387-74901-3

Prinz, M. & Mildner A. (2011). Microglia in the CNS: Immigrants from another world. *GLIA* Vol. 59, pp. 177-187.

Read, K. D. & Braggio, S. (2010). Assessing brain free fraction in early drug discovery. *Expert Opinion on Drug Metabolism and Toxicology*. Vol. 6, pp. 337-344.

Reichel, A. (2009). Addressing Central Nervous System (CNS) Penetration in Drug Discovery: Basics and Implications of the Evolving New Concept. *Chemistry & Biodiversity.* Vol. 6, pp. 2030-2049.

Rooy, I.; Cakir-Tascioglu, S.; Hennink, W. E.; Storm, G.; Schiffelers, R. M. & Mastrobattista, E. (2010). In vivo Methods to Study Uptake of Nanoparticles into the Brain. *Pharmaceutical Research.* DOI: 10.1007/s11095-010-0291-7.

Shayanfar, A.; Soltani, S.& Jouyban, A. (2011). Prediction of Blood–Brain Distribution: Effect ofIonization. *Biological and Pharmaceutical Bulletin.* Vol. 34, pp. 266-271.

Smith, Q. R. & Allen, D. D. (2003). In situ Brain Perfusion Technique. *Springer protocols.* Vol. 89, pp. 209-218.

Ueno, M. (2009). Mechanisms of the penetration of blood-borne substances into the brain. *Current Neuropharmacology.* Vol. 7, pp. 142-149.

2

Diagnostic Accuracy and Interpretation of Urine Drug Testing for Pain Patients: An Evidence-Based Approach

Amadeo Pesce[1], Cameron West[1], Kathy Egan-City[1] and William Clarke[2]
[1]*Millennium Research Institute,*
[2]*Johns Hopkins School of Medicine,*
USA

1. Introduction

Pain is a complex disease. The complexities and co-morbidities of this disease include depression, anxiety, addiction, and other psychological diagnoses that lead to difficulties in management and aberrant behavior such as not taking medications as prescribed, taking additional medications, or illicit drugs. In the effort to provide the highest standard of care for their patients, pain physicians are required to continually assess patients for addiction and, if necessary, refer them to addictionologists for additional treatment (Chou et al., 2009).

1.1 Chronic opioid therapy

In this chapter we will refer to pain patients as those persons being treated with chronic opioid therapy for non-cancer-related pain. It is this patient population that has been associated with opiate abuse and diversion, and therefore monitoring these patients for drug use in a manner analogous to therapeutic drug monitoring is necessary. One of the most frequent complaints by patients seeing pain physicians is back pain, which is often associated with failed back surgery (Manchikanti et al., 2004; Michna et al., 2007). Currently opiate medications are one of the treatments of choice used by physicians to provide pain relief. These medications can induce euphoria as well as pain relief; because of this, opiates are frequently abused by this population, as well as the general population (National Survey on Drug Use and Health: Detailed Tables - Prevalence Estimates, Standard Errors, P Values, and Sample Sizes, 1995-2006; Webster & Dove, 2007). Additionally, these medications are associated with physical as well as psychological dependence and can pose addiction risks (Webster & Dove, 2007).

1.2 Pain treatment

One of the treatments of choice for chronic pain involves strong medications such as opioids, as well as additional or adjuvant medications (Chou et al., 2009; Trescot et al., 2006). Side effects of opioids include sedation, dizziness, nausea, vomiting, and constipation. Living day to day with any or all of these symptoms is challenging at the least and is compounded by the underlying pain these patients suffer from. Naturally, patients often attempt to minimize the side effects by taking less of the medication when side effects are particularly debilitating or unpleasant. "Chronic pain patients often adjust their dose of prescribed medication in response to changing levels of activity with no malicious or maladaptive intent. Although they may state that their pattern of use of medications is stable, this is often a statement made "on average" rather than a precise pattern of use. This is particularly evident with short-acting medications used in the treatment of breakthrough pain." (Gourlay & Heit, 2010b)

UDT is used to give confidence to both the physician and the patient that the patient is following the medication regimen and is therefore getting the most benefit from their treatment. In addition, the side effects of these medications often result in their misuse, underuse, and/or mixing of medications that are not prescribed (Manchikanti et al., 2004). This can also result in the social problems of abuse, misuse, or diversion of these medications. These factors require of pain physicians that they be particularly attentive to their prescribing practices. Adding to the complexity of managing pain patients is the fact that these medications are controlled substances and cannot be purchased over the counter, and so have high street value (Katz et al., 2003; National Prescription Drug Threat Assesment, 2009). This in turn requires of the physician that he or she determine whether patients under their care are compliant with their medication regime, binging on their medications, or diverting them for financial gain (Manchikanti et al., 2005, 2006a, 2006b).

1.3 Complications of pain treatment

Further compounding the situation, alcohol use is of major concern to the physician because alcohol-drug interactions can cause morbidity (Harmful Interactions: Mixing Alcohol with Medicines, 2007). Although physicians prohibit patient alcohol use during treatment with opiates or benzodiazepines, verbal contracts are commonly broken and therefore alcohol use must be monitored with (UDT) to manage the high risk of alcohol-drug reactions and mortality (Chou et al., 2009; Trescot et al., 2006). In addition, for reasons involving inadequate pain control, sleep deprivation, and psychological pathology, this patient population commonly takes other medications not prescribed by treating physicians as well as illicit drugs (Manchikanti et al., 2005, 2006a, 2006b). To respond to these potential problems, physicians traditionally relied upon behavioral assessment and pill counts to aid them in making treatment decisions. UDT has augmented these tools by providing physicians with objective, scientifically measurable outcomes to help them make decisions (Gourlay et al., 2010; Hammett-Stabler & Webster, 2008; Nafziger & Bertino, 2009; Reisfield et al., 2007). A detailed protocol of how to appropriately prescribe these controlled substances for this population is discussed in the book *Universal Precautions*, by Gourlay and Heit (Gourlay et al., 2005).

2. Urine drug testing

Traditionally, UDT has been associated with forensic testing, often referred to as workplace testing, to detect illicit drug use in employees. Workplace UDT has traditionally focused on identifying use of abused drugs including amphetamines (methamphetamine), cocaine, marijuana, phencyclidine (PCP), and heroin (opiates) (Federal Register - Mandatory Guidelines and Proposed Revisions to Mandatory Guidelines for Federal Workplace Drug Testing Programs [Federal Register], 2004). This type of testing is oriented toward determining positive results; that is, identifying the presence of an illicit substance. The reasoning behind this focus is obvious; a positive result for a prohibited substance is a cause for a consequence such as job dismissal (Federal Register, 2004). Testing for these drugs usually follows scheduled guidelines established by the Substance Abuse and Mental Health Services Administration (SAMHSA) (Federal Register, 2004). Analytically, the testing involves qualitative immunoassay screening followed by confirmation by mass spectrometry. Testing for patients on chronic opioid therapy is a different paradigm as both positive and negative results are important. It also requires assays that are more sensitive and can determine both the parent drug and one or more of its metabolites.

2.1 Immunoassays

Immunoassays are tests that are based on the ability of an antibody to bind with a drug (Feldkamp, 2010). Antibodies are made in such a way that they bind with a specific drug, such as morphine. In one approach, manufacturers of point of care (POC) devices embed test strips with antibodies and install them in devices designed to interact with urine specimens (Amedica Drug Screen Test Cup). A urine specimen with the drug in it (in this example, morphine) will displace the drug-indicator molecule on the test strip causing the morphine drug indicator line to disappear or change color. These test strips are then visually inspected by the person administering the test. The absence or presence of a line or the change in color, such as on a home pregnancy test, indicates whether the result is positive or negative. The immunoassay antibody binding reaction can be measured in other, more sophisticated ways than using test strips, such as reference laboratory analytical instruments (Olympus Au640 Product Information; Siemens V-Twin Analyzer Product Information; Thermo Fisher Mgc-240 Analyzer Product Information). However, the fundamental property of immunoassays is always the binding reaction of the antibody to the test drug (analyte).

2.2 Limitations of immunoassay

The qualitative immunoassay model of testing is only a partial UDT solution for the pain population (Gourlay et al., 2010; Hammett-Stabler & Webster, 2008; Nafziger & Bertino, 2009; Reisfield et al., 2007). There are a number of reasons for this. First, doctors treating patients for pain are concerned with negative as well as positive results. This is because a negative result can mean that a patient is not taking a prescribed medication. Second, workplace UDT assays do not fit the clinical medication regimen used in the treatment of pain patients and do not take into account the variable dosing often employed by pain patients as they try to balance their need for pain relief against the side effects of these medications (Gourlay & Heit, 2010a). In analytical terms this means that the cutoff for detection and quantitation (concentration of drug present) must be low enough to capture minimal use of the drug. Thirdly, the physicians need to have an exact indication of the medications the patients are taking. For example, a positive opiate test does not indicate whether the patient is on codeine, hydrocodone, morphine, or hydromorphone. That is, it measures the class not the particular drug. Each of these are specific medications the physician may choose to treat the patient with, so in order to establish compliance it is necessary to determine exactly which medication has been ingested and assure the patient is not taking additional opiates which could create an unsafe situation (Cone et al., 2008). Finally, if an immunoassay screening method is used, the antibody must detect all drugs of that particular class. Recent advances in designing opiate and benzodiazepine classes of drugs have resulted in agents which do not react well with the traditional antibodies. and are used in much lower concentrations than the earlier-designed drugs (Fraser, 2001). This complicates identification of these new agents by immunoassay.

3. Drugs observed in pain patients

Table 1 lists both licit and illicit drugs as well as alcohol and the frequency observed in the pain patient population tested by Millennium Laboratories. These observations are similar to those reported by Cone (Cone et al., 2008). The medications most commonly found in the urine of this population are clearly hydrocodone and oxycodone, followed by morphine and hydromorphone; codeine is not frequently prescribed for this population. Benzodiazepines are the next most prescribed group. Other opioid medications such as fentanyl, meperidine, tramadol, and propoxyphene are less frequently used. Use of the muscle relaxants carisoprodol is commonly seen. Marijuana is by far the most prevalent among the illicit drugs, followed by cocaine and methamphetamine. From the table it is clear that alcohol use is about 10% as measured by the presence of alcohol's metabolites ethyl glucuronide (EtG) and ethyl sulfate (EtS) (Crews et al., 2011a; Dahl et al., 2002; Helander & Beck, 2005; Helander et al., 1996; Schmitt et al., 1997; Stephanson et al., 2002; Wojcik & Hawthorne, 2007; Wurst et al., 2006; Wurst et al., 2004). These data show that in order to provide appropriate monitoring and decrease risk and mortality for this population, a broad test menu is needed. These same drugs are often abused and frequently found to be present though they had not been prescribed by the treating physician. Table 2 shows the frequency of these non-prescribed drugs in the pain patient population.

3.1 Need for urine drug testing

Many physicians prescribing opioids for non-cancer pain patients follow guidelines established by the American Pain Society (Chou et al., 2009). These guidelines specify the regular or periodic use of UDT as a component of treatment, including administering UDT upon assessing potential risk for substance abuse, misuse or addiction (Atluri & Sudarshan, 2003; Ives et al., 2006; Madras et al., 2009). Guidelines also suggest that doctors use UDT to monitor patient adherence to prescribed treatments and further state that periodic UDT is warranted because "the therapeutic benefits of these medications are not static and can be affected by changes in the underlying pain condition, coexisting disease, or in psychological or social circumstances" (Chou et al., 2009). In observation of these recommendations, many physicians use POC devices to obtain a real time, in-office assessment of patient compliance, illicit drug use and possible diversion (Manchikanti et al., 2006b, 2010).

3.2 Point of care testing

As mentioned previously, these POC devices are qualitative immunoassays that test for various drug classes as well as a few specific drugs. A typical POC device can measure 12 drugs or drug classes (Amedica Drug Screen Test Cup). The most commonly monitored agents are barbiturates, benzodiazepines, opiates, oxycodone, propoxyphene, methadone, tricyclic antidepressants and the illicit drugs methamphetamine, marijuana, cocaine, methylenedioxymethamphetamine (MDMA), and phencyclidine (PCP). The physicians use these screens to immediately detect adherence to regimen or non-adherence to the prescribed drug therapy. At that point they can elicit a more complete drug history, initiate a conversation assessing the need for additional medications not prescribed, or confront the

Drug Class	N Positive	% Positive	Mean (ng/mL)	Median (ng/mL)	Range (ng/mL)	Cutoff (ng/mL)
Alcohol	10,594	*10.0%*				
Ethyl Glucuronide	8,602	81.2%	59,827.9	7,220.1	500.47 - 5,942,830	500
Ethyl Sulfate	6,644	62.7%	18,660.7	3,546.1	500.17 - 1,565,150	500
Ethanol (Screen)	2,410	22.7%	735.1 mg/dL	68.6 mg/dL	20 - 151,316 mg/dL	20 mg/dL
Total Specimens Tested	**106,014**					
Amphetamines	7,005	*4.2%*				
Amphetamine	6,045	86.3%	8,471.2	2,790.2	100.31 - 409,816	100
Methamphetamine	1,178	16.8%	18,217.8	3,263.8	105.12 - 453,763	100
MDA	961	13.7%	1,771.1	844.5	101 - 416,68.9	100
MDMA	74	1.1%	5,328.2	1,260.6	120.14 - 40,395.3	100
Total Specimens Tested	**167,533**					
Barbiturates	4,797	*3.6%*				
Barbiturates (Screen)	4,797	100.0%	927.8	904.0	200 - 15,886	200
Total Specimens Tested	**133,032**					
Benzodiazepines	60,160	*35.6%*				
α-Hydroxyalprazolam	26,954	44.8%	479.9	177.3	20 - 55,249.1	20
Oxazepam	18,475	30.7%	2,036.0	617.4	40 - 203,128	40
7-Amino-Clonazepam	16,466	27.4%	674.6	287.0	20.01 - 47,501.7	20
Temazepam	15,647	26.0%	5,552.3	851.9	50 - 752,950	50
Nordiazepam	12,758	21.2%	693.9	281.5	40 - 25,864.3	40
Lorazepam	6,390	10.6%	1,583.1	681.2	40.09 - 63,170.8	40
Total Specimens Tested	**168,980**					
Buprenorphine	6,308	*6.0%*				
Buprenorphine	5,841	92.6%	313.0	75.1	10.01 - 58,691.5	10
Norbuprenorphine	4,237	67.2%	639.8	279.0	20 - 13,615.1	20
Total Specimens Tested	**104,972**					
Cannabinoids	11,752	*11.3%*				
cTHC	11,752	100.0%	579.6	153.1	15 - 25,960.3	15
Total Specimens Tested	**104,453**					
Carisoprodol	13,302	*16.4%*				
Meprobamate	13,188	99.1%	36,884.0	16,190.5	100.18 - 1,244,200	100
Carisoprodol	5,379	40.4%	2,931.9	455.0	100.1 - 648,442	100
Total Specimens Tested	**80,990**					
Cocaine	4,951	*3.0%*				
Cocaine metabolite	4,951	100.0%	12,372.5	627.1	50.05 - 342,160	50
Total Specimens Tested	**166,501**					

Table 1. Drug and Metabolite Prevalence, Positivity, and Concentrations. N = 184,049 patient specimens. Test dates: 10/01/09–4/29/10.

Drug Class	N Positive	% Positive	Mean (ng/mL)	Median (ng/mL)	Range (ng/mL)	Cutoff (ng/mL)
Fentanyl	13,141	*14.1%*				
Norfentanyl	11,589	88.2%	626.8	236.6	8 - 47,354.9	8
Fentanyl	9,283	70.6%	109.4	36.1	2 - 33,050.7	2
Total Specimens Tested	**93,526**					
Meperidine	6,310	*7.3%*				
Normeperidine	4,247	67.3%	1,456.3	339.5	50 - 276,993	50
Meperidine	2,522	40.0%	34,321.8	13,533.4	50.18 - 616,862	50
Total Specimens Tested	**86,344**					
Methadone	12,415	*11.0%*				
EDDP	12,109	97.5%	7,871.9	4,117.3	100.05 - 251,835	100
Methadone	11,792	95.0%	5,265.1	2,409.4	100.11 - 260,433	100
Total Specimens Tested	**113,073**					
Opiates	116,683	*64.6%*				
Hydrocodone	59,346	50.9%	2,564.4	859.9	50 - 477,876	50
Hydromorphone	51,205	43.9%	836.0	240.4	50 - 204,633	50
Oxymorphone	49,688	42.6%	5,760.2	1,298.6	50 - 1,512,220	50
Oxycodone	41,603	35.7%	11,207.3	2,124.5	50 - 5,947,380	50
Morphine	21,400	18.3%	29,611.8	9,600.3	50.06 - 1,995,940	50
Codeine	3,686	3.2%	4,752.0	828.4	50.01 - 233,036	50
6-Acetylmorphine	465	0.4%	1,108.8	275.7	10.01 - 24,069.1	10
Total Specimens Tested	**180,487**					
Phencyclidine	23	*0.02%*				
Phencyclidine	23	100.0%	539.4	87.5	10.89 - 3,718.53	10
Total Specimens Tested	**104,137**					
Propoxyphene	6,397	*4.8%*				
Norpropoxyphene	6,395	100.0%	5,524.3	2,026.9	100 - 167,037	100
Propoxyphene	2,780	43.5%	1,919.5	583.6	100 - 178,006	100
Total Specimens Tested	**133,992**					
Tapentadol	277	*0.4%*				
Tapentadol	277	100.0%	11,557.1	6,870.3	52.05 - 492,895	50
Total Specimens Tested	**66,797**					
Tramadol	6,521	*12.1%*				
Tramadol	6,521	100.0%	19,288.0	8,191.4	100 - 601,928	100
Total Specimens Tested	**54,111**					

Table 1. (continued). Drug and Metabolite Prevalence, Positivity, and Concentrations. N = 184,049 patient specimens. Test dates: 10/01/09–4/29/10.

DRUG CATEGORY	OCCURRENCES	% of TOTAL
Benzodiazepine	14,559	28.32%
Illicit Drugs	6,769	13.17%
Natural and Semi-Synthetic Opioids	13,241	25.75%
Other	11,514	22.39%
Stimulants	954	1.86%
Synthetic Opioids	4,379	8.52%
TOTALS	**51,416**	**100.00%**
Total Creatinine Tests	69,888	
Total RADAR C Positives	51,416	
% POSITIVE	**73.57%**	
Benzodiazepine	***14,559***	
7-Amino-Clonazepam	3,864	
Alpha-Hydroxyalprazolam	5,543	
Lorazepam	1,079	
Nordiazepam	1,907	
Oxazepam	1,803	
Temazepam	363	
Illicit Drugs	***6,769***	
6-MAM (Heroin metabolite)	165	
Cocaine metabolite	1,710	
Methamphetamine	320	
MDMA	17	
cTHC (Marijuana metabolite)	4,546	
Phencyclidine	11	
Natural and Semi-Synthetic Opioids	***13,241***	
Buprenorphine	809	
Codeine	692	
Hydrocodone	5,138	
Hydromorphone	1,789	
Morphine	1,317	
Norbuprenorphine	73	
Oxycodone	2,618	
Oxymorphone	805	
Other	***11,514***	
Carisoprodol	735	
Ethyl Glucuronide	5,320	
Ethyl Sulfate	4,820	
Meprobamate	639	
Stimulants	***954***	
Amphetamine	954	
Synthetic Opioids	***4,379***	
EDDP (Methadone metabolite)	1,381	
Fentanyl	729	
Meperidine	29	
Methadone	271	
Norfentanyl	204	
Normeperidine	55	
Norpropoxyphene	898	
Propoxyphene	25	
Tapentadol	17	
Tramadol	770	

Table 2. Incidence of Non-prescribed Use of Prescription Medications and Illicit Drugs.

patient about illicit drug use. Point of care devices are extremely useful because they provide physicians with immediate information, particularly on initial patient intake. Of course, like many CLIA-waived (or simple) test devices, they do have limitations, inasmuch as they require that a person visually inspect them in order to interpret the results. For this reason as well as the fact that these units are not 100% accurate, manufacturers of POC devices recommend that doctors not confront patients without first confirming the POC results (Table 3) (Amedica Drug Screen Test Cup). Table 3 lists a number of known drugs or agents that cause false positive results in POC immunoassays. In contrast with POC immunoassay tests, which only show a positive or negative result, laboratory-based immunoassays are often semi-quantitative (Feldkamp, 2010). This means that a positive result for morphine will also indicate approximately how much morphine is in the specimen. These immunoassays have quality control and proficiency testing surveys that make the results more objective and reliable than those obtained using POC devices (American Proficiency Institute 2011 Catalog of Programs, 2011; College of American Pathologists 2011 Surveys and Anatomic Pathology Education Programs, 2011).

POCT Kit Abbreviation	Drug or Drug Class	Target Drugs[1]	Compounds That May Cause A False Positive[1]
THC	Marijuana	Marijuana and Marinol (contains THC),	Prilosec, Protonix , efavirenz, NSAIDs
COC	Cocaine	Cocaine	Unknown/Infrequent
OPI300[2]	Opiates	Codeine, morphine, hydrocodone, hydromorphone. Also, poppy seeds that contain morphine.	Oxycodone
AMP	Amphetamines	Amphetamine, Adderall. Occasionally: benzphetamine, selegiline, Vicks Nasal Inhaler[4]	Phenylpropanolamine, ephedrine, pseudoephedrine, ranitidine, phentermine
MET	Methamphetamine	Methamphetamine. Occasionally: benzphetamine, selegilene, Vicks Nasal Inhaler[4]	Adderal, phenylpropanolamine, ephedrine, pseudoephedrine, ranitidine, phentermine
PCP	Phencyclidine	Phencyclidine	Venlafaxine, dextromethorphan, diphenhydramine
MDMA	Methylenedioxymethamphetamine	Methylenedioxy-methamphetamine	Phenylpropanolamine, ephedrine, pseudoephedrine, ranitidine, phentermine
BAR	Barbiturates	Butalbital, phenobarbital, secobarbital, amobarbital and other barbiturates	Unknown/Infrequent

BZO	Benzodiazepines	Oxazepam, nordiazepam, temazepam, alprazolam and other benzodiazepines to varying degrees	Oxaprozin, sertaline
MTD	Methadone	Methadone	Verapamil, quetiapine
TCA	Tricyclic Antidepressants	Amitriptyline, nortriptyline, imipramine, desipramine, doxepin and other tricyclics to varying degrees.	Cyclobenzaprine, carbamazepine, diphenhydramine
OXY[3]	Oxycodone	Oxycodone and oxymorphone	Codeine, morphine, hydrocodone and hydromorphone

Table 3. False Positive Results: Immunoassay Cross Reactants.

[1] While most immunoassays are highly selective for their target compounds, cross reactive compounds and adulterants, particularly when present at high concentrations may result in a false positive. Additional cross reactants have been reported and cross reactivity may vary between immunoassay manufacturers and lot to lot. The manufacturers of point of care test devices recommend that positive results should be confirmed by mass spectrometry.

[2] OPI300 is an assay to detect codeine, morphine, hydrocodone and hydromorphone. Oxycodone may give a positive at higher concentrations.

[3] OXY is an assay to detect Oxycodone. Other opiates, esp. codeine, morphine, hydrocodone and hydromorphone may give a positive result at higher concentrations.

[4] Adderall contains amphetamine. Benzphetamine (Didrex) is metabolized to d-amphetamine and d-methamphetamine. Selegiline (Eldepryl) is metabolized to l-amphetamine and l-methamphetamine. Vick's Inhaler contains l-methamphetamine.

3.3 Determining appropriate UDT cutoffs

Sensitivity of detection currently used in many immunoassays may not be appropriate for the pain patient. This is because manufacturers set cutoffs for assays to identify overdose in emergency unit settings (Fraser & Zamecnik, 2003; Fraser, 2001; Hattab et al., 2000; Wingert, 1997). There is a need to establish appropriate cutoffs for patients on clinical doses of their medications rather than the high concentrations encountered in overdose situations. Specifically, studies have been conducted that better identify the appropriate cutoff for the pain patient population (Pesce et al., 2011).

One definition of appropriate cutoff levels is one that captures 97.5% or more of the population on a specific drug (Pesce et al., 2011). An example of the importance of setting appropriate cutoffs is for the drug clonazepam (West et al., 2010b). When measured by immunoassay using a nominal cutoff of 200 ng/mL, only 28% of the patients on the drug were determined to be compliant. When the same samples were measured by LC-MS/MS technique using a cutoff of 200 ng/mL, the group was found to be 70% compliant. Finally, when the LC-MS/MS cutoff was lowered to 40 ng/mL the group was 87% compliant. This study showed that first the immunoassay was insensitive in that the nominal 200 ng/mL cutoff did not apply to clonazepam, and second, a lower cutoff was needed to appropriately categorize compliance. Other studies have shown the need for lower cutoffs for pain medications (Mikel et al., 2009; Pesce et al., 2010a). As the consequences to the patient of dismissal from a practice can be very large and even life-changing (e.g., loss of insurance, loss of job or income), it is essential that physicians do not unjustifiably dismiss even a single patient who is compliant with their medication regimens. This can be avoided by using appropriate cutoffs.

In an attempt to better define appropriate cutoffs for the pain patient population, the quantitative urine drug test results were examined for the prescription medications listed in Table 4. Using the criterion that the cutoffs should capture 97.5% of the examined population and employing the LC-MS/MS cutoffs listed in Table 4 showed it was possible to meet this standard (Pesce et al., 2011). One limitation of this approach is that the time after last dose and the dose itself were not known for these subjects. Regardless of the limitations of the study, the lower cutoffs provide results that can clearly identify compliance more accurately than other methods.

Drug	Analytical Cutoff (ng/mL)	Lower 2.5%	
		Estimated New Cutoff (Raw, ng/mL)	CR Normalized Cutoff (µg/g creatinine)
7-Amino-Clonazepam	10	19	15
Alpha-Hydroxyalprazolam	10	15	11
Amphetamine	50	76	59
Buprenorphine	5	7	5
Carisoprodol	50	56	35
Codeine	25	29	15
Fentanyl	1	2	2
Hydrocodone	25	41	31
Hydromorphone	25	34	26
Lorazepam	20	30	25
Meperidine	25	88	28
Meprobamate	50	92	113
Methadone	50	89	74
Morphine	25	59	52
Oxycodone	25	45	46
Oxymorphone	25	44	38
Propoxyphene	50	60	42
Tapentadol	25	42	58
Tramadol	50	147	70

Table 4. Medication Cutoff Values. Modified with permission from Pesce et al., 2011.

As stated earlier, illicit drug use is common in this population (Madras et al., 2009; Schuckman et al., 2008). It stands to reason that identifying the appropriate illicit drug cutoffs for UDT is equally important. Using the same criterion as stated above, cutoffs for marijuana, cocaine, and methamphetamine have also been determined (Table 5) (West et al., 2011a). The lowering of these illicit drug cutoffs consistent with the latest SAMHSA guidelines in which the cocaine and amphetamine cutoffs were lowered to capture more illicit drug users (Federal Register, 2004).

Drug	Lower 2.5%	
	Raw (ng/mL)	CR Normalized (ng/mg CR)
Cocaine	29.6	17
Marijuana	9.5	6.2
Methamphetamine	56.1	33.5

Table 5. Illicit Drug Cutoff Values. Modified with permission from West et al., 2011a.

3.4 Confirmatory testing: mass spectrometry

Physicians dealing with pain patients not following the treatment plan or using illicit or non-prescribed medications, have difficulty with these situations (Jung & Reidenberg, 2007). The doctor must be absolutely confident that the test data from both the POC and laboratory conducting further testing is correct. By having positive results obtained in their offices as well as confirmatory laboratory data, physicians can confidently discuss expectations and behavioral changes with patients. Questions about laboratory mix-up of specimens or laboratory error can be dismissed.

Many laboratories performing UDT on the pain patient population typically test specimens by immunoassay and then follow this with confirmation by mass spectrometry (Cone et al., 2008). Mass spectrometry is an analytical technique that separates molecules based on their weight (mass) and fragmentation pattern. Identification is based on the fact that each drug has a specific mass and breakdown in the same way that each person has a specific fingerprint. A mass spectrometry instrument is usually coupled to a chromatographic column, in which the test drug, for example morphine, is separated from other components in the urine before submitting the sample into the mass spectrometer. The mass spectrometer identifies the test drug by its position in the chromatogram, the specific weight of the molecule, and by its fragmentation pattern. This technology is virtually foolproof. Mass spectrometry techniques are divided into two methods: gas chromatography-mass spectrometry (GC-MS) and liquid chromatography-tandem mass spectrometry (LC-MS/MS). Of the two, the newer LC-MS/MS is considered the gold standard, for reasons we will describe later (Siuzdak, 2006).

In cases where the physician wants the results immediately (within hours), confirmatory mass-spectrometry methods used at the most modern diagnostic laboratories provide results within 24-30 hours. As stated above, the major limitations of immunoassays are inappropriate cutoffs (sensitivity), varying specificity for individual drugs, and cross-reactivity with other agents producing both false-negative and false-positive results (Manchikanti et al., 2008). The term cross reactivity is used to describe the reaction of an antibody with a chemical that is not the original immunizing drug. The reaction is poor because the affinity is much worse than the original drug. By poor we mean that at the same concentration of the original drug the test compound does not bind as well. However, as the concentration of the test compound is increased it eventually saturates the antibody binding site giving a positive test result.

3.5 Test menu requirement

As mentioned earlier a broader clinical laboratory UDT menu is necessary to accurately monitor the pain patient population. Smaller hospitals as well as physician offices cannot meet this requirement. One reason for this is that immunoassays require separate analytical channels for each assay and this limits the number of tests a smaller laboratory may have in its menu (Olympus Au640 Product Information; Siemens V-Twin Analyzer Product Information; Thermo Fisher Mgc-240 Analyzer Product Information). Another reason is that certain drug tests may not exist for the laboratory's specific instruments, and the addition of another instrument is financially prohibitive, particularly if that instrument is a mass spectrometer (Agilent Technologies, Inc.). Many physicians treating the pain patient population send specimens to reference laboratories specifically designed to provide the required test menu to meet these needs. Tests for new drugs (i.e., tapentadol) (Nucynta - Tapentadol, 2010) or new illicit substances (i.e., K2, spice) (Sobolevsky et al., 2010; Vardakou et al., 2010) encountered in the pain patient population can be rapidly set up and validated on LC-MS/MS instrumentation. Therefore, this analytical technique is supplementing screening by immunoassay. Because of the limitations of immunoassays, confirmatory testing is essential for accurate clinical assessment of medication usage. With confirmatory testing, physicians have specific evidence of what medications a patient is or isn't taking. This assures the doctor that he or she is not discharging a patient inappropriately, and that care is appropriate and not limited.. The laboratories with the most advanced technology can eliminate the immunoassay step saving both the patient and the insurer money.

3.6 Mass spectrometry as the gold standard for testing

At this point in time, mass spectrometry is considered the method of choice for UDT analysis in pain management. This is because mass spectrometry offers the chromatographic separation and mass fragmentation patterns that are specific for the test medications such as opiates and benzodiazepines (Mohsin et al., 2007). In addition, this analytic approach uses isotope dilution to quantify the amount of drug in the urine specimen; isotope dilution is considered the gold standard for determining how much of a drug is in a specimen (quantitation) (Federal Register, 2004). This ability to quantify the amount of drug in urine has been proposed as a method of detecting drug abuse (Pesce et al., 2010c). However, it is important to note that it is not possible to relate the quantitative excretion of a drug to the drug dosage (Nafziger & Bertino, 2009). Quantitation of drugs using immunoassay technology is problematic, particularly if the antibody reagent cross reacts with multiple structurally related drugs; if the urine drug sample contains more than one drug in a class (i.e., hydrocodone and hydromorphone), the antibody reaction will vary with each drug present in the solution. This means that the assay cannot distinguish between the two drugs and give a reliable calculation of the amount of either drug present (Feldkamp, 2010).

Of the two commonly used mass spectrometry methods, LC-MS/MS offers several advantages over GC-MS (Mikel et al., 2010). These include the ability to discriminate a larger number of drugs in each test run, the very small amount of urine specimen required (as little as 25 microliters, or one drop), and the ability to use a sample that is neither derivatized nor extracted. This in turn has made possible the analysis of hundreds of urine specimens per day for a single mass spectrometer. Advances in the automated handling of specimens and bar coding allow for the accurate processing of thousands of samples per day. This method of analysis can provide physicians with results more rapidly than by GC-MS (Mikel et al., 2010).

4. Interpretation of UDT results

The accurate interpretation of test results requires an understanding of the usefulness and limitations of immunoassays (Gourlay et al., 2010; Hammett-Stabler & Webster, 2008; Manchikanti et al., 2010; Nafziger & Bertino, 2009; Reisfield et al., 2007), a knowledge of opiate metabolism, and awareness of the expected ratios of the parent drug and its metabolites in urine (Reisfield et al., 2007). In addition, small amount of impurities in medications detectable by mass spectrometry can complicate the interpretation of UDT results. For example, codeine is present in morphine preparations and hydrocodone is present in oxycodone preparations (Evans et al., 2009; West et al., 2009, 2011b). Physicians who aren't aware of the presence of these impurities may wrongly dismiss a patient because he or she tested positive for codeine or hydrocodone when it was not prescribed. The presence of both parent drug and its metabolite in a urine sample readily measured by mass spectrometry can reassure the physician that the patient is taking the medication and that it is being metabolized appropriately. Also, for some drugs such as carisoprodol, fentanyl, or buprenorphine, only the metabolite may be observed. It is imperative that physicians prescribing these medications use a reference laboratory that is able to measure both the parent drug and its corresponding metabolite and be able to present interpretive results for the physician (Heltsley et al., 2010).
Creatinine is a metabolic breakdown product that is present in urine. The amount of creatinine excreted into urine is nearly constant for any individual. Reference laboratories calculate the amount of drug excreted per gram of creatinine, which allows the monitoring of excreted medication or illicit drug over time. This information is useful to physicians in certain circumstances because some drugs, such as nordiazepam remain in the system long after a person stops taking them. A UDT result that is not corrected for creatinine may show that the patient is more positive for the drug than on a previous test, even though the patient has in fact stopped taking it. Except for changes in the patient's renal status, or loss from adipose tissue due to dieting, this conflicting result may be due to the second urine being more concentrated than the first. A creatinine-corrected value will correct for a patient's hydration on the day of the test and show a decrease in the amount of nordiazepam in the urine, thus supporting the patient's claim that he or she has stopped taking the drug. It is important that reference laboratories not only provide creatinine-corrected results but that they give doctors or staff help in interpreting the data (Cone et al., 2009). It is also important for the physician to know if a patient has attempted to obscure UDT results by diluting a urine specimen. To accomplish this, he or she must have a grasp of creatinine and specific gravity UDT validity tests (Wu, 2001). Laboratory staff who interface with clients should provide this information when questions arise.

5. Monitoring ethanol use in pain patients

As stated earlier, alcohol (ethanol) use among pain patients is a significant problem because of the risk for drug-drug interaction with opioid medication. For doctors to understand UDT ethanol results, it is essential that they understand ethanol metabolism and the formation of the ethanol byproducts ethyl glucuronide and ethyl sulfate (Crews et al., 2011a; Crews et al., 2011b; Dahl et al., 2002; Helander & Beck, 2005; Helander et al., 1996; Rosano & Lin, 2008; Schmitt et al., 1997; Stephanson et al., 2002; Wojcik & Hawthorne, 2007; Wurst et al., 2006; Wurst et al., 2004). This is because false positive ethanol results can result from fermentation of glucose from diabetic patient samples (Crews et al., 2011b). Crews et al. reported that about 1/3 of the ethanol positive samples were due to fermentation. Misinterpretation of these results can have grave consequences as doctors may establish a contract with a patient that he or she abstain from any alcohol use while being treated with opioid medication; therefore, a positive finding for alcohol use can result in dismissal from the practice (Federal Register, 2004).

6. When to use UDT

Urine drug testing must be tailored to fit the pain patient's clinical history. For the intake visit, the patient is advised as to the necessity for UDT and is typically requested to provide a urine specimen. If the patient fails to do this, he or she may be immediately dismissed from the practice. In some practices, the urine specimen is tested by a POC device at the time of the appointment and the results are compared to the patient reported history. If necessary, discrepancies are discussed. As a matter of course, a portion of the POC urine sample is sent to the reference laboratory to confirm the POC test results, test for additional medications, and, at the discretion of the physician, to test for the prescribed medications, non-prescribed medications and illicit drugs at lower cutoff levels than those provided by the POC test.

For many established pain patients, quarterly or semi-annual UDT is considered appropriate. It is best if this is done on a random basis. The strongest recommendation for doing UDT is adding additional medications to the regimen or changing medications. Urine drug testing may also be administered if a patient changes their behavior or exhibits addiction tendencies such as complaining of running out of medications early (Chou et al., 2009; Trescot et al., 2006). Testing may be conducted as frequently as every office visit for some patients who exhibit unusual behavior, have a history of abuse, or if illicit or non-prescription drugs were found to be present on a previous test. Gourlay, D. & Heit, H. (2010a).

7. Purposes and costs of UDT

As stated earlier, the purpose of UDT (as well as the relative costs) may be broken down into three components: testing prescribed medications for compliance; testing for non-prescribed medications; and testing for illicit drugs. At the time when the forensic model of drug testing was instituted the vast majority of people who died from drugs died from the use of illicit drugs. At this point in time more people die from prescription medications than by illicit drugs (Hall et al., 2008; Krausz et al., 1996; Okie, 2010). There are now 13 or more classes of drugs that are used to treat pain. Pain patients are on an average using three of these drugs (Kuehn, 2007; Okie, 2010). Therefore, for every 100 patients, 300 confirmations by mass spectroscopy are required. This is more than a 100-fold increase in the number of tests needed to serve this patient population compared to workplace testing. This represents a radical change in UDT model from the forensic model used at the time when the purpose of drug testing was to root out the one or two percent of drug-using professional drivers. It is important that legislators and payors for UDT services understand the shift from the forensic UDT model to the clinical model. Currently the insurance reimbursement codes and categories do not accurately reflect the costs associated with these new clinical drug testing requirements (*Cpt Current Procedural Technology*, 2010).

7.1 Cost effectiveness of UDT

It is also important to discuss the cost-effectiveness of UDT. The National Institute on Drug Abuse (NIDA) states that the cost of not treating an addict is $56,000/year. An example of

effective treatment for heroin addiction is the methadone maintenance program, which has an average cost of $4,700/per patient/per year (Principles of Drug Addiction Treatment: A Research-Based Guide, 2009). Based on these figures, every dollar invested in drug treatment programs yields a return of about 12 times this amount. The goal then should be detecting untreated drug abuse. Urine drug testing helps accomplish this goal.
There are two aspects of drug abuse in the pain patient population; one is the use of illicit drugs, and the other more prevalent aspect is abuse of the prescribed and non-prescribed medications. Combined, these two facets of abuse may approach 20-30% of the patients on chronic opioid therapy. Using this percentage of patients and factoring the $56,000/patient cost, this means that on average each of these patients may actually be costing society and insurers $16,800 more annually than what is estimated by only calculating costs of office visits and medications. If clinical UDT is performed 2-4 times per year for each patient reimbursed at $500 per UDT, this represents a cost of $1000-$2000 per patient per year. This is in contrast to the $16,800 referenced above. It seems clear that using UDT to detect these patients should significantly reduce the cost of care as well as the costs to society (Wall et al., 2000).

7.2 Social costs of drug abuse

In light of the fact that providing the highest standard of care is one of the basic tenets of the medical profession, it is important to note that several studies have shown that untreated opioid-abusing patients have significantly higher societal cost (Wall et al., 2000) and mortality rate (between 2 and 10 times) than the comparative general population (Hall et al., 2008; Oyefeso et al., 1999). Based on this data alone, the use of UDT should be justified for pain patients.

8. Conclusions

8.1 When and how to test

Pain is a complex disease and chronic opioid therapy is one of the treatments of choice. Urine drug testing is one of the ways to measure patient adherence to the treatment regimen. At the intake office visit it is important for the physician to be able to make immediate assessment of the patient to validate their reported history and to determine the overt presence of illicit drugs or non-prescribed medications. Either a POC device or in-office immunoassay analyzer should be used for this purpose. A portion of the patient's urine specimen should be sent to a reference laboratory for analysis using lower cutoffs and a much extended test menu such as those listed in Tables 1 and 2. As stated earlier, this will give the physician further confidence that the patient's history is valid and provide measurable evidence for informed clinical decision making. In addition, alcohol use, which cannot easily be detected by the POC devices, can be identified as a risk factor.

8.2 Ongoing testing

At subsequent visits UDT will provide the physician with evidence of patient compliance with prescribed medications (West et al., 2010a) and eliminate the potential for abuse of non-prescribed medications or illicit drugs (Pesce et al., 2010b). For this purpose, depending upon clinical judgment, the test menu does not have to be quite as extensive. Tests for rarely-observed illicit drugs such as MDMA and PCP may not be included. Similarly, tests for rarely-prescribed or removed medications such as propoxyphene may not be included. If intake visit UDT showed that the patient was observed to be taking a non-prescribed medication or illicit drug then subsequent visit UDT's should include tests for those agents. Because of the potential for morbidity from alcohol-medication interactions, it may be necessary to continue to monitor certain patients for ethanol and its metabolites.

8.3 Minimum analytical requirements

When monitoring for opioid medication compliance, the testing method should be able to differentiate between codeine, morphine, hydrocodone, norhydrocodone, and hydromorphone. The test should also be able to differentiate between oxycodone, noroxycodone, and oxymorphone. This will allow the physician to determine that the opiate the patient is taking is in fact the one being prescribed and that the patient is metabolizing the medication properly (Pesce et al., 2010a). A similar case can be made for the testing of benzodiazepines. The method should be able to detect at low concentrations and differentiate between alpha-hydroxyalprazolam, 7-aminoclonazepam, lorazepam, nordiazepam, temazepam, and oxazepam. This will allow the doctor to see that the patient is taking the prescribed benzodiazepine and allay any concerns about doctor shopping. Frequency of UDT should be based on the physician's observations of the patient's behavior as well as suggested guidelines. For those patients whose behavior is not of concern, some guidelines suggest UDT between two and four times per year on a random basis (Chou et al., 2009; Trescot et al., 2006). For those patients with non-compliant behavior or a history of addiction, testing should be done as often as every office visit (Chou et al., 2009; Trescot et al., 2006).

9. References

Agilent Technologies, Inc. 5301 Stevens Creek Blvd, Santa Clara, CA 95051, USA. Thermo Fisher Scientific. 81 Wyman St, Waltham, MA 02454, USA.

Amedica Drug Screen Test Cup. Hayward, CA: Amedica Biotech, Inc.

American Proficiency Institute 2011 Catalog of Programs. Traverse City, MI: American Proficiency Institute, 2011.

Atluri, S. & Sudarshan, G. (2003). Evaluation of Abnormal Urine Drug Screens among Patients with Chronic Non-Malignant Pain Treated with Opioids. *Pain Physician,* Vol.6, No.4, pp.407-409,

Chou, R., Fanciullo, G., Fine, P., Adler, J., Ballantyne, J., Davies, P., Donovan, M., Fishbain, D., Foley, K., Fudin, J., Gilson, A., Kelter, A., Mauskop, A., O'Connor, P., Passik, S., Pasternak, G., Portenoy, R., Rich, B., Roberts, R., Todd, K. & Miaskowski, C. (2009). Clinical Guidelines for the Use of Chronic Opioid Therapy in Chronic Noncancer Pain. *The Journal of Pain,* Vol.10, No.2, (February 2009), pp.113-130, 1526-5900

College of American Pathologists 2011 Surveys and Anatomic Pathology Education Programs. Northfield, IL: College of American Pathologists, 2011.

Cone, E., Caplan, Y., Black, D., Robert, T. & Moser, F. (2008). Urine Drug Testing of Chronic Pain Patients: Licit and Illicit Drug Patterns. *Journal of Analytical Toxicology,* Vol.32, No.8, (October 2008), pp.530-543, ISSN 1945-2403

Cone, E., Caplan, Y., Moser, F., Robert, T., Shelby, M. & Black, D. (2009). Normalization of Urinary Drug Concentrations with Specific Gravity and Creatinine. *Journal of Analytical Toxicology,* Vol.33, No.1, (January-February 2009), pp.1-7, ISSN 1945-2403

Cpt Current Procedural Technology. (2010). (Professional ed.), American Medical Association, Chicago, IL

Crews, B., Latyshev, S., Mikel, C., Almazan, P., West, R., Pesce, A. & West, C. (2011a). Improved Detection of Ethyl Glucuronide and Ethyl Sulfate in a Pain Management Population Using High-Throughput Lc-Ms/Ms. *Journal of Opioid Management,* Vol.6, No.6, (Novenber-December 2010), pp.415-421, ISSN 1551-7489

Crews, B., West, R., Gutierrez, R., Latyshev, S., Mikel, C., Almazan, P., Pesce, A., West, C. & Rosenthal, M. (2011b). An Improved Method of Determining Ethanol Use in a Chronic Pain Population. *Journal of Opioid Management,* Vol.In Press, (n.d.), ISSN 1551-7489

Dahl, H., Stephanson, N., Beck, O. & Helander, A. (2002). Comparison of Urinary Excretion Characteristics of Ethanol and Ethyl Glucuronide. *Journal of Analytical Toxicology,* Vol.26, No.4, (May-June 2002), pp.201-204, ISSN 1945-2403

Evans, M., Kriger, S., Gunn, J. & Schwilke, E. (2009). Anomalous Opiate Detection in Compliance Monitoring. *Practical Pain Management,* Vol.9, No.7, (September 2009), pp.54-55,

Federal Register - Mandatory Guidelines and Proposed Revisions to Mandatory Guidelines for Federal Workplace Drug Testing Programs. Substance Abuse and Mental Health Services Administration. Rockville, MD: Department of Health and Human Services, 2004;69(71).

Feldkamp, C.S. (2010). Immunological Reactions, In: *Clinical Chemistry: Theory, Analysis, and Correlation,* L. A. Kaplan and A. J. Pesce, pp. 151-179, Mosby, St. Louis

Fraser, A. & Zamecnik, J. (2003). Impact of Lowering the Screening and Confirmation Cutoff Values for Urine Drug Testing Based on Dilution Indicators. *Therapeutic Drug Monitoring,* Vol.25, No.6, (December 2003), pp.723-727, ISSN 1536-3694

Fraser, A.D. (2001). Psychotropic Agents: The Benzodiazepines, In: *The Clinical Toxicology Laboratory: Contemporary Practice of Poisoning Evaluation,* L. C. Shaw, T. C. Kwong, T. G. Rosano, P. J. Orsolak, B. A. Wolf and B. Magnani, pp. 211-221, American Association for Clinical Chemistry, Inc., Washington, DC

Gourlay, D. & Heit, H. (2010a). The Art and Science of Urine Drug Testing. *The Clinical Journal of Pain,* Vol.26, No.4, (May 2010), pp.358, ISSN 0749-8047

Gourlay, D., Heit, H. & Almahrezi, A. (2005). Universal Precautions in Pain Medicine: A Rational Approach to the Treatment of Chronic Pain. *Pain Medicine,* Vol.6, No.2, (March-April 2010), pp.107-112, ISSN 1526-4637

Gourlay, D., Heit, H. & Caplan, Y. Urine Drug Testing in Clinical Practice: The Art and Science of Patient Care. California Academy of Family Physicians. Stamford, CT: PharmaCom Group, Inc., 2010.

Gourlay, D. & Heit, H.A. (2010b). The Art and Science of Urine Drug Testing. *Clin J Pain,* Vol.26, No.4, pp.358,

Hall, A., Logan, J., Toblin, R., Kaplan, J., Kraner, J., Bixler, D., Crosby, A. & Paulozzi, L. (2008). Patterns of Abuse among Unintentional Pharmaceutical Overdose Fatalities. *JAMA,* Vol.300, No.22, (December 2008), pp.2613-2620, ISSN 1538-3598

Hammett-Stabler, C. & Webster, L. A Clinical Guide to Urine Drug Testing: Augmenting Pain Management and Enhancing Patient Care. University of Medicine and

Dentistry of New Jersay - Center for Continuing and Outreach Education. Stamford, CT: PharmaCom Group, Inc, 2008.

Harmful Interactions: Mixing Alcohol with Medicines. National Institute on Alcohol Abuse and Alcoholism. Bethesda, MD: National Institutes of Health, 2007.

Hattab, E., Goldberger, B., Johannsen, L., Kindland, P., Ticino, F., Chronister, C. & Bertholf, R. (2000). Modification of Screening Immunoassays to Detect Sub-Threshold Concentrations of Cocaine, Cannabinoids, and Opiates in Urine: Use for Detecting Maternal and Neonatal Drug Exposures. *Annals of Clinical and Laboratory Science,* Vol.31, No.1, (January 2000), pp.85-91, ISSN 1550-8080

Helander, A. & Beck, O. (2005). Ethyl Sulfate: A Metabolite of Ethanol in Humans and a Potential Biomarker of Acute Alcohol Intake. *Journal of Analytical Toxicology,* Vol.29, No.5, (July-August 2005), pp.270-274, ISSN 1945-2403

Helander, A., Beck, O. & Jones, A. (1996). Laboratory Testing for Recent Alcohol Consumption: Comparison of Ethanol, Methanol, and 5-Hydroxytryptophol. *Clinical Chemistry,* Vol.42, No.4, (April 1996), pp.618-624, ISSN 1530-8561

Heltsley, R., Zichterman, A., Black, D., Cawthon, B., Robert, T., Moser, F., Caplan, Y. & Cone, E. (2010). Urine Drug Testing of Chronic Pain Patients. Ii. Prevalence Patterns of Prescription Opiates and Metabolites. *Journal of Analytical Toxicology,* Vol.34, No.1, (January-February 2010), pp.32-38, ISSN 1945-2403

Ives, T., Chelminski, P., Hammett-Stabler, C., Malone, R., Perhac, J., Potisek, N., Shilliday, B., DeWalt, D. & Pignone, M. (2006). Predictors of Opioid Misuse in Patients with Chronic Pain: A Prospective Cohort Study. *BMC Health Services Research,* Vol.6, No.1, (April 2006), pp.46, ISSN 1472-6963

Jung, B. & Reidenberg, M. (2007). Physicians Being Deceived. *Pain Medicine,* Vol.8, No.5, (July-August 2007), pp.433-437, ISSN 1526-4637

Katz, N., Sherburne, S., Beach, M., Rose, R., Vielguth, J., Bradley, J. & Fanciullo, G. (2003). Behavioral Monitoring and Urine Toxicology Testing in Patients Receiving Long-Term Opioid Therapy. *Anesthesia and Analgesia,* Vol.97, No.4, (October 2003), pp.1097-1102, ISSN 1526-7598

Krausz, M., Degkwit, P., Haasen, C. & Verthein, U. (1996). Opioid Addiction and Suicidality. *Crisis,* Vol.17, No.4, pp.175-181,

Kuehn, B.M. (2007). Opioid Prescriptions Soar: Increase in Legitimate Use as Well as Abuse. *JAMA,* Vol.297, No.3, pp.249-251, 0098-7484 1538-3598

Madras, B., Compton, W., Avula, D., Stegbauer, T., Stein, J. & Clark, H. (2009). Screening, Brief Interventions, Referral to Treatment (Sbirt) for Illicit Drug and Alcohol Use at Multiple Healthcare Sites: Comparison at Intake and 6 Months Later. *Drug and Alcohol Dependence,* Vol.99, No.1-3, (January 2009), pp.280-295, ISSN 1879-0046

Manchikanti, L., Atluri, S., Trescot, A. & Giordano, J. (2008). Monitoring Opioid Adherence in Chronic Pain Patients: Tools, Techniques, and Utility. *Pain Physician,* Vol.11, No.2, (March 2008), pp.S155-S180, ISSN 1533-3159

Manchikanti, L., Cash, K., Damron, K., Manchukonda, R., Pampati, V. & McManus, C. (2006a). Controlled Substance Abuse and Illicit Drug Use in Chronic Pain Patients: An Evaluation of Multiple Variables. *Pain Physician,* Vol.9, No.3, (July 2006), pp.215-226, ISSN 1533-3159

Manchikanti, L., Damron, K., McManus, C. & Barnhill, R. (2004). Patterns of Illicit Drug Use and Opioid Abuse in Patients with Chronic Pain at Initial Evaluation: A Prospective, Observational Study. *Pain Physician,* Vol.7, No.4, (October 2004), pp.431-437, ISSN 1533-3159

Manchikanti, L., Malla, Y., Wargo, B., Cash, K., Pampati, V., Damron, K., McManus, C. & Brandon, D. (2010). Protocol for Accuracy of Point of Care (Poc) or in-Office Urine Drug Testing (Immunoassay) in Chronic Pain Patients: A Prospective Analysis of Immunoassay and Liquid Chromatography Tandem Mass Spectometry (Lc/Ms/Ms). *Pain Physician,* Vol.13, No.1, (January 2010), pp.E1-E22, ISSN 1533-3159

Manchikanti, L., Manchukonda, R., Pampati, V., Damron, K., Brandon, D., Cash, K. & McManus, C. (2006b). Does Random Urine Drug Testing Reduce Illicit Drug Use in Chronic Pain Patients Receiving Opioids? *Pain Physician,* Vol.9, No.2, (April 2006), pp.123-129, ISSN 1533-3159

Manchikanti, L., Manchukonda, R., Pampati, V. & Damron, K.S. (2005). Evaluation of Abuse of Prescription and Illicit Drugs in Chronic Pain Patients Receiving Short-Acting (Hydrocodone) or Long-Acting (Methadone) Opioids. *Pain Physician,* Vol.8, No.3, pp.257-261,

Michna, E., Jamison, R., Pham, L., Ross, E., Janfaza, D., Nedeljkovic, S., Narang, S., Palombi, D. & Wasan, A. (2007). Urine Toxicology Screening among Chronic Pain Patients on Opioid Therapy: Frequency and Predictability of Abnormal Findings. *The Clinical Journal of Pain,* Vol.23, No.2, (February 2007), pp.173-179, ISSN 1536-5409

Mikel, C., Almazan, P., West, R., Crews, B., Latyshev, S., Pesce, A. & West, C. (2009). Lc-Ms/Ms Extends the Range of Drug Analysis in Pain Patients. *Therapeutic Drug Monitoring,* Vol.31, No.6, (December 2009), pp.746-748, ISSN 1536-3694

Mikel, C., Pesce, A. & West, C. (2010). A Tale of Two Drug Testing Technologies: Gc-Ms and Lc-Ms/Ms. *Pain Physician,* Vol.13, No.1, pp.91-92,

Mohsin, S., Yang, Y. & Zumwalt, M. Quantitative Analysis of Opiates in Urine Using Rrht Lc/Ms/Ms. Santa Clara, CA: Agilent Technologies, Inc., 2007.

Nafziger, A. & Bertino, J., Jr. (2009). Utility and Application of Urine Drug Testing in Chronic Pain Management with Opioids. *The Clinical Journal of Pain,* Vol.25, No.1, (January 2009), pp.73-79, ISSN 1536-5409

National Prescription Drug Threat Assesment. U.S. Department of Justice. Johnstown, PA: National Drug Intelligence Center, 2009.

National Survey on Drug Use and Health: Detailed Tables - Prevalence Estimates, Standard Errors, P Values, and Sample Sizes. Substance Abuse and Mental Health Services Administration. Rockville, MD: Department of Health and Human Services, 1995-2006.

Nucynta - Tapentadol. (2010). December 3, 2010, Available from: <www.nucynta.com>

Okie, S. (2010). A Flood of Opioids, a Rising Tide of Deaths. *The New England Journal of Medicine,* Vol.363, No.21, (November 2010), pp.1981-1985, ISSN 1533-4406

Olympus Au640 Product Information. Brea, CA: Beckman Coulter, Inc. Lab Systems and Routine Testing.

Oyefeso, A., Ghodse, H., Clancy, C., Corkery, J. & Goldfinch, R. (1999). Drug Abuse-Related Mortality: A Study of Teenage Addicts over a 20-Year Period. *Social Psychiatry and Psychiatric Epidemiology,* Vol.34, No.8, (August 1999), pp.437-441, ISSN 1433-9285

Pesce, A., Rosenthal, M., West, R., West, C., Crews, B., Mikel, C., Almazan, P. & Latyshev, S. (2010a). An Evaluation of the Diagnostic Accuracy of Liquid Chromatography-Tandem Mass Spectrometry Versus Immunoassay Drug Testing in Pain Patients. *Pain Physician,* Vol.13, No.3, pp.273-281,

Pesce, A., West, C., Rosenthal, M., West, R., Crews, B., Mikel, C., Almazan, P., Latyshev, S. & Horn, P. (2010b). Marijuana Correlates with Use of Other Illicit Drugs in a Pain Patient Population. *Pain Physician,* Vol.13, No.3, pp.283-287,

Pesce, A., West, C., West, R., Crews, B., Mikel, C., Almazan, P., Latyshev, S., Rosenthal, M. & Horn, P. (2010c). Reference Intervals: A Novel Approach to Detect Drug Abuse in a Pain Patient Population. *Journal of Opioid Management,* Vol.6, No.5, (September-October 2010), pp.341-350, ISSN 1551-7489

Pesce, A., West, C., West, R., Crews, B., Mikel, C., Rosenthal, M., Almazan, P. & Latyshev, S. (2011). Determination of Medication Cutoff Values in a Pain Patient Population. *Journal of Opioid Management,* Vol.In Press, (n.d.), ISSN 1551-7489

Principles of Drug Addiction Treatment: A Research-Based Guide. National Institue on Drug Abuse. Bethesda, MD: Department of Health and Human Services, 2009.

Reisfield, G., Salazar, E. & Bertholf, R. (2007). Rational Use and Interpretation of Urine Drug Testing in Chronic Opioid Therapy. *Annals of Clinical and Laboratory Science,* Vol.37, No.4, (Autumn 2007), pp.301-314, ISSN 1550-8080

Rosano, T. & Lin, J. (2008). Ethyl Glucuronide Excretion in Humans Following Oral Administration of and Dermal Exposure to Ethanol. *Journal of Analytical Toxicology,* Vol.32, No.8, (October 2008), pp.594-600, ISSN 1945-2403

Schmitt, G., Droenner, P., Skopp, G. & Aderjan, R. (1997). Ethyl Glucuronide Concentration in Serum of Human Volunteers, Teetotalers, and Suspected Drinking Drivers. *Journal of Forensic Sciences,* Vol.42, No.6, (November 1997), pp.1099-1102, ISSN 1556-4029

Schuckman, H., Hazelett, S., Powell, C. & Steer, S. (2008). A Validation of Self-Reported Substance Use with Biochemical Testing among Patients Presenting to the Emergency Department Seeking Treatment for Backache, Headache, and Toothache. *Substance Use and Misuse,* Vol.43, No.5, (n.d.), pp.589-595, ISSN 1433-9285

Siemens V-Twin Analyzer Product Information. Hermosa Beach, CA: Siemens Healthcare Diagnostic, Inc.

Siuzdak, G. (2006). *The Expanding Role of Mass Spectrometry in Biotechnology* (2nd ed.), MCC Press, San Diego, CA

Sobolevsky, T., Prasolov, I. & Rodchenkov, G. (2010). Detection of Jwh-018 Metabolites in Smoking Mixture Post-Administration Urine. *Forensic Science International,* Vol.200, No.1-3, (July 2010), pp.141-147, ISSN 1872-6283

Stephanson, N., Dahl, H., A., H. & Beck, O. (2002). Direct Quantification of Ethyl Glucuronide in Clinical Urine Samples by Liquid Chromatography-Mass

Spectrometry. *Therapeutic Drug Monitoring,* Vol.24, No.5, (October 2002), pp.645-651, ISSN 1536-3694

Thermo Fisher Mgc-240 Analyzer Product Information. Franklin, MA: Thermo Fisher Scientific.

Trescot, A., Boswell, M., Atluri, S., Hansen, H., Deer, T., Abdi, S., Jasper, J., Singh, V., Jordan, A., Johnson, B., Cicala, R., Dunbar, E., Helm, S., II, Varley, K., Suchdev, P., Swicegood, J., Calodney, A., Ogoke, B., Minore, W. & Manchikanti, L. (2006). Opioid Guidelines in the Management of Chronic Non-Cancer Pain. *Pain Physician,* Vol.9, No.1, (January 2006), pp.1-40, ISSN 1533-3159

Vardakou, I., Pistos, C. & Spiliopoulou, C. (2010). Spice Drugs as a New Trend: Mode of Action, Identification and Legislation. *Toxicology Letters,* Vol.197, No.3, (September 2010), pp.157-162, ISSN 1879-3169

Wall, R., Rehm, J., Fischer, B., Brands, B., Gliksman, L., Stewart, J., Medved, W. & Blake, J. (2000). Social Costs of Untreated Opioid Dependence. *Journal of Urban Health,* Vol.77, No.4, (December 2000), pp.688-722, ISSN 1468-2869

Webster, L. & Dove, B. (2007). *Avoiding Opioid Abuse While Managing Pain: A Guide for Practitioners,* Sunrise River Press, North Branch, MN

West, R., Crews, B., Mikel, C., Almazan, P., Latyshev, S., Pesce, A. & West, C. (2009). Anomalous Observations of Codeine in Patients on Morphine. *Therapeutic Drug Monitoring,* Vol.31, No.6, (December 2009), pp.776-778, ISSN 1536-3694

West, R., Pesce, A., Crews, B., Mikel, C., Rosenthal, M., Almazan, P., Latyshev, S. & West, C. (2011a). Determination of Illicit Drug Cutoff Values in a Pain Patient Population. *Clinica Chimica Acta,* Vol.In Press, (n.d.), ISSN 1873-3492

West, R., Pesce, A., Mikel, C., Rosenthal, M., Latyshev, S., Crews, B. & Almazan, P. (2010a). Observations of Medication Compliance by Measurement of Urinary Drug Concentrations in a Pain Management Population. *Journal of Opioid Management,* Vol.6, No.4, (July-August 2010), pp.253-257, ISSN 1551-7489

West, R., Pesce, A., West, C., Crews, B., Mikel, C., Almazan, P., Rosenthal, M. & Latyshev, S. (2010b). Comparison of Clonazepam Compliance by Measurement of Urinary Concentration by Immunoassay and Lc-Ms/Ms in Pain Management Population. *Pain Physician,* Vol.13, No.1, pp.71-78,

West, R., West, C., Crews, B., Almazan, P., Latyshev, S., Rosenthal, M., Pesce, A. & Mikel, C. (2011b). Anomalous Observations of Hydrocodone in Patients on Oxycodone. *Clinica Chimica Acta,* Vol.412, No.1-2, (January 2011), pp.29-32, ISSN 1873-3492

Wingert, W. (1997). Lowering Cutoffs for Initial and Confirmation Testing for Cocaine and Marijuana: Large-Scale Study of Effects on the Rates of Drug-Positive Results. *Clinical Chemistry,* Vol.43, No.1, (January 1997), pp.100-103, ISSN 1530-8561

Wojcik, M. & Hawthorne, J. (2007). Sensitivity of Commercial Ethyl Glucuronide (Etg) Testing in Screening for Alcohol Abstinence. *Alcohol and Alcoholism,* Vol.42, No.4, (July-August 2007), pp.317-320, ISSN 1464-3502

Wu, A.H.B. (2001). Urine Adulteration before Testing for Drugs of Abuse, In: *The Clinical Toxicology Laboratory: Contemporary Practice of Poisoning Evaluation,* L. C. Shaw, T. C. Kwong, T. G. Rosano, P. J. Orsolak, B. A. Wolf and B. Magnani, pp. 157-171, American Association for Clinical Chemistry, Inc., Washington, DC

Wurst, F., Dresen, S., Allen, J., Wiesbeck, G., Graf, M. & Weinmann, W. (2006). Ethyl Sulphate: A Direct Ethanol Metabolite Reflecting Recent Alcohol Consumption. *Addiction,* Vol.101, No.2, (February 2006), pp.204-211, ISSN 1360-0443

Wurst, F., Wiesbeck, G., Metzger, J., Weinmann, W. & Graf, M. (2004). On Sensitivity, Specificity, and the Influence of Various Parameters on Ethyl Glucuronide Levels in Urine - Results from the Who/Isbra Study. *Alcoholism, Clinical and Experimental Research,* Vol.28, No.8, (August 2004), pp.1220-1228, ISSN 1530-0277

3

Experimental and Computational Methods Pertaining to Surface Tension of Pharmaceuticals

Abolghasem Jouyban[1] and Anahita Fathi-Azarbayjani[2]
[1]*Drug Applied Research Center and Faculty of Pharmacy, Tabriz University of Medical Sciences, Tabriz,*
[2]*Faculty of Medicine, Urmia University of Medical Sciences, Urmia, Iran*

1. Introduction

The molecules of a fluid experiences attractive forces exerted on it by all its neighboring molecules. In the bulk of the liquid, molecules are attracted equally in all directions resulting in a net force of zero. Molecules at or near the surface experience attractive force which tends to pull them to the interior. Surface chemistry deals with thermodynamic and kinetic parameters that take place between two different coexisting phases at equilibrium. Surface tension, γ is free energy of the surface at any air/fluid interface defined as force per unit length or energy per unit area. The latter term, also called surface energy, is more useful in thermodynamics and it applies to solids as well as liquid surfaces. The surface free energy of a liquid is measured by its surface tension and the surface free energy of a solid can be revealed by contact angle measurements. The surface tension measurement depends very markedly upon the presence of impurities in the liquid, temperature and pressure changes (Buckton, 1988).

Surface tension is a phenomenon that we see in our everyday life. Human biological fluids, e.g. serum, urine, gastric juice, amniotic liquid, cerebrospinal and alveolar lining liquid contain numerous low-and high-molecular weight surfactants, proteins and lipids that adsorb at liquid interface. The physicochemical processes that take place in these interfaces are extremely important for the vital function of body organs and have a great impact on pharmacodynamic parameters of drug molecules (Kazakov et al., 2000; Trukhin et al., 2001). Drug substances are usually administered as part of a formulation in combination with excipients that have varied and specialized pharmaceutical functions. The design of drug formulation is based on the principles of pharmacokinetic, biopharmaceutic and pharmaceutical technology. The pharmaceutical industry has directed its attention mainly to the quality and processability of active pharmaceutical products which is reflected in various physicochemical parameters. The drug and pharmaceutical materials require extensive characterization and testing of their stability, physico-chemical properties, effectiveness, palatability and ease of administration to ensure drug efficacy. Among the important characteristics are the drug dissolution and solubility in gastrointestinal tract, intestinal absorption, drug distribution and drug-plasma protein binding. By applying special surface treatments such as contact angle and surface tension measurements to pharmaceutical compounds, drug distribution, dissolution behavior and release pattern in various body fluids can be improved (Hancock et al., 1997; Ho et al., 2010).

Surface tension can influence the development, prediction and performance of pharmaceutical products and help to solve industrial problems and improve products quality. Due to the importance of this phenomenon in drug formulations, there is a growing need for specific interfacial consideration that can be used routinely to solve pharmaceutical problems and improve product quality and stability. In order to meet challenges and develop new and better performing pharmaceutical products, knowledge of surface tension and its measurements techniques is of utmost importance. Amongst many techniques used for characterizing the surface energies of pharmaceuticals are the surface tension measurements, contact angle and wettability tests (Buckton, 1988; Chamarthy et al., 2009; Puri et al., 2010). The objective of this chapter is to introduce experimental and computational methods of surface tension measurment in the pharmaceutical industry.

2. Standard methods and instrumentations of surface tension measurement

Surface tension is a very complicated property of a liquid and it depends upon many variables such as temperature, composition of the solution, measurement time, materials of the apparatus and viscosity of the liquid. When a new surface is being formed, surface active chemicals diffuse to the surface and align. During this process, the surface tension is changing rapidly and continuously. Dynamic surface tension measurements allows track of these changes. When the process reaches equilibrium, static surface tension is obtained by measuring the maximum force at a liquid/gas interface on a sample where the net forces on the line is zero during the test time. Pure fluids and solvents have a single surface tension value and are measured with these devices (Drelich et al. 2002, Thiessen and Man, 1999).

There are a number of commonly available methods for measuring surface tension of liquids. Each has its advantages and limitations. The choice of a method depends on the nature of system to be studied and its stability, the degree of accuracy required, the condition under which its tension is to be measured and possibly on the ability of the instrument to automate the measurements. Realistically the surface tension values of a liquid will vary depending upon the method used (Thiessen and Man, 1999). The following section describes the most used methods for measuring static and dynamic surface and interfacial tension of liquid mixtures as well as semi solids and solids (a summary of the methods is shown in Table 1).

2.1 Wilhelmy plate method

The Wilhelmy plate consists of a thin glass, platinum plate or pre-wetted paper, usually on the order of a few centimeters square, attached to an electrobalance via thin metal wire and is used to measure equilibrium interfacial tension at an air-liquid or liquid-liquid interface (Figure 1). The metal plate must be cleaned from organic contaminants or test solutions, therefore the plate is flamed before the experiment to avoid contamination and to help maintain good wetting of the plate by the test liquid. The plate is then immersed and retracted into and out of the test solution contained in a beaker on a mechanical stage. During these cycles the force acting on the plate vs. depth of immersion are recorded. The meniscus formed at the solid–liquid interface is characterized by the contact angle. Two contact angles are measured, an advancing contact angle and a receding contact angle and the surface tension is calculated from the resulting force. The wetting force is monitored with time and this method is specially suited to check static surface tension value which in some cases is more than 4 h, hence the measurements are assumed to represent equilibrium. The main drawback of this method is that the surface age (time taken from surface formation till measurement) is not taken into account. When working with viscous liquids it takes time for a viscous material to flow from the dipped portion of the plate. Thus the surface tension will decrease initially till it reaches a pleatue once the excess liquid has flowed from the plate, therefore this method is not suited for highly viscous solutions (Avranas and Taspoulos, 2000; Krishnan et al., 2005; Santos and Castanho, 2004). The static wetting force on the plate is used to calculate the static surface tension (γ) using the Wilhelmy equation:

$$\gamma = \frac{F}{l.\cos\theta} \tag{1}$$

where F is the difference in wetting force upon immersion and withdrawal in mN/m, l is the wetted perimeter of the Wilhelmy plate and θ is the advancing or receding contact angle between the liquid phase and the plate. The contact angle θ of most liquids against platinum plate or clean glass is often assumed to be zero. This method does not require other correction factors such as fluid density. This method can be used to measure the contact angle and wetting properties of solid surfaces, where the platinum ring plate is replaced by the test surface (Avranas and Tasopoulos, 2000; Krishnan et al., 2005; Santos and Castanho, 2004; Sipahi, 2001; Tan et al., 2005).

The static contact angle, θ, is an important parameter in many industries including pharmaceutics. Contact angle measurements span every pharmaceutical field, from fluid dynamic to powder and tablet (Muster and Prestidge, 2002), adhesion and spray-drying of various drug delivery systems (Millqvist-Fureby et al., 1999) to the detection of impurities in the solutions of surface active compounds (Al-Maaieh and Aburub, 2007). It is of particular interest in powders, because the formulations are dependent on the contact angle. Contact angle measurements can be performed using various methods including Wilhelmy plate method, capillary rise method, goniometer and sessile drop method (Dingles and Harris, 2005). Among the interfacial tensiometry methods, the Wilhelmy plate method has been extensively developed and used by scientists in the pharmaceutical industry. The equipment used in this method is commercially available at several companies. With this technique it is possible to measure and control interfacial properties in granulation and tabletting, (Dreu et al., 2005) polymeric surfactants, emulsions and foams, protein-phospholipid interaction (Oritz et al., 2003), interfacial tension of topical skin formulations (Vejnovic et al., 2010), bioadhesive forces between mucosal tissue and microsphere drug delivery system (Vasir et al., 2003).

2.2 Du Noüy ring method

Du Noüy ring method is a traditional method used to measure static surface or interfacial tension. The measurement simply requires the ring to be wetted by the liquid and then pulled through the interface while measuring the force exerted on the ring (see Figure 1). Wetting properties of the surface or interface have little influence on this measuring technique. As in the case of Wilhelmy plate, the ring, with a diameter of 2-3 cm, is usually made up of platinum or iridium is submerged into liquid and then pulled through the liquid-air interface. Maximum pull exerted on the ring by the surface is measured which is directly proportional to the surface tension value at equilibrium (Bodour and Miller-Maier, 1998). The ring is submerged into the solution and then slowly pulled through the liquid-air interface to detach from the interface with a force that is correlated to the surface tension. With this method, it is possible to measure the interfacial tension at both liquid-air and liquid-liquid interfaces. Surface tension can be calculated using the equation below:

$$\gamma = \frac{F}{p\cos\theta} f \tag{2}$$

where p is the perimeter of the three-phase contact line, f is the correction factor (because additional volume of liquid is lifted during the detachment of the ring from the interface) between each measurement. The platinum wire ring was rinsed three times with water, later with acetone as was blow dried (Drelich et al., 2002).

One major difference between the Du Noüy ring method and Wilhelmy's plate is the way in which the surface tension measurement is carried out. The ring moves through the interface whereas the plate is static at the interface, therefore there is no disturbance at the interface and this method is the recommended geometry for studying time dependent characteristics. Both ring and plate geometries can be used with the force balance type of tensiometer. A single instrument is normally capable of performing either Wilherlmy plate or du Noüy ring measurements (Thiessen and Man, 1999).

The surface tension measured by du Noüy method has been utilized in pharmaceutical research, for example, in the measurement of emulsion stability (Ishii et al., 1988; Takamura et al., 1984) and development of a dissolution media to simulate the physiological environment of the gastric region (Luner et al., 2001). This method can be used for characterization of pharmaceutical formulations such as plasticizer and polymer coating and surface tension calculation of various surfactant solutions and their CMC values (Palma et al., 2002) at the point of intersection of the interfacial tension value versus surfactant concentration plot (de la Maza, 1998; Korhonen et al., 2004; Zelkó et al., 2002).

2.3 Maximum bubble pressure method

The maximum bubble pressure method involves flow of a gas bubble (typically air or nitrogen) at a constant rate and blows them through a capillary with a known diameter which is submerged in the sample liquid. The pressure inside of the gas bubble increases until the bubble becomes hemispherical and its radius corresponds to the radius of the capillary. Beyond this the bubble is unstable and grows explosively until it detaches itself from the capillary and a new bubble is formed. The method is based on the continuous measurement of the applied pressure versus bubble rate formed at the end of the capillary. Figure 1 shows each step of bubble formation and corresponding change of bubble radius. The dynamic surface tension can be directly calculated by Young-LaPlace equation:

$$\gamma = \frac{\Delta P_{\max} R}{2} \tag{3}$$

where ΔP_{max} is the maximum pressure difference and R is the capillary radius (Drelich et al., 2002; Hallowell and Hirt, 1994; Fainerman et al., 2006). This method is one of the most popular techniques to measure the dynamic surface tension of various surfactants around and above their CMC value where adsorption is rapid (Christov et al., 2006). In the maximum bubble pressure method, a single interfacial tension value is drawn from each bubble formed. This device is the only available method capable of measuring surface tension in milliseconds time range. This method is particularly useful in measuring surface tension of highly concentrated surfactant solutions (Mischuk et al., 2000) and molten metals (Drelich et al., 2002).

2.4 Drop volume/weight method

Among the conventional methods of surface tension measurement, drop shape techniques have proven to be reliable and easy to handle. This method weighs the mass of the liquid drop or the volume of the drop that falls off a capillary tip of known diameter when pumped very slowly. The weight of the drop falling off the capillary correlates with the interfacial tension and is measured by balancing it against a known gravitational force through the following equation:

$$W = V\Delta\rho g = 2\pi r f \tag{4}$$

where $\Delta\rho$ is the difference in the density of the heavy phase and the light phase, g is the gravitational constant (g=9.81652 m/s^2), r is the radius of the capillary tip and f denotes the empirical drop correction factor introduced by Harkins and Brown. The correction factor is required because only a portion of the drop falls from the capillary tip during detachment and this corrects the deviation of the drop volume from its ideal value (Drelich et al., 2002; Gunde et al., 2001). Impurity of active pharmaceutical solutions (Al-Maaieh and Aburub 2007), emulsion stability (Rangsansarid and Fukada, 2007), potency of local anesthetics (Matsuki et al., 1998), stability of biphasic aqueous systems (Mishima et al., 1998) and surface active properties of drugs (Deo et al., 2004) have been evaluated using this technique.

2.5 Pendant drop method

Most of surface tension measurement techniques have limitations and only a few are suitable for protein solutions and high viscous solutions such as polymers blends. As discussed earlier, the Wilhelmy plate technique requires the establishment of a zero contact angle of the liquid at the plate which is difficult to guarantee with systems involving protein solutions and polymeric solutions with high viscosity. Du Noüy ring method, the drop volume technique or the maximum bubble method also lack dynamic control (Chen et al., 1999). In general, the equilibrium static methods such as sessile drop, spinning drop or a pendant drop method are most commonly used for measuring surface tension of molten metals and viscous solutions (Arashiro and Demarquette, 1999).

The pendent drop technique is capable of producing highly accurate static as well as dynamic interfacial tensions and contact angle measurements. This method is mostly used for the surface tension measurements of metals, alloys and polymers. In this method geometry of the drop is analyzed optically. The increased accuracy and simplicity of this ground based method allow ultra low surface tension, temperature and time dependence of interfacial tension as well as surface tension measurements at elevated pressures (Chen et al., 1999).

A typical pendant drop apparatus (see Figure 1) consists of three parts:

1. An experimental compartment, which includes a microsyringe to produce a pendent drop of a solution at the tip of a capillary, to measure the maximum volume of the drop at reservoir conditions (pressure and temperature).
2. A viewing system to visualize the drop; this part consist of an accurate video system and magnification factor for the image in both the x and y direction.
3. A data acquisition system to compute the surface tension from the digital image of the pendant drop (via Laplace's equation).

The accuracy of the surface tension measurements is highly dependent on the imaging system. Images of the drop can be captured automatically at certain frequencies over a period of several hours depending on the time duration of the test. These digitized pendant drop images can be stored on the computer to calculate the surface tension values as a function of the length of time (Arashiro and Demarquette, 1999; Gunde et al., 2001; Semmler and Kohler, 1999).

This method involves the determination of the profile of a drop of one liquid suspended in another liquid at mechanical equilibrium. This is done by the balance between gravity and surface forces. The equation of Bashforth and Adams which is based on Laplace's equation relates the drop profile to the interfacial tension. This is the most widely used method to date which is given below:

$$\gamma = \frac{\Delta \rho g D_e^2}{H} \tag{5}$$

where g is gravitational constant, $\Delta\rho$ is the difference in densities between tile drop and its surroundings and D is the equatorial diameter of the drop at the apex and H is the shape factor that contains the properties of the fluid (Arashiro and Demarquette, 1999; Dingle et al., 2005; Hernández-Baltazar and Gracia-Fadrique, 2005).

Dynamic surface tension of biological fluids (Trukhin et al., 2001), surfactants and protein complexes (Krägel et al., 2003) and surface tension of viscous solutions are some of the examples which employ this method to measure surface tension.

2.6 Sessile drop method

The sessile drop method is based on the analysis of the profile of the drop placed on a solid substrate (see Figure 1). The solid may be a flat horizontal plate, a tilted plate, a vertical plate, or the walls of a thin tube (capillary). This method for contact angle determination is, in principle, simple, but great care must be taken to make accurate measurements. When the contact angle is small, a sessile drop is difficult to observe, therefore it is recommended that substrates used in sessile drop measurements be poorly wetted by the drop and should have a contact angle greater than 90 degrees. The liquid is contained in a syringe from which a droplet is deposited onto the substrate, and a high resolution camera captures the image. The drop can then be analyzed either by eye (using a protractor) or using image analysis software to calculate contact angle, surface and interfacial tension, wettability and absorption (Allen, 2003; Dingle and Harris, 2005).

The sessile drop technique can be used to measure contact angle between solid, liquid and vapor phases and characterize the solid surface properties by solving Young's equation:

$$\cos\theta_c = \frac{\gamma_{SL} - \gamma_{SV}}{\gamma_{LV}} \tag{6}$$

where equilibrium contact angle, cos θ_c is related to the interfacial energy of the three involved surfaces; solid-liquid, γ_{SL}, solid-vapor, γ_{SV} and liquid-vapor γ_{LV}. If θ is less than 90°, the liquid is said to wet the solid. A zero contact angle represents complete wetting. If θ is greater than 90° then it is said to be non-wetting (Bachmann et al., 2000; Dingle and Harris, 2005; Muster and Prestidge, 2002).

The most widely employed method for contact angle studies is to measure the angle of a sessile drop resting on a flat solid surface using a goniometer-microscope equipped with an angle-measuring eyepiece or a video camera equipped with a suitable magnifying lens, interfaces with a computer and an image-analysis software to determine the tangent value precisely on the captured image. Contact angles are obtained at intervals over a period of time. The sessile drop method for contact angle determination is, in principle, simple, but great care must be taken to make accurate measurements. The error associated with this instrument varies based on user expertise. This method employs a single point on the contact line to measure the surface tension, therefore it is not a suitable technique in studying rough and heterogenous surfaces. To obtain reproducible and accurate measurements with rough surfaces it is advantageous to use the Wilhelmy plate method. An advantage of of the sessile drop method is that, the large solid surface allows multiple droplet evaluation. Reproducibility of the surface measured contact angle values will reflect the heterogeneity of the surface's energy properties (Allen, 2003; Dingle and Harris, 2005; Drelich et al., 2002; Ho et al., 2010).

Contact angle is one of the most widely used techniques in the surface characterization and wettability of pharmaceuticals formulations. The sessile drop technique is commonly used for estimating contact angle of pharmaceutical powders (Buckton, 1993), drug-carrier adhesion (Podczeck et al., 1996), compaction and granulation (Puri et al., 2010), emulsion stability (Hansen and Fagerheim, 1998), human biological fluids (Noordman et al., 1999) and dynamic wettability properties of contact lens hydrogels (Ketelson et al., 2005).

2.7 Spinning drop method

Spinning drop method is based on the profile analysis of rotating liquid drop or thread where a drop of the less dense phase is put into another heavy phase contained in a horizontal tube. The tube is then spun about its longitudinal axis causing the lower density fluid to centrifuge to the center and form an elongated drop (see Figure 1). The diameter of a drop within a heavy phase is measured while the tube is spun at a constant speed. For each speed of rotation the drop attains equilibrium where the shape of the drop is a balance between interfacial tension and the pressure difference between the phases. With this method the interfacial tension can easily be calculated from Vonnegut's Equation:

$$\gamma = \frac{1}{4} r^3 \Delta\rho\omega^2 \tag{7}$$

where r denotes the radius of the cylindrical drop, $\Delta\rho$ is the density difference between the drop and the surrounding fluid and ω is the rotational velocity (Drelich et al., 2002; Hu and Joseph, 1994; Seifert and Wendorff, 1992).

This technique has many advantages when compared to the other methods. The centrifugal force used for determining the shape of the interface can be changed at will, however pendant drop and the sessile drop use gravity as the deforming force. This technique is ideal for measuring ultralow interfacial tensions down to 10^{-6} mN/m. Time and temperature-dependent surface tension can be studied using this technique (Seifert and Wendorff, 1992).

Design and manufacturing of a spinning drop device are simple in principle and this method is widely used to study the interfacial tensions of many systems, e.g., polymer melts, organic solvents (Jon et al., 1986; Schoolenberg et al., 1998) and surfactants and emulsions (El-Aaseer et al., 1984; Martin and Velankar, 2008).

2.8 Capillary rise method

The origin of this method dates to one century ago, however it is still a subject of interest due to the widespread application in the pharmacy and it is considered the standard method for determining the surface tension and wettability of a liquid. This method is capable of very good accuracy in measurement when suitable precautions are taken. But in practice it suffers from the fact that the calibration of the capillary diameter is tedious. This method is based on measuring the penetration time needed for a liquid to rise to a certain height when the end of a capillary is immersed into the solution (see Figure 1). According to the rising speed, the contact angle may be calculated (Ramírez-Flores et al., 2010; Xue et al., 2006).

The Lucas- Washburn elucidated the dynamics of capillary rise by using the Poiseuille equation for capillary penetration of liquids using the pressure difference across the invading liquid meniscus. When the meniscus is ideally 'hemi-cylindrical' concave in shape, the height at which the solution reaches inside the capillary is related to the surface tension. The wicking of a solvent vertically through a powder is described by Washburn equation:

$$x^2 = \frac{r\gamma\cos\theta}{2\eta}t \tag{8}$$

where t is the time required for solvent to rise x millimeters above the solvent through the MPs, γ and η are the surface tension and viscosity of the solvent, cos θ is the cosine of the contact angle and r is the internal radius of the capillary (Norris et al., 1999; Ramírez-Flores et al., 2010; Xue et al., 2006).

The wetting of small particles and porous materials is a very important phenomenon in pharmaceutical technologies for wettability studies of drug powder and drug manufacturing with related processes. There are a number of available methods, however capillary rise method is a routine measurement for contact angle study of powder and porous materials (Ramírez-Flores et al., 2010; Galet et al., 2010; Xue et al., 2006). Contact angle method for powders can be classified into those which require compaction, and those which utilize penetration of liquid through an uncompacted bed. Powder penetration technique can be measured with the capillary rise method. However it has been found that this method tends to overestimate the contact angle value. An alternative method is to measure the contact angle on a compacted powder surface with the use of sessile drop technique. Disadvantage of the sessile drop method is that compaction may change the characteristics of the powder surface; also it requires the compact powder to be fully wetted by the test liquid. These problems may cause this method to underestimate the angle value. In such circumstances, Wilhelmy plate method allows calculation of contact angle without the need to pre-saturate the powder (Buckton et al., 1995).

2.9 Atomic force microscopy

Many engineered surfaces and pharmaceutical products cannot be melted, dissolved, or fractured; therefore their surface/interfacial tension cannot be determined through any of the conventional techniques. These conventional techniques are applicable to macroscopic solids with flat and homogenous surface and inert substrate, whereas for microscale surfaces with increased surface-to-volume ratio, or sensitive substrates another method needs to be employed. Atomic force microscopy (AFM) is a well-known tool capable of surface characterization at the atomic scale. This technique can be used to produce high resolution images and can offers contact angle studies for macroscopic surfaces and adhesion force measurements for microscopic and submicroscopic surfaces (Cuenot et al., 2004; Drelich et al., 2004). AFM can also provide information on other surface properties such as stiffness, friction, or elasticity (Alonso and Goldmann, 2003). Atomic force microscope works by scanning the samples surface using a fine tip attached to a cantilever in the equipment. The AFM can be operated in the contact (tip touching the sample) and tapping modes (tip oscillating rapidly above the sample). Thus, a topological or force map of the surface can be constructed which allows us to determine the structural information and surface properties such as surface tension (Edwardson and Henderson 2004; Handojo et al., 2009). The force required to pull the tip off the substrate surface is called pull-off or adhesion force (F) which is directly related to the surface tension of the sample (Drelich et al., 2004):

$$\gamma = \frac{F}{2c\pi R} \tag{9}$$

where R is the radius of the particle (probing tip) and c is a constant which depends on the model of the AFM (Drelich et al., 2004).

Atomic force microscopy allows imaging and measurement of biological and biomaterial samples, ligand-receptor interaction, protein adsorption and folding (Alonso and Goldmann, 2003; Edwardson and Henderson, 2004). This device is fast becoming a valuable tool in the pharmaceutical industry and is used in formulation and surface characterization of liposome vesicles (Maeda et al., 2002), microparticle preparation and biomaterials (Méndez-Vilas et al., 2006), surface characterization of parenteral nutrition bags (Realdon et al., 2003), wetting properties of human hair (Dupres et al., 2004) and other applications are discussed elsewhere (Santos and Castanho, 2004).

2.10 Oscilating jet method

The oscillating jet method consists of forcing a stream of liquid under constant pressure through an orifice. By adjusting the osciallation frequency, the liquid vibrates to forms a jet having a series of stationary waves which depends chiefly on the characteristics of the orifice, its position, wave number, rate of flow and the surface tension of the liquid (Chang and Franses, 1995; Defay and Pétré, 1962; Stückrad et al., 1993; Thomas and Potter, 1975). Surface tension can be calculated using Bohr equation:

$$\gamma = \frac{2\times 10^3 \rho f^2 (1+1.542b^2 / r^2)\psi}{3r\lambda^2 + 5\pi^2 r^3} \tag{10}$$

where γ is the surface tension on the wave surface (mN/m), f is the flow rate (m^3/sec), ρ is the density of solution (kg/m3), λ is the wavelength of oscillation (m), r is the stream radius (m) , b/r is the wave amplitude, and Ψ differs from unity by about 1 part in 1000 (Thomas and Potter, 1975; Zhang and Zao, 1989).

This method can be employed to measure surface tension versus surface age (dynamic surface tension) for surface age varying between 0.1 and 0.001 second of surfactant solutions and surface elastisity (Defay and Hommelen, 1958; Warszynski et al., 1998). Oscillating bubble method is a similar method in which surface is periodically changed and the resulting surface tension variation is measured. Results have shown that surface tension measurements obtained using these methods are similar in value (Lunkenheimer et al., 1990).

2.11 Other methods of surface tension measurement

Laser light-scattering method is a non-invasive technique which is able to measure low values of surface tension without perturbing the interfacial thermal equilibrium (Jon et al., 1986; Huang, 1997). This method takes advantage of microscopic interfacial roughness caused by thermal fluctuations of a liquid surface and can be used to measure soft matter systems including microemulsions and bilayer lipid membranes (Cicuta and Hopkinson, 2004).

Langmuir trough methods can be used to study monolayers of surfactants and lipid solutions. In this method lipid solution is applied dropwise at the water surface with a micro liter syringe. This technique allows accurate measurement of surface and interfacial pressure and measurement of dilatational rheology of interfacial film and like Wilhelmy method this technique is independent of contact angle. Langmuir method can be used to measure equilibrium and dynamic surface tension of alveolar surfactant and lipid monolayers (Aveyard et al., 2000; Hills, 1985).

Pulsating bubble surfactometer can be used for studying the dynamic surface tension behavior of surfactants under constant or pulsating area. This method employs a sensitive transducer to determine the pressure difference across the bubble surface. A known area is pulsated sinosoidally resulting in a range of radius from which the surface tension is calculated. This method has been used for the interfacial measurement of soaps, surfactants and protein solutions and lung surfactant drugs (Chang et al., 1996; Coltharp and Franses, 1996).

The inclined plate method involves flowing a thin layer of surfactant solution over an inclined plate method. Surfactant molecules in the bulk adsorb at the interface and surface tension can be obtained from the flow rate of surfactant solution. However, since a Wilhelmy plate is used to measure the surface tension of the flowing surfactant solution, the lag time may introduce some errors during measurement, therefore, proper care is needed to orient the plate parallel to the flowing solution (Chang and Franses, 1995).

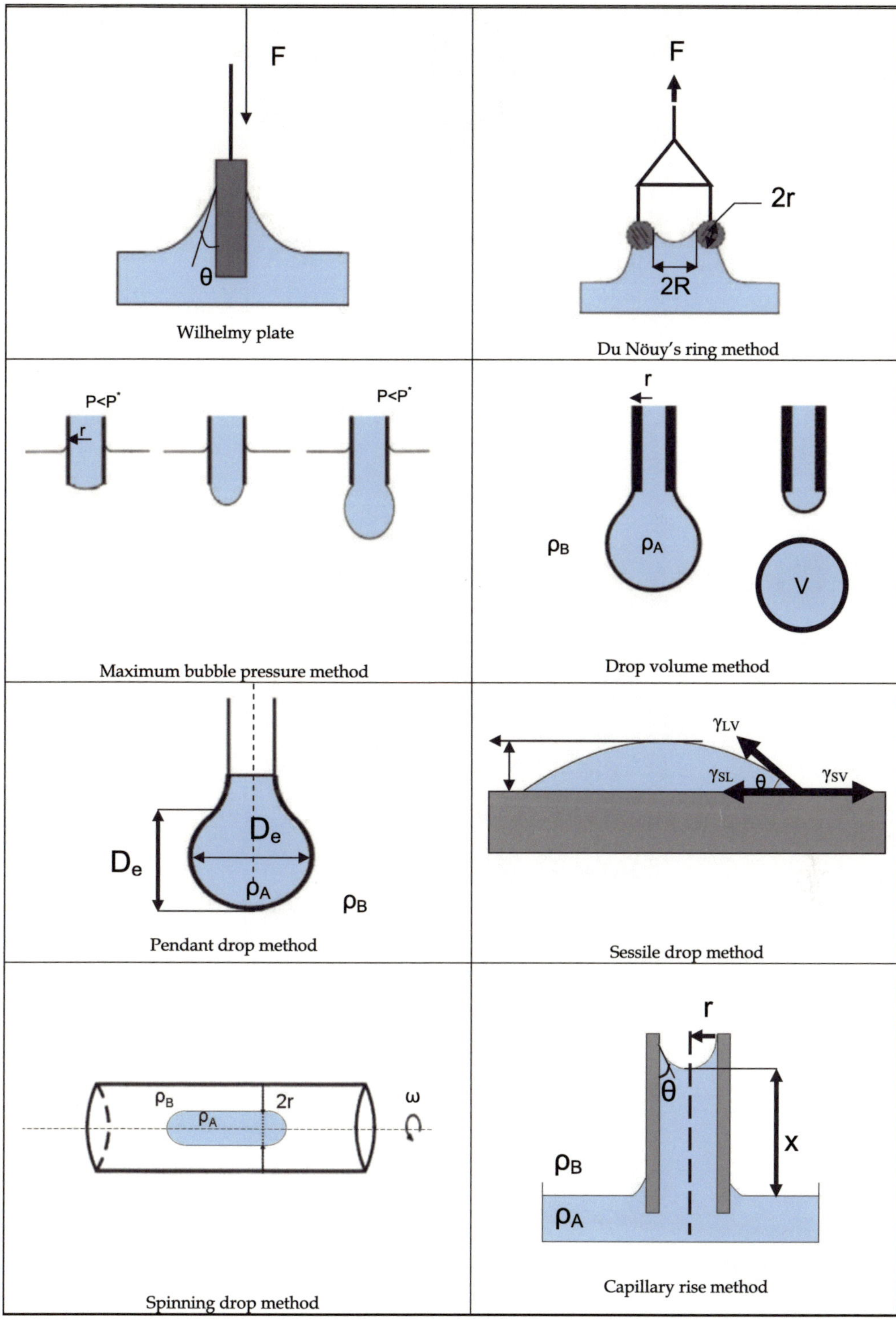

Fig. 1. Schematic illustration of standard methods of surface tension measurement.

Method involves measure of γ with:	Method	Accuracy mN/m	Suitability for surfactant solutions	Suitability for two-liquid systems	Suitability for viscous liquids	Suitability for contact angle measurement	Commercial availability	Instrument type
Microbalance	Wilhelmy plate	~0.1	Limited	Good	Good	Good	Yes	Manual
	Du Noüy ring	~0.1	Limited	Reduced accuracy	Not recommended	Not applicable	Yes	Manual
Capillary pressure	Maximum bubble pressure	0.1-0.3	Very good	Very good	Not recommended	Not applicable	Yes	Automatic
Equilibrium between capillary and gravity	Capillary rise	<<0.1	Very good	Very good, But experimentally difficult	Not recommended	Good	Not	Manual
	Drop volume/weight	0.1-0.2	Limited	Good	Not recommended	Not applicable	Yes	Automatic
Gravity-distorted drop	Pendant drop	~0.1	Very good	Very Good	Not recommended	Not applicable	Yes	Manual/ Automatic
	Sessile drop	~0.1	Good	Very Good	Good	Good	Not	Manual/ Automatic
Centrifugal forces	Spinning drop	0.1	Good	Very Good	Good	Not applicable	Yes	Manual
Resonance frequency	Atomic Force Microscopy	0.1	Good	Very Good	Good	Good	Yes	Automatic

*Drelich et al., 2002
*Thiessen and Man, 1999
*Fainerman et al., 2006
* Xue et al., 2006

Table 1. Accuracy and suitability of classic techniques used in surface tension measurement.

3. Computational methods of surface tension measurements

Modeling of physicochemical properties such as surface tension is needed in the pharmaceutical research. Experimental data on surface tension of liquid mixtures are very scarce in the literature, therefore theoretical methods of their prediction are found to be very useful. Reliable methods of surface tension prediction are useful in design of new materials and will undoubtfuly save laborious experimental measurement time. Surface tension of a liquid mixture is not a simple function of the surface tension of pure components, and is based on the assumption that the composition of the bulk phase is different from the composition of the adjacent vapor-liquid interface. There are various computational techniques in which the surface tension is evaluated through its thermodynamic definition or with the use of empirical equations. Most models require surface tension of the pure components. Models differ in the way in which the molar surface area and the activitycoefficients of the components are calculated (Bezerra et al., 2010; Pandey and Srivastava,2010). Evaluation of the performance of the models is calculated through average absolute deviation, AAD (%) for M data points using equation 11:

$$AAD(\%) = 100\left[\sum_{i=1}^{M}\frac{\left|\left(\gamma_{\exp}-\gamma_{calc}\right)/\gamma_{\exp}\right|}{M}\right] \quad (11)$$

With this, the reported experimental values of surface tension obtained using experimental methods are compared with predicted surface tension values from the proposed model.
The following topics present some literature models proposed for correlation and prediction of surface tension of liquid mixtures and solid surfaces.

3.1 Surface thermodynamic theory

The thermodynamic methods are based on the fact that surface layer between the bulk liquid and vapor phases has its own composition which affect the surface tension of the mixture. The number of the surface active molecules that reside on the surface can be calculated by the Gibbs adsorption equation:

$$\Gamma = -\frac{1}{RT}\frac{D\gamma}{d\ln c} \quad (12)$$

where Γ is the surface excess or surface concentration in moles per unit area of surface, c is the concentration of the substance in the bulk solution, γ is the surface tension, differential $d\gamma/dc$ show the change in surface tension with change in concentration, R is the gas constant and T is the temperature (Ramírez-Verduzco et al., 2006). Butler developed an application of Gibbs energy based on the assumption that the surface layer can be treated thermodynamically as a separate phase from the bulk phase. Some important thermodynamic-based equations were developed from the Butler equation and have been studied for their ability to correlate the surface tension of non-ideal mixtures. Sprow and Prausnitz developed an equation to correlate the surface tension of binary and multicomponent liquid mixtures by employing UNIFAC to calculate the activity coefficients of the individual components at the interface and in the bulk of the liquid. The predictive method of Sprow and Prausnitz was applied to 4 systems including binary and ternary

systems of water, ethyl butyrate/propionate and methanol at a constant temperature with an AAD value of less than 3.0 % (Kijevcanin et al., 2004; Rafati and Ghasemian, 2008).
Shereshefsky (1967) presented a model for the surface tension of binary solutions which is able to compute the excess properties and free energy changes in the surface region. This model was applied to 100 aqueous and 200 non-aqueous binary solutions at constant temperature. The agreement between the calculated and the experimental data is found to be very good with AAD of ~ 1.8% for aqueous and ~ 0.6% for non-aqueous systems (Tahery et al., 2005).
Guggenheim (1945) derived an equation for the surface tension as a function of heat for ideal solutions. Hildebrand and Scott extended this model for mixtures with dissimilar molecules. Eberhart (1966) employed a statistical thermodynamic approach and developed a one-parameter equation for binary liquid mixtures with good accuracy (Tahery et al., 2005).
A two-parameter equation was developed based on Wilson theory (Fu et al., 1986). This model was trained for a large number of systems and was able to correlate the data of 251 binary systems with an ADD of 0.5%. Li and co-workers extended that model and used the UNIFAC group contribution method to propose another two-parameter model to calculate the surface tension of binary mixtures (Kijevcanin et al., 2004; Li et al., 1990; Tahery et al., 2005).
Li and Lu have developed a predictive model for the surface tension of real mixtures on the basis of Davis theory and tested it against molecular dynamics simulation of the surface tension of the Lennard-Jones fluid. The proposed method was found to be suitable for obtaining surface tension values (Davis, 1975; Li and Lu, 2001).
The gradient theory of fluid interfaces is applied to compute the surface tension of various binary and ternary mixtures made up of gas (carbon dioxide, nitrogen or methane) and hydrocarbons. This model employs the Helmholtz energy density of the bulk homogeneous fluid and the influence parameters of the interfacial inhomogeneous fluid to correlate the surface tension of various pure fluids, binary mixtures and binary and ternary mixtures of gas and liquid hydrocarbons with good results. This method is predictive and is able to estimate surface tension values of gas mixtures with satisfactory results (Lin et al., 2007; Miqueu, 2004).

3.2 Empirical and correlative theories

MacLeod proposed an empirical method based on the temperature-independent constant K, between density ρ, and surface tension γ:

$$\gamma^{1/4} = K.\rho \tag{13}$$

Sugden slightly modified MacLeod's original expression to give a constant which he called the parachor (Sugden, 1924). Escobeo and Mansoori generated a model based on statistical mechanics for the prediction of surface tension of pure solvent using the equation of state. This model is shown to represent the experimental surface tension data of 94 pure solvent within 1.1 AAD% across all temperature ranges (Escobedo and Mansoori, 1996). Later they extended the same conformal solution theory to the case of mixtures of organic liquids. This equation was applied to 55 binary mixtures and the AAD was 0.5 % (Escobedo and Mansoori, 1998). However these equations are complicated and require critical temperature, critical pressure as well as critical compressibility and acentric factor. Therefore this model requires complex computational procedures which may not be suitable in pharmaceutical research.

There are a few models where the surface tension of the pure liquid is not required. Panday and co workers have extended Brick-Bird corresponding-state model, Goldsack-Sarvas volume fraction statistics and Sanchez method to multicomponent systems. These approaches require the values of thermal expansivity, isothermal compressibility and critical constants of pure components (Pandey et al., 2008).
Redlich-Kister equation expresses the excess energy thermodynamic properties which consist of a function of the mole fraction of each component and an interaction parameter (Redlich and Kister, 1948). An extension of this model was proposed which is able to correlate surface tension with the composition of the conjugate liquid (Fleming and Vinatieri, 1979).
Studies concerning temperature effect on the surface tension of aqueous and non-aqueous solutions are limited. Some of the models require many experimental parameters leading to low precision and accuracy in surface tension prediction. The Jouyban-Acree model was proposed based on the extension of the Redlich-Kister model as:

$$\ln \gamma_{m,T} = f_1 \ln \gamma_{1,T} + f_2 \ln \gamma_{2,T} + \frac{f_1 f_2}{T} \sum_{i=0}^{2} K_i \left(f_1 - f_2\right)^i \quad (14)$$

where $\gamma_{m,T}$, $\gamma_{1,T}$, $\gamma_{2,T}$ are the surface tension of the mixture and solvents 1 and 2, respectively and f_1 and f_2 are the volume fractions of the solvents and K_i are the model constant calculated using a no intercept least square method. This model is able to correlate surface tension of binary and ternary mixtures at various temperatures with AAD of 4.1 and 1.4 % respectively (Jouyban et al., 2004a; 2004b). This equation can be extended to correlate different physicochemical properties of solvent mixtures; including acid dissociation constant, dielectric constant, and drug solubility in water-cosolvent mixtures (Jouyban et al., 1999; 2002; 2004a).
Neural network (NN) modeling in quantitative structure-property relationship (QSPR) studies allows prediction of various physicochemical properties from the molecular structure. Reliable methods for prediction of basic physicochemical properties would save time consuming experimental studies. Kauffman and Jurs reported a predictive NN model for surface tension of 213 common organic solvents using 8 descriptors. The root mean square error of the test sets were 2.89 mN/m (Taskinen and Yliruusi, 2003; Kauffman and Jurs, 2001).

3.3 Surface tension of immiscible fluids and solids

Surface tension calculation of immiscible fluids is possible by introducing repulsion between the neighboring particles of different fluids which has been employed in the macro-scale particle method. However equation of state is also possible for this type of measurement (Zhou et al., 2008).
Determination of the surface tension of solids is crucial in pharmaceutical powders and tableting. Amongst the various approaches to estimate the contact angle of solids is the Young equation (see equation 6). This method requires an ideal, flat and homogenous surface, whereas real measurements are carried out on rough and heterogeneous surfaces, on which the typical contact angle measured is an advancing contact angle which is larger than Young's equilibrium contact angle. The surface tension of a solid cannot be easily estimated from the Young's equation because of the two unknown parameters γ_{SV}, γ_{SL}. In order to calculate these quantities, equation of state (EQS) was proposed (Li and Neumann,

1990). However many researchers have criticized this equation for its thermodynamic analysis (Johnson and Dettre, 1989; Lee, 1993). Another approach is the geometrical methods for measuring surface tension of solids including Owen Wendt and van Oss theory. These methods decompose the surface tension into different components (Owens and Wendt, 1969; van Oss et al., 1986). Ahadian and colleagues compared the surface tension of 41 artificial solid surfaces as predicted by the equation of state and compared it to the values obtained by van Oss theory and Owen Wendt equation. Results indicate that equation of state was capable of good predictability, whereas the geometric methods are limited to higher range surface tension value of solid surfaces (Ahadian et al.,2007).

4. Conclusion

Measurements of surface rheological characteristics are of great importance for the pharmaceutical industry. Many of pharmaceutical processes depend on the cohesive and adhesive interactions between the materials used during the preparation of the product. Understanding and determination of surface free energies of both liquid and solid surfaces plays a key role in characterization of materials during their development, formulation and manufacturing of pharmaceutical applications. The chemical activity, adsorption, dissolution, and bioavailability of a drug may depend on the surface of the molecule.

There are several experimental approaches that one can employ to evaluate interfacial tension and large differences can exist among measurement methods. While one method may be proven useful for a number of applications, there are several restrictions that detract from its applicability in a specific system. The choice of the method depends on the nature of the interface, the rheology of the liquid(s), the range of temperature and pressure, ease of analysis, accuracy, precision, surface age, cost and convenience of the probing instrument. Most equilibrium methods may be used to measure dynamic tension, and there are certain methods by which one can measure solely dynamic tension. Most methods involve measurement of forces, interface shapes, pressure differences, or flow rates. Commonly used methods for measuring interfacial tension of various solutions as well as solid systems are mentioned in this chapter.

To facilitate an in-depth process understanding, a combination of experimental and computational design may be integrated in interfacial tension of compounds. Providing a simple method of correlating and predicting the interfacial properties of materials would be of great interest for pharmaceutical technology. There are various computational techniques in which the surface tension is evaluated through its thermodynamic definition or empirical equations. These methods require input data and several adjustable parameters obtained from multicomponent system and the pure component. Some of these equations on a thermodynamic basis are the two-parameter model for liquid mixtures. With these methods calculation of the free-energy between the two systems is a challenge to be accurately determined and these methods are difficult to implement at relatively high temperature due to stability problems. Empirical equations may be used to correlate and predict surface tension using one or two parameters. Some of these models may have limited range of applicability and may require a lot of experimental data. For practical use it is very important that the surface tension of multicomponent system can be predicted from the composition of the conjugate phases and some predictable physical parameters without any adjustable parameters.

In essence, an attempt has been made in this chapter to review and examine the performance of computational and experimental techniques in which surface tension are evaluated.

5. Acknowledgment

This work is dedicated to the spirit of Professor Fathollah Fathi-Azarbayjani, for believing that great things are born from tiny sparks of inspiration.

6. References

Ahadian, S.; Moradian, S.; Sharif, F.; Amani Tehran, M. & Mohseni, M. (2007). Application of artificial neural network (ANN) in order to predict the surface free energy of powders using the capillary rise method. *Colloids and Surfaces A: Physicochemical and Engineering Aspects*, Vol. 302, pp. 280-285.

Al-Maaieh, A. & Aburub, A. (2007). Surface activity of a non-micelle forming compound containing a surface-active impurity. *International Journal of Pharmaceutics*, Vol. 334, pp. 125–128.

Allen, J.S. (2003). An analytical solution for determination of small contact angles from sessile drops of arbitrary size. *Journal of Colloid and Interface Science*, Vol. 261, pp. 481–489.

Alonso, J.L. & Goldmann, W.H. (2003). Feeling the forces: atomic force microscopy in cell biology. *Life Sciences*, Vol. 72, pp. 2553–2560.

Arashiro, E.Y. & Demarquette, N.R. (1999). Use of the pendant drop method to measure interfacial tension between molten polymers. *Materials Research*, Vol. 2, pp. 23-32.

Aveyard, R.; Clint, J.H.; Nees, D. & Quirke, N. (2000). Structure and collapse of particle monolayers under lateral pressure at the octane/aqueous surfactant solution interface. *Langmuir*, Vol. 16, pp. 8820-8828.

Avranas, A. & Tasopoulos, V. (2000). Aqueous solutions of sodium deoxycholate and hydroxypropylmethylcellulose: dynamic surface tension measurements. *Journal of Colloid and Interface Science*, Vol. 221, pp. 223–229.

Bachmann, J.; Ellies, A. & Hartge, K.H. (2000). Development and application of a new sessile drop contact angle method to assess soil water repellency. *Journal of Hydrology*, Vol. 231–232, pp. 66–75.

Bezerra, E.S.; Santos, J.M.T. & Paredes, M.L.L. (2010). A new predictive model for liquid/air surface tension of mixtures: Hydrocarbon mixtures. *Fluid Phase Equilibria*, Vol. 288, pp. 55–62.

Bodour, A.A.; & Miller-Maier, R.M. (1998). Application of a modified drop-collapse technique for surfactant quantitation and screening of biosurfactant-producing microorganisms. *Journal of Microbiological Methods*, Vol. 32, pp. 273–280.

Buckton, G. (1988). The assessment, and pharmaceutical importance, of the solid/liquid and the solid/vapour interface: A review with respect to powders. *International Journal of Pharmaceutics*, Vol. 44, pp. 1-8.

Buckton, G. (1993). Assessment of the wettability of pharmaceutical powders. *Journal of Adhesion Science and Technology*, Vol. 7, pp. 205–219.

Buckton, G.; Darcy, P. & McCarthy, D. (1995). The extent of errors associated with contact angles, 3. The influence of surface roughness effects on angles measured using a

Wilhelmy plate technique for powders. *Colloids and Surfaces A: Physicochemical and Engineering Aspects*, Vol. 95, pp. 27-35.

Chamarthy, S.P.; Pinal, R. & Carvajal, M.T. (2009). Elucidating raw material variability - importance of surface properties and functionalities in pharmaceutical powders. *AAPS PharmSciTech*, Vol. 10, pp. 780–788.

Chang, C.-H.; Coltharp, K.A.; Park, S.Y. & Franses, E.I. (1996). Surface tension measurements with the pulsating bubble method. *Colloids and Surfaces A: Physicochemical and Engineering Aspects*, Vol. 114, pp. 185 197.

Chang, C.-H. & Franses, E.I. (1995). Adsorption dynamics of surfactants at the air/water interface: a critical review of mathematical models, data, and mechanisms. *Colloids and Surfaces A: Physicochemical and Engineering Aspects*, Vol. 100, pp. 1-45.

Chen, P.; Policova, Z.; Pace-Asciak, C.R. & Neumann, A.W. (1999). Study of molecular interactions between lipids and proteins using dynamic surface tension measurements: A review. *Colloids and Surfaces B: Biointerfaces*, Vol.15, pp. 313–324.

Christov, N.C.; Danov, K.D.; Kralchevsky, P.A.; Ananthapadmanabhan, K.P. & Lips, A. (2006). Maximum bubble pressure method: Universal surface age and transport mechanisms in surfactant solutions. *Langmuir*, Vol. 22, pp. 7528-7542.

Cicuta, P. & Hipkinson, I. (2004). Recent developments of surface light scattering as a tool for optical-rheology of polymers monolayers. *Colloids and Surfaces A: Physicochemical Engineering Aspects*, Vol. 233, pp. 97-107.

Coltharp, K.A. & Franses, E.I. (1996). Equilibrium and dynamic surface tension behavior of aqueous soaps: Sodium octanoate and sodium dodecanoate (sodium laurate). *Colloids and Surfaces Physicochemical and Engineering Aspects*, Vol. 108, pp. 225 242

Cuenot, S.; Fétigny, C.; Demoustier-Champagne, S. & Nysten, B. (2004). Surface tension effect on the mechanical properties of nanomaterials measured by atomic force microscopy. *Physical Review B*, Vol. 69, pp. 1-5.

Currie, P.K. & van Nieuwkoop, J. (1982). Buoyancy effects in the spinning-drop interfacial tensiometer. *Journal of Colloid Interface Science*, Vol. 87, pp. 301-316.

Davis, H.T. (1975). Statistical mechanics of interfacial properties of polyatomic fluids. 1. Surface tension. *Journal of Chemical Physics*, Vol. 62, pp. 3412–3415.

de la Maza, A.; Coderch, L.; Gonzalez, P. & Parra, J.L. (1998). Subsolubilizing alterations caused by alkyl glucosides in phosphatidylcholine liposomes. *Journal of Controlled Release*, Vol. 52, pp. 159–168.

Defay, R. & Hommelen, J.R. (1958). I. Measurement of dynamic surface tensions of aqueous solutions by the oscillating jet method. *Journal of Colloid Science*, Vol.13, pp. 553-564.

Defay, R. & Pétré, G. (1962). Correcting surface tension data obtained by the oscillating jet method. *Journal of Colloid Science*, Vol. 17, pp. 565-569.

Deo, N.; Somasundaran, T. & Somasundaran, P. (2004). Solution properties of amitriptyline and its partitioning into lipid bilayers. *Colloids and Surfaces B: Biointerfaces*, Vol. 34, pp. 155–159.

Dingle, N.M. & Harris, M.T. (2005). A robust algorithm for the simultaneous parameter estimationof interfacial tension and contact angle from sessile drop profiles. *Journal of Colloid and Interface Science*, Vol. 286, pp. 670–680.

Drelich, J.; Fang, C. & White, C.L. (2002). Measurment of interfacial tension in fluid-fluid systems, in: *Encyclopedia of Surface and Colloid Science*, Hubbard AT, pp. 3152-3166, Marcel Dekker, ISBN: 9780824707965, New York.

Dreu, R.; Šircab, J.; Pintye-Hodi, K.; Burjan, T.; Planinšek, O. & Srčič, S. (2005). Physicochemical properties of granulating liquids and their influence on microcrystalline cellulose pellets obtained by extrusion-spheronisation technology. *International Journal of Pharmaceutics*, Vol. 291, pp. 99–111.

Dupres, V.; Camesano, T.; Langevin, D.; Checco, A. & Guenoun, P. (2004). Atomic force microscopy imaging of hair: Correlations between surface potential and wetting at the nanometer scale. *Journal of Colloid and Interface Science*, Vol. 269, pp. 329–335.

Eberhart, J.G. (1966). Surface tension of binary liquid mixtures. *Journal of Physical Chemistry*, Vol. 70, pp. 1183–1186.

Edwardson, J.M. & Henderson, R.M. (2004). Atomic force microscopy and drug discovery. *Drug Discovery Today*, Vol. 9, pp. 64-71.

El-Aasser, M.S.; Lack, C.D.; Choi, Y.T.; Min, T.I.; Vanderhoff, J.W. & Fowkes, F.M. (1984). Interfacial aspects of miniemulsions and miniemulsion polymers. *Colloids and Surfaces*, Vol. 12, pp. 79-97.

Escobedo, J. & Mansoori, G.A. (1996). Surface tension prediction for pure fluids, *AIChE Journal*, Vol. 42, pp. 1425-1433.

Escobedo, J. & Mansoori, G.A. (1998). Surface tension prediction for liquid mixtures. *AIChE Journal*, Vol. 44, pp. 2324-2332.

Fainerman, V.B.; Mys, V.D.; Makievski, A.V. & Miller, R. (2006). Application of the maximum bubble pressure technique for dynamic surface tension studies of surfactant solutions using the Sugden two-capillary method. *Journal of Colloid and Interface Science*, Vol. 304, pp. 222–225.

Fleming, P.D. & Vinatieri, J.E. (1979). Quantitative interpretation of phase volume behaviour of multicomponent systems near critical points. *AIChE Journal*, Vol. 25, pp. 493–502.

Fu, J.; Li, B. & Wang, Z. (1986). Estimation of fluid-fluid interfacial tension of multicomponent mixtures. *Chemical Engineering Science*, Vol. 41, pp. 2673–2679.

Galet, L.; Patry, S. & Dodds, J. (2010). Determination of the wettability of powders by the Washburn capillary rise method with bed preparation by a centrifugal packing technique. *Journal of Colloid and Interface Science*, Vol. 346, pp. 470–475.

Guggenheim, E.A. (1945). The principle of corresponding states. *Journal of Chemical Physics*, Vol. 13, pp. 253-261.

Gunde, R;. Kumar, A.; Lehnert-Batar, S.; Mäder, R. & Windhab E.J., (2001). Measurement of the surface and interfacial tension from maximum volume of a pendant drop. *Journal of Colloid and Interface Science*, Vol. 244, pp. 113–122.

Hallowell, C.P. & Hirt, D.E. (1994). Unusual characteristics of the maximum bubble pressure method using a Teflon capillary. *Journal of Colloid and Interface Science*, Vol. 168, pp. 281-288.

Hancock, B.C.; York, P. & Rowe, R.C. (1997). The use of solubility parameters in pharmaceutical dosage form design. *International Journal of Pharmaceutics*, Vol. 148, pp. 1- 21.

Handojo, A.; Zhai, Y.; Frankel, G. & Pascall, M.A. (2009). Measurement of adhesion strengths between various milk products on glass surfaces using contact angle measurement and atomic force microscopy. *Journal of Food Engineering*, Vol. 92, pp. 305–311.

Hernández-Baltazar, E. & Gracia-Fadrique, J. (2005). Elliptic solution to the Young–Laplace differential equation. *Journal of Colloid and Interface Science*, Vol. 287, pp. 213–216.

Hills, B. (1985). Alveolar liquid lining: Langmuir method used to measure surface tension in bovine and canine lung extracts. *Journal of Physiology*, Vol. 359, pp. 65-79.

Ho, R.; Hinder, J.; Watts, J.F.; Dilworth, S.E.; Williams, D.R. & Heng, J.Y.Y. (2010). Determination of surface heterogeneity of d-mannitol by sessile drop contact angle and finite concentration inverse gas chromatography. *International Journal of Pharmaceutics*, Vol. 387, pp. 79–86.

Hu, H.H. & Joseph, D.D. (1994). Evaluation of a liquid drop in a spinning drop tensiometer. *Journal of Colloid and Interface Science*, Vol. 162, pp. 331-339.

Huang, Y.-X. (1997). Laser light scattering studies on thermodynamics of C8-lecithin and monovalent salt solutions. *Journal of Chemical Physics*, Vol. 107, pp. 9141-9145.

Ishii, F.; Takamura, A. & Ogata, H. (1988). Compatibility of intravenous fat emulsions with prodrug amino acids. *Journal of Pharmarmacy Pharmacology*, Vol. 40, pp. 89-92.

Johnson, R.E. & Dettre, R.H. (1989). An evaluation of Neumann's "surface equation of state". *Langmuir*, Vol. 5, pp. 293–295.

Jon, D.I.; Rosano, H.L. & Cummins, H.Z. (1986). Toluene/water/1-propanol interfacial tension measurements by means of pendant drop, spinning drop, and laser light-scattering methods. *Journal of Colloid and Interface Science*, Vol. 114, pp. 330-341.

Jouyban, A.; Chan, H.K.; Clark, B.J. & Acree, W.E. (2002). Mathematical representation of apparent dissociation constants in aqueous-organic solvent mixtures. *International Journal of Pharmaceutics*, Vol. 246, pp. 135-142.

Jouyban, A.; Fathi Azarbayjani, A.; Barzegar-Jalali, M. & Acree, W.E. (2004a). Correlation of surface tension of mixed solvents with solvent composition. *Pharmazie*, Vol. 59, pp. 937-941.

Jouyban, A.; Fathi-Azarbayjani, A. & Acree, W.E. (2004b). Surface tension calculation of mixed solvents with respect to solvent composition and temperature by using Jouyban-Acree model. *Chemical and Pharmaceutical Bulletin*, Vol. 52, pp. 1219-1222.

Jouyban, A.; Soltanpour, Sh. & Chan, H.K. (2004). A simple relationship between dielectric constant of mixed solvents with solvent composition and temperature. *International Journal of Pharmaceutics*, Vol. 269, pp. 353-360.

Jouyban, A.; Valaee, L.; Barzegar-Jalali, M.; Clark, B.J. & Acree, W.E. (1999). Comparison of various cosolvency models for calculating solute solubility in water-cosolvent mixtures. *International Journal of Pharmaceutics*, Vol. 177, pp. 93-101.

Kauffman, G.W. & Jurs, P.C. (2001). Prediction of surface tension, viscosity, and thermal conductivity for common organic solvents using quantitative structure–property relationships. *Journal of Chemical Information and Computer Science,* Vol. 41, pp. 408–418.

Kazakov, V.N.; Vozianov, A.F.; Sinyachenko, O.V.; Trukhin, D.V.; Kovalchuk, V.I. & Pison, U. (2000). Studies on the application of dynamic surface tensiometry of serum and cerebrospinal liquid for diagnostics and monitoring of treatment in patients who have rheumatic, neurological or oncological diseases. *Advances in Colloid and Interface Science*, Vol. 86, pp.1-38.

Ketelson, H.A.; Meadows, D.L. & Stone, R.P. (2005). Dynamic wettability properties of a soft contact lens hydrogel. *Colloids and Surfaces B: Biointerfaces*, Vol. 40, pp. 1–9.

Kijevcanin, M.Lj.; Ribeiro, I.S.A.; Ferreira, A.G.M. & Fonseca, I.M.A. (2004). Water + esters + methanol: Experimental data, correlation and prediction of surface and interfacial tensions at 303.15K and atmospheric pressure. *Fluid Phase Equilibria*, Vol. 218, pp. 141–148.

Krägel, J.; O'Neill, M.; Makievski, A.V.; Michel, M.; Leser, M.E. & Miller, R. (2003). Dynamics of mixed protein-/surfactant layers adsorbed at the water/air and water/oil interface. *Colloids and Surfaces B: Biointerfaces*, Vol. 31 pp. 107-114.

Krishnan, A.; Liu, Y.-H.; Cha, P.; Woodward, R.; Allara, D. & Vogler, E.A. (2005). An evaluation of methods for contact angle measurement. *Colloids and Surfaces B: Biointerfaces*, Vol. 43, pp. 95–98.

Korhonen, M.; Hirvonen, J.; Peltonen, L.; Antikainen, O.; Yrjänäinen, L. & Yliruusi, J. (2004). Formation and characterization of three-component-sorbitan monoester surfactant, oil and water-creams. *International Journal of Pharmaceutics*, Vol. 269, pp. 227–239.

Lee, L.-H. (1993). Scope and limitations of the equation of state approach for interfacial tensions. *Langmuir*, Vol. 9, pp. 1898–1905

Li, Z.B. & Lu, B.C.Y. (2001). On the prediction of surface tension for multicomponent mixtures. *Canadian Journal of Chemical Engineering*, Vol. 79, pp. 402–411.

Li, D. & Neumann, A.W. (1990). A reformulation of the equation of state for interfacial tensions. *Journal of Colloid Interface Science*, Vol. 137, pp.304-307.

Li, Z.B.; Shen, S.Q.; Shi, M.R. & Shi, J. (1990). Prediction of the surface tension of binary and multicomponent liquid mixtures by the unifac group contribution method. *Thermochimica Acta*, Vol. 169, pp. 231–238.

Lin, H.; Duan, Y.-Y. & Min, Q. (2007). Gradient theory modeling of surface tension for pure fluids and binary mixtures. *Fluid Phase Equilibria*, Vol. 254, pp. 75–90.

Luner, P.E. & Van Der Kamp, D. (2001). Wetting characteristics of media emulating gastric fluids. *International Journal of Pharmaceutics*, Vol. 212, pp. 81–91.

Lunkenheimer, K.; Serrien, G. & Joos, P. (1990). The adsorption kinetics of octanol at the air/solution interface measured with the oscillating bubble and oscillating jet methods. *Journal of Colloid and Interface Science*, Vol. 134, pp. 407-411.

Maeda, N.; Senden, T.J. & di Meglio, J.-M. (2002). Micromanipulation of phospholipid bilayers by atomic force microscopy. *Biochimica et Biophysica Acta*, Vol. 1564, pp. 165- 172.

Martin, J.D. & Velankar, S.S. (2008). Unusual behavior of PEG/PPG/Pluronic interfaces studied by a spinning drop tensiometer. *Journal of Colloid and Interface Science*, Vol. 322, pp. 669–674.

Matsuki, H.; Shimada, K.; Kaneshina, S.; Kamaya, H. & Ueda, I. (1998). Difference in surface activities between uncharged and charged local anesthetics: Correlation with their anesthetic potencies. *Colloids and Surfaces B: Biointerfaces*, Vol. 11, pp. 287–295.

Méndez-Vilas, A.; Donoso, M.G.; Gonz´alez-Carrasco, J.L. & González-Martín, M.L. (2006). Looking at the micro-topography of polished and blasted Ti-based biomaterials using atomic force microscopy and contact angle goniometry. *Colloids and Surfaces B: Biointerfaces*, Vol. 52, pp. 157–166.

Millqvist-Fureby, A.; Malmsten, M. & Bergenståhl, B. (1999). Spray-drying of trypsin-surface characterisation and activity preservation. *International Journal of Pharmaceutics*, Vol. 188, pp. 243–253.

Miqueu, C.; Mendiboure, B. ; Graciaa, C. & Lachaise, J. (2004). Modelling of the surface tension of binary and ternary mixtures with the gradient theory of fluid interfaces. *Fluid Phase Equilibria*, Vol. 218, pp. 189–203.

Mishchuk, N.A. Fainerman, V.B. Kovalchuk, V.I.R. Miller, R. Dukhin, S.S. (2000). Studies of concentrated surfactant solutions using the maximum bubble pressure method. *Colloids and Surfaces A: Colloids and Surfaces A: Physicochemical and Engineering Aspects*, Vol. 175, pp. 207–216.

Mishima, K.; Matsuyama, K.; Ezawa, M.; Taruta, Y.; Takarabe, S. & Nagatani, M. (1998). Interfacial tension of aqueous two-phase systems containing poly (ethylene glycol) and dipotassium hydrogenphosphate. *Journal of Chromatography B*, Vol. 711, pp. 313–318.

Muster, T.H. & Prestidge, C.A. (2002). Application of time-dependent sessile drop contact angles on compacts to characterise the surface energetics of sulfathiazole crystals. *International Journal of Pharmaceutics*, Vol. 234, pp. 43–54.

Noordmans, J.; Wormeester, H. & Busscher, H.J. (1999). Simultaneous monitoring of protein adsorption at the solid–liquid interface from sessile solution droplets by ellipsometry and axisymmetric drop shape analysis by profile. *Colloids and Surfaces B: Biointerfaces*, Vol. 15, pp. 227–233.

Norris, D.A.; Puri, N.; Labib, M.E. & Sinko, P.J. (1999). Determining the absolute surface hydrophobicity of microparticulates using thin layer wicking. *Journal of Controlled Release*, Vol. 59, pp. 173–185.

Ortiz, S.E.M.; Sánchez, C.C.; Rodríguez Niño, M.R.; Añon, M.C. & Rodríguez Patino, J.M. (2003). Structural characterization and surface activity of spread and adsorbed soy globulin films at equilibrium. *Colloids and Surfaces B: Biointerfaces*, Vol. 32, pp. 57-67.

Owens, D.K. & Wendt, R.C. (1969). Estimation of the surface free energy of polymers. *Journal of Applied Polymer Science*, Vol. 13, pp. 1741–1747.

Palma, S.; Lo Nostro, P.; Manzo, R. & Allemandi, D. (2002). Evaluation of the surfactant properties of ascorbyl palmitate sodium salt. *European Journal of Pharmaceutical Sciences*, Vol. 16, pp. 37–43.

Pandey, J.D.; Chandra, P.; Srivastava, T.; Soni, N.K. & Singh, A.K. (2008). Estimation of surface tension of ternary liquid systems by corresponding-states group-contributions method and Flory theory. *Fluid Phase Equilibria*, Vol. 273, pp. 44–51.

Podczek, F.; Newton, J.M. & James, M.B. (1996). The influence of physical properties of the materials in contact on the adhesion strength of particles of salmeterol base and salmeterol salts to various substrate materials. *Journal of Adhesion Science and Technology*, Vol. 10, pp. 257-268.

Puri, V.; Dantuluri, A.K.; Kumar, M.; Karar, N. & Bansal, A.K. (2010). Wettability and surface chemistry of crystalline and amorphous forms of a poorly water soluble drug. *European Journal of Pharmaceutical Sciences*, Vol. 40 pp. 84–93.

Rafati, A.A. & Ghasemian, E. (2008). Study of surface tension and surface properties of binary alcohol/n-alkyl acetate mixtures. *Journal of Colloid and Interface Science*, Vol. 328, pp. 385–390.

Ramírez-Flores, J.C.; Bachmann, J. & Marmur, A. (2010). Direct determination of contact angles of model soils in comparison with wettability characterization by capillary rise. *Journal of Hydrology*, Vol. 382, pp. 10–19.

Ramírez-Verduzco, L.F.; Romero-Martínez, A. & Trejo, A. (2006). Prediction of the surface tension, surface concentration, and the relative Gibbs adsorption isotherm of binary liquid systems. *Fluid Phase Equilibria*, Vol. 246, pp. 119–130.

Rangsansarid, J. & Fukada, K. (2007). Factors affecting the stability of O/W emulsion in BSA solution: Stabilization by electrically neutral protein at high ionic strength. *Journal of Colloid and Interface Science*, Vol. 316, pp. 779–786.

Realdon, N.; Zennaro, L.; Perin, F.; Bettero, A.; Bortoluzzi, S.; Rigo, A. & Ragazzi, E. (2003). Surface characterisation of bags for total parenteral nutrition by tensiometry and atomic force microscopy. *International Journal of Pharmaceutics*, Vol. 265, pp. 27–35.

Redlich, O. & Kister, A.T. (1948). Algebraic representation of thermodynamic properties and the classification of solutions. *Industrial and Chemistry Engineering Research,* Vol. 40, pp. 341–348.

Santos, N.C. & Castanho, M.A.R.B. (2004). An overview of the biophysical applications of atomic force microscopy. *Biophysical Chemistry*, Vol. 107, pp. 133–149.

Schoolenberg, G.E.; During, F. & Ingenbleek, G. (1998). Coalescence and interfacial tension measurements for polymer melts: experiments on a PS-PE model system. *Polymer,* Vol. 39, pp. 765-772.

Seifert, A.M. & Wendorff, J.H. (1992). Spinning drop experiments on interfacial phenomena: Theoretical background and experimental evidence. *Colloid Polymer Science,* Vol. 270, pp. 962-971.

Semmler, A. & Kohler, H.-H. (1999). Surface properties of Alkylpyridinium Chlorides and the applicability of the pendant drop technique. *Journal of Colloid and Interface Science,* Vol. 218, pp. 137–144.

Shereshefsky, J.L. (1967). A theory of surface tension of binary solutions. 1. Binary liquid mixtures of organic compounds. *Journal of Colloid and Interface Science,* Vol. 24, pp. 317–322.

Sipahi, C.; Anil, N. & Bayramli, E. (2001). The effect of acquired salivary pellicle on the surface free energy and wettability of different denture base materials. *Journal of Dentistry,* Vol. 29, pp. 197-204.

Stückrad, B.; Hiller, W.J. & Kowalewski, T.A. (1993). Measurement of dynamic surface tension by the oscillating droplet method. *Experiments in Fluids,* Vol. 15, pp. 332-340.

Sugden S., (1924). The influence of the orientation of surface molecules on the surface tension of pure liquids. *Journal of Chemical Society Transaction,* Vol. 125, pp. 1167–1177.

Tahery, R.; Modarress, H. & Satherley, J. (2005). Surface tension prediction and thermodynamic analysis of the surface for binary solutions. *Chemical Engineering Science,* Vol. 60, pp. 4935 – 4952.

Takamura, A.; Ishii, F.; Noro, S.; Tanifuji, M. & Nakajima, S. (1984). Study of intravenous hyperalimentation: effect of selected amino acids on the stability of intravenous fat emulsions. *Journal of Pharmaceutical Science,* Vol. 73, pp. 91-94.

Tan, S.N.; Fornasiero, D.; Sedev, R. & Ralston, J. (2005). Marangoni effects in aqueous polypropylene glycol foams. *Journal of Colloid and Interface Science,* Vol. 286, pp. 719–729.

Taskinen, J. & Yliruusi, J. (2003). Prediction of physicochemical properties based on neural network modeling. *Advanced Drug Delivery Reviews,* Vol. 55, pp. 1163–1183.

Thiessen, D.B. & Man, K.F. (1999). Surface tension measurements, CRC Press, Retrieved from <http://www.engnetbase.com>

Thomas, W.D.E. & Potter, L. (1975). Solution/Air Interfaces I. An oscillating jet relative method for determining dynamic surface tensions. *Journal of Colloid and Interface Science*. Vol. 50. pp. 397-412.

Trukhin, D.V.; Sinyachenko, O.V.; Kazakov, V.N.; Lylyk, S.V.; Belokon, A.M. & Pison, U. (2001). Dynamic surface tension and surface rheology of biological liquids. *Colloids and Surfaces B: Biointerfaces*, Vol. 21, pp. 231-238.

van Oss, C.J.; Good, R.J. & Chaudhury, M.K. (1986). The role of van der Waals forces and hydrogen bonds in "hydrophobic interactions" between biopolymers and low energy surfaces. *Journal of Colloid and Interface Science*, Vol. 111, pp. 378–390.

Vasir, J.K.; Tambwekar, K. & Garg, S. (2003). Bioadhesive microspheres as a controlled drug delivery system. *International Journal of Pharmaceutics*, Vol. 255, pp. 13–32.

Vejnovic, I.; Simmler, L. & Betz, G. (2010). Investigation of different formulations for drug delivery through the nail plate, *International Journal of Pharmaceutics*, Vol. 386, pp. 185-194.

Warszunski, P.; Wantke, K.-D. & Fruhner, H. (1998). Surface elasticity of oscillating spherical interfaces, *Colloids and Surfaces A*, Vol. 139, pp. 137–153.

Xue, H.T.; Fang, Z.N.; Yang, Y.; Huang, J.P. & Zhou, L.W. (2006). Contact angle determined by spontaneous dynamic capillary rises with hydrostatic effects: Experiment and theory. *Chemical Physics Letters*, Vol. 432, pp. 326–330.

Zelkó, R.; Orbán, Á.; Süvegh, K.; Riedl, Z. & Rácz, I. (2002). Effect of plasticizer on the dynamic surface tension and the free volume of Eudragit systems. *International Journal of Pharmaceutics,* Vol. 244, pp. 81-86.

Zhang, L.-H. & Zhao, G.-X. (1989). Dynamic surface tension of the aqueous solutions of cationic-anionic surfactant mixtures. *Journal of Colloid and Interface Science*, Vol. 127, pp. 353-361.

Zhou, G.; Ge, W. & Li, J. (2008). A revised surface tension model for macro-scale particle methods. *Powder Technology*, Vol. 183, pp. 21–26.

4

Multi-Well Engineered Heart Tissue for Drug Screening and Predictive Toxicology

Alexandra Eder, Arne Hansen and Thomas Eschenhagen
Department of Experimental Pharmacology and Toxicology, University Medical Centre Hamburg-Eppendorf, Germany

1. Introduction

Drug development is time- and cost-intensive and, overall, inefficient. Only one out of an estimated 10.000 new chemical entities (NCEs) finally enters the market. The later the failure occurs, the higher are the costs. It is for this reason that preclinical development aims at identifying the potential for failure as early as possible and with high sensitivity. On the other hand, high sensitivity generally also means low specificity, suggesting that many potentially successful NCEs are currently excluded from further development. Common reasons for exclusion are adverse drug reactions (ADR). Among the various ADRs, cardiac toxicities and arrhythmias play an important role, because they represent about 21% of all ADRs (Lasser et al., 2002) and are frequently lethal. The single most important mechanism in this context is the prolongation of cardiac repolarization bearing a proarrhythmic potential. These interferences can be visualized by standard ECGs as a prolongation of the QT-interval. Such a prolongation is called "long QT-syndrome" (LQT-syndrome) and is associated with *Torsade-de-Pointes* (TdP) arrhythmias and sudden cardiac death. In the past, several prominent drugs had to be withdrawn from the market due to TdP in humans, e.g. astemizole, terfenadine, cisapride, sparfloxacin, grepafloxacin and recently clobutinol (Silomat). Moreover, numerous drugs are still on the market that are associated with the potential to cause LQT and TdP, including widely prescribed drugs such as the antibiotic erythromycin.

Given the fatal consequences of LQT and TdP in healthy patients without any cardiac disposition, the regulatory bodies (FDA, EMEA and others) have decided some years ago to require testing for LQT to be an obligatory part of preclinical development of any NCE. Several tests have been developed and some of them are routinely used. The three major (but by far not exclusive) tests in the field are the HERG test, rabbit Purkinje fibers and telemetry in dogs. These tests have different advantages and disadvantages and are generally employed subsequently. The HERG test can be considered an obligatory test for all NCEs and it is unlikely that any company further develops a compound that showed major inhibitory activity in this test (of a single ion channel activity). However, examples exist of successful drugs on the market that are potent inhibitors of the HERG current without ever giving rise to TdP arrhythmia (e.g. verapamil, azithromycin). Thus, the predictive value of the HERG test is limited. Reasons lie, among others, in its inability to give an integrated readout of effects of drugs on the electrophysiology of the intact cardiac myocyte or the intact heart as a multicellular organ consisting of a functional syncytium of cardiac myocytes and all other cardiac cell types that make up normal heart tissue (e.g. fibroblasts, endothelial cells and smooth muscle cells).

1.1 Cardiac tissue engineering

Over the past decade, techniques have been developed to generate cardiac tissue-like 3-dimensional constructs *in vitro* (Eschenhagen & Zimmermann, 2005). The field of cardiac tissue engineering opened the possibility for many applications. Artificial hart constructs may serve as means for cell-based cardiac repair and as improved *in vitro* models for predictive toxicology and target validation, taking advantage of a more physiological cellular environment. Previous studies used different approaches to construct engineered tissues: Cell seeding onto solid, preformed scaffolds (Carrier et al., 1999; Engelmayr et al., 2008; Leor et al., 2000; Li et al., 2000; Ott et al., 2008; Radisic et al., 2004), matrix-free generation of tissues from stackable cell sheets (Shimizu et al., 2002) or the generation of constructs in preformed casting moulds using hydrogels such as collagen I, matrigel, fibronectin or fibrin (Bian et al., 2009; Eschenhagen et al., 1997; Huang et al., 2007; Naito et al., 2006; Zimmermann et al., 2002). The hydrogel technique has been shown to be suitable for both, cardiac repair *in vivo* (Zimmermann et al., 2006) and target validation *in vitro* (El-Armouche et al., 2007). Circular engineered heart tissues (EHTs) were made by casting neonatal rat heart cells, collagen I and matrigel into circular casting moulds and develop a high degree of cellular differentiation, longitudinal orientation, intercellular coupling and force generation (Zimmerman et al., 2002). It turned out that several factors improve tissue quality and force generation of EHT such as phasic (Fink et al., 2000) or auxotonic stretch, increased ambient oxygen concentration during culture and supplementation with insulin (Zimmermann et al., 2006). Others demonstrated beneficial effects of electrical stimulation (Radisic et al., 2004). The possibility to generate cardiac myocytes from human embryonic stem cells (Kehat et al., 2001) or induced pluripotent stem cells (Zhang et al., 2009) have opened the realistic and exciting perspective to use these techniques for the validation of hypotheses and testing drugs in healthy and diseased human heart muscles (Zimmermann & Eschenhagen 2007).

The current techniques to generate engineered cardiac tissues are either not suitable for this purpose (stacked cell sheet technique) or exhibit drawbacks that limit their usefulness. Extensive handling steps preclude routine execution of large series in an at least medium through put scale and are always a source of variability. Furthermore, the EHT technique in the ring format requires relatively high numbers of cells and turned out to be difficult to miniaturize.

In this chapter we describe a new EHT technique that was driven by the intention to miniaturize the EHT-format for multi-well-testing and automated evaluation and to determine the suitability of EHTs for drug screening and predictive toxicology. The main results have been published in a recent original paper (Hansen et al. 2010). An essentiel change was to use fibrin(ogen) instead of collagen I as a matrix. Fibrinogen is part of the blood clotting cascade. It is a glycoprotein with a size of 340 kDa. Physiologically it achieves plasma concentrations of 1.5 to 4 g/l and can be relative easily purified from different species. An important mechanical property is its nonlinear elasticity. Due to this, fibrin polymers have a high elastic modulus under shear stress combined with a beneficial softness in comparison to other filamentous biopolymers (Janmey et al., 2009). The final properties of fibrin are mainly governed by the concentrations of fibrinogen and thrombin. Additionally fibrin properties can be affected by the introduction of bonds by plasma transglutaminase (factor XIII; Janmey et al., 2009). In contrast to other extracellular matrices, the *in vitro* polymerisation of fibrin is very close to the *in vivo* fibrin polymer. Fibrin gels are fully degradable by fibrinolytic enzymes like plasmin. All together, the mechanical and biological properties, its availability from autologous sources in addition to the possibility to covalently bind growth or other factors (Hubbell 2003) make fibrin an interesting compound for tissue engineering approaches.

2. Methods

2.1 Cell isolation

Total heart cells (excluding the atria) were isolated from neonatal Wistar rats (postnatal day 0 to 3) by a fractionated DNase/Trypsin digestion protocol as previously described (Eschenhagen & Zimmermann, 2005). The resulting cell populations were immediately subjected to FBME generation. Experimental procedures were reviewed and approved by Ethics Committee, Hamburg University.

2.2 Manufacturing teflon spacers and sylgard posts racks

For the generation of fibrin-based mini-EHTs (FBMEs), Teflon spacer and silicone post racks were used. The Teflon spacers were important for the casting molds. They had the following geometry (Figure: 1B): length 12 mm, width 3 mm, height 13.5 mm. Sylgard 184 silicone elastomer (Dow Corning) was used for the production of silicone post racks, which were needed for culturing the FBMEs. The silicone post racks were made in custom-made Teflon casting molds. According to the manufacture's instructions, the 2-component Sylgard 184 was degassed under vacuum conditions before casting. The final silicone post racks consisted of 4 pairs of posts, having a little plate at their end. The racks had the following geometry (Figure 1A): length/width of rack: 79x18.5 mm, length of posts 12 mm, diameter 1 mm, plate diameter 2 mm, distance (center-center) 8.5 mm. They were initially self-made and currently industrial-made. Silicone post racks can be autoclaved and reused for several times.

2.3 Generation of fibrin-based mini-EHTs

The reconstitution mixture for the generation of fibrin-based mini-EHTs was prepared on ice as follows (final concentration): 4.1×10^6 cells/ml, 5 mg/ml bovine fibrinogen (Sigma F4753, stock solution: 200 mg/ml in 0.9% NaCl supplemented with 0.5 µg/mg aprotinin), 3 U/ml bovine thrombin (Sigma T7513, stock solution: 100 U/ml). To ensure isotonic conditions, one additional fibrinogen and thrombin volume of 2x DMEM was added. Ordinary 24-well cell culture plates were used as casting molds. After 1.6 ml of sterile 2% agarose (Invitrogen 15510-027) in PBS was pipetted into each well, the Teflon spacers could be placed. After the agarose was solidified, the Teflon spacers were removed. The silicone posts racks were placed onto the cell culture dish with each pair of silicone posts reaching into one of the preformed casting molds (geometry: 12x3x4 mm). The reconstitution mix was carefully resuspended. For each FBME 100 µl of the mixture was mixed briefly with an appropriate volume of thrombin and pipetted into an agarose slot. To ensure complete polymerization of the fibrinogen, the constructs were placed into a humidified cell culture incubator (37 °C, 7% CO_2, 40% O_2) for 2 hours. Before transferring the silicone posts racks to a new medium-filled culture plate, every construct was covered with DMEM (300 µl) to ease the removal. FBMEs were maintained in 37 °C, 7% CO_2, 40% O_2 in a humidified cell culture incubator. Media was changed on Mondays, Wednesdays and Fridays. FBME medium consisted of DMEM (Biochrom F0415) supplemented with 10% horse serum (Gibco 26050), 2% chick embryo extract (self-made), 1% penicillin/streptomycin (Gibco 15140), insulin (Sigma I9278, 10 µg/ml) and aprotinin (Sigma A1153, 33 µg/ml).

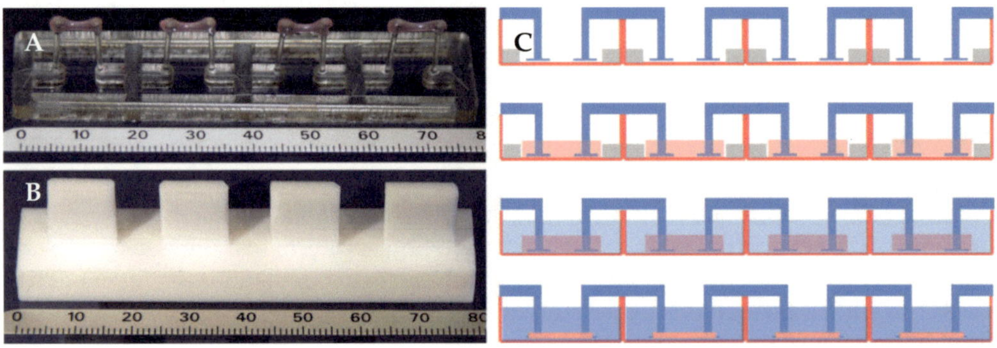

Fig. 1. Illustration of the experimental setup for casting and cultivation and photography of a silicone post rack with four FBMEs. Silicone post rack with four FBMEs (turned upside down, scale in millimetres; A). Teflon spacer for the generation of agarose casting molds (turned upside down, scale in millimetres; B). Illustration of FBME generation (C). First lane: Casting molds are made using Teflon spacers and agarose in a 24-well cell culture dish. Silicone posts racks are placed onto the culture dish, with each pair of posts reaching into a mold. Second lane: Mastermix is pipetted into each mold. Third lane: After 2 h the fibrin is polymerized and the silicone posts are embedded in the hydrogel. FBMEs can be transferred into a new medium-filled 24-well culture plate. Fourth lane: FBMEs are maintained in culture for 15 to 30 days (Hansen et al. 2010).

2.4 Video-optical analyses

The setup for video-optical analyses consisted of a cell culture incubator-like unit, in which gas conditions, humidity and temperature could be controlled. This device was equipped with a glass roof for monitoring purposes. A Basler CCD-camera (Type A 602f-2) was attached to an XYZ-device (IAI Corporation) and positioned above the glassroof in a PC-controlled manner. Light-emitting diodes (LEDs) were placed underneath the cell culture dish. Illumination of a single LED was synchronized with the video-optical recording procedure in order to minimize heating of the cell culture medium by LED waste heat. Figure 2A shows a schematic picture of the whole setup and 2B shows a 24 well cell culture plate with six silicone posts racks and with one FBME in every well (view from above). For the video-optical analyses a customized software package developed by Consulting Team Machine Vision (ctmv.de; Pforzheim, Germany) was used. This software is based on figure recognition and is able to identify the FBME's shape in a fully automated manner. In brief, the system automatically places measuring points at the top and bottom end of the contracting muscle strip. Due to the contraction, the distance in between the moving silicone posts changes. These changes are determined and recorded by the software over time. Based on post geometry, elastic modulus of the Sylgard 184 (2.6 kPa) and the delta value of post distance (post deflection), the developed force was calculated based on a recently published equation (Vandenburgh et al. 2008). The recorded contractions are filtered and identified as such by certain peak criteria (e.g. threshold value, minimal force and minimum relaxation). Besides average force, the software calculates values for frequency, fractional shortening, contraction- and relaxation time (bpm, T1 and T2, respectively) based on the recognized contraction peaks. T1 and T2 were determined at 20% of peak maximum. Reports with an overview of the environmental information (temperature, gas, humidity) in the cell culture like unit plus all calculated parameters are automatically generated after each run. These underlie two levels of quality control: pictures are taken at the beginning and the end of each recording. Blue squares indicate top and bottom end of each respective FBME where the software placed the points for the measurement (Figure 2D). Contractions are recorded as force development over time. Identified peaks, which are included in the calculation, are marked with green squares (Figure 2C). The effort to analyse a 24-well plate with contracting muscle strips is limited to defining the XYZ-coordinates for each well once before starting a series of measurements.

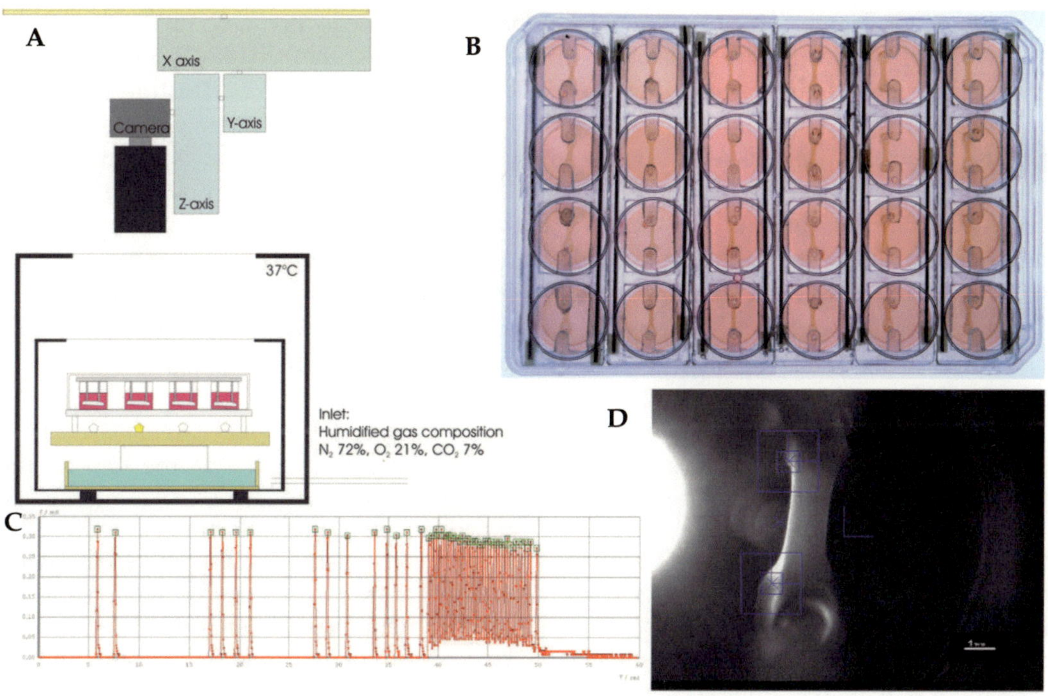

Fig. 2. Illustration of the experimental setup for video-optical recordings of FBME, a 24 well cell culture dish with FBMEs, a magnified view of a single FBME as recorded by the video camera and an example of a contraction pattern (one FBME for 60 s). A shows a schematic picture of the experimental setup for video-optical recordings. In B a 24 well cell culture dish with FBMEs is shown (view from above). The original contraction pattern of one FBME over time (60 s, C). Image of a contractile muscle strip from an automatically generated report (D). Blue squares indicate positions automatically recognized by the software at top and bottom end of the FBME. Green squares mark the recognized contraction peaks which are included for the calculation of several parameters (Hansen et al. 2010).

3. Results

3.1 General aspects of the new technique

We developed a new technique for the generation and evaluation of contractile cardiac tissue from neonatal rat heart cells *in vitro* (Hansen et al. 2010). In this method, isolated heart cells are mixed with fibrinogen, thrombin and medium and pipetted into rectangular casting moulds made from 2%-agarose in ordinary 24-well cell culture plates. Due to the polymerisation of the fibrin, the gel is fixed to both silicone posts. After 2 h at 37 °C the constructs can be transferred to new culture dishes and maintained under cell culture conditions for several days. Figure 1C demonstrates this procedure in a schematic way. During cultivation, the cells inside the gel spread along the force lines and form extensive cell-cell contacts, the hydrogel is remodelled and degraded. These processes are accompanied by marked condensation of the constructs and deflection of the silicone posts towards each other. The initial length of a FBME directly after casting is 8.5 mm and the mean final length 6.5 mm. The post deflection differs between individual FBMEs, likely reflecting their degree of cardiac tissue development. In consequence, each FBME is exposed to an "individually optimized preload". With this simplified method, 48-72 FBMEs can be routinely generated out of one cell preparation (30 rat hearts). Figure 2B illustrates a typical 24 well plate with silicone posts racks and FBMEs. Fibrin is affected by proteases in the culture medium. To decrease degradation, the protease inhibitor aprotinin at a concentration of 33 µg/ml is added to the medium. This inhibitor markedly reduces fibrinolysis but cannot entirely stop it. To further protect the hydrogel from proteolysis tranexamic acid, another protease inhibitor, can be added to the medium. The combination of both inhibitors results in improved stability and allows longer cultivation periods. Tranexamic acid-treated FBMEs have a markedly increased diameter (final width 1.3 to 1.4 mm [Figure 2C and 8D] instead of 0.2 to 1.0 mm in its absence [Figure 4A]).

3.2 Morphology and beating activity

Directly after casting, FBMEs appeared as a soft fibrin-block fixed at the end of the silicone posts and exhibiting the dimensions of the casting moulds (12x3xx mm). Within this clot, the heart cells were round and amorphous but homogeneously distributed throughout the gel (Figure 3A). During the first days after casting, cells spread, elongated along force lines, started to beat as single cells and finally in the form of synchronously beating areas on day 4 to 5. The further development was characterized by matrix remodelling and degradation. This lead to a marked reduction of the size (from 3 mm to 1-2 mm width in the presence and 0.2-1 mm in the absence of tranexamic acid) and increased cell-density. Between day 5 and day 7 the cardiomyocytes formed small groups (Figure 3B through E). Coherent beating of the muscle construct started around day 7 to 9. By day 10 the generated force was sufficient to rhythmically deflect the silicone posts. Measurements were routinely performed between day 14 to 16. At this point the cardiomyocytes finally appeared as spindle-shaped cells with an approximately length of 100 to 200 µm and a diameter of 10 to 20 µm (Figure 3F).

Hematoxylin/eosin-stained paraffin sections of mature FBMEs (day 15) showed a dense network of longitudinally aligned cells throughout the gel (Figure 4A). No clear evidence for cell density gradient from peripheral to central areas of the gel could be found, arguing against a significant inhomogeneity of oxygen and nutrient supply.

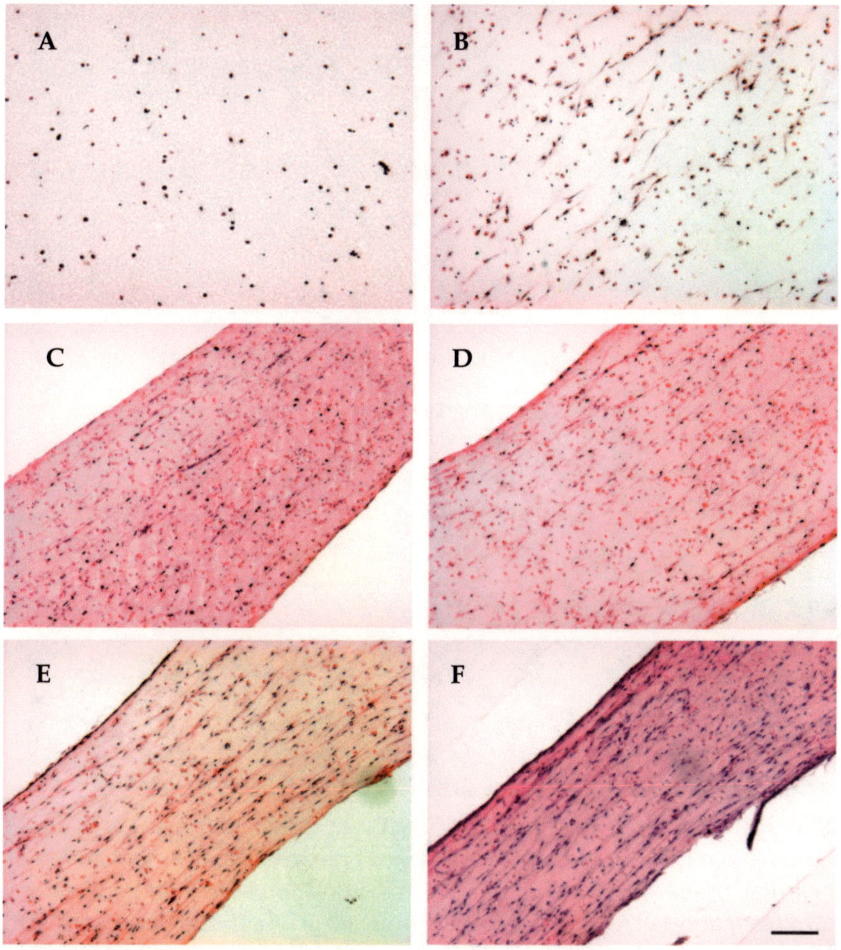

Fig. 3. Histological analysis of FBMEs. FBMEs were cultured with aprotinin plus tranexamic acid. For histological analysis they were fixed with formaldehyde at indicated time points, embedded with paraffin and the sections were HE-stained (10x magnification). A Day 0: cells are present as single, round and amorphous cell suspension in fibrin matrix; B day 3: cells spread out along force lines. C day 6, D day 9: degradation of extracellular matrix, cells spread and align with neighbouring cells. E day 12, F day 15: extended degradation of extracellular matrix, the cellular density is increased; cells align and show orientation along force lines. Scale bar 100 µm (Hansen et al. 2010).

Whole-mount FBMEs were also analysed by immunofluorescent staining. The pictures showed a dense network of regularly cross striated, α-actinin-positive, longitudinally aligned cardiomyocytes. The elongated cells had well developed sarcomeric structures reaching into the periphery of the cytoplasm. Cardiomyocytes were also characterized by connexion-43 positive structures, the gap junctions. In contrast to the *in vivo* situation connexion-positivity was mostly localized on lateral parts of the cell membrane, but not clustered at the border to connecting cells. Moreover, the immunfluorescence showed lectin-positive endothelial cells intermingled with cardiomycytes and forming primitive tube-like structures (Figure 4).

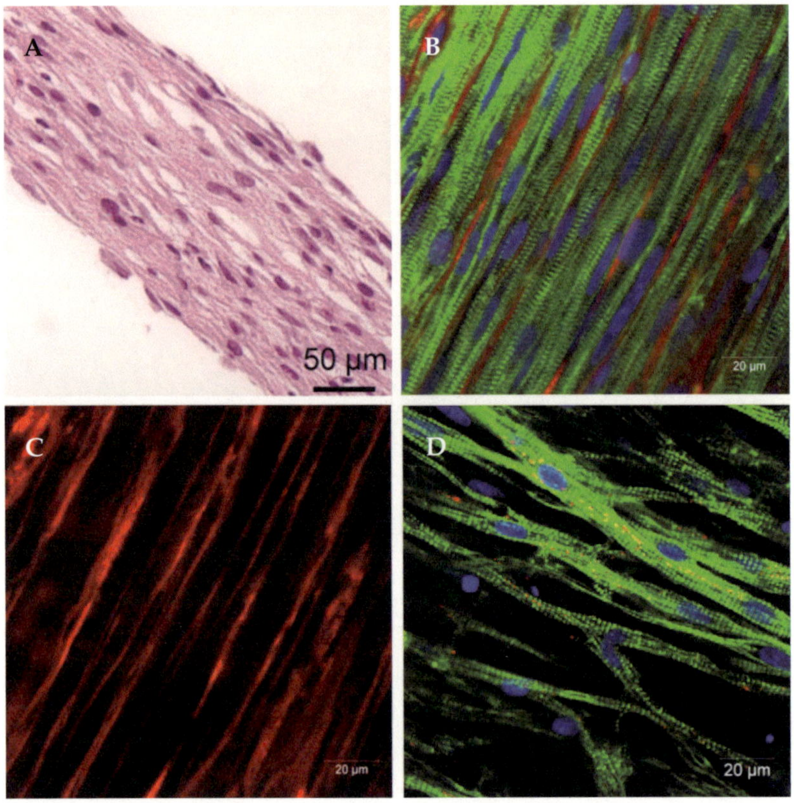

Fig. 4. Histological analysis of FBMEs (day 15, without tranexamic acid). A, HE-stained paraffin section. Note the almost complete absence of extracellular matrix and well-developed cardiac tissue structure. B, Merged immunofluorescence staining for α-actinin (green), lectin (red) and DRAQ5 (blue; 63x magnification). C, Lectin-positive structures alone (63x magnification). D, Connexin-43 (red), phalloidin (green) and DRAQ5 (blue; 63x magnification). Scale bar 50 µm (A) and 20 µM (B-D; Hansen et al. 2010).

3.3 DNA/RNA content, histone H3 phosphorylation and caspase-3 activity

To further investigate cell survival in FBMEs during culture, the histological data were supported by measurements on a molecular biological level. The DNA/RNA content, histone H3 phosphorylation as well as the caspase-3-activity were analysed. The DNA content dropped by 20% between day 0 and day 3. Thereafter it remained stable for at least two weeks (Figure 5A). Investigations of histone H3 phosphorylation as a marker of proliferative activity and caspase-3 activity as a marker for apoptosis in FBMEs were well in line with these observations. Histone H3 phosphorylation level was initially very low and further decreased over time (Figure 5C). Caspase-3 activity was high directly after cell preparation and dropped during culture even below detectable levels (Figure 5D). After an initial drop of the RNA-content during the first three days of 50% it remained, like the DNA content, more or less stable for at least two weeks (Figure 5B). In summary, these data suggest that some of the cells died within the first three days after casting, likely as a consequence of cell damage during the isolation procedure. Thereafter the cell population remained essentially stable in FBMEs.

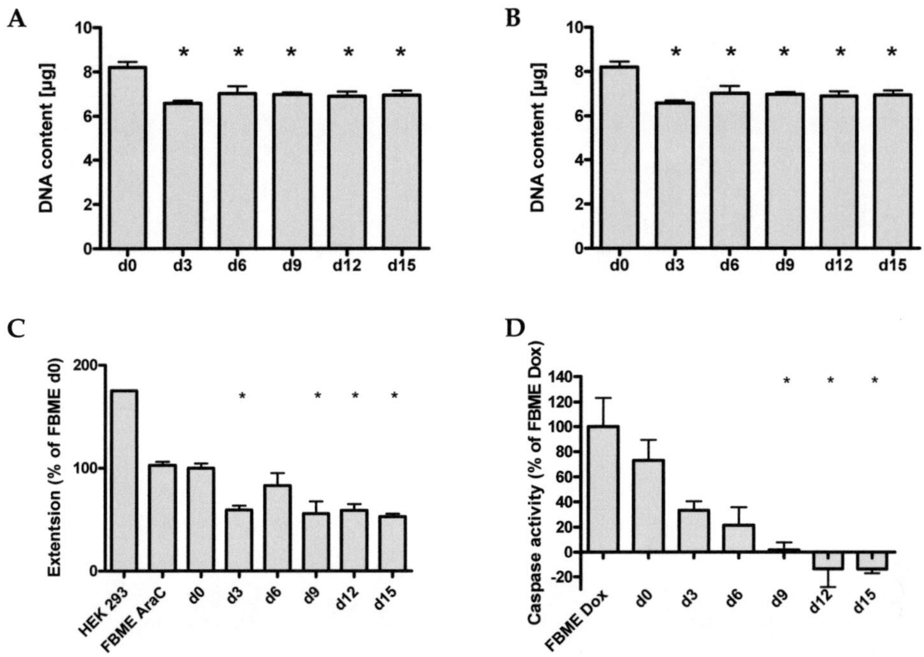

Fig. 5. DNA and total RNA content of FBMEs. A DNA content of FBMEs over time (n=4). B Total RNA content over time (n=4). * $p<0.05$ vs. d0 (Student's t test). Bars show means +/- SD. C, D Concentration of phosphorylated histone H3 (C) and caspase-3 activity (D) in FBMEs over time of cultivation. Day 0 represents freshly solidified FBMEs 2 h after casting. Proliferating HEK293 cells and AraC-treated FBMEs served as positive and negative controls for proliferation, respectively. Doxorubicin-treated FBMEs served as positive controls for caspase-3 activity. Bars show mean +/-SEM, n=4. * $p<0.05$ vs. d0 (Student's t test; Hansen et al. 2010).

3.4 Cardiac marker gene expression over time

To get an idea about cardiomyocyte maturation in FBMEs, transcript levels of known cardiac marker genes (α-actinin, SR Ca^{2+}-ATPase [SERCA], α- and β-myosin heavy chain [α-/β-MHC], Na^{+}/Ca^{2+}-exchanger [NCX], titin) were analysed over time. To avoid bias due to the effect of the drop of overall cell count after preparation, all values were normalized to the mRNA concentration of the cardiac myocyte-specific protein calsequestrin 2. Values were additionally compared to intact adult (ARH) and neonatal rat hearts (NRHT; Figure 6). In the first phase (day 0 to day 6), which represents the time when the single cells spread, formed clusters and started to beat, the transcript levels seemed to be relatively stable. In the second phase (day 9 to day 12) the expression levels reached their maximum concomitantly with the start of rhythmical deflection of the silicone posts by the FBMEs. In the third phase (day 12 to day 15) transcript levels generally decreased. Some cardiac markers (α-actinin, SERCA, α-MHC) reached a comparable level to native myocardium on day 15. Other (β-MHC, titin and NCX) remained several fold higher, indicating higher remodelling activity.

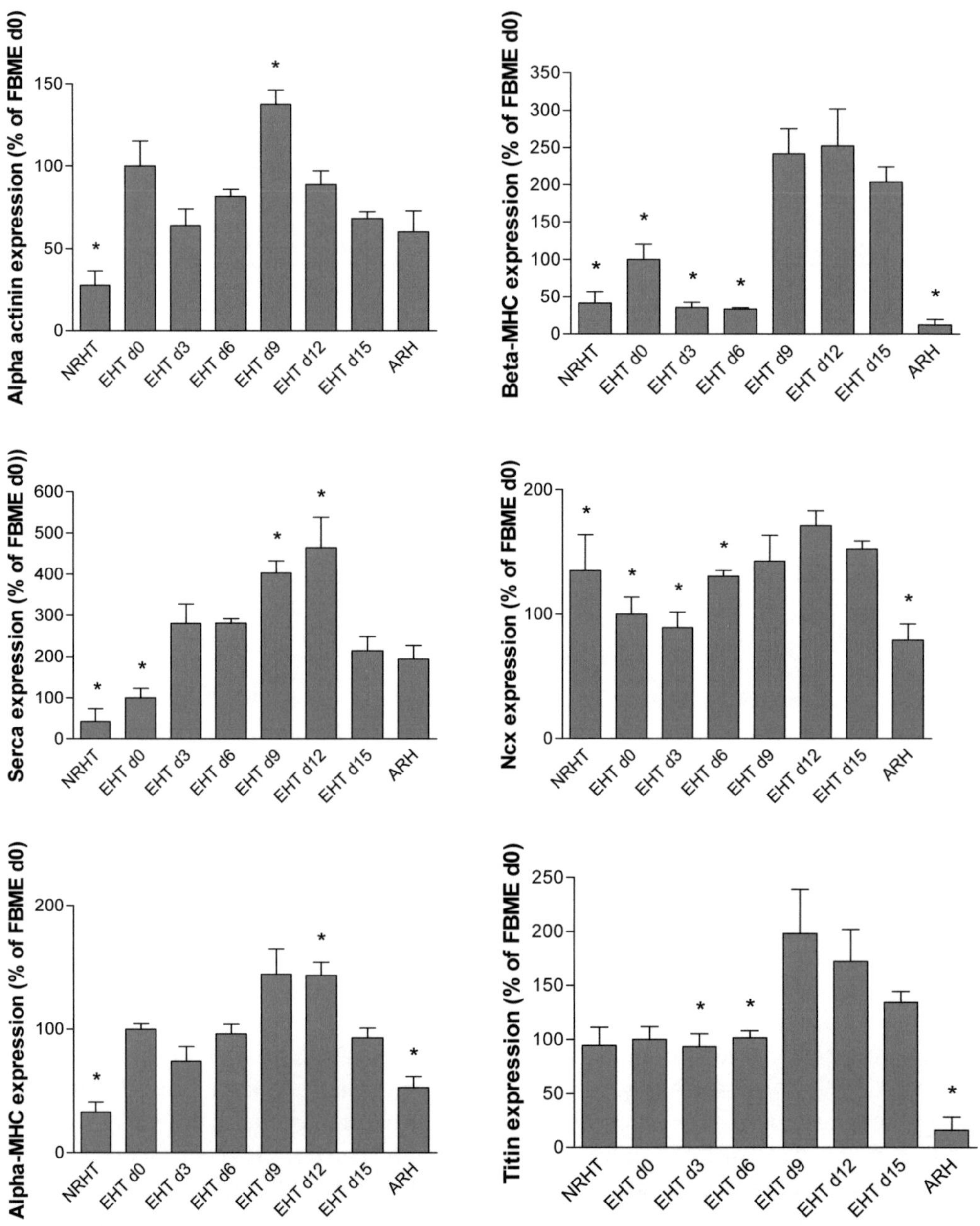

Fig. 6. RT-qPCR of FBMEs in comparison to neonatal (NRHT) and adult rat heart (ART). ΔΔCT values were generated by normalisation to the mRNA of cardiac specific protein calsequestrin 2 (average CT values for normalisation were as follows: d0: 20.8, d3: 20.4, d6: 20.6, d9: 21.3, d12: 21.6, d15: 20.5). Figures show relative expression compared to day 0. Each bar represents results from 4 biological replicates (each measured 3 times). * $p<0.05$ vs. day 15 (Student's t test). Bars show means +/- SEM (Hansen et al. 2010).

3.5 Non quantitative ion channel expression profile

Ion channels play an important role as targets of proarrhythmic drugs. To determine whether the principal ion channel subunits known from human hearts are expressed in rat FBMEs transcripts of 23 ion channel α-subunits (7 calcium channels, 6 sodium channels, 10 potassium channels) were amplified from total RNA of FBMEs and a nonfailing human heart sample by RT-PCR (35 cycles). 22/23 transcripts were amplified from both sources, one channel (CacnA1I) was neither amplified in FBMEs nor in the nonfailing human heart (Figure 7).

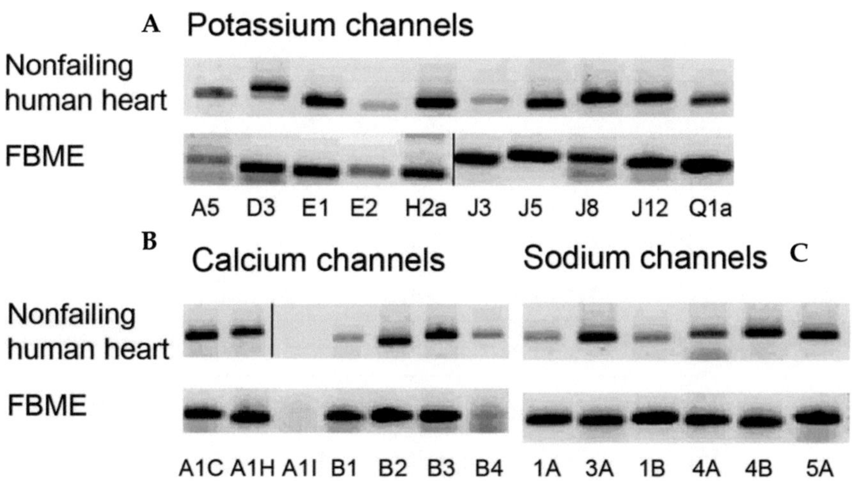

Fig. 7. Agarose gel of the PCR-products of 23 ion channel subunits. The ion channel profile of FBMEs was compared to the expression profile of a nonfailing human heart. Potassium channels (A), calcium channel (B) and sodium channels (C) showed qualitatively similar results (descriptions indicate the related gene for each channel subunit; for further information see table 1; Hansen et al. 2010).

3.6 Robustness and reproducibility of the new method

To determine robustness and reproducibility or the assay, we generated 6 independent series of FBMEs (1-2 24-well plates each, total number 192 FBMEs) and analysed them under standard conditions (culture medium with insulin, aprotinin and tranexamic acid; measurements done by video-optical recordings). Two FBMEs could not be transferred from the casting moulds, 4 FBMEs were not recognized by the software and 17 did not beat during the recording time (60 s) at day 15. Thus, the total success rate was 89% (169/192; Figure 8). Contraction parameters were examined and compared among different series. These results showed that the average force per series (day 15) was between 0.11 and 0.22 mN (series SD 7.6%), the contraction time (T1=time to peak) ranged between 66 and 81 ms (series SD 41%), relaxation time (T2=time to 80% relaxation) between 67 and 88 ms (series SD 25%), frequency between 162 and 20 beats per minute (series SD 109%), construct diameter between 1.3 and 1.4 mm (series SD 9.9%) and length between 5.6 and 6.7 mm (series SD 16.7%). The relatively large size in FBME diameter in these examinations could be attributed to the use of tranexamic acid.

Family	Abbre-viation	Description
KCN	A5	Voltage-gated channel subunit Kv1.5
	D3	Voltage-gated channel subunit Kv4.3
	E1	Potential voltage-gated channel subunit beta (KvLQT1; ERG; function: I_{Ks} or $_{Kr}$)
	E2	Potential voltage-gated channel subunit beta (minK-related peptide 1; KvLQT1; ERG; function: I_{Ks} or I_{Kr})
	H2a	I_{Kr} producing rapid voltage-gated channel subunit beta (ether-a-go-go-related gene (ERG) channel 1)
	J3	G protein-activated inward rectifier channel 1 (Kir3.1)
	J5	G protein-activated inward rectifier channel 4 (Kir3.4)
	J8	ATP-sensitive inward rectifier channel 8 (Kir6.1)
	J12	ATP-sensitive inward rectifier channel 12 (Kir2.2)
	Q1a	I_{Ks} producing slow voltage-gated channel subunit alpha (KvLQT1)
CACN	A1C	Voltage-dependent subunit alpha-1C (L-type)
	A1H	Voltage-dependent subunit alpha-1H (T-type)
	A1I	Voltage-dependent subunit alpha-1I (T-type)
	B1	Voltage-dependent subunit beta-1 (L-type)
	B2	Voltage-dependent subunit beta-2 (L-type)
	B3	Voltage-dependent subunit beta-3 (L-type)
	B4	Voltage-dependent subunit beta-4 (L-type)
SCN	1A	Voltage-gated channel protein type-1 subunit alpha
	3A	Voltage-gated channel protein type-3 subunit alpha
	1B	Voltage-gated channel subunit beta-1
	4A	Voltage-gated channel protein type 4 subunit alpha
	4B	Voltage-gated channel subunit beta-4
	5A	Voltage-gated channel protein type-5 subunit alpha

Table 1. Overview of the analysed ion channels shown in figure 7.

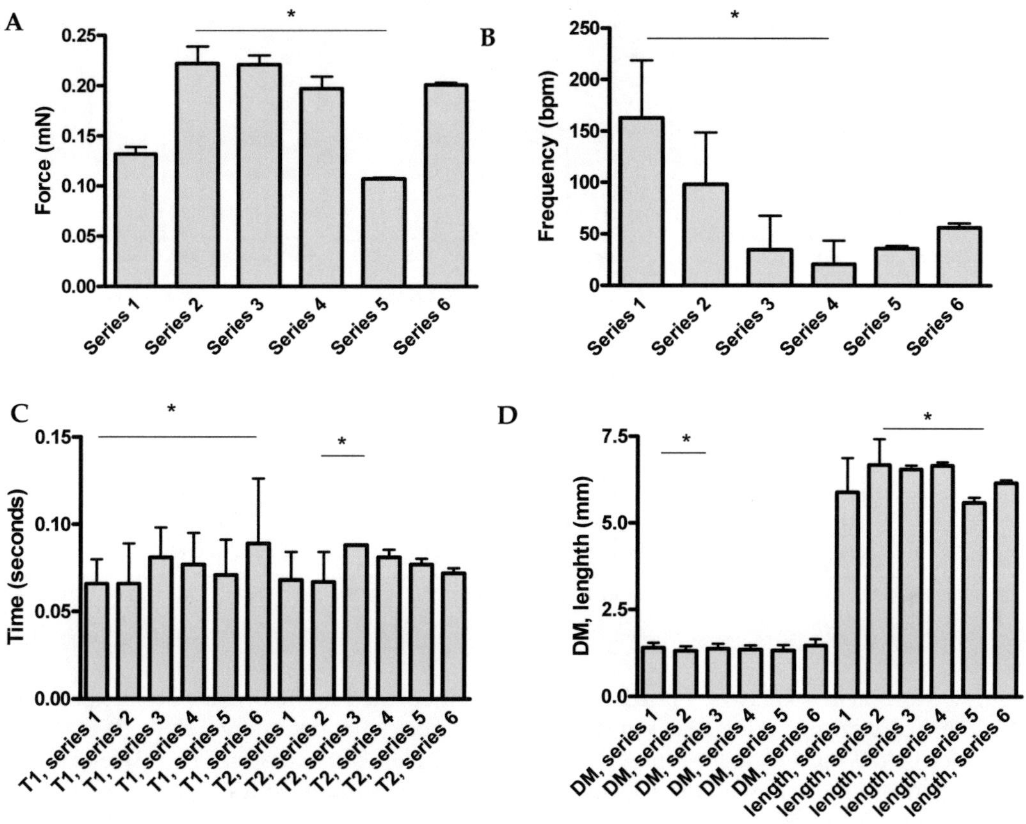

Fig. 8. Reproducibility of the assay. FBMEs were generated at 6 different time points (series 1-6) and spontaneous activity was recorded on day 15. Parameters of contractility (A: force, B: frequency, C: contraction time T1, relaxation time T2) and construct dimensions (D) were averaged and compared. Minimal and maximal values were used to test for significant differences and are indicated with * $p<0.05$ (Student's t test). Bars show means +/- SD. Analysed FBMEs for each series were: Series 1: n=21, series 2: n=24, series 3: n=20, series 4: n=18, series 5: n=39, series 6: n=47 (Hansen et al. 2010).

3.7 Cardiotoxic and proarrhythmic effects of drugs

To determine whether the new method could be used for the detection of cardiotoxic and proarrhythmic drug effects, well characterized compounds with known cardiotoxic and repolarization-inhibitory effects were tested. The cardiotoxic drug doxorubicin was applied in different concentrations (0.1-1.000 nmol/L) for up to 96 h. Doxorubicin-treated FBMEs showed time- and concentration-dependent changes in contractile force. Very low concentrations of doxorubicin (1-10 nmol/L) led to a trend towards an increase in contractile force, 100 nmol/L induced a transient increase in contractile force after 24 h which was followed by a decrease at 72 and 96 h (Figure 9). In the presence of 1 µmol/L doxorubicin all FBMEs stopped to beat after 3 days.

To examine a repolarization-inhibitory effect on FBMEs, the experimental I_{Ks}-blocker chromanol 293B as well as the clinically used drugs quinidine and erythromycin were

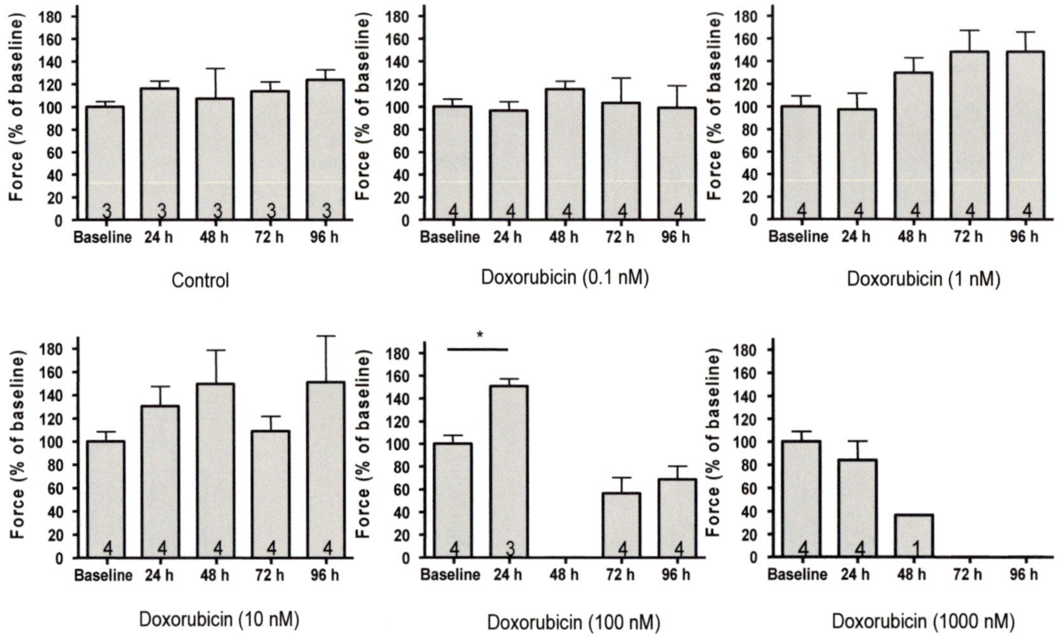

Fig. 9. Doxorubicin toxicity on FBMEs. FBMEs were incubated in the presence of doxorubicin (0.1-1000 nM, starting at day 13 of culture), average forces were determined daily. While doxorubicin at 0.1 µM increased force after 24 hours, higher concentrations (1 µM) lead to a time-dependent reduction in force development. * $p<0.05$ (Student's t test). Bars show means +/- SEM, number of evaluated (beating) constructs as indicated (Hansen et al. 2010).

tested. All three compounds induced a concentration-dependent delay in relaxation time (T2; Figure 10). In the presence of chromanol 293B, FBMEs already showed a prolongation of T2 at a concentration of 1 µmol/L. At 100 µmol/L chromanol, T2 was 7-fold longer than control, resulting in a "church-like" configuration of the twith (Figure 10). Quinidine and erythromycin, both associated with arrhythmias in clinical applications, also extended the relaxation time at high concentrations (100 µmol/L). Time of contraction was not affected by any of the compounds.

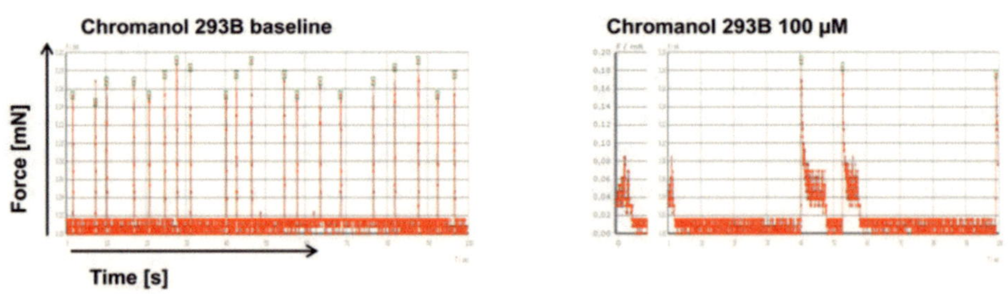

Fig. 10. Chromanol 293B-induced "church-like" contraction pattern. Cutout of the original contraction recordings in the presence and absence of Chromanol 293B (100 µM; modified from: Hansen et al. 2010).

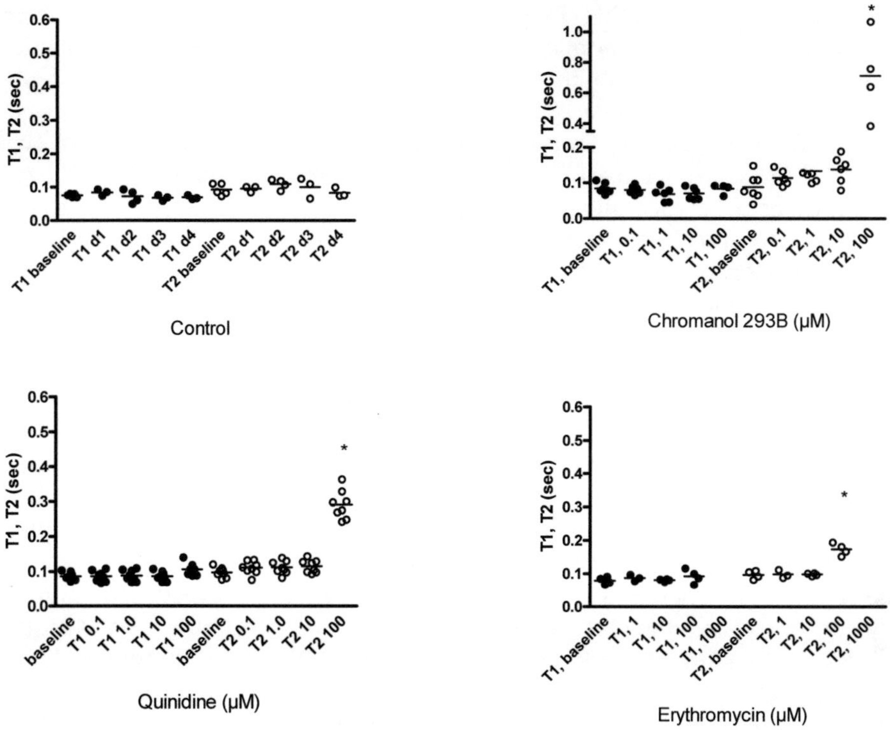

Fig. 11. Effect of repolarisation inhibitors on FBME contraction (T1) and relaxation time (T2). FBMEs were incubated with increasing concentrations of the indicated compounds (1-2 h) and evaluated before application of drug (baseline) and after each concentration. Note the absence of effect of all compounds on T1 and the concentration-dependent increase in T2 with chromanol, quinidine and erythromycin (at 1000 µM of erythromycin FBMEs discontinued contractile activity). A typical alteration of contraction peak morphology with increasing concentrations of quinidine, chromanol and erythromycin is shown in supplementary figure 5. * $p<0.05$ (Student's t test). Bars show means +/- SEM, each spot represents one analysed FBME (Hansen et al. 2010).

4. Conclusion

In this book chapter we describe a recently developed method (Hansen et al. 2010) to generate miniaturized, fibrin-based EHTs (FBMEs) in a 24-well format and determine their contractile activity in an automated manner. This technique turned out to be robust and highly reproducible. Its main advantages are its simplicity in terms of handling, the standard 24-well format, its robustness and the high content automated readout of contractile activity. Compared to previously EHT-protocols (Eschenhagen et al. 1997, Zimmermann et al. 2002), three major changes were introduced. (i) Collagen I was replaced by fibrinogen and thrombin. Due to the fast fibrin-polymerisation, the heart cells were homogenously distributed throughout the entire hydrogel. Polymerisation occurs in minutes and allows transfer of the constructs from the casting moulds to a new medium-filled culture dish after two hours. Moreover, fast solidification allowed 50% higher cell concentration ($0.6x10^6$/150 µl versus $2.5x10^6$/900 µl), because it prevents accumulation of cells at the bottom of the casting moulds with detrimental consequences. Fibrin has additional advantages for future applications, such as transplantations. It is available from autologoues sources and has the ability to couple covalently growth-promoting, angiogenic or other interesting factors (Hubble 2003). (ii) The original ring-format was changed to a stripe-format. This step was very important because it allowed miniaturization (volume reduced from 900 to 150 µl), the use of standard 24-well plates and automation. The silicone racks with 4 pairs of posts each allow simple transfer of FBMEs from one plate to another and thus reduce the number of nonstandardized handling steps to a minimum. Moreover, the silicone posts subject the growing muscle construct to an individually optimized preload and allow them to perform contractile work against the elastic properties of the post. (iii) Video-optical measurements of contractile parameters further improved the whole technique. They superseded the manual transfer for measurements as it was required in former EHT-protocols. Additionally, video-optical recordings allowed simple, reproducible, standardized measurements of large series in a short spell.

The new stripe-format was inspired by a previously described method for generating skeletal muscle tissues (Vandenburgh et al. 2008). Turning the silicone posts up side down was the major difference to this method and simplified handling. In this way the quality of the constructs could be determine with an ordinary microscope or even by eye and opened the possibility for automated video-optical recordings from above the plate. This experimental setup, in combination with fibrin, has several important features. (i) It is simple and not longer addicted to some kind of special dish because standard 24-well cell culture plates can be used. In the beginning silicone posts racks were self-made, which turned out to relevantly limit reproducibility. We therefore have the racks industrial made now, which makes the method robust and highly reproducible (Figure 8). (ii) FBMEs exhibit an excellent cardiac tissue development (Figure 4). Several factors are likely to contribute to these beneficial effects. As outlined above, the fast polymerisation of fibrin allowed higher cell concentrations and lead to homogenous cell distribution throughout the hydrogel. Another reason was that cell survival appeared very high in the current fibrin-based format. Moreover, proliferative activity (of non-myocytes) was very low (Figure 5), making the system stable over prolonged periods. The stable mRNA expression pattern of cardiac markers (α-actinin, α-MHC, titin, calsequestrin 2 and SERCA) may be an additional hint for a relatively stable system. Interestingly, the fetal gene marker β-MHC showed a several fold decrease within in the first six days. This phase was associated with cell spreading and contractions on a cellular level. Later, between day 6 and day 9 there was a ~5-fold increase of the β-MHC mRNA expression, coinciding with the beginning of macroscopic contractions. A third positive effect of the described new technique is the optimized mechanical load on the cardiomyocytes. The mechanical load is produced by the resistance of the silicon posts and adapted individually for each FBME. If the tonic (diastolic force) of the construct is high, post deflection by the FBMEs is stronger and *vice versa*. Furthermore, the FBMEs can perform contractile work against an elastic resistance. These circumstances mimic in some ways the *in vivo* situation in which the beating heart needs to work against the afterload induced by the total peripheric resistance. This kind of optimized "auxotonic" load in contrast to motorized phasic stretch improves tissue development as shown earlier in other EHT-studies (Zimmermann et al. 2006).

Regarding the development of a drug screening, miniaturization, reduction of nonstandardized steps during the procedure and an automated, objective readout were very important. The miniaturization to a 24-well format reduced the cell number by a factor of

~4. Additionally, pilot experiments could show that a further miniaturization to a 96-well format would be possible. At this point the 24-well format turned out to be a good compromise between miniaturization and ease of handling. FBMEs do not longer need to be manually transferred as single tissues because the entire silicon racks were handled. In contrast to that, circular EHTs needed to be manually transferred from the casting mould to a motorized stretcher and finally from the stretcher to the organ bath for the measurements. Compared to this method, the video-optical recordings were simple and robust. To confirm the calculated forces, isometric measurements were exemplarily done in the organ bath in parallel and showed that the calculated forces were roughly in the range of the measured ones (0.3 vs. 0.9 mN). The threefold difference could indicate a systematic error, but more likely reflects optimized conditions in the organ bath (preload optimization, electrical pacing and isometric versus auxotonic contraction). A force of 0.9 mN (organ bath) and a diameter of 0.2 mm (Figure 4A; without tranexamic acid) results in a relative force development of 28.7 mN/mm^2. This is still lower than values in an intact muscle (50 mN/mm^2), but point in the right direction. The development of a software which works by automated figure recognition was important in two aspects. On the one hand, it is time-saving since it calculates all important contractile parameters automatically. On the other hand, it provides an objective readout.

Initial experiments to determine the suitability of FBMEs to detect either cardiotoxic or proarrhythmic effects looked promising. The known cardiotoxic drug doxorubicin suppressed contractile activity at the highest concentration (1.000 nmol/L) and increased force at lower concentrations (100 nmol/L) and earlier time points (24 h). This may be due to the reactive oxygen species-generating effect of this compound, which at later time points and/or higher concentrations turned into toxicity.

Three known proarrhythmic drugs caused a concentration-dependent prolongation of relaxation time in FBMEs. Chromanol 293B is an experimental I_{Ks}-blocker with an IC_{50}-value of 8 µmol/L in H9c2 cells (Lo et al. 2005). A concentration of 100 µmol/L was needed to fully block I_{Ks} in these cells. This correspond well to the relaxation-prolonging effect in FBMEs, which was visible at 10 µmol/L and marked at 100 µmol/L (Figure 10) matching quite well the published data (Lo et al. 2005). Quinidine, known as a class IA antiarrhythmic drug according to Vaughan-Williams classification (Vaughan-Williams 1975), also blocks I_{Ks} and I_{Kr} with EC_{50} values of 10 µmol/L and 300 nmol/L, respectively (Lo et al. 2005; Redfern et al. 2003). In FBMEs, quinidine prolonged relaxation time at 100 µmol/L. This is not an entirely different range in comparison with the determined IC_{50} for quinidine on I_{Ks} but far away from I_{Kr}-IC_{50}. This argues again for the role of I_{Ks} in FBME-repolarisation. Erythromycin, a clinically used antibiotic, which is associated with *Torsades-de-Pointes* arrhythmias and increased lethality in men (Ray et al. 2004), inhibits I_{Kr} but not I_{Ks} in dogs (Antzelevitch et al. 1996) and increases action potential duration in rat ventricular cardiomyocytes (IC_{50} 60 µmol/L; Hanada et al. 2003). In FBMEs erythromycin caused an increase in relaxation time at concentrations of 100 µmol/L and above. Even though the channel subunits for both I_{Kr} and I_{Ks} are expressed on mRNA-level in FBMEs (Figure 7), their role in repolarisation of rat cardiomyocytes is still controversial (Regan et al. 2005). In any case, the observation that the prototype proarrhythmic drugs specifically affected relaxation time in FBMEs indicates that this parameter may be useful as a surrogate of repolarisation. However, the detailed mechanisms behind the cardiotoxic and proarrhythmic effects are still unclear and need to be further investigated in follow up studies.

The presented technique still has a number of important limitations with regard to drug screening. (i) The cell preparation cannot be fully standardized. In particular, the age of newborn rats varies from 0-3 days and has significant impact of the quality of FBMEs, most likely explaining part of the variability between series (Figure 6). (ii) The system is not well suited to determine acute positive or negative inotropic effects because measurements are done under spontaneous beating, leading to confounding effects of concomitant negative or positive chronotropic effects. We are working on a system which allows measurements to be done under continuous pacing. (iii) Histological observations showed spindle-shaped cardiomyocytes and a predominantly lateral orientation of connexion-43-postive gap junctions. This suggests that cardiomyocytes, despite functional, molecular and morphological indices of advanced maturation, do not reach an adult phenotype. (iv) Our assay system exclusively monitors alterations in contractile activity and does not directly determine calcium transients or action potential duration. We believe that relaxation time is a good surrogate parameter of action potential, but the direct proof is still lacking. (v) Finally, rodents are known to be poor models for detecting proarrhythmic drug effects because mechanisms governing their action potential differ considerably from that in humans. For example, I_{Kr} plays a relatively minor role in rodents, but a major one in humans (Regan et al. 2005). Our present results suggest that proarrhythmic drug effects can still be monitored in this system, but much more work is necessary to determine which ion channel or combination of ion channels have to be blocked to see changes in relaxation time and/or arrhythmias in FBMEs.

Thus, validation of the new system will require testing of a large number of drugs that are known to cause cardiac arrhythmias in humans and those that are known to be free of arrhythmic side effects, including those that have effects on HERG but are not associated with *Torsades-de-Pointes* arrhythmias. Moreover, a number of randomly chosen new chemical entities should be analysed to obtain an estimate how many non selected compounds give a signal. These studies are currently under way.

5. References

Antzelevitch, C.; Sun, Z. Q.; Zhang, Z. Q. & Yan, G. X (1996). Cellular and ionic mechanisms underlying erythromycin-induced long QT intervals and torsade de pointes. *Journal of the American College of Cardiology*; 28:1836-48

Bian, W.; Liau, B.; Badie, N. & Bursac, N. (2009). Mesoscopic hydrogel molding to control the 3D geometry of bioartificial muscle tissues. *Nature Protocols*; 4:1522-34

Carrier, R. L.; Papadaki, M.; Rupnick, M.; Schoen, F.J.; Bursac, N.; Langer, R.; Freed, L. E. & Vunjak-Novakovic, G. (1999). Cardiac tissue engineering: cell seeding, cultivation parameters, and tissue construct characterization. *Biotechnology Bioengineerening*; 64:580–589

El-Armouche A, Singh J, Naito H, Wittköpper K, Didié M, Laatsch A, Zimmermann WH, Eschenhagen T. (2007). Adenovirus-delivered short hairpin RNA targeting PKCalpha improves contractile function in reconstituted heart tissue. *Journal of Molecular Cell Cardiology*; 43:371-6

Engelmayr, G. C. Jr; Cheng, M.; Bettinger C. J.; Borenstein J.T.; Langer, R. & Freed L. E. (2008). Accordion-like honeycombs for tissue engineering of cardiac anisotropy. *Nature Materials.*; 7:1003–1010

Eschenhagen, T.; Fink, C.; Remmers, U.; Scholz, H.; Wattchow, J.; Weil J.; Zimmermann, W.; Dohmen, H. H.; Schafer, H.; Bishopric, N.; Wakatsuki, T. & Elson, E. L. (1997). Three-dimensional reconstitution of embryonic cardiac myocytes in a collagen matrix: a new heart muscle model system. *The FASEB Journal*; 11:683–694

Eschenhagen, T. & Zimmermann, W.H. (2005). Engineering myocardial tissue. *Circulation Research.*; 97:1220-31

Fink, C.; Ergün, S.; Kralisch, D.; Remmers, U.; Weil, J. & Eschenhagen, T. (2000). Chronic stretch of engineered heart tissue induces hypertrophy and functional improvement. *The FASEB Journal*; 14:669-79

Hanada, E.; Ohtani, H.; Hirota, M.; Uemura, N.; Nakaya, H.; Kotaki, H.; Sato, H.; Yamada, Y. & Iga, T. (2003). Inhibitory effect of erythromycin on potassium currents in rat ventricular myocytes in comparison with disopyramide. *The Journal of Pharmacy and Pharmacology*; 55:995-1002

Hansen, A.; Eder, A.; Bönstrup, B.; Flato, M.; Mewe, M.; Schaaf, S.; Aksehirlioglu, B.; Schwörer, A.; Uebeler, J. & Eschenhagen T. (2010). Development of a drug screening platform based on engineered heart tissue. *Circulation Research*; 107(1):35-44.

Huang, Y.C.; Khait, L. & Birla, R. K. (2007). Contractile three-dimensional bioengineered heart muscle for myocardial regeneration. *Journal of Biomedical Material Research Part A*; 80:719–731

Hubbell, J. A. (2003). Materials as morphogenetic guides in tissue engineering. *Current Opinion in Biotechnology*; 14:551-8

Janmey, P. A.; Winer, J. P. & Weisel, J.W. (2009). Fibrin gels and their clinical and bioengineering applications. *Journal of the Royal Society Interface*; 6:1-10

Kehat, I.; Kenyagin-Karsenti, D.; Snir, M.; Segev, H.; Amit, M.; Gepstein, A.; Livne, E.; Binah, O.; Itskovitz-Eldor, J. & Gepstein, L. (2001). Human embryonic stem cells can differentiate into myocytes with structural and functional properties of cardiomyocytes. *Journal of Clinical Investigation*; 108:407-14

Lasser, K. E.; Allen, P. D.; Woolhandler, S. J.; Himmelstein, D. U.; Wolfe, S. M. & Bohr D. H. (2002). Timing of new black box warnings and withdrawals for prescription medications. *JAMA*; 287(17):2215-20

Leor, J.; Aboulafia-Etzion, S.; Dar, A.; Shapiro, L.; Barbash, I. M.; Battler, A.; Granot, Y. & Cohen, S. (2000). Bioengineered cardiac grafts a new approach to repair the infarcted myocardium? *Circulation*; 102:III56–IIII61

Li, R. K.; Yau, T. M.; Weisel, R. D.; Mickle, D. A.; Sakai, T.; Choi, A. & Jia, Z. Q. (2000). Construction of a bioengineered cardiac graft. *Journal of Thoracic and Cardiovascular Surg*ery;119:368–375

Lo, Y. C.; Yang, S. R.; Huang, M.H.; Liu, Y. C. & Wu, S. N. (2005). Characterization of chromanol 293B-induced block of the delayed-rectifier K+ current in heart-derived H9c2 cells. *Life Sciences*;76:2275-2286

Naito, H.; Melnychenko, I.; Didie, M.; Schneiderbanger, K.; Schubert, P.; Rosenkranz, S.; Eschenhagen, T. & Zimmermann, W. H. (2006). Optimizing engineered heart tissue for therapeutic applications as surrogate heart muscle. *Circulation*; 114:I72–I78

Ott, H.C.; Matthiesen, T. S.; Goh, S. K.; Black, L. D.; Kren, S. M.; Netoff, T. I. & Taylor, D. A. (2008). Perfusion-decellularized matrix: using nature's platform to engineer a bioartificial heart. *Nature Medicine*; 14:213–221

Radisic, M.; Park, H.; Shing, H.; Consi, T.; Schoen, F. J.; Langer, R.; Freed, L. E. & Vunjak-Novakovic, G. (2004). Functional assembly of engineered myocardium by electrical stimulation of cardiac myocytes cultured on scaffolds. *PNAS*; 101:18129–18134

Ray, W. A.; Murray, K. T.; Meredith, S.; Narasimhulu, S. S.; Hall K. & Stein C. M. (2004). Oral erythromycin and the risk of sudden death from cardiac causes. *The New England Journal of Medicine*; 351(11):1089-96

Redfern, W. S.; Carlsson, L.; Davis, A. S.; Lynch, W. G.; MacKenzie I.;Palethorpe, S.; Siegl, P. K.; Strang, I.; Sullivan, A. T.; Wallis, R.; Camm, A. J. & Hammond, T. G. (2003). Relationship between preclinical cardiac electrophysiology, clinical QT interval prolongation and torsade de pointes for a broad range of drugs: evidence for a provisional safety margin in drug development. *Cardiovascular Research*; 58(1):32-45.

Regan, C. P.; Cresswell, H. K.; Zhang, R. & Lynch J. J. (2005). Novel method to assess cardiac electrophysiology in the rat. *Journal of Cardiovascular Pharmacology*; 46(1):68-75.

Shimizu, T.; Yamato, M.; Isoi, Y.; Akutsu, T.; Setomaru, T.; Abe, K.; Kikuchi, A.; Umezu, M. & Okano, T. (2002). Fabrication of pulsatile cardiac tissue grafts using a novel 3-dimensional cell sheet manipulation technique and temperature-responsive cell culture surfaces. *Circulation Research*; 90:e40

Vandenburgh, H.; Shansky, J.; Benesch-Lee, F.; Barbata, V.; Reid, J.; Thorrez, L.; Valentini, R. & Crawford, G. (2008). Drug-screening platform based on the contractility of tissue-engineered muscle. *Muscle Nerve*; 37:438-447

Vaughan-Williams E., M. (1975). Classificationof antidysrhythmic drugs. Pharmacology & therapeutics; 1(1):115-38.

Zhang, J.; Wilson, G. F.; Soerens, A. G.; Koonce, C. H.; Yu, J.; Palecek S. P.; Thomson J. A. & Kamp, T. J. (2009). Functional cardiomyocytes derived from human induced pluripotent stem cells. *Circulation Research*; 104:e30-41

Zimmermann, W. H.; Schneiderbanger, K.; Schubert, P.; Didie, M.; Munzel, F.; Heubach, J. F.; Kostin, S.; Neuhuber, W. L. & Eschenhagen, T. (2002). Tissue engineering of a differentiated cardiac muscle construct. *Circulation Research*; 90:223–230

Zimmermann, W. H.; Melnychenko, I.; Wasmeier, G.; Didié, M.; Naito, H.; Nixdorff, U.; Hess, A.; Budinsky, L.; Brune, K.; Michaelis, B.; Dhein, S.; Schwoerer, A.; Ehmke, H. & Eschenhagen, T. (2006). Engineered heart tissue grafts improve systolic and diastolic function in infarcted rat hearts. *Nature Medicine*; 12:452-8

Zimmermann, W. H. & Eschenhagen, T. (2007). Embryonic stem cells for cardiac muscle engineering. *Trends in Cardiovascular Medicine*; 17:134-40

5

Prediction of Partition Coefficients and Permeability of Drug Molecules in Biological Systems with Abraham Model Solute Descriptors Derived from Measured Solubilities and Water-to-Organic Solvent Partition Coefficients

William E. Acree, Jr.[1], Laura M. Grubbs[1] and Michael H. Abraham[2]
[1]*University of North Texas,*
[2]*University College London,*
[1]*United States*
[2]*United Kingdom*

1. Introduction

Modern drug testing and design includes experimental *in vivo* and *in vitro* measurements, combined with *in silico* computations that enable prediction of the drug candidate's ADMET (adsorption, distribution, metabolism, elimination and toxicity) properties in the early stages of drug discovery. Recent estimates place the discovery and development cost of a small drug molecule close to US $1.3 billion, from the time of inception to the time when the drug finally reaches the market place. Only 20 % of conceived drug candidates proceed to clinical trial stage testing, and of the compounds that enter clinical development less than 10 % receive government approval. Reasons for the low success rate include unsatisfactory efficacy, poor solubility, poor bioavailability, unfavorable pharmacokinetic properties, toxicity concerns and drug-drug interactions, degradation and poor shelf-life stability. Unfavorable pharmacokinetic and ADME properties, toxicity and adverse side effects account for up to two-thirds of drug failures. Traditional ADME analyses relied heavily on whole animal assays and the more labor intensive biochemical studies. High throughput screening methods, fast ADMET profiling assays, and computational approaches have allowed the pharmaceutical industry to identify quickly the less promising drug candidates in the very early development stage so that time and valuable resources are not spent pursuing compounds that have little probability of reaching the general population.

Of the fore-mentioned properties, the drug's aqueous solubility will likely be one of the first properties measured. Aqueous solubility is a major indicator of the drug's solubility in physiological gastrointestinal fluids and is a major indicator of the drug's oral bioavailability. Approximately 40 % of the proposed new pharmaceutical candidates are rejected in the very early stages of drug discovery because of their poor aqueous solubility resulting in bioavailability problems (Lukyanov and Torchilin, 2004; Keck *et al.*, 2008). The number of failures due to poor solubility is likely to increase in future years because the new drug candidates generally have higher molecular weights and more complicated molecular structures than their predecessors. Moreover, drug molecules that are insoluble in water are difficult to study with existing *in vitro* biological assays, often give unreliable biological test results, and may precipitate from solution during storage or upon dilution. The importance of aqueous solubility in drug design is further evidenced by the fact that the editors of one prominent computational journal (Llinàs *et al.*, 2008) challenged readers to develop *in silico* methods to predict the intrinsic solubilities of 32 crystalline drug like molecules in water from an experimental data set of accurately measured solubilities of 100 compounds. Only a few of the more successful approaches were actually published (Wang, *et al.* 2009; Hewitt *et al.*, 2009). Similar challenges have been published regarding the prediction and measurement of the hydration free energies of functionally diverse neutral drug-like molecules (Nicholls *et al.*, 2008; Guthrie, 2009). Aqueous solubility is the reference media to predict the absorption and bioavailability of orally administered drugs. More than 85 % of the drugs sold in the US and in Europe are administered orally.

Amidon and coworkers (1995) proposed a biopharmaceutical classification scheme (BCS) to categories drugs and drug candidates into four groups based on their combined solubility and permeability properties. The classification scheme is depicted in Figure 1a. Drug candidates in Class I exhibit high solubility and high permeability, which is preferred from both a bioavailability and drug delivery standpoint. A drug candidate is considered highly soluble when the highest dose strength is soluble in 250 ml water over a pH range 1 to 7.5. A drug candidate possesses high permeability when the extent of absorption in humans is determined to be 90% of an administered dose, based on the mass balance or in comparison to an intravenous dose. Drug candidates in Class II have low solubility and high permeability, hence, the dissolution rate becomes the governing parameter for bioavailability. These drugs exhibit variable bioavailability and need enhancement in the dissolution rate for improvement in bioavailability. Drug candidates in Class III have high solubility and low permeability. Permeation through the intestinal membrane represents the rate-determining step for Class III drug candidates, with the bioavailability being independent of drug release from the dosage form. Class IV drug candidates possess both low solubility and low permeability. Drugs in this category are generally not suitable for oral drug delivery unless one employs a special drug delivery technology (such as a nano-suspension). Wu and Benet (2005) examined the biopharmaceutical classification scheme as a predictive method for assessing drug disposition. The authors found that drugs in Classes I and II of BCS were metabolized and eliminated. Drugs in the latter two classes were eliminated unchanged from the body by renal and/or biliary elimination. On the basis of these findings the authors suggested the Biopharmaceutics Drug Disposition Classification System (BDDCS) where the extent of metabolism has replaced permeability as a classification criterion (see Figure 2b). Aqueous solubility is an important consideration in both drug classification systems. Adverse drug solubility can sometimes be overcome by structural modifications (e.g., prodrugs) or by adding an organic cosolvent, surfactant, hydrophilic macromolecular and/or an inclusion host compound (such as a modified cyclodextrin) to the drug formulation or application vehicle. Knowledge of the drug's solubility in different organic solvents aids in the selection of an appropriate organic cosolvent and provides valuable information regarding drug's molecular interactions with other organic molecules.

	Solubility	Low Solubility
High Permeability	**Class I** High Solubility High Permeability	**Class II** Low Solubility High Permeability
Low Permeability	**Class III** High Solubility Low Permeability	**Class IV** Low Solubility Low Permeability

a)

	High Solubility	Low Solubility
Extensive Metabolism	**Class I** High solubility Highly Metabolized	**Class II** Low solubility Highly Metabolized
Poor Metabolism	**Class III** High solubility Poorly Metabolized	**Class IV** Low solubility Poorly Metabolized

b)

Fig. 1. Properties used in the Biopharmaceutical Classification Scheme (a) and Biopharmaceutics Drug Disposition Classification System (b)

Lipophilicity is another of the physical properties that is measured in the early stages of drug testing to predict the transport of molecules from the gastrointestinal track into the epithelial cells that line the inner and outer surfaces of the body. Most common drugs cross cellular barriers by transcellular pathways (across epithelial cells) that require the drug to enter the outer portion of the lipid bilayer of the cell membrane. The drug then diffuses to the inner lipid layer and travels across the cell before crossing the cell membrane once again to exit. Lipophilicity was introduced to describe a compound's affinity to be in lipid-like environment. Several solvent systems have been suggested as a surrogate to represent the lipid membrane against water. For convenience and economical reasons, the partition coefficient of the drug candidate between 1-octanol and a series of aqueous buffers has become the standard measure of lipophilicity. The *intrinsic lipophilicity* (logarithm of the water-to-octanol partition coefficient, log $P_{o/w}$) describes the equilibrium distribution of molecular drug candidate (unionized form of the molecule) between water and the aqueous buffer, and is independent of pH. The *effective lipophilicity* (logarithm of the water-to-octanol distribution coefficient) reflects the concentration ratio of the neutral drug molecule plus all ionized forms that may be present in the aqueous buffered solution at the given pH. The effective lipophilicity is often quoted at the physiological pH of 7.4. The intrinsic and effective lipophilicities are equivalent if the drug candidate contains no ionizable or protonatable functional groups. Experimental techniques employed to measure water-to-octanol partition coefficients include the traditional shake-flask method, as well as several methods based on reversed-phase liquid chromatography (hplc), counter-current chromatography and centrifugal partition chromatography (Sangster, 1989; Berthod *et al.*, 1992; Menges *et al.*, 1990; Berthod *et al.*, 1988; McDuffie, 1981; Veith *et al.*, 1979). Ribeiro and coworkers (2010) recently discussed the advantages and limitations associated with using the water-to-octanol partitioning system as a surrogate for biological membranes. The authors noted that there is a considerable difference between the homogeneous macroscopic 1-octanol solvent system and the highly-ordered microscopic structure of a lipid layer. Chromatographic retention data determined using an immobilized artificial membrane (IAM) stationary phase was suggested as a more appropriate method for measuring the lipophilicity of drug candidates and for quantifying drug-membrane interactions.

Solubility and water-to-organic solvent partition coefficients are fairly easy to measure as the equilibrated solutions contain only the dissolved drug candidate and the solubilizing solvent media. Blood-to-tissue partition coefficients, plasma-to-milk partition coefficient, percentage of human intestinal absorption and the steady-state volume of distribution are much harder to measure. The analytical methodology employed to measure these latter properties must be able to distinguish and quantify the drug from all of the many other molecules present in the biological sample. It is not easy, even with today's modern instrumentation, to design chemical analysis methods that are specific to a given molecule. Moreover, measurements involving human and/or animal tissues are expensive and are subject to larger experimental uncertainties. Replicate studies involving the same animal species have shown that the measured values can depend on gender, age and eating habits. This chapter will discuss the prediction of the blood-to-tissue partition coefficients, plasma-to-milk partition coefficients, human intestinal absorption based on the Abraham solvation parameter model and solute descriptors calculated from measured solubilities and partition coefficients.

2. Abraham solvation parameter model

The Abraham general solvation model is one of the more useful approaches for the analysis and prediction of the adsorption, distribution and toxicological properties of potential drug candidates. The method relies on two linear free energy relationships (lfers), one for transfer processes occurring within condensed phases (Abraham, 1993a,b; Abraham *et al.*, 2004):

$$SP = c + e \cdot \mathbf{E} + s \cdot \mathbf{S} + a \cdot \mathbf{A} + b \cdot \mathbf{B} + v \cdot \mathbf{V} \tag{1}$$

and one for processes involving gas-to-condensed phase transfer

$$SP = c + e \cdot \mathbf{E} + s \cdot \mathbf{S} + a \cdot \mathbf{A} + b \cdot \mathbf{B} + l \cdot \mathbf{L} \tag{2}$$

The dependent variable, SP, is some property of a series of solutes in a fixed phase, which in the present study will include the logarithm of drug's water-to-organic solvent and blood-to-tissue partition coefficients, the logarithm of the drug's molar solubility in an organic solvent divided by its aqueous molar solubility, the logarithm of the drug's plasma-to-milk partition coefficient, percent human intestinal absorption and the logarithm of the kinetic constant for human intestinal absorption, and the logarithm of the human skin permeability coefficient. The independent variables, or descriptors, are solute properties as follows: **E** and **S** refer to the excess molar refraction and dipolarity/polarizability descriptors of the solute, respectively, **A** and **B** are measures of the solute hydrogen-bond acidity and basicity, **V** is the McGowan volume of the solute and **L** is the logarithm of the solute gas phase dimensionless Ostwald partition coefficient into hexadecane at 298 K. The first four descriptors can be regarded as measures of the tendency of the given solute to undergo various solute-solvent interactions. The latter two descriptors, **V** and **L**, are both measures of solute size, and so will be measures of the solvent cavity term that will accommodate the dissolved solute. General dispersion interactions are also related to solute size, hence, both **V** and **L** will also describe the general solute-solvent interactions. Solute descriptors are available for more than 4,000 organic, organometallic and inorganic solutes. No single article lists all of the numerical values; however, a large compilation is available in one published review article (Abraham *et al.*, 1993a), and in the supporting material that has accompanied several of our published papers (Abraham *et al.*, 2006a; Abraham *et al.*, 2009a; Mintz *et al.*, 2007). Solute descriptors can be obtained by regression analysis using various types of experimental data, including water-to-solvent partitions, gas-to-solvent partitions, solubility data and chromatographic retention data as discussed below and elsewhere (Abraham *et al.*, 2010; Zissimos *et al.*, 2002a,b). For a number of partitions into solvents that contain large amounts of water at saturation, an alternative hydrogen bond basicity parameter, $\mathbf{B^o}$, is used for specific classes of solute: alkylpyridines, alkylanilines, and sulfoxides.

Equations 1 and 2 contain the following three quantities: (a) measured solute properties; (b) calculated solute descriptors; and (c) calculated equation coefficients. Knowledge of any two quantities permits calculation of the third quantity through the solving of simultaneous equations and regression analysis. Solute descriptors are calculated from measured partition coefficient ($P_{solute,system}$), chromatographic retention factor (k′) and molar solubility ($C_{solute,solvent}$) data for the solutes dissolved in partitioning systems and in organic solvents having known equation coefficients. Generally partition coefficient, chromatographic retention factor and molar solubility measurements are fairly accurate, and it is good practice to base the solute descriptor computations on observed values having minimal experimental uncertainty. The computation is depicted graphically in Figure 1 by the unidirectional arrows that indicate the direction of the calculation using the known equation coefficients that connect the measured and solute descriptors. Measured $P_{solute,system}$ and $C_{solute,solvent}$ values yield solute descriptors. The unidirectional red arrows originating from the center solute descriptor circle represent the equation coefficients that have been reported for blood-to-brain partition coefficient, blood-to-tissue partition coefficients, percentage of human intenstinal absorption, Draize eye scores, and aquatic toxicity Abraham model linear free energy relationships. Plasma-to-milk partition ratio predictions are achieved (Abraham *et al.*, 2009b) through an artificial neural network with five inputs, 14 nodes in the hidden layer and one node in the output layer. Linear analysis of the plasma-to-milk partition ratios for 179 drugs and hydrophobic environmental pollutants revealed that drug molecules preferentially partition into the aqueous and protein phases of milk. Hydrophobic environmental pollutants, on the other hand, partition into the fat phase. Prediction of the fore-mentioned ADMET and biological properties does require a prior knowledge of the Abraham solute descriptors for the drug candidate of interest. There are also commercial software packages (ADME Boxes, 2010) and several published estimation schemes (Mutelet and Rogalski, 2001; Arey *et al.*, 2005; Platts *et al.*, 1999; Abraham and McGowan, 1987) for calculating the numerical values of solute descriptors from molecular structural information if one is unable to find the necessary partition, chromatographic and/or solubility data. For any fully characterized system/process (those with calculated values for the equation coefficients) further values of SP can be estimated for solutes with known values for the solute descriptors.

The usefulness of Eqns. 1 and 2 in the characterization of solvent phases is that the coefficients *e, s, a, b, l* and *v* are not just curve-fitting constants. The coefficients reflect particular solute-solvent interactions that correspond to chemical properties of the solvent phase. The excess molar refraction, **E**, is defined from the solute refractive index, and hence the *e* coefficient gives a measure of general solute-solvent dispersion interactions. The **V** and **L** descriptors were set up as measures of the endoergic effect of disrupting solvent-solvent bonds. However, solute volume is always well correlated with polarizability and so the *v* and *l* coefficients will include not only an endoergic cavity effect but also exoergic solute-solvent effects that arise through solute polarizability. The **S** descriptor is a measure of dipolarity and polarizability and hence the *s* coefficient will reflect the ability of a solvent to undergo dipole-dipole and dipole-induced dipole interactions with the solute. The **A** descriptor is a measure of solute hydrogen bond acidity, and hence the *a* coefficient will reflect the complementary solvent hydrogen bond basicity. Similarly the *b* coefficient will be a measure of solvent hydrogen bond acidity. All this is straightforward for gas-to-solvent partitions because there are no interactions to consider in the gas phase. For partition between solvents, the coefficients in Eqn. 1 then refer to differences between the properties of the two phases.

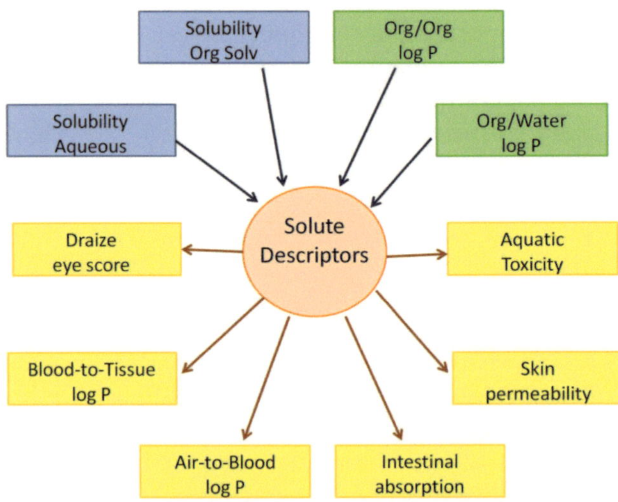

Fig. 2. Outline illustrating the calculation of Abraham model solute descriptors from experimental partition coefficient and solubility data, and then using the calculated values to estimate biological activities and partitioning, such as blood-to-tissue partition coefficients, Draize eye scores, aquatic toxicities and air-to-blood partition coefficients.

The Abraham model equation coefficients encode chemical information, and several methods have been suggested to assess the chemical similarity between different partitioning processes/systems. Abraham and Martins (2004) calculated the five-dimensional distance between the coefficients as points in five-dimensional space by straightforward geometry

$$\text{Distance} = \sqrt{(e_i - e_j)^2 + (s_i - s_j)^2 + (a_i - a_j)^2 + (b_i - b_j)^2 + (v_i - v_j)^2} \quad (3)$$

where the subscripts "i" and "j" denote the two partitioning processes being compared. For comparison purposes, the authors suggested that for a good chemical model the calculated distance should be less than about 0.5 - 0.8. The water-to-isobutanol and water-to-octanol partitioning systems were the two chemical systems that the authors found closest to human skin permeability, with calculated distances of 1.2 and 1.9, respectively. The chemical interactions that govern skin permeability were quite different from the chemical interactions governing solute partitioning between water and isobutanol, and between water and 1-octanol. Ishiharma and Asakawa (1999) suggested a different comparison method based on calculating the cosine of the angle (cos θij) between the coefficients

$$Cos\ \Theta_{ij} = \frac{e_i e_j + s_i s_j + a_i a_j + b_i b_j + v_i v_j}{\sqrt{e_i^2 + s_i^2 + a_i^2 + b_i^2 + v_i^2}\ \sqrt{e_j^2 + s_j^2 + a_j^2 + b_j^2 + v_j^2}} \tag{4}$$

which are now regarded as lines in five-dimensional space. The angle between the two lines, θ_{ij}, yields information regarding how the two compared processes are in terms of their chemical similarity. As θ_{ij} approaches zero (or alternatively as cos θ_{ij} approaches unity) the two lines coincide, and the correlation between the two partitioning processes/systems approaches unity. Analysis of the Abraham model coefficients for the solubility of gases and vapors in biological phases (blood, brain, fat, heart, kidney, liver, lung and muscle) and organic solvents (alcohols, amides, olive oil, chloroform, diethyl ether, butanone), and equation coefficients for biological activity (nasal pungency thresholds, eye irritation thresholds, odor detection and anesthesia) using Eqns. 3 and 4 (along with Principal Component Analysis) found N-methylformamide to be an excellent model for both eye irritation thresholds in humans and nasal pungency thresholds in humans (Abraham *et al.*, 2009a). The receptor site controlling both biological responses must be protein-like in character. The study further showed that no organic solvent is a suitable model (or surrogate) for blood, brain, heart, kidney, liver, lung and muscle. Two relatively nonpolar solvents (olive oil and chloroform) were found to be suitable models for fat, which is not too surprising given that fat is about 80 % lipid.

3. Experimental methods for measuring thermodynamic and kinetic solubilities

Recent advances in automated chemical synthesis and combinatorial chemistry have generated large numbers of new chemical compounds that need to be screened for possible biological activity and desired ADMET properties. The conventional experimental methods that were once used in the pharmaceutical industry to measure solubility and water-to-organic solvent partition coefficients are inadequate to handle large numbers of new compound because of low throughput capacity and the amount of compound required for the experimental determination. Large quantities of highly purified compounds are not usually available in the initial stages of drug discovery and drug testing. To meet the demands imposed by the increased compound numbers, the pharmaceutical industry has developed miniaturized and automated sample preparation platforms, combined with rapid chemical analysis methods based on nephelometric, uv/visible absorption and/or chromatographic measurements. The experimental protocol used depends on whether one needs to measure the kinetic or thermodynamic solubility.

High throughput kinetic aqueous solubility assays are based on the detection of precipitation of compounds in aqueous or aqueous buffered solutions. Typically, small known aliquots of the stock solution are added incrementally to the aqueous (or aqueous buffered solution) at predetermined time intervals until the solubility limit is reached. The resulting precipitation can be detected optically by nephlometric or laser monitoring methods, and the kinetic solubility is defined as the solute concentration immediately preceding the point at which precipitation was first detected. Kinetic solubility thus represents the maximum solubility of the fastest precipitation species of the given compound into the desired solubilizing solvent media. Numerous modifications of kinetic assays have been suggested in recent years. The suggested modifications differ in the dilution and detection method. For example, Lipinski *et al.* (2001) added small aliquots of a stock solution of the drug (dissolved in dimethyl sulfoxide, DMSO) to the aqueous solvent media every minute until precipitation occurred. The DMSO in solution did increase with each added aliquot and may result in a higher measured aqueous solubility. Dimethyl sulfoxide is known to increase the solubility by helping to solvate the more lipophilic drug compounds. Solubility enhancement by dimethyl sulfoxide can be reduced if the samples are first serially diluted in dimethyl sulfoxide before the aliquots are added to the aqueous solvent system. Special 96-well plates have been designed to facilitate high throughput solubility measurements. The method depicted in Figure 3 allows one to quickly measure the aqueous solubility and aqueous-buffered solubility of 12 different drug candidates. The eight DMSO-diluted concentrations (1 mM to 100 mM) of each drug candidate are placed in the specified well of the drug's respective column. In the 12 x 9 cell matrix, the drug is identified by column number and the concentration is identified by row number. A predetermined aliquot volume from each of the DMSO diluted sample wells is transferred to the corresponding cell in the aqueous plate and aqueous-buffered plate. The volume of DMSO-diluted sample is the same for each transferred aliquot. Each cell in the aqueous plate and aqueous-buffered plate contains an identical volume of solvent. The cell contents are examined for precipitation immediately after the passage of the defined time interview, or alternatively, one can remove the solid and determine the concentration of dissolved drug by standard spectroscopic and/or chromatographic methods.

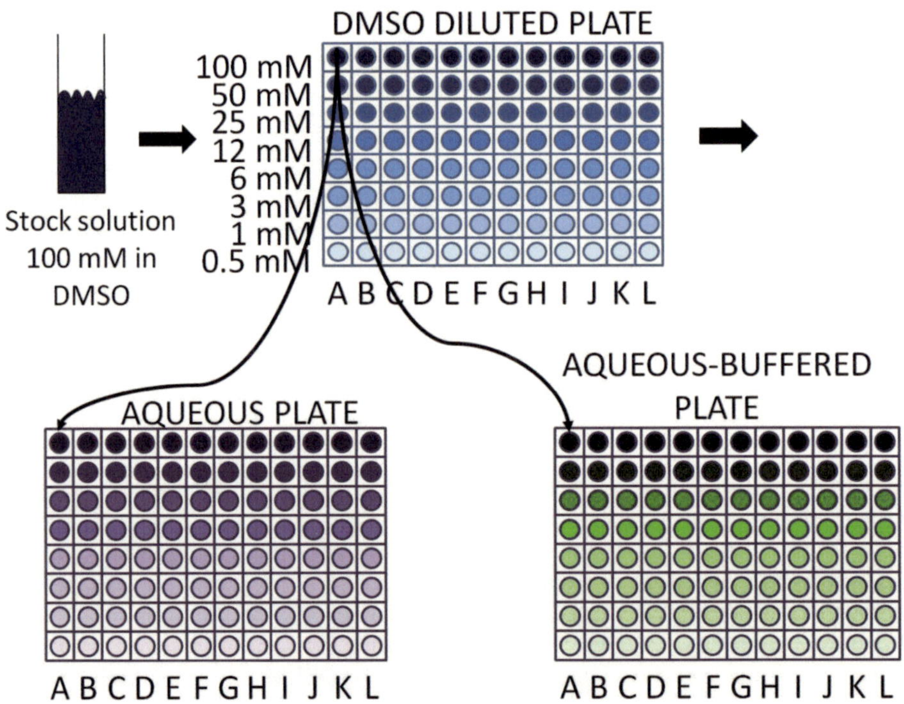

Fig. 3. Outline of a high throughput method for measuring drug solubility in water and in an aqueous-buffered solution using a 96-well plate.

Kinetic methods often overestimate the thermodynamic drug solubility because of the increased solubilization effect caused by the presence of dimethyl sulfoxide in the aqueous solvent and by the fact that one has not allowed sufficient time for equilibrium to be achieved. Thermodynamic solubility is defined as the concentration in solution of a compound in equilibrium with an excess of solid material being present in solution at the conclusion of the dissolution process. Thermodynamic solubility is considered the "true" solubility of a compound. Experimental methods for determining thermodynamic solubility may be grouped into categories, one that extends the experimental protocols of exiting kinetic solubility determinations to longer "equilibration times" and the other that conducts solubility studies on solid compounds obtained from dried stock solutions to remove the enhancement effects caused by having the added dimethyl sulfoxide present in the final equilibrated solution. The rationale behind the longer equilibration times is that sufficient time will now be afforded for the first-precipitated crystalline phase to convert to the more thermodynamically stable crystalline phase. Sugano and coworkers (2006) reported a significant decrease in solubility with equilibration time for more than half of the 26 model compounds studied.

The preceding discussion focused on aqueous kinetic and thermodynamic solubility measurements. There is no reason that the basic high throughput experimental methodologies cannot be applied to organic solvents and to aqueous-organic solvent mixtures. Measured drug solubility in organic solvents, in combination with the Abraham general solvation model, provides valuable information in regarding the molecule's hydrogen-bonding character and dipolarity. Solubility ratios are substituted into Eqns. 1 and 2 to give the following mathematical correlations:

$$\log\left(C_{A,organic} / C_{A,water}\right) = c + e\cdot\mathbf{E} + s\cdot\mathbf{S} + a\cdot\mathbf{A} + b\cdot\mathbf{B} + v\cdot\mathbf{V} \quad (5)$$

$$\log\left(C_{A,organic} / C_{A,gas}\right) = c + e\cdot\mathbf{E} + s\cdot\mathbf{S} + a\cdot\mathbf{A} + b\cdot\mathbf{B} + l\cdot\mathbf{L} \quad (6)$$

where $C_{A,organic}$ and $C_{A,water}$ denote the molar solubility of the solute (component A) in the anhydrous "dry" organic solvent and in water, respectively, and $C_{A,gas}$ is the molar gas phase concentration of the solute above the crystalline phase at the system temperature. This later quantity is calculable as $C_{A,gas} = P_A{}^o\, V/RT$, from the solute's vapor pressure above the crystalline phase, $P_A{}^o$.

The solubility ratio in Eqn. 5 represents a hypothetical partitioning process for transferring the solute from water to the anhydrous organic solvent as depicted in Figure 4. Also depicted in Figure 4 are the gas-to-water and gas-to-organic solvent partitioning processes, along with their respective concentration ratios. The hypothetical water-to-organic solvent partitioning process should not be confused with the direct practical organic solvent/water partitioning system that corresponds to the equilibrium solute partitioning between a water-saturated organic phase and an aqueous phase saturated with the organic solvent. For solvents that are partially miscible with water, such as 1-butanol and ethyl acetate, partition coefficients calculated as the ratio of the molar solute solubilities in the organic solvent and water are not the same as those obtained from direct partition between water (saturated with the organic solvent) and organic solvent (saturated with water). Solubility ratios and practical partition coefficients, however, are nearly identical for solvents like linear alkanes, cycloalkanes, chloroform, carbon tetrachloride and dichloromethane, which are almost "completely" immiscible with water. Tables 1 and 2 give the equation coefficients for the Abraham model solubility ratio correlations (Eqns. 5 and 6) for the different organic solvents that have been reported to date.

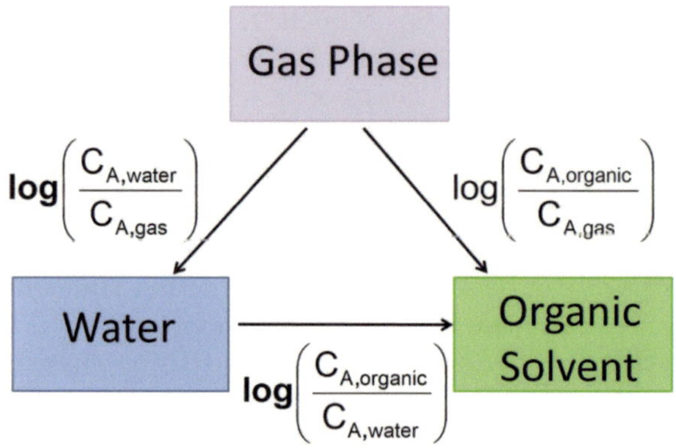

Fig. 4. Solubility ratios describing the various solute transfer processes.

Dry Solvent	c	e	s	a	b	v
Olely alcohol	-0.096	0.148	-0.841	-0.438	-4.040	4.125
Dichloromethane	0.319	0.102	-0.187	-3.058	-4.090	4.324
Trichloromethane	0.191	0.105	-0.403	-3.112	-3.514	4.395
Tetrachloromethane	0.199	0.523	-1.159	-3.560	-4.594	4.618
1,2-Dichloroethane	0.183	0.294	-0.134	-2.801	-4.291	4.180
1-Chlorobutane	0.222	0.273	-0.569	-2.918	-4.883	4.456
Butane	0.297	-0.005	-1.584	-3.188	-4.567	4.562
Pentane	0.369	0.386	-1.568	-3.535	-5.215	4.514
Hexane	0.361	0.579	-1.723	-3.599	-4.764	4.344
Heptane	0.325	0.670	-2.061	-3.317	-4.733	4.543
Octane	0.223	0.642	-1.647	-3.480	-5.067	4.526
Nonane	0.240	0.619	-1.713	-3.532	-4.921	4.482
Decane	0.160	0.585	-1.734	-3.435	-5.078	4.582
Undecane	0.058	0.603	-1.661	-3.421	-5.120	4.619
Dodecane	0.114	0.668	-1.664	-3.545	-5.006	4.459
Hexadecane	0.087	0.667	-1.617	-3.587	-4.869	4.433
Cyclohexane	0.159	0.784	-1.678	-3.740	-4.929	4.577
Methylcyclohexane	0.246	0.782	-1.982	-3.517	-4.293	4.528
Isooctane	0.318	0.555	-1.737	-3.677	-4.864	4.417
Benzene	0.142	0.464	-0.588	-3.099	-4.625	4.491
Toluene	0.143	0.527	-0.720	-3.010	-4.824	4.545
Fluorobenzene	0.139	0.152	-0.374	-3.030	-4.601	4.540
Chlorobenzene	0.065	0.381	-0.521	-3.183	-4.700	4.614
Bromobenzene	-0.017	0.436	-0.424	-3.174	-4.558	4.445
Iodobenzene	-0.192	0.298	-0.308	-3.213	-4.653	4.588
Nitrobenzene	-0.152	0.525	0.081	-2.332	-4.494	4.187
Benzonitrile	0.155	0.337	-0.036	-1.544	-4.614	3.990
Olive oil	-0.035	0.574	-0.798	-1.422	-4.984	4.210
Carbon disulfide	0.047	0.686	-0.943	-3.603	-5.818	4.921
Isopropyl myristate	-0.605	0.930	-1.153	-1.682	-4.093	4.249
Triolein	0.385	0.983	-2.083	-2.007	-3.452	4.072

Dry Solvent	c	e	s	a	b	v
Methanol	0.276	0.334	-0.714	0.243	-3.320	3.549
Ethanol	0.222	0.471	-1.035	0.326	-3.596	3.857
Propan-1-ol	0.139	0.405	-1.029	0.247	-3.767	3.986
Butan-1-ol	0.165	0.401	-1.011	0.056	-3.958	4.044
Pentan-1-ol	0.150	0.536	-1.229	0.141	-3.864	4.077
Hexan-1-ol	0.115	0.492	-1.164	0.054	-3.978	4.131
Heptan-1-ol	0.035	0.398	-1.063	0.002	-4.343	4.317
Octan-1-ol	-0.034	0.489	-1.044	-0.024	-4.235	4.218
Decan-1-ol	-0.058	0.616	-1.319	0.026	-4.153	4.279
Propan-2-ol	0.099	0.343	-1.049	0.406	-3.827	4.033
Isobutanol	0.127	0.253	-0.976	0.158	-3.882	4.114
sec-Butanol	0.188	0.354	-1.127	0.016	-3.568	3.968
tert-Butanol	0.211	0.171	-0.947	0.331	-4.085	4.109
3-Methyl-1-butanol	0.073	0.360	-1.273	0.090	-3.770	4.273
Pentan-2-ol	0.115	0.455	-1.331	0.206	-3.745	4.201
Ethylene glycol	-0.270	0.578	-0.511	0.715	-2.619	2.729
2,2,2 -Trifluoroethanol	0.395	-0.094	-0.594	-1.280	-1.274	3.088
Diethyl ether	0.350	0.358	-0.820	-0.588	-4.956	4.350
Tetrahydrofuran	0.207	0.372	-0.392	-0.236	-4.934	4.447
1,4-Dioxane	0.098	0.350	-0.083	-0.556	-4.826	4.172
Dibutyl ether	0.176	0.394	-0.985	-1.414	-5.357	4.524
Methyl *tert*-butyl ether	0.341	0.307	-0.817	-0.618	-5.097	4.425
Methyl acetate	0.351	0.223	-0.150	-1.035	-4.527	3.972
Ethyl acetate	0.328	0.369	-0.446	-0.700	-4.904	4.150
Butyl acetate	0.248	0.356	-0.501	-0.867	-4.973	4.281
Propanone	0.313	0.312	-0.121	-0.608	-4.753	3.942
Butanone	0.246	0.256	-0.080	-0.767	-4.855	4.148
Cyclohexanone	0.038	0.225	0.058	-0.976	-4.842	4.315
Dimethylformamide	-0.305	-0.058	0.343	0.358	-4.865	4.486
Dimethylacetamide	-0.271	0.084	0.209	0.915	-5.003	4.557
Diethylacetamide	0.213	0.034	0.089	1.342	-5.084	4.088
Dibutylformamide	0.332	0.302	-0.436	0.358	-4.902	3.952
N-Methylpyrolidinone	0.147	0.532	0.225	0.840	-4.794	3.674
N-Methyl-2-piperidone	0.056	0.332	0.257	1.556	-5.035	3.983
N-Formylmorpholine	-0.032	0.696	-0.062	0.014	-4.092	3.405
N-Methylformamide	0.114	0.407	-0.287	0.542	-4.085	3.471
N-Ethylformamide	0.220	0.034	-0.166	0.935	-4.589	3.730
N-Methylacetamide	0.090	0.205	-0.172	1.305	-4.589	3.833
N-Ethylacetamide	0.284	0.128	-0.442	1.180	-4.728	3.856
Formamide	-0.171	0.070	0.308	0.589	-3.152	2.432
Acetonitrile	0.413	0.077	0.326	-1.566	4.391	3.364
Nitromethane	0.023	-0.091	0.793	-1.463	-4.364	3.460
Dimethylsulfoxide	-0.194	0.327	0.791	-1.260	-4.540	3.361
Tributylphosphate	0.327	0.570	-0.837	-1.069	-4.333	3.919

Dry Solvent	c	e	s	a	b	v
Propylene carbonate	0.004	0.168	0.504	-1.283	-4.407	3.421
Gas-water	-0.994	0.577	2.549	3.813	4.841	-0.869

Table 1. Coefficients in Eqn. 5 for Correlating Solute Solubility in Dry Organic Solvents at 298 K

Dry Solvent	c	e	s	a	b	l
Olely alcohol	-0.268	-0.392	0.800	3.117	0.978	0.918
Dichloromethane	0.192	-0.572	1.492	0.460	0.847	0.965
Trichloromethane	0.157	-0.560	1.259	0.374	1.333	0.976
Tetrachloromethane	0.217	-0.435	0.554	0.000	0.000	1.069
1,2-Dichloroethane	0.017	-0.337	1.600	0.774	0.637	0.921
1-Chlorobutane	0.130	-0.581	1.114	0.724	0.000	1.016
Butane	0.291	-0.360	0.091	0.000	0.000	0.959
Pentane	0.335	-0.276	0.000	0.000	0.000	0.968
Hexane	0.292	-0.169	0.000	0.000	0.000	0.979
Heptane	0.275	-0.162	0.000	0.000	0.000	0.983
Octane	0.215	-0.049	0.000	0.000	0.000	0.967
Nonane	0.200	-0.145	0.000	0.000	0.000	0.980
Decane	0.156	-0.143	0.000	0.000	0.000	0.989
Undecane	0.113	0.000	0.000	0.000	0.000	0.971
Dodecane	0.053	0.000	0.000	0.000	0.000	0.986
Hexadecane	0.000	0.000	0.000	0.000	0.000	1.000
Cyclohexane	0.163	-0.110	0.000	0.000	0.000	1.013
Methylcyclohexane	0.319	-0.215	0.000	0.000	0.000	1.012
Isooctane	0.264	-0.230	0.000	0.000	0.000	0.975
Benzene	0.107	-0.313	1.053	0.457	0.169	1.020
Toluene	0.121	-0.222	0.938	0.467	0.099	1.012
Fluorobenzene	0.181	-0.621	1.432	0.647	0.000	0.986
Chlorobenzene	0.064	-0.399	1.151	0.313	0.171	1.032
Bromobenzene	-0.064	-0.326	1.261	0.323	0.292	1.002
Iodobenzene	-0.171	-0.192	1.197	0.245	0.245	1.002
Nitrobenzene	-0.275	0.001	1.861	1.119	0.000	0.925
Benzonitrile	-0.062	-0.402	1.939	2.007	0.000	0.880
Olive oil	-0.159	-0.277	0.904	1.695	-0.090	0.876
Carbon disulfide	0.101	0.251	0.177	0.027	0.095	1.068
Triolein	0.147	0.254	-0.246	1.520	1.473	0.918
Methanol	-0.039	-0.338	1.317	3.836	1.396	0.773
Ethanol	0.017	-0.232	0.867	3.894	1.192	0.846
Propan-1-ol	-0.042	-0.246	0.749	3.888	1.078	0.874
Butan-1-ol	-0.004	-0.285	0.768	3.705	0.879	0.890
Pentan-1-ol	-0.002	-0.161	0.535	3.778	0.960	0.900
Hexan-1-ol	-0.014	-0.205	0.583	3.621	0.891	0.913

Dry Solvent	c	e	s	a	b	l
Heptan-1-ol	-0.056	-0.216	0.554	3.596	0.803	0.933
Octan-1-ol	-0.147	-0.214	0.561	3.507	0.749	0.943
Decan-1-ol	-0.139	-0.090	0.356	3.547	0.727	0.958
Propan-2-ol	-0.048	-0.324	0.713	4.036	1.055	0.884
Isobutanol	-0.034	-0.387	0.719	3.736	1.088	0.905
sec-Butanol	-0.003	-0.357	0.699	3.595	1.247	0.881
tert-Butanol	0.053	-0.443	0.699	4.026	0.882	0.907
3-Methyl-1-butanol	-0.052	-0.430	0.628	3.661	0.932	0.937
Pentan-2-ol	-0.031	-0.325	0.496	3.792	1.024	0.934
Ethylene glycol	-0.887	0.132	1.657	4.457	2.355	0.565
2,2,2-Trifluoroethanol	-0.092	-0.547	1.339	2.213	3.807	0.645
Diethyl ether	0.288	-0.379	0.904	2.937	0.000	0.963
Tetrahydrofuran	0.189	-0.347	1.238	3.289	0.000	0.982
1,4-Dioxane	-0.034	-0.354	1.674	3.021	0.000	0.919
Dibutyl ether	0.153	-0.406	0.758	2.152	-0.610	1.008
Methyl *tert*-butyl ether	0.231	-0.536	0.890	2.623	0.000	0.999
Methyl acetate	0.129	-0.447	1.675	2.625	0.213	0.874
Ethyl acetate	0.182	-0.352	1.316	2.891	0.000	0.916
Butyl acetate	0.147	-0.414	1.212	2.623	0.000	0.954
Propanone	0.127	-0.387	1.733	3.060	0.000	0.866
Butanone	0.112	-0.474	1.671	2.878	0.000	0.916
Cyclohexanone	-0.086	-0.441	1.725	2.786	0.000	0.957
Dimethylformamide	-0.391	-0.869	2.107	3.774	0.000	1.011
Dimethylacetamide	-0.308	-0.736	1.802	4.361	0.000	1.028
Diethylacetamide	-0.075	-0.434	1.911	4.801	0.000	0.899
Dibutylformamide	-0.002	-0.239	1.402	4.029	0.000	0.900
N-Methylpyrolidinone	-0.128	-0.029	2.217	4.429	0.000	0.777
N-Methyl-2-piperidone	-0.264	-0.171	2.086	5.056	0.000	0.883
N-Formylmorpholine	-0.437	0.024	2.631	4.318	0.000	0.712
N-Methylformamide	-0.249	-0.142	1.661	4.147	0.817	0.739
N-Ethylformamide	-0.220	-0.302	1.743	4.498	0.480	0.824
N-Methylacetamide	-0.197	-0.175	1.608	4.867	0.375	0.837
N-Ethylacetamide	-0.018	-0.157	1.352	4.588	0.357	0.824
Formamide	-0.800	0.310	2.292	4.130	1.933	0.442
Acetonitrile	-0.007	-0.595	2.461	2.085	0.418	0.934
Nitromethane	-0.340	-0.297	2.689	2.193	0.514	0.728
Dimethylsulfoxide	-0.556	-0.223	2.903	5.036	0.000	0.719
Tributylphosphate	0.097	-0.098	1.103	2.411	0.588	0.844
Propylene carbonate	-0.356	-0.413	2.587	2.207	0.455	0.719
Gas-water	-1.271	0.822	2.743	3.904	4.814	-0.213

Table 2. Coefficients in Eqn. 6 for Correlating Solute Solubility in Dry Organic Solvents at 298 K

Three specific conditions must be met in order to use the Abraham solvation parameter model to predict saturation solubilities. First, the same solid phase must be in equilibrium with the saturation solutions in the organic solvent and in water (i.e., there should be no solvate or hydrate formation). Second, the secondary medium activity coefficient of the solid in the saturated solutions must be unity (or near unity). This condition generally restricts the method to those solutes that are sparingly soluble in water and nonaqueous solvents. Finally, for solutes that are ionized in aqueous solution, $C_{A,water}$, refers to the solubility of the neutral form. The second restriction may not be as important as initially believed. The Abraham solvation parameter model has shown remarkable success in correlating the solubility of several very soluble crystalline solutes. For example, Eqns 5 and 6 described the molar solubility of benzil in 24 organic solvents to within overall standard deviations of 0.124 and 0.109 log units, respectively. Standard deviations for acetylsalicylic acid dissolved in 13 alcohols, 4 ethers and ethyl acetate were 0.123 and 0.138 log units. Benzil (Acree and Abraham, 2002) and acetylsalicylic acid (Charlton *et al.*, 2003) exhibited solubilities exceeding 1Molar in several of the organic solvents studied. In the case of acetylsalicylic acid it could be argued that the model's success relates back to when the equation coefficients were originally calculated for the dry solvents. The databases used in the regression analyses contained very few carboxylic acid solutes (benzoic acid, 2-hydroxybenzoic acid and 4-hydroxybenzoic acid). Most of the experimental data for carboxylic acids and other very acidic solutes was in the form of saturation solubilities, which were also in the 1 to 3 Molar range. Such arguments do not explain why equations (5) and (6) described the measured benzil solubility data. The benzil solubilities were measured after most of the equation coefficients were first determined.

4. High throughput experimental methods for measuring water-to-octanol partition coefficients

Each administered drug has to pass several membrane barriers in order to be delivered to the desired target site for therapeutic action. Orally administered drugs have to be absorbed into the intestine. Transdermally administered drugs need to penetrate human skin. Drugs intended to act in the central nervous system must cross the blood-brain brain barrier (BBB). This barrier is formed by the endothelial cells of the cerebral capillaries and restricts the transport of many compounds into the brain from the blood stream. The cellular architecture of the human intestine, human skin and human brain are quite different; however, the principle of transcellular absorption is the same. The dissolved drug must be transferred from an aqueous environment into the membrane phase, must diffuse across the membrane, and afterwards must partition back into an aqueous-phase compartment. The water-to-octanol partition coefficient, $P_{o/w}$, is widely regarded in the pharmaceutical industry as a quantitative measure for assessing a drug molecule's affinity for the membrane phase. Considerable attention has been afforded to developing high throughput experimental methodologies that either directly measure $P_{o/w}$ values, or that enable accurate estimation of $P_{o/w}$ from other conveniently measured properties. Poole and Poole (2003) reviewed the direct and indirect separation for obtaining water-to-octanol partition coefficients, with emphasis on the high throughput methods.

As selected examples of experimental methods that have been developed in recent years, Faller and coworkers (2005) designed a rather novel high throughput method to measure lipophilicity based on the diffusion of organic compounds between to aqueous phase compartments separated by a thin 1-octanol liquid layer coated on a polycarbonate filter. The apparatus is shown in Figure 5. The molar concentration of the compound in the aqueous acceptor compartment, $C_{acceptor,end}$ is measured at the end of the defined time endpoint, tend. The apparent membrane permeability, P_{app}, is calculated from $C_{acceptor,end}$ by

$$P_{app} = -\left(\frac{V_{acceptor}V_{donor}}{V_{acceptor}+V_{donor}}\right)\left(\frac{1}{A\,t_{end}}\right)\ln\left(1-\frac{C_{acceptor,end}}{C_{equ}}\right) \quad (7)$$

$$C_{equ} = \left(\frac{V_{donor}}{V_{donor}+V_{acceptor}}\right) C_{donor,initial} \quad (8)$$

where $V_{acceptor}$ and V_{donor} denote the aqueous phase volumes in the acceptor and donor compartments, respectively, $C_{donor,initial}$ refers to the initial compound concentration in the donor phase, and A is the membrane accessible surface area times porosity. The water-to-octanol partition coefficient, $P_{o/w}$, is derived from the measured apparent permeability using a calibration curve constructed from measured permeabilities of standard compounds of known $P_{o/w}$ values. The assay has been used to measure water-to-hexadecane partition coefficients (Wohnsland and Faller, 2001) and can be performed using 96-well microtiter plates.

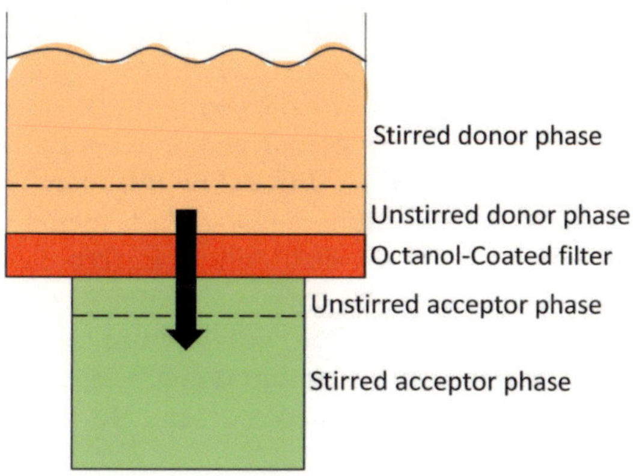

Fig. 5. High throughput experimental method for measuring water-to- octanol partition coefficients based on the diffusion of a solute betweentwo aqueous phase compartments.

Gao *et al.* (2005) developed a miniaturized method involving the dispersion of colloidal stable porous silica-encapsulated magnetic nanoparticles into water and/or an aqueous-buffered solution. Prior to dispersion, the nanoparticles are preloaded with a known amount of 1-octanol. Equilibrium is quickly established between the drug dissolved in the aqueous (or aqueous-buffered) solution and the small octanol droplets on the nanoparticles. The paramagnetic properties of the nanoparticles facilitate magnetic-induced phase separation. Once the magnetic particles are removed, the uv/visible absorbance of the solution is recorded. The log $P_{o/w}$ (or log Do/w in the case of an ionic solute) is calculated as

$$\log P_{o/w} = \log\left[\left(\frac{Abs_{before}-Abs_{after}}{Abs_{after}}\right)\left(\frac{V_{aqueous}}{V_{octanol}}\right)\right] \quad (9)$$

where Abs_{before} and Abs_{after} refer to the measured uv/visible absorbance of the aqueous solution prior and after partitioning, respectively, and $V_{aqueous}/V_{octanol}$ is the ratio of the aqueous phase volume divided by the volume of the octanol phase.

Henchoz and coworkers (2010) determined the water-to-octanol partition coefficients of 21 acidic and 29 basic pharmaceutical compounds using microemulsion electrokinetic capillary chromatography (MEEKC) coupled with uv absorption and mass spectrometric detection. The method involves measuring the retention factor of the investigated compound

$$k_{solute} = \frac{(t_{r,solute} - t_{r,eof})}{(1 - \frac{t_{r,solute}}{t_{r,mc}})t_{r,eof}} \tag{10}$$

where $t_{r,solute}$, $t_{r,eof}$ and $t_{r,mc}$ are the retention/migration times of the investigated drug compound, a highly hydrophilic neutral marker (such as dimethyl sulfoxide) and a highly lipophilic pseudostationary phase marker (such as dodecanophenone or 1-phenyldodecane). The migration times of the two markers define the migration window. The log $P_{o/w}$ of the drug molecules are obtained from a calibration curve

$$\log k_{solute} = \text{slope} \cdot \log P_{o/w} + \text{intercept} \tag{11}$$

established with the measured retention factors of standard compounds with known log $P_{o/w}$ values. The proposed method was validated using a set of 35 well-balanced reference compounds that contained neutral, acidic ($pK_a > 3.6$) or basic ($pK_a < 5.5$) compounds with log $P_{o/w}$ values ranging from 0.7 to 4.8. The acidic compounds were analyzed at a pH = 2, while the neutral and basic compounds were analyzed at pH = 10. The authors found that the log $P_{o/w}$ values based on MEEKC method differed by less than 0.5 log units from the log $P_{o/w}$ values determined by the more traditional shake-flask method. The method allowed log $P_{o/w}$ measurement in less than 20 minutes, which is acceptable for quick screening methods. The authors further noted that the MEEKC method could be easily automated, consumed very little sample and solvent, and did not require a highly purified drug sample.

Logarithms of the water-to-organic solvent partition coefficients represent another solute property that has been successfully correlated by Eqn. 12 of the Abraham solvation parameter model.

$$\text{Log } P = c + e \cdot \mathbf{E} + s \cdot \mathbf{S} + a \cdot \mathbf{A} + b \cdot \mathbf{B} + v \cdot \mathbf{V} \tag{12}$$

In Table 3 we have compiled the equation coefficients that have been reported describing the various water-to-organic solvent partitioning systems that have been studied. In the case of the alkane and chloroalkane (dichloromethane, trichloromethane, tetrachloromethane, 1,2-dichloroethane and 1-chlorobutane) solvents, one will note that the equation coefficients for describing log P are identical to the coefficients for correlating the log molar solubility ratios, log $(C_{A,organic}/C_{A,water})$ values. As noted previous the molar solubility ratios describe a "hypothetic partitioning" processes for solute transfer to an anhydrous "dry" organic solvent. Solubility ratios and practical partition coefficients are nearly identical for solvents that are almost "completely" immiscible with water.

Water-organic solvent based biphasic systems are widely used in liquid-liquid extraction and in calculating Abraham model solute descriptors in accordance with Eqn. 12. For compounds that react with water, or for compounds that have very low aqueous solubilities, water-based

Wet Solvent	c	e	s	a	b	v
Butan-1-ol[a]	0.376	0.434	-0.718	-0.097	-2.350	2.682
Pentan-1-ol[a]	0.185	0.367	-0.732	0.105	-3.100	3.395
Hexan-1-ol[a]	-0.006	0.460	-0.940	0.142	-3.284	3.792
Heptan-1-ol[a]	0.041	0.497	-0.976	0.030	-3.438	3.859
Octan-1-ol[a]	0.088	0.562	-1.054	0.034	-3.460	3.814
Nonan-1-ol[a]	-0.041	0.562	-1.103	0.090	-3.540	3.922
Decan-1-ol[a]	-0.136	0.542	-0.989	0.046	-3.722	3.996
Isobutanol[a]	0.249	0.480	-0.639	-0.050	-2.284	2.758
Olely alcohol [a]	-0.096	0.148	-0.841	-0.438	-4.040	4.125
Dichloromethane	0.319	0.102	-0.187	-3.058	-4.090	4.324
Trichloromethane	0.191	0.105	-0.403	-3.112	-3.514	4.395
Tetrachloromethane	0.199	0.523	-1.159	-3.560	-4.594	4.618
1,2-Dichloroethane	0.183	0.294	-0.134	-2.801	-4.291	4.180
1-Chlorobutane	0.222	0.273	-0.569	-2.918	-4.883	4.456
Butane	0.297	-0.005	-1.584	-3.188	-4.567	4.562
Pentane	0.369	0.386	-1.568	-3.535	-5.215	4.514
Hexane	0.361	0.579	-1.723	-3.599	-4.764	4.344
Heptane	0.325	0.670	-2.061	-3.317	-4.733	4.543
Octane	0.223	0.642	-1.647	-3.480	-5.067	4.526
Nonane	0.240	0.619	-1.713	-3.532	-4.921	4.482
Decane	0.160	0.585	-1.734	-3.435	-5.078	4.582
Undecane	0.058	0.603	-1.661	-3.421	-5.120	4.619
Dodecane	0.114	0.668	-1.664	-3.545	-5.006	4.459
Hexadecane	0.087	0.667	-1.617	-3.587	-4.869	4.433
Cyclohexane	0.159	0.784	-1.678	-3.740	-4.929	4.577
Methylcyclohexane	0.246	0.782	-1.982	-3.517	-4.293	4.528
Isooctane	0.318	0.555	-1.737	-3.677	-4.864	4.417
Benzene	0.142	0.464	-0.588	-3.099	-4.625	4.491
Toluene	0.143	0.527	-0.720	-3.010	-4.824	4.545
Fluorobenzene	0.139	0.152	-0.374	-3.030	-4.601	4.540
Chlorobenzene	0.065	0.381	-0.521	-3.183	-4.700	4.614
Bromobenzene	-0.017	0.436	-0.424	-3.174	-4.558	4.445
Iodobenzene	-0.192	0.298	-0.308	-3.213	-4.653	4.588
Nitrobenzene	-0.152	0.525	0.081	-2.332	-4.494	4.187
Diethyl ether[a]	0.248	0.561	-1.016	-0.226	-4.553	4.075
Diisopropyl ether[a]	0.472	0.413	-0.745	-0.632	-5.251	4.059
Dibutyl ether	0.252	0.677	-1.506	-0.807	-5.249	4.815
o-Nitrophenyl octyl ether	0.121	0.600	-0.459	-2.246	-3.879	3.574
Ethyl acetate[a]	0.441	0.591	-0.699	-0.325	-4.261	3.666
Butyl acetate[a]	-0.475	0.428	-0.094	-0.241	-4.151	4.046
PGDP[b]	0.256	0.501	-0.828	-1.022	-4.640	4.033
Methyl isobutyl ketone	0.383	0.801	-0.831	-0.121	-4.441	3.876
Olive oil	-0.035	0.574	-0.798	-1.422	-4.984	4.210

Carbon disulfide	0.047	0.686	-0.943	-3.603	-5.818	4.921
Isopropyl myristate	-0.605	0.930	-1.153	-1.682	-4.093	4.249
Triolein	0.385	0.983	-2.083	-2.007	-3.452	4.072

[a] Correlation uses the Bo solute descriptor.

[b] Propylene glycol dipelargonate.

Table 3. Coefficients in Eqn. 12 for Correlating Solute Water-to-Organic Solvent log P values at 298 K

Wet Solvent	c	e	s	a	b	l
Butan-1-ol	-0.095	0.262	1.396	3.405	2.565	0.523
Pentan-1-ol	-0.107	-0.001	1.188	3.614	1.671	0.721
Hexan-1-ol	-0.302	-0.046	0.880	3.609	1.785	0.824
Heptan-1-ol	-0.159	0.018	0.825	3.539	1.425	0.830
Octan-1-ol	-0.198	0.002	0.709	3.519	1.429	0.858
Nonan-1-ol	-0.197	0.141	0.694	3.616	1.299	0.827
Decan-1-ol	-0.302	0.233	0.741	3.531	1.177	0.835
Isobutanol	-0.095	0.262	1.396	3.405	2.565	0.523
Olely alcohol	-0.268	-0.392	0.800	3.117	0.978	0.918
Dichloromethane	0.192	-0.572	1.492	0.460	0.847	0.965
Trichloromethane	0.157	-0.560	1.259	0.374	1.333	0.976
Tetrachloromethane	0.217	-0.435	0.554	0.000	0.000	1.069
1,2-Dichloroethane	0.017	-0.337	1.600	0.774	0.637	0.921
1-Chlorobutane	0.130	-0.581	1.114	0.724	0.000	1.016
Butane	0.291	-0.360	0.091	0.000	0.000	0.959
Pentane	0.335	-0.276	0.000	0.000	0.000	0.968
Hexane	0.292	-0.169	0.000	0.000	0.000	0.979
Heptane	0.275	-0.162	0.000	0.000	0.000	0.983
Octane	0.215	-0.049	0.000	0.000	0.000	0.967
Nonane	0.200	-0.145	0.000	0.000	0.000	0.980
Decane	0.156	-0.143	0.000	0.000	0.000	0.989
Undecane	0.113	0.000	0.000	0.000	0.000	0.971
Dodecane	0.017	0.000	0.000	0.000	0.000	0.989
Hexadecane	0.000	0.000	0.000	0.000	0.000	1.000
Cyclohexane	0.163	-0.110	0.000	0.000	0.000	1.013
Methylcyclohexane	0.318	-0.215	0.000	0.000	0.000	1.012
Isooctane	0.264	-0.230	0.000	0.000	0.000	0.975
Benzene	0.107	-0.313	1.053	0.457	0.169	1.020
Toluene	0.121	-0.222	0.938	0.467	0.099	1.012
Fluorobenzene	0.181	-0.621	1.432	0.647	0.000	0.986
Chlorobenzene	0.064	-0.399	1.151	0.313	0.171	1.032
Bromobenzene	-0.064	-0.326	1.261	0.323	0.292	1.002
Iodobenzene	-0.171	-0.192	1.197	0.245	0.245	1.002
Nitrobenzene	-0.296	0.092	1.707	1.147	0.443	0.912
Benzonitrile	-0.067	-0.257	1.848	2.009	0.227	0.870

Diethyl ether	0.206	-0.169	0.873	3.402	0.000	0.882
Dipropyl ether	0.065	-0.202	0.776	3.074	0.000	0.948
Diisopropyl ether	0.114	-0.032	0.685	3.108	0.000	0.941
Dibutyl ether	0.369	-0.216	0.026	2.626	-0.499	1.124
Ethyl acetate	0.130	0.031	1.202	3.199	0.463	0.828
Butyl acetate	-0.664	0.061	1.671	3.373	0.824	0.832
Methyl isobutyl ketone	0.244	0.183	0.987	3.418	0.323	0.854
Olive oil	-0.156	-0.254	0.859	1.656	0.000	0.873
Carbon disulfide	0.101	0.251	0.177	0.027	0.095	1.068
Triolein	0.147	0.254	-0.246	1.520	1.473	0.918

Table 4. Coefficients in Eqn. 2 for Correlating Solute Gas-to-Organic Solvent log K values at 298 K

partitioning systems may not be appropriate. Poole and coworkers (Karunasekara and Poole, 2010; Qian and Poole, 2007; Ahmed and Poole, 2006a,b) have reported Abraham model correlations for several totally organic biphasic systems, such as heptane + formamide, hexane + acetonitrile, heptane + methanol, heptane + N,N-dimethylformamide, heptane + 2,2,2-trifluoroethanol, and heptane + 1,1,1,3,3,3-hexafluoroisopropanol. The organic-based biphasic systems allow one to calculate solute descriptors for compounds that might not otherwise be possible with water-based partitioning systems. For example, the biphasic hexane + acetonitrile, heptane + N,N-dimethylformamide, and heptane + 2,2,2-trifluoroethanol systems were used, in combination with chromatographic retention factors, to determine a complete set of descriptors for organosilicon compounds (Atapattu and Poole, 2009; Ahmed *et al.*, 2007), many of which react with water. Abraham model equation coefficients are tabulated in Table 5 for seven organic solvent-to-organic solvent partitioning systems.

Partitioning system	c	e	s	a	b	v
Formamide-to-heptane	0.083	0.559	-2.244	-3.250	-1.614	2.384
N,N-Dimethylformamide-to-heptane	0.065	0.030	-1.405	-2.039	-0.806	0.721
2,2,2-Trifluoroethanol-to-heptane	0.160	0.856	-1.538	-1.325	-2.965	1.190
1,1,1,3,3,3-Hexafluoroisopropanol-to-heptane	-0.225	0.720	-1.357	-0.577	-2.819	1.161
Methanol-to-heptane	-0.056	0.164	-0.620	-1.337	-0.957	0.507
Ethylene glycol-to-heptane	0.343	0.000	-1.247	3.807	-2.194	2.065
Acetonitrile-to-hexane	0.097	0.189	-1.332	-1.649	-0.966	0.773

Table 5. Coefficients in Eqn. 12 for Correlating Solute Organic Solvent-to-Organic Solvent log P values at 298 K

5. Calculation of Abraham solute descriptors from measured solubility and partition coefficient data

The application of Eqn. 1 and Eqn. 2 requires a knowledge of the descriptors (or properties) of the solutes: **E**, **S**, **A**, **B**, **V** and **L**. The descriptors **E** and **V** are quite easily obtained. **V** can be calculated from atom and bond contributions as outlined previously (Abraham and McGowan, 1987). The atom contributions are in Table 6; note that they are in $cm^3\ mol^{-1}$. The bond contribution is 6.56 cm^3 mol^{-1} for each bond, no matter whether single, double, or triple, to be subtracted. For complicated molecules it is time consuming to count the number of bonds, Bn, but this can be calculated from the algorithm given by Abraham (1993a)

$$Bn = Nt - 1 + R \tag{13}$$

where Nt is the total number of atoms in the molecule and R is the number of rings.
Once **V** is available, **E** can be obtained from the compound refractive index at 20°C. If the compound is not liquid at room temperature or if the refractive index is not known the latter can be calculated using the freeware software of Advanced Chemistry Development (ACD). An Excel spreadsheet for the calculation of **V** and **E** from refractive index is available from the authors. Since **E** is almost an additive property, it can also be obtained by the summation of fragments, either by hand, or through a commercial software program (ADME Boxes, 2010). There remain the descriptors **S**, **A**, **B**, and **L** to be determined.
Partition coefficients and/or solubilities can be used to obtain all the four remaining descriptors (Abraham *et al.*, 2004). Suppose there are available solubilities for a given compound in water and a number of solvents. Then solubility ratios, log ($C_{A,organic}/C_{A,water}$), can be obtained as shown in Eqn. 5 and Eqn. 6. If three solubility ratios are available for three solvent systems shown in Table 1, we have three equations and three unknowns (**S**, **A**, and **B**) so that the latter can be determined. Of more practical use is a situation where several solubility ratios are known. Then if we have, say, six solubility ratios and three equations, the three unknowns can be obtained as the descriptors that give the best fit to the six equations. The Solver add-on program to Excel can be set up to carry out such a calculation automatically. However, it is possible to increase the number of equations by the stratagem of converting the water-to-solvent solubility ratios into gas to solvent solubility ratios, $C_{A,organic}/C_{A,gas}$

$$C_{A,organic}/C_{A,water} * C_{A,water}/C_{A,gas} = C_{A,organic}/C_{A,gas} \tag{14}$$

The ratio $C_{A,water}/C_{A,gas}$ is the gas-to-water partition coefficient, usually denoted as K_w. A further set of equations is available for gas-to-solvent solubility ratios, Table 2. Thus six water-to-solvent solubility ratios can be converted into six gas-to-solvent solubility ratios, leading to a set of 12 equations. If $\log K_w$ is not known, it can be used as another parameter to be determined. This increases the number of unknowns from four (**S, A, B, L**) to five (**S, A, B, L**, $\log K_w$) but the number of equations is increased from six to twelve. In addition, two equations are available for gas to solvent partitions themselves, see the last entries in Tables 1 and 2, making for the present case no fewer than fourteen equations.
As an example, we use data on solubilities of trimethoprim in eight solvents (Li *et al.*, 2008) converted from mol fraction to mol dm^{-3}. The solubility in water was not given, but is known to be $2.09 * 10^{-3}$ in mol dm^{-3} (Howard and Meylan, 1997). The eight observed solubility ratios, $C_{A,organic}/C_{A,water}$, are in Table 7, as log (ratio). We took log K_w as another parameter to be determined, leading to no less than 18 equations: the eight original equations from solubilities in the eight solvents that led to $C_{A,organic}/C_{A,water}$, the corresponding eight equations for $C_{A,organic}/C_{A,gas}$, and two equations for $C_{A,water}/C_{A,gas}$ (*ie* K_w). With **E** fixed at 1.892 and **V** fixed at 2.1813, the best fit values of the descriptors were **S** = 2.52, **A** = 0.44, **B** = 1.69, **L** = 11.81 and log K_w = 14.49; these yielded the calculated log (ratios) in Table 7. For all 18 values, the Average Error = -0.002, the Absolute Average Error = 0.092, the RMSE = 0.107, and the SD = 0.110 log unit. Not only do the original solubilities allow the derivation of descriptors for trimethoprim, but the latter, in turn, allow the prediction of solubility ratios and hence actual solubilities in all the solvents listed in Table 1.

Exactly the same procedure is adopted if actual partition coefficients are experimentally available, rather than solubilities. The relevant equations are now those in Table 3 and Table 4. Of course if both solubilities and actual partition coefficients have both been experimentally determined, a combination of equations from Tables 1 and 2 and from Tables 3 and 4 can be used. Even though partition coefficients refer to partition into wet solvents, descriptors obtained from partition coefficients using equations in Table 3 and Table 4 can still be used to predict solubility ratios and solubilities in dry solvents for all the solvents listed in Table 1.

C	16.35	N	14.39	O	12.43
Si	26.83	P	24.87	S	22.91
Ge	31.02	As	29.42	Se	27.81
Sn	39.35	Sb	37.74	Te	36.14
Pb	43.44	Bi	42.19		
H	8.71	He	6.76	B	18.32
F	10.48	Ne	8.51	Hg	34.00
Cl	20.95	A	1.90		
Br	26.21	Kr	2.46		
I	34.53	Xe	3.29		
		Rn	3.84		

Table 6. Atom contributions to the McGowan volume, in $cm^3 mol^{-1}$

Water-to-solvent	calc	obs
Methanol	1.35	1.48
Ethanol	0.98	0.94
Propanol	0.75	0.80
Butanol	0.53	0.68
2-Propanol	0.61	0.51
2-Butanol	0.65	0.62
Tetrahydrofuran	1.18	1.02
Propanone	0.90	0.94
Gas to water	14.48	14.49
Gas-to-solvent	calc	obs
Methanol	15.81	15.97
Ethanol	15.48	15.43
Propanol	15.23	15.29
Butanol	15.02	15.18
2-Propanol	15.14	15.01
2-Butanol	15.18	15.11
Tetrahydrofuran	15.70	15.51
Propanone	15.34	15.43
Gas to water	14.53	14.49

Table 7. Solubility ratios for trimethoprim, as log (ratio)

Although we have set out the determination of descriptors from experimental measurements, it is still very helpful to use the ACD software (ADME Boxes, 2010) to calculate the descriptors at the same time. Occasionally there may be erroneous solubility measurements, or solubilities may be affected through solvate formation, and the calculated descriptors afford a useful check on the obtained descriptors from experiment measurements.

6. Abraham solvation parameter model: prediction of blood-to-brain and blood-to-iissue partition coefficient

Successful drug development requires efficient delivery of the drug to the target site. The drug must cross various cellular barriers by passive and/or transporter-mediated uptake. Drug delivery to the brain is particularly challenging as there are two physiologically barriers - the blood-brain barrier (BBB) and the blood-cerebrospinal fluid barrier (BCSFB) - separating the brain from its blood supply controlling the transport of chemical compounds. The BBB is a continuous layer of microvessel endothelial cells, connected by highly-developed tight junctions, which effectively restrict paracellular transport of molecules irrespective of their molecular size. Tight junctions provide significant transendothelial electrical resistance to the brain microvessel endothelial cells and serves to further impede the penetration of the BBB. The electrical resistance between the endothelial cells is on the order of 1500 - 2000 Ω/cm^2, as compared to and electrical resistance of 3.33 Ω/cm^2 found in other body tissues (Alam *et al.*, 2010). Under normal conditions the BBB acts as a barrier to toxic agents and safeguards the integrity of the brain. A compound may circumvent the BBB and gain access to the brain by the nose-to-brain route. The compound is transported to the brain via an olfactory pathway following absorption across the nasal mucosa.

Alternatively, compounds may permeate from the blood into the cerebrospinal fluid and permeate into the brain interstitial fluid. The BCSFB separates the blood from the cerebrospinal fluid (CSF) that runs in the subarachnoid space surrounding the brain. The BCSFB is located at the choroid plexus, and it is composed of epithelial cells held together at their apices by tight junctions, which limit paracellular flux. Hence compounds penetrate the barrier transcellularly. The CSF-facing surface of the epithelial cells, which secrete CSF into the ventricles, is increased by the presence of microvilli. The capillaries in the choroid plexus allow free movement of molecules via fenestractions and intracellular gaps. Transport across the BCSFB is not an accurate measure of transport across the BBB as the two barriers are anatomically different. However, as Begley *et al.* (2000) point out, for many compounds there is a permanently maintained concentration gradient between brain interstitial fluid and the CSF.

The transport of compounds into the brain can take place through 'passive' transport or 'active' transport. Nearly all the calculational models for transport into the brain deal with passive transport, although it is now known that many compounds are prevented from crossing the BBB through efflux mechanisms especially involving P-glycoprotein. The use of wildtype mice and knockout mice (the latter deficient in Pgp) has shown conclusively that for a number of drugs the brain to plasma distribution is much lower for the wildtype mice than for knockout mice. We will focus on passive transport, but it must be appreciated that any analysis might well include compounds that are actually subject to active transport and will appear as outliers in the analyses.

The steady-state distribution of a compound between the blood (or plasma) and brain, and the rate of permeation of a compound from blood (or from an aqueous saline solution) through the blood brain barrier, are two quantitative measures of drug uptake in the brain.

The logarithm of the blood-to-brain concentration ratio, log BB, is a thermodynamic quantity defining the extent of blood penetration. The log BB is mathematically given by

$$\log BB = \left(\frac{C_{solute,brain}}{C_{solute,blood}}\right) \quad (15)$$

the ratio of the solute concentration in brain tissue divided by the solute's concentration in blood (or serum or plasma) at steady-state conditions. The blood/brain distribution ratio can be experimentally determined by intravenous administration of a single injection of ^{14}C-radioactive isotope labeled test substance in rats. The animal is sacrificed at a specified time endpoint after equilibrium is achieved. The brain and blood are immediately harvested, and the concentration in each biological sample is quantified from the measured radioactivity. Isotopic labeling provides a convenient means to distinguish the injected test substance from all other chemicals that might be present in the body. Radioactive counting methods do not distinguish between the radioactive isotope in the injected test substance and any degradation products that might have been formed before the animal was sacrificed. The distribution experiments are usually carried out over a long time scale, possibly hours, and concentrations in blood and brain obtained as a function of time. The ratio, as Eq. 15, will change with time and only if it reaches a constant value can the ratio be taken as an equilibrium value. This is very time consuming indeed, as only one measurement can be made with each rat. Despite these shortcomings, radioactive labeling is one of the more popular methods for not only determining the blood-to-brain distribution coefficient, but other blood-to-tissue partition coefficients as well.

Blood-to-brain and blood-to-tissue partition coefficients have also been measured for volatile organic compounds using the *in vitro* vial method (see Figure 6). A known amount of animal sample is placed in a glass vial of known volume. The vial is then sealed and a minute known quantity of the volatile organic compound (VOC) is introduced by syringe through the rubber septum. After equilibration a sample of the headspace vapor phase is withdrawn from the glass vial for gas chromatographic analysis. The gas-to-tissue partition coefficient is computed from mass balance considerations as the total amount of solute added, the concentration of the vapor phase, the headspace volume and amount of tissue sample are all known. The blood-to-tissue partition coefficient, $P_{tissue/blood}$, is calculated as

$$P_{tissue/blood} = P_{tissue/air} x P_{air/blood} = \left(\frac{C_{solute,tissue}}{C_{solute,air}}\right) x \left(\frac{C_{solute,air}}{C_{solute,blood}}\right) \quad (16)$$

the product of the measured air-to-tissue partition coefficient, $P_{tissue/air}$, times the measured blood-to-air partition coefficient, $P_{air/blood}$. The *in vitro* partition coefficient data are important and are used as required input parameters in pharmacokinetic models developed to determine the disposition of volatile organic compounds that individuals inhale in the workplace and in the environment.

Abraham and coworkers (2006a) reported correlation models for the air-to-brain ($P_{brain/air}$) and blood-to-brain ($P_{brain/blood}$) partition coefficients for VOCs in humans and rats

$$\text{Log } P_{brain/air}(in\ vitro) = -0.987 + 0.263\mathbf{E} + 0.411\mathbf{S} + 3.358\mathbf{A} + 2.025\mathbf{B} + 0.591\mathbf{L}$$
$$\left(N = 81, R^2 = 0.923, SD = 0.346, RMSE = 0.333, F = 179.0\right) \quad (17)$$

$$\text{Log BB} = \text{Log P}_{\text{brain/blood}}(\textit{in vitro}) = -0.057 + 0.017\mathbf{E} - 0.536\mathbf{S} - 0.323\mathbf{A} - 0.335\mathbf{B} + 0.731\mathbf{V}$$
$$(\text{N} = 78, \text{R}^2 = 0.725, \text{SD} = 0.203, \text{RMSE} = 0.196, \text{F} = 37.9) \quad (18)$$

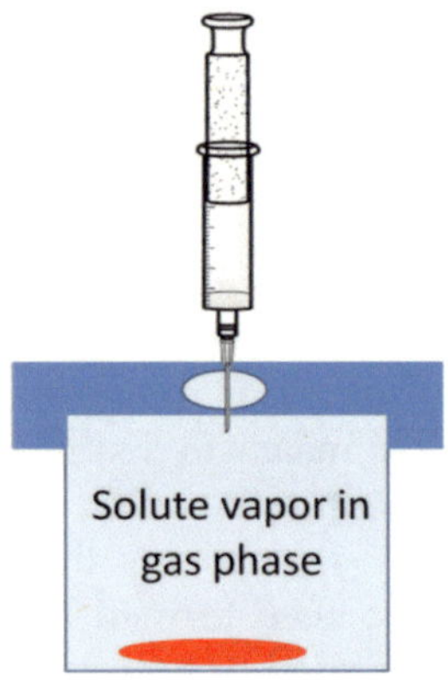

Fig. 6. Equilibrium vial technique depicting removal of the equilibrated headspace vapor above the animal/human tissue

In Eqns. 17 and 18, N is the number of data points in the regression analysis, R^2 represents the squared correlation coefficient, SD denotes the standard deviation and RMSE corresponds to the root mean square error. Note that in a multiple linear regression equation, the denominator in the definition of SD is N - P - 1 and in the definition of RMSE it is N - P, where P is the number of independent variables in the equation. The derived correlations provided a reasonably accurate mathematical description of the observed partition coefficient data as evidenced by the high squared correlation coefficients and reasonably small standard deviations. Both correlations were validated using training set and test set analyses. In comparing calculated biological data to observed values one must remember that the measured values do have larger experimental uncertainties. A reasonable estimated uncertainty for the measured log $P_{brain/air}$ would be about 0.2 log units based on independent values from different laboratories. Rat and human partition coefficient data for each given VOC were averaged (if both values were available), and the average values were combined into a single regression analysis. In a comparison of experimental human and rat partition coefficient data for 17 common compounds, the authors had shown that the two sets of data (human versus rat) differed by only 0.062 log units, which is likely less than the experimental uncertainty associated with the measured experimental values. For the compounds studied, human and rat partition coefficient data were identical for all practical purposes. The authors also showed that blood-to-brain and plasma-to-brain partition coefficients were sufficiently close and could be combined into a single Abraham model correlation

$$\log \text{P}_{\text{brain/(blood,plasma)}} = -0.028 + 0.003\,\mathbf{E} - 0.485\,\mathbf{S} - 0.117\,\mathbf{A} - 0.408\,\mathbf{B} + 0.703\,\mathbf{V}$$
$$(\text{N} = 99, \text{R}^2 = 0.703, \text{SD} = 0.197, \text{RMSE} = 0.191, \text{F} = 44.1) \quad (19)$$

Eqs. (18) and (19), are not substantially different, and the statistics are almost the same. It is a moot point as to whether further values of blood to brain partition coefficients should best be predicted through Eqn. 18 or 19. We recommend that Eqn. 18 be used to predict blood-to-brain partition coefficients of VOC because it refers specifically to blood rather than to blood or plasma.

A follow-up study (Abraham *et al.*, 2006b) considered the partitioning behavior of drugs and drug candidates (measured by *in vivo* experimental methods), as well as the VOC *in vitro* partition coefficient data discussed above. The Abraham model correlation for the *in vivo* log $P_{brain/blood}$ data

$$\log BB = \log P_{brain/blood}(in\ vivo) = 0.547 + 0.221\mathbf{E} - 0.604\mathbf{S} - 0.641\mathbf{A} - 0.681\mathbf{B} + 0.635\mathbf{V} - 1.216\mathbf{Ic}$$
$$\left(N = 233, R^2 = 0.75, SD = 0.33, F = 113\right) \quad (20)$$

differs from the correlation equation for the VOCs (see Eqn. 18). In particular, the c-coefficients differ appreciably 0.547 (SD = 0.078) as against -0.024 (SD=0.069), which suggests that there is a systematic difference between the *in vivo* and *in vitro* distributions. The authors went on to show that the difference resulted in part because the two sets of compounds (drugs versus VOCs) inhabit different areas in chemical space. The *in vivo* drug compounds had much larger solute descriptors, and included compounds having a carboxylic acid functional group. The independent variable **Ic** was needed as an indicator descriptor for carboxylic acids (**Ic** = 1 for carboxylic acids, **Ic** = 0 for noncarboxylic acid solutes).

The blood-to-brain partition coefficient provides valuable information regarding a compound's ability to penetrate the blood-brain barrier. Cruciani *et al.* (2000) noted that compounds having log BB values greater than 0.0 (concentration in the brain exceeds concentration in the blood) should cross the barrier, whereas compounds having log BB less than -0.3 tended not to cross the barrier. Li and coworkers (2005) used a slightly different classification scheme (see Figure 7) of dividing compounds into BBB-penetrating (BBB+) or BBB-non-penetrating (BBB-) according to whether the log BB value was ≥ -1 or ≤ -1, respectively. Many times an actual numerical log BB is not needed in the decision making process, and in such cases, an indication of BBB+ or BBB- is often sufficient. Zhao *et al.* (2007) proposed a fairly simple decision tree for classifying drug candidates as BBB+ or BBB- based on their Abraham solute descriptors (See Figure 7). Solute acidity and solute basicity were the two most important properties governing BBB penetration, with solute excess molar refraction playing a much smaller role. The proposed classification scheme correctly predicted the BBB penetration of 90 % of the 1093 compounds considered.

As noted above permeation of a compound from blood (or from an aqueous saline solution) through the blood brain barrier can be used to indicate drug uptake in the brain. The membrane permeability-surface area product, PS, is a kinetic parameter used in describing initial rate of unidirectional transfer

$$k_{in} = F(1 - e^{-PS/F}) \quad (21)$$

where k_{in} is the measured transfer constant and F is the perfusion fluid flow expressed in milliliters per second per gram. For solutes that bind rapidly and reversibly to plasma proteins, Eqn. 21 is modified as follows

$$k_{in} = F(1 - e^{-fu\,PS/F}) \quad (22)$$

assuming that the unbound and bound forms of the drug are in equilibrium in the fluid. In Eqn. 22, fu is the fraction of the unbound drug in the perfusion fluid. In a typical experiment, the drug (dissolved in blood or in an aqueous saline solution) is perfused into the internal carotid artery and the rate of drug uptake is determined by a radioisotope assay method. The animals are sacrificed at various time intervals. The time scale needed to perform the perfusion study is very short - typically no more than a few minutes. Because of the small time scale, perfusion measurements are less subject to degradation effects than are log BB measurements, although the same difficulties over passive and active transport still exist.

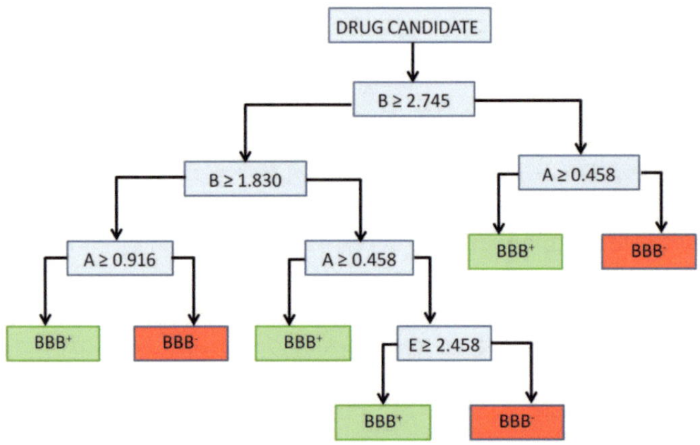

Fig. 7. Decision tree for predicting whether drugs pass through the BBB based on their Abraham solute descriptors. BBB+ indicates BBB penetrating whereas BBB- denotes BBB non-penetration. The right-handside of any decision branch is no penetration (red box), and the left-handside is yes penetration (green box). (The right-hand side of any decision branch is yes, and the left-hand side is no.)

Abraham (2004) derived the following mathematical correlation

$$\log PS = -0.716 - 0.974\mathbf{S} - 1.802\mathbf{A} - 1.603\mathbf{B} + 1.893\mathbf{V}$$
$$\left(N = 30,\ R^2 = 0.868,\ SD = 0.52,\ F = 42\right) \tag{23}$$

by regression analysis of the experimental log PS data for 30 neutral compounds from protein-free saline solution buffered at pH of 7.4. The contribution of the e $\cdot$ **E** term was not significant and was removed from Eqn. 23. The negative equation coefficients in Eqn. 23 indicate that an increase in compound polarity of any kind, that is dipolarity/polarizability, hydrogen-bonding acidity or hydrogen-bonding basicity, results in a decrease in the rate of permeation. Increased solute size (**V** solute descriptor), on the other hand, results in a greater permeation rate.

The Abraham model correlations that have been presented thus far pertain to neutral molecules. The basic model has been extended to include processes between condensed phases involving ions and ionic species

$$SP = c + e\cdot\mathbf{E} + s\cdot\mathbf{S} + a\cdot\mathbf{A} + b\cdot\mathbf{B} + v\cdot\mathbf{V} + j_+\cdot\mathbf{J}^+ + j_-\cdot\mathbf{J}^- \tag{24}$$

by adding one new term for cations and one new term for anions. $\mathbf{J}^+$ is used whenever a cation is the solute, $\mathbf{J}^-$ whenever an anion is the solute, and neither is used whenever the solute is a nonelectrolyte. It is very important to note that the two new ionic descriptors are used together with the descriptors originally chosen for nonelectrolytes. This ensures that values of **S**, **A** and **B** for ions and ionic species are on the same scale as those for nonelectrolytes. Solute descriptors have been reported for many simple cations and anions, for carboxylates, for phenoxides, and for protonated amines and protonated pyridines. The j_+ and j_- equation coefficients have been determined (Abraham and Acree, 2010a,b,c,d) for several of the organic solvents listed in Table 1. Abraham (2011) recently reanalyzed the published log PS data in terms of Eqn. 24 to yield the following correlation model

$$\log PS = -1.268 - 0.047\mathbf{E} - 0.876\mathbf{S} - 0.719\mathbf{A} - 1.571\mathbf{B} + 1.767\mathbf{V} + 0.469\mathbf{J}^+ + 1.663\mathbf{J}^- \quad (N = 88, R^2 = 0.810, SD = 0.534, F = 48.8) \tag{25}$$

The 88 log PS values in Eqn. 25 were for compounds that existed in the saline perfusate entirely (or almost entirely) as neutral molecules or entirely (or almost entirely) as charged species, and which underwent perfusion by a passive process. Abraham showed that log PS values for carboxylate anions are about two log units less than those for the neutral carboxylic acids, and that log PS values for protonated base cations are about one log unit less than those for the neutral bases.

7. Abraham solvation parameter model: prediction of blood-to-tissue and gas-to-tissue partition coefficients

Air-to-blood partitioning is a major determinant governing the uptake of chemical vapors into the blood and their subsequent elimination from blood to exhaled air. Air partitioning processes are becoming increasing more important in the pharmaceutical industry given the large numbers of drugs and vaccines that are now administered by inhalation aerosols and nasal delivery devices. Inhalation drug delivery is appealing given the large surface area for drug absorption, the high blood flow to and from the lung, and the absence of first pass metabolism that is characteristic of the lung. Inhalation drug delivery results in both a rapid clearance action and a rapid onset of therapeutic action, and a reduction in the number of undesired side effects. Eixarch and coworkers (2010) proposed the development of a pulmonary biopharmaceutical classification system (pBCS) that would classify drugs according to their ability to reside in the lung or to be transferred to the bloodstream. The classification scheme would need to consider factors associated with the lung's biology (metabolism, efflux transporters, clearance) and with the drug formulation/physicochemical properties (solubility, lipophilicity, protein binding, particle size, aerosol physics). Blood-to-tissue partitionings govern the distribution throughout the rest of the body once the drug has entered the bloodstream.

Abraham model correlations have been developed to describe the air-to-tissue and blood-to-tissue partition coefficients of drugs and volatile organic compounds (VOCs). The derived mathematical equations include:

Muscle (Abraham *et al.*, 2006c):

$$\log K_{muscle/air}(\textit{in vitro}) = -1.039 + 0.207\mathbf{E} + 0.723\mathbf{S} + 3.242\mathbf{A} + 2.469\mathbf{B} + 0.463\mathbf{L} \quad (N = 114, R^2 = 0.944, SD = 0.267, F = 363) \tag{26}$$

$$\log P_{muscle/blood}(in\ vitro) = -0.185 - 0.209\mathbf{E} - 0.593\mathbf{S} - 0.081\mathbf{A} - 0.168\mathbf{B} + 0.741\mathbf{V}$$
$$\left(N = 110,\ R^2 = 0.537,\ SD = 0.207,\ F = 24\right) \quad (27)$$

$$\log P_{muscle/blood}(in\ vivo)\ 0.082 - 0.059\mathbf{E} + 0.010\mathbf{S} - 0.248\mathbf{A} + 0.028\ B + 0.110\mathbf{V} - 1.022\mathbf{Ic}$$
$$\left(N - 60,\ R^2 = 0.745,\ SD = 0.253,\ F = 25.9\right) \quad (28)$$

Fat (Abraham and Ibrahim, 2006):

$$\log K_{fat/air}(in\ vitro) = -0.052 + 0.051\mathbf{E} + 0.728\mathbf{S} + 1.783\mathbf{A} + 0.332\mathbf{B} + 0.743\mathbf{L}$$
$$\left(N = 129,\ R^2 = 0.958,\ SD = 0.194,\ F = 562.8\right) \quad (29)$$

$$\log P_{fat/blood}(in\ vitro) = 0.474 + 0.016\mathbf{E} - 0.005\mathbf{S} - 1.577\mathbf{A} - 2.246\mathbf{B} + 1.560\mathbf{V}$$
$$\left(N = 126,\ R^2 = 0.847,\ SD = 0.304,\ F = 132.7\right) \quad (30)$$

$$\log P_{fat/blood}(in\ vivo) = 0.077 + 0.249\mathbf{E} - 0.215\ \mathbf{S} - 0.902\mathbf{A} - 1.523\mathbf{B} + 1.234\mathbf{V} - 1.013\mathbf{Ic}$$
$$\left(N = 50,\ R^2 = 0.811,\ SD = 0.33\ F = 30.7\right) \quad (31)$$

Liver (Abraham *et al.*, 2007a):

$$\log K_{liver/air}(in\ vitro) = -0.943 + 0.836\mathbf{S} + 2.836\mathbf{A} + 2.081\mathbf{B} + 0.561\mathbf{L}$$
$$\left(N = 124,\ R^2 = 0.927,\ SD = 0.256,\ F = 376.8\right) \quad (32)$$

$$\log P_{liver/blood}(in\ vitro) = -0.095 - 0.366\mathbf{S} - 0.357\mathbf{A} - 0.180\mathbf{B} + 0.730\mathbf{V}$$
$$\left(N = 125,\ R^2 = 0.583,\ SD = 0.228,\ F = 41.9\right) \quad (33)$$

$$\log P_{liver/blood}(in\ vivo) = 0.292 - 0.296\mathbf{S} - 0.334\mathbf{A} + 0.181\mathbf{B} + 0.337\mathbf{V} - 0.597\mathbf{Ic}$$
$$\left(N = 85,\ R^2 = 0.522,\ SD = 0.420,\ F = 17.3\right) \quad (34)$$

Lung (Abraham *et al.*, 2008a):

$$\log K_{lung/air}(in\ vitro) = -1.250 + 0.639\mathbf{E} + 1.038\mathbf{S} + 3.661\mathbf{A} + 3.041\mathbf{B} + 0.420\mathbf{L}$$
$$\left(N = 44,\ R^2 = 0.968,\ SD = 0.250,\ F = 231.8\right) \quad (35)$$

$$\log P_{lung/blood}(in\ vitro) = -\ 0.143 - 0.383\mathbf{B} + 0.308\mathbf{V}$$
$$\left(N = 43,\ R^2 = 0.264,\ SD = 0.190,\ F = 7.2\right) \quad (36)$$

Correlations obtained by regression analysis of experimental drug partition coefficient data are denoted as "*in vivo*", and correlations pertaining to volatile organic compound partitioning are indicated as "*in vitro*". Human and rat partition coefficient data were combined into data set used in the regression analyses. The independent variable **Ic** was needed as an indicator descriptor for carboxylic acids (**Ic** = 1 for carboxylic acids, **Ic** = 0 for noncarboxylic acid solutes) for the *in vivo* correlations involving drug molecules. The *in vivo* data sets included partition coefficient data for drug molecules such as nalidixic acid and valproic acid. No carboxylic acid solutes were contained in the *in vitro* data sets. The poor R^2 statistics noted in several of the blood-to-tissue correlations are due, at least in part, to the small spread in the log P values and the increased experimental uncertainties as noted below. Each derived correlation was validated by training set and test set analyses. Based on the validation computations the derived correlations are expected to predict the log $K_{tissue/air}$ and log $P_{tissue/blood}$ values of additional compounds to within about 0.2 to 0.3 log units.

As an informational note, the experimental data sets for the *in vitro* Abraham model correlations were determined using the equilibrium vial method. The gas-to-tissue partition coefficient of the VOC was calculated from the measured vapor phase composition in the headspace above the given tissue. The measured *in vitro* gas-to-tissue partition coefficients were converted to the corresponding blood-to-tissue values, $P_{tissue/blood}$ values, through Eqn. 16. The $P_{tissue/blood}$ include the experimental uncertainty in both the $K_{tissue/air}$ and $P_{blood/air}$ values. Should the *in vitro* experimental air-to-blood partitioning data not be available for the conversion, one can estimate the needed $P_{blood/air}$ values from the three correlation models

$$\log K_{blood/air}(\text{human}) = -1.18 + 0.39\mathbf{E} + 0.97\mathbf{S} + 3.80\mathbf{A} + 2.69\mathbf{B} + 0.41\mathbf{L} \quad (N = 155,\ R^2 = 0.34,\ \text{RSME} = 0.332,\ F = 474) \tag{37}$$

$$\log K_{blood/air}(\text{rat}) = -0.75 + 0.56\mathbf{E} + 1.06\mathbf{S} + 3.64\mathbf{A} + 2.41\mathbf{B} + 0.29\mathbf{L} \quad (N = 127,\ R^2 = 0.91,\ SD = 0.29,\ \text{RMSE} = 0.286,\ F = 242) \tag{38}$$

$$\log K_{blood/air}(\text{human or rat}) = -1.069 + 0.456\mathbf{E} + 1.083\mathbf{S} + 3.738\mathbf{A} + 2.580\mathbf{B} + 0.376\mathbf{L} \quad (N = 196.\ R^2 = 0.938,\ SD = 0.324,\ \text{RMSE} = 0.319,\ F = 572.8) \tag{39}$$

reported by Abraham and coworkers (2005). For any fully characterized system/process (those with calculated values for the equation coefficients) further values of SP (see Eqns. 1 and 2) can be estimated for solutes with known values for the solute descriptors. Solute descriptors can be obtained by regression analysis of measured drug solubilities in organic solvents and measured water-to-solvent and organic solvent-to-organic solvent partition coefficients as discussed above.

8. Abraham solvation parameter model: prediction of water-to-skin and blood-to-skin partition coefficients and skin permeability coefficients

Human skin is an important permeation barrier that controls the entry of chemicals into the body. The barrier properties of skin depend primarily on the outer skin cells, which are called the stratum corneum. The stratum corneum consists of multiple non-living layers of densely packed keratin-filled cells embedded in a lipid-rich extracellular matrix containing a mixture of ceramides, fatty acids, cholesterol and triglycerides (Monteiro-Riviere *et al.*, 2001). The multiple layers are 7 – 16 micrometers in total thickness in most regions of the human body; however, in the palms of the hands and soles of the feet a much total layer thickness of 400 - 600 micrometers is found (Holbrook and Odland, 1974) For a chemical to be absorbed into the body after dermal exposure, it must first dissolve in the stratum corneum and then diffuse through the remaining epidermis sub-layers and into the dermis layer, from where it will eventually enter the blood stream. Passive diffusion is the mechanism by which chemicals move through the stratum corneum. Passage through the remaining sub-layers of the skin is more rapid.

Penetration of a compound into the skin is controlled by the compound's chemical structure and physicochemical properties. Lipophilicity and hydrogen-bonding character play a major role in a compound's skin absorption profile. In general, substances possessing the greater lipophilicity are more readily absorbed by the skin than compounds with lesser lipophilicity. Dermal absorption generally increases with increasing water-to-octanol partition coefficient from log $P_{OtOH/water}$ = -1 to log $P_{OtOH/water}$ = 3.5. Highly lipophilic compounds (those with log $P_{OtOH/water} > 5$) pass easily through the stratum corneum, but are generally too water-insoluble to pass through the remaining epidermis sub-layers to enter the blood stream. There has been increasing experimental evidence that ionized species can contribute to transdermal absorption (Netzlaff *et al.*, 2006; Abraham and Martins, 2004; Michaels *et al.*, 1975). When the penetrating compound can exist in both ionized and unionized forms, it is the unionized form that penetrates faster through the lipid regions. Some contribution of the ionized form to the overall permeability, however, is expected. The solubilizing vehicle and formulation ingredients can alter the skin penetration of a compound by affecting the barrier properties of the skin by a range of mechanisms including hydration, delipidization, fluidization and desmosome disruption in the stratum corneum, or by changing the partitioning of the compound into the stratum corneum.

Skin partitioning is important in the pharmaceutical industry as many medications are applied topically to the skin in ointments, in creams, in lotions and gels, and in skin patches. Once applied, the medication often needs to find its way into the blood system for delivery to the desired target site. Abraham and Martins (2004) developed a mathematical correlation between the water-to-skin partition coefficient, K_{sc}, and the Abraham solute descriptors

$$\begin{aligned}\text{Log } K_{sc} &= 0.341 + 0.341\mathbf{E} - 0.206\mathbf{S} - 0.024\mathbf{A} - 2.178\mathbf{B} + 1.850\mathbf{V} \\ &\left(N = 45, SD = 0.216, R^2 = 0.926, F = 97\right)\end{aligned} \tag{40}$$

based on an experimental database containing 45 solutes, including several linear alcohols (*e.g.* methanol through 1-decanol) and several fairly large steroidal molecules (*e.g.* testosterone, progesterone, hydrocortisone, corticosterone, and aldosterone) and steroid esters (*e.g.* hydrocortisone-21 acetate, hydrocortisone-21 pentanoate, cortisone-21 acetate, cortisone-21 octanoate). Careful examination of Eqn. 40 reveals that the water-to-skin partition coefficient increases with increasing solute size, and decreasing with increasing solute polarity and solute hydrogen-bonding character.

Abraham and Ibrahim (2007) compiled experimental data on the distribution coefficients of drugs from blood or plasma to rat skin and rabbit skin. The authors analyzed the experimental log P_{skin} data in accordance with Eqn. 1 of the Abraham model

$$\begin{aligned}\log P_{skin} &= -0.253 - 0.189\mathbf{A} - 0.620\mathbf{B} + 0.713\mathbf{V} - 0.683\mathbf{I}_{\mathbf{acid}} + 0.059\mathbf{I}_{\mathbf{rabbit}} \\ &\left(N = 59, SD = 0.26, R^2 = 0.733, F = 29\right)\end{aligned} \tag{41}$$

The e · **E** and s · **S** terms were not statistically significant and were eliminated from the final derived correlation model. The poor R^2 statistics for Eqn. 41 is due, at least in part, to the small spread in the values of log P_{skin}, from log P_{skin} = -0.82 to log P_{skin} = 1.61, for a range of only 2.43 log units. Carboxylic acids were found to be systematically retained in blood or plasma more than calculated. An indicator descriptor, $\mathbf{I_{acid}}$, was needed to describe the log Pskin data of solutes containing a carboxylic acid functional group. The $\mathbf{I_{acid}}$ descriptor equals unity for carboxylic acid solutes, and takes the value of $\mathbf{I_{acid}}$ = 0 for all other compounds. The second indicator descriptor in Eqn. 41 was needed to combine the rat skin ($\mathbf{I_{rabbit}}$ = 0) and rabbit skin ($\mathbf{I_{rabbit}}$) partitioning data into a single correlation model. The 0.059 $\mathbf{I_{rabbit}}$ term amounts to a 0.059 log unit offset, which is likely less than the experimental uncertainty in the measured log P_{skin} data. If the 0.059 $\mathbf{I_{rabbit}}$ term is omitted, the squared correlation coefficient decreases to R^2 = 0.608.

Theoretical models of passive diffusion are based on Fick's law of diffusion and the conversation of particle numbers. Fick's law of diffusion states that a chemical diffuses from a region of higher concentration to a region of lower concentration with a magnitude that is directly proportional to the chemical's concentration gradient. When applied to trans-stratum corneum diffusion, the amount of chemical passing through a unit area of the stratum corneum per unit time (J) is given by

$$J = -\frac{K_{p,sc} D \Delta C}{h} \tag{42}$$

where $K_{p,sc}$ is the chemical's solvent-to-stratum corneum partition coefficient, D represents the chemical's diffusivity in the stratum corneum lipid matrix and h is the apparent skin thickness (*i.e.*, the diffusion pathlength). Under the assumption of constant donor concentration and sink conditions (zero receptor phase concentration) Eqn. 42 simplifies to

$$J_{SS} = \frac{K_{p,sc} D C_{donor}}{h} \tag{43}$$

The permeability coefficient, k_p, is the coefficient of proportionality between the steady-state flux J_{SS} and the donor concentration, C_{donor}.

Skin permeability experiments are generally performed *in vitro* using a Franz diffusion cell (shown in Figure 8). A freshly excised skin sample is mounted on the receptor compartment of the Franz cell with the stratum corneum facing upwards into the donor compartment and the dermis facing the receptor compartment. The latter compartment is filled with the receptor solution (often a phosphate saline solution buffered at pH of 7.4), and maintained at a constant temperature of 37 °C with a water jacketed cell under constant stirring. The donor compartment is filled with the vehicle solution containing the dissolved chemical of interest. At appropriate time intervals, aliquots of the receptor medium are withdrawn for analysis, and immediately replaced with an equal volume of fresh medium. Alternative diffusion cell designs and mathematical procedures for calculating the drug's diffusivity and permeability coefficient from the experimental permeation results are described in greater detail elsewhere (Friend, 1992; Hathout *et al.*, 2010). For *in vitro* skin penetration studies, the skin retention of a drug can be assessed by the use of radiolabeled drugs (usually carbon-14 or tritium labeled). Skin samples should be exposed to the drug for no more than a maximum of 24 hours because of deterioration of skin integrity with time.

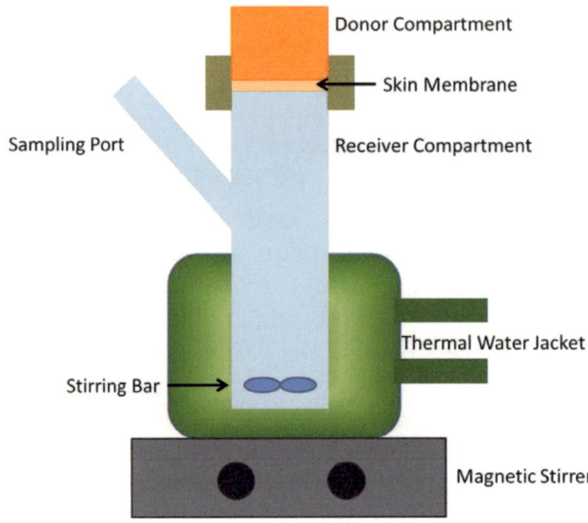

Fig. 8. Franz diffusion cell used to measure skin permeability coefficients

The parallel artificial membrane permeability assay (PAMPA) has been suggested as a high throughput screening method for rapid determination of passive transport permeability in connection with gastrointestinal (GI) absorption (Sugano *et al.*, 2002), blood-brain barrier penetration (Mensch *et al.*, 2010 and skin permeation (Ottaviani *et al.*, 2006). In the PAMPA method a 96-well filter plate coated with a liquid membrane is used to separate the donor and receptor compartments. Artificial membrane selection depends on the transport property to be determined. Ottaviani *et al.* (2006) found a reasonably accurate mathematical correlation between human skin permeability coefficient, k_p, and the effective permeability coefficient, k*eff*, for a set of 31 compounds

$$\log k_p = 1.34 \log k_{eff} + 0.28 \quad (N = 31, SD = 0.42, R^2 = 0.81, F = 31) \tag{44}$$

tested through an artificial membrane consisting of 70 % silicone and 30 % isopropyl myristate. The authors further noted that presence of isopropyl myristate as only a hydrogen-bond acceptor group in the artificial membrane was in accord with previous results demonstrating that stratum corneum lipids were better hydrogen-bond acceptors than hydrogen-bond donors.

Abraham and Martins (2004) reported an Abraham model correlation for human skin permeability coefficients from aqueous solution, k_p,

$$\text{Log } k_p(\text{cm}/\text{s}) = -5.426 - 0.106\mathbf{E} - 0.473\mathbf{E} - 0.473\mathbf{A} - 3.000\mathbf{B} + 2.296\mathbf{V} \quad (N = 119, SD = 0.461, R^2 = 0.832, F = 112) \tag{45}$$

based on a database containing 119 experimental values at a common temperature of 37 °C. The authors adjusted the experimental data for ionization by assuming that the measured permeability coefficient was a simple addition of terms in Eqn. 46

$$k_p = f_{neutral} k_{p,neutral} + f_{ionic} k_{p,ionic} \tag{46}$$

where, k_p, $k_{p,ionic}$, and $k_{p,neutral}$ represent the overall permeation coefficient, that due to the ionic species, and that due to the neutral species; f_{ionic} and $f_{neutral}$ denote the fraction of ionic and neutral species at a given pH. For ionizable acids the skin permeability coefficient of the neutral molecule, $k_{p,neutral}$, was so much larger than the skin permeability coefficient of the ionic form, $k_{p,ionic}$, that the experimental unadjusted values of k_p was adjusted to give $k_{p,neutral}$ from the fraction of the neutral form present under the experimental conditions of pH. For ionizable bases the ratio of $k_{p,neutral}$ to $k_{p,ionic}$ was assumed to be 17.5, and this value was used to obtain $k_{p,neutral}$ values from experimental unadjusted values of k_p. If the experimental pH is near to the basic pK_a, such an adjustment will be very close to the adjustment that assumes negligible permeation of ionizable species. But as the difference in ($pH - pK_a$) becomes larger, the adjustment will be smaller than that of negligible permeation of ionic species. To account for the temperature differences, the authors adjusted experimental log k_p values by 0.20 units from 32 °C to 37 °C, and by 0.48 units from 25 °C to 37 °C. The main factors that influence log k_p are hydrogen bond basicity (b · B term) that decreases log k_p, and solute volume (v · **V** term) that increases log k_p. Solute dipolarity/polarizability (s · S term) and hydrogen bond acidity (a · **A** term) make minor contributions, both in the sense of lowering log k_p.

9. Conclusion

The Abraham solvation parameter model provides an in silico method for estimating ADMET properties of potential drug molecules in the early stages of drug discovery. To date mathematical expressions have been reported for predicting water-to-organic solvent partition coefficients and solubilities in more than 70 organic solvents, air-to-tissue and blood-to-tissue partition coefficients for 5 human and rat tissues, water-to-human skin and blood-to-rat/rabbit skin partitions, human skin permeability coefficients, and rat (Zhao *et al.*, 2003) and human (Zhao *et al.*, 2002) intestinal absorption. Expressions are also available for estimating Draize rabbit eye test scores for pure liquids and eye irritation thresholds in humans (Abraham *et al.*, 2003), odor detection thresholds and nasal pungency of volatile organic compounds (VOCs) (Abraham *et al.*, 2007b), and the minimum alveolar concentration (MAC) for inhalation anesthetics in rats (Abraham *et al.*, 2008b). The number of derived Abraham model correlations is expected in future years as more experimental data becomes available. Predictive applications require as input parameters the numerical values of the drug candidate's solute descriptors, which are easily calculable from measured solubility and partition coefficient data.

10. References

Abraham, M. H. & McGowan, J. C. (1987) The use of characteristic volumes to measure cavity terms in reversed phase liquid chromatography. *Chromatographia* 23 (4) 243–246.

Abraham, M. H. (1993a) Scales of solute hydrogen-bonding: their construction and application to physicochemical and biochemical processes. *Chemical Society Reviews* 22 (2),73-83.

Abraham, M. H. (1993b) Application of solvation equations to chemical and biochemical processes. *Pure and Applied Chemistry* 65 (12), 2503-2512.

Abraham, M. H.; Hassanisadi, M.; Jalali-Heravi, M.; Ghafourian, T.; Cain, W. S. & Cometto-Muniz, J. E. (2003) Draize rabbit eye test compatibility with eye irritation thresholds in humans: a quantitative structure-activity relationship analysis. *Toxicological Sciences* 76 (2), 384-391.

Abraham, M. H. (2004) The factors that influence permeation across the blood-brain barrier. *European Journal of Medicinal Chemistry* 39 (3), 235-240.

Abraham, M. H.; Ibrahim, A. & Zissimos, A. M. (2004) Determination of sets of solute descriptors from chromatographic measurements. *Journal of Chromatography, A* 1037 (1-2), 29-47.

Abraham, M. H. & Martins, F. (2004) Human skin permeation and partition: General linear free-energy relationship analyses. *Journal of Pharmaceutical Sciences* 93 (6), 1508-1523.

Abraham, M. H.; Ibrahim, A. & Acree, W. E. Jr., (2005) Air-to-blood distribution of volatile organic compounds: a linear free energy analysis. *Chemical Research in Toxicology* 18 (5), 904-911.

Abraham, M. H. & Ibrahim, A. (2006) Air to fat and blood to fat distribution of volatile organic compounds and drugs: Linear free energy analyses. *European Journal of Medicinal Chemistry* 41 (12), 1430-1438.

Abraham, M. H.; Ibrahim, A. & Acree, W. E (2006a) Air to brain, blood to brain and plasma to brain distribution of volatile organic compounds: linear free energy analyses. *European Journal of Medicinal Chemistry* 41 (4), 494-502.

Abraham, M. H.; Ibrahim, A.; Zhao, Y. & Acree, W. E., Jr. (2006b) A data base for partition of volatile organic compounds and drugs from blood/plasma/serum to brain, and an LFER analysis of the data. *Journal of Pharmaceutical Sciences* 95 (10), 2091-2100.

Abraham, M. H.; Ibrahim, A. & Acree, W. E., Jr. (2006c) Air to muscle and blood/plasma to muscle distribution of volatile organic compounds and drugs: linear free energy analyses. *Chemical Research in Toxicology* 19 (6), 801-808.

Abraham, M. H. & Ibrahim, A. (2007) Blood or plasma to skin distribution of drugs: a linear free energy analysis. *International Journal of Pharmaceutics* 329 (1-2) 129-134.

Abraham, M. H.; Ibrahim, A. & Acree, W. E., Jr. (2007a) Air to liver partition coefficients for volatile organic compounds and blood to liver partition coefficients for volatile organic compounds and drugs. *European Journal of Medicinal Chemistry* 42 (6), 743-751.

Abraham, M. H.; Sanchez-Moreno, R.; Cometto-Muniz, J. E. & Cain, W. S. (2007b) A quantitative structure-activity analysis on the relative sensitivity of the olfactory and the nasal trigeminal chemosensory systems. *Chemical Senses* 32 (7), 711-719.

Abraham, M. H.; Ibrahim, A. & Acree, W. E, Jr. (2008a) Air to lung partition coefficients for volatile organic compounds and blood to lung partition coefficients for volatile organic compounds and drug. *European Journal of Medicinal Chemistry* 43 (3), 478-485.

Abraham, M. H.; Acree, W. E., Jr.; Mintz, C. & Payne, S. (2008b) Effect of anesthetic structure on inhalation anesthesia: implications for the mechanism. *Journal of Pharmaceutical Sciences* 97 (6), 2373-2384.

Abraham, M. H.; Acree, W. E., Jr. & Cometto-Muniz, J. E. (2009a) Partition of compounds from water and from air into amides. *New Journal of Chemistry* 33 (10), 2034-2043.

Abraham, M. H.; Gil-Lostes, J. & Fatemi, M. (2009b) Prediction of milk/plasma concentration ratios of drugs and environmental pollutants. *European Journal of Medicinal Chemistry* 44 (6), 2452-2458.

Abraham, M. H. & Acree, W. E., Jr. (2010a) Equations for the transfer of neutral molecules and ionic species from water to organic phases. *Journal of Organic Chemistry* 75 (4), 1006-1015.

Abraham, M. H. & Acree, W. E., Jr. (2010b) Solute descriptors for phenoxide anions and their use to establish correlations of rates of reaction of anions with iodomethane. *Journal of Organic Chemistry* 75 (9), 3021-3026.

Abraham, M. H. & Acree, W. E., Jr. (2010c) The transfer of neutral molecules, ions and ionic species from water to ethylene glycol and to propylene carbonate; descriptors for pyridinium cations. *New Journal of Chemistry* 34 (10), 2298-2305.

Abraham, M. H. & Acree, W. E., Jr. (2010d) The transfer of neutral molecules, ions and ionic species from water to wet octanol. *Physical Chemistry Chemical Physics* 12 (40), 13182-13188.

Abraham, M. H.; Smith, R. E.; Luchtefeld, R.; Boorem, A. J.; Luo, R. & Acree, W. E., Jr. (2010) Prediction of solubility of drugs and other compounds in organic solvents. *Journal of Pharmaceutical Sciences* 99 (3), 1500-1515.

Abraham, M. H. (2011) The permeation of neutral molecules, ions and ionic species: brain permeation as an example. *Journal of Pharmaceutical Sciences*, 100, (5), 1690-1701.

Acree, W. E., Jr. & Abraham, M. H. (2002) Solubility of crystalline nonelectrolyte solutes in organic solvents: mathematical correlation of benzil solubilities with the Abraham general solvation model. *Journal of Solution Chemistry* 31 (4), 293-303

ADME Boxes, version*, Advanced Chemistry Development, 110 Yonge Street, 14th Floor, Toronto, Ontario, M5C 1T4, Canada.

Ahmed, H.; Poole, C. F. & Kozerski, G. E. (2007) Determination of descriptors for organosilicon compounds by gas chromatography and non-aqueous liquid-liquid partitioning. *Journal of Chromatography, A* 1169 (1-2), 179-192.

Ahmed, H. & Poole, C. F. (2006a) Distribution of neutral organic compounds between n-heptane and methanol or N,N-dimethylformamide. *Journal of Separation Science* 29 (14), 2158-2165.

Ahmed, Hamid & Poole, Colin F. (2006b) Model for the distribution of neutral organic compounds between n-hexane and acetonitrile. *Journal of Chromatography, A* 1104 (1-2), 82-90.

Alam, M. I.; Beg, S.; Samad, A.; Baboota, S.; Hohli, K.; Ali, J.; Ahuja, A. & Akbar, M. (2010) Strategy for effective brain drug delivery. *European Journal of Pharmaceutical Science* 40 (5), 385-403.

Amidon, G. L.; Lennenas, H.; Shah, V. P. & Crison, J. R. (1995) A theoretical basis for a biopharmaceutic drug classification: the correlation in vitro drug product dissolution and in vivo bioavailability. *Pharmaceutical Research* 12 (3), 413-420.

Arey, J. S.; Green, W. H., Jr. & Gschwend, P. M. (2005) The electrostatic origin of Abraham's solute polarity parameter. *Journal of Physical Chemistry B* 109 (15), 7564-7573.

Atapattu, S. N. & Poole, C. F. (2009) Determination of descriptors for semivolatile organosilicon compounds by gas chromatography and non-aqueous liquid-liquid partition. *Journal of Chromatography, A* 1216 (45), 7882-7888.

Begley, D. J.; Khan, E. U.; Rollinson, C. & Abbott, J. (2000) in 'The blood-brain barrier and drug delivery to the CNS, Ed by Befley, D.J.; Bradbury, M. W. & Kreuter, J., Marcel Dekker, New York, 2000.

Berthod, A.; Han, Y. Il. & Armstrong, D. W. (1988) Centrifugal partition chromatography. V. Octanol-water partition coefficients, direct and indirect determination. *Journal of Liquid Chromatography* 11 (7), 1441-1456.

Berthod, A.; Menges, R. A. & Armstrong, D. W. (1992) Direct octanol-water partition coefficient determination using co-current chromatography. *Journal of Liquid Chromatography* 15 (15-16), 2769-2785.

Charlton, A. K.; Daniels, C. R.; Acree, W. E., Jr. & Abraham, M. H. (2003) Solubility of crystalline nonelectrolyte solutes in organic solvents: mathematical correlation of acetylsalicylic acid solubilities with the Abraham general solvation model. *Journal of Solution Chemistry* 32 (12), 1087-1102.

Cruciani, G.; Pastor, M. & Guba, W. (2000) VolSurf: a new tool for the pharmacokinetic optimization of lead compounds. *European Journal of Pharmaceutical Sciences* 11 (Suppl. 2), S29-S39.

Eixarch, H.; Haltner-Ukomadu, E.; Beisswenger, C. & Bock, U. (2010) Drug delivery to the lung: permeability and physicochemical characteristics of drugs as the basis for a pulmonary Biopharmaceutical Classification System (pBCS). *Journal of Epithelial Biology and Pharmacology* 3, 1-14.

Faller, B.; Grimm, H. P.; Loeuillet-Ritzler, F.; Arnold, S. & Briand, X. (2005) High-throughput lipophilicity measurement with immobilized artificial membranes. *Journal of Medicinal Chemistry* 48 (7), 2571-2576.

Friend, D. R. (1992) *In vitro* skin permeation techniques. *Journal of Controlled Re*lease 18, 235-248.

Gao, X.; Yu, C. H.; Tam, K. Y. & Tsang, S. C. (2005) New magnetic nano-absorbent for the determination of n-octanol/water partition coefficients. *Journal of Pharmaceutical and Biomedical Analysis* 38 (2), 197-203.

Guthrie J. P. (2009) A blind challenge for computational solvation free energies: introduction and overview. *Journal of Physical Chemistry B* 113 (14) 4501-4507.

Hathout, R. M.; Woodman, T. J.; Mansour, S.; Mortada, N. D.; Geneidi, A. S. & Guy, R. H. (2010) Microemulsion formulations for the transdermal delivery of testosterone. *European Journal of Pharmaceutical Sciences* 40 (3), 188-196.

Henchoz, Y.; Romand, S.; Schuppler, J.; Rudaz, S.; Veathey, J.-L. & Carrupt, P. A. (2010) High-throughput log P determination by MEEKC coupled with UV and MS detections. *Electrophoresis*, 31 (5), 952-964.

Hewitt, M.; Cronin, M. T. D.; Enoch, S. J.; Madden, J. C.; Roberts, D. W. & Dearden, J. C. (2009) In silico prediction of aqueous solubility: the solubility challenge. *Journal of Chemical Information and Modeling* 49 (11), 2572–2587.

Holbrook K A. & Odland G F. (1974) Regional differences in the thickness (cell layers) of the human stratum corneum: an ultrastructural analysis. *The Journal of Investigative Dermatology* 62 (4), 415-422.

Howard, P. H. & Meylan, W. M. (1997) Handbook of Physical properties of Organic Chemicals, CRC Press, Boca Raton, 1997.

Ishihama, Y. & Asakawa, N. (1999) Characterization of the lipophilicity scales using vectors from solvation energy descriptors. *Journal of Pharmaceutical Sciences* 88 (12), 1305-1312.

Karunasekara, T. & Poole, C. F. (2010) Model for the partition of neutral compounds between n-heptane and formamide. *Journal of Separation Science* 33 (8), 1167-1173.

Keck, C.; Kobierski, S.; Mauludin, R. & Muller, R. H. (2008) Second generation of drug nanocrystals for delivery of poorly soluble drugs: smartcrystal technology. *Dosis*, 2 (24), 124-128 .

Li, H.; Yap, C. W.; Ung, C. Y.; Xue, Y.; Cao, Z. W. & Chen, Y. Z. (2005) Effect of selection of molecular descriptors on the prediction of blood-brain barrier penetrating and nonpenetrating agents by statistical learning methods. *Journal of Chemical Information and Modeling* 45 (5) 1376-1384.

Li, Q.-S.; Li, Z. & Wang, S. (2008) Solubility of trimethoprim (TMP) in different organic solvents from (278 to 333) K. *Journal of Chemical and Engineering Data* 53 (1), 286-287.

Lipinski, C. A.; Lombardo, F.; Dominy, B. W. & Feeney, P. J. (2001) Experimental and computational approaches to estimate solubility and permeability in drug discovery and development settings. *Advances in Drug Delivery Reviews* 46 (1-3), 3-26.

Llinàs, A.; Glen, R. C. & Goodman, J. M. (2008) Solubility challenge: can you predict solubilities of 32 molecules using a database of 100 reliable measurements. *Journal of Chemical Information and Modeling* 48 (7), 1289–1303.

Lukyanov, A. N. & Torchilin, V. P. (2004) Micelles from lipid derivatives of water-soluble polymers as delivery systems for poorly soluble drugs. *Advanced Drug Delivery Reviews* 56 (9), 1273-1289.

McDuffie, B. (1981) Estimation of octanol/water partition coefficients for organic pollutants using reverse-phase HPLC *Chemosphere* 10 (1), 73-83.

Menges, R. A.; Bertrand, G. L. & Armstrong, D. W. (1990) Direct measurement of octanolwater partition coefficients using centrifugal partition chromatography with a back-flushing technique. *Journal of Liquid Chromatography* 13 (15), 3061-3077.

Mensch, J.; Jaroskova, L.; Anderson, W.; Mells, A.; Mackle, C.; Verreck, G.; Brewster, M. E. & Augustinjns, P. (2010) Application of PAMPA-models to predict BBB permeability including efflux ratio, plasma protein binding and physicochemical parameters. *International Journal of Pharmaceutics* 395, 182-197.

Michaels A. S, Chandrasekaran S. K, & Shaw J. E. (1975).Drug permeation through human skin: theory and *in vitro* experimental measurement. *AIChE Journal* 21 (5), 985–996.

Mintz, C.; Clark, M.; Acree, W. E., Jr. & Abraham, M. H. (2007) Enthalpy of solvation correlations for gaseous solutes dissolved in water and in 1-octanol based on the Abraham model. *Journal of Chemical Information and Modeling* 47 (1), 115-121.

Monteiro-Riviere, N. A.; Inman, A. O.; Mak, V.; Wertz, P. & Riviere, J. E. (2001) Effect of selective lipid extraction from different body regions on epidermal barrier function. *Pharmaceutical Research* 18 (7) 992-998.

Mutelet, F. & Rogalski, M. (2001) Experimental determination and prediction of the gas-liquid n-hexadecane partition coefficients. *Journal of Chromatography A* 923 (102), 153-163.

Netzlaff, F.; Schaefer, U. F.; Lehr, C.-M.; Meiers, P.; Stahl, J.; Kietzmann, M. & Niedorf, F. (2006) Comparison of bovine udder skin with human and porcine skin in percutaneous permeation experiments. *ATLA, Alternatives to Laboratory Animals* 34 (5), 499-513.

Nicholls, A.; Mobley, D. L.; Guthrie, J. P.; Chodera, J. D.; Bayly, C. I.; Cooper, M. D. & Pande, V. S. (2008) Predicting small-molecule solvation free energies: an informal blind test for computational chemistry. *Journal of Medical Chemistry* 51 (4) 769-779.

Ottaviani, G.; Martel, S. & Carrupt, P.-A. (2006) Parallel artificial membrane permeability assay: A new membrane for the fast prediction of passive human skin permeability. *Journal of Medicinal Chemistry* 49 (6), 3948-3954.

Platts, J. A.; Butina, D.; Abraham, M. H. & Hersey, A. (1999) Estimation of molecular linear free energy relation descriptors using a group contribution approach. *Journal of Chemical Information and Computational Science* 39 (5), 835-845.

Poole, S. K. & Poole, C. F. (2003) Separation methods for estimating octanol-water partition coefficients. *Journal of Chromatographty B* 797 (1-2), 3-19.

Qian, J. & Poole, C. F. (2007) Distribution of neutral organic compounds between n-heptane and fluorine-containing alcohols. *Journal of Chromatography, A* 1143 (1-2), 276-283.

Ribeiro, M. M. B.; Melo, M. N.; Serrano, I. D.; Santos, N. C. & Castanho, M. A. R. B. (2010) Drug-lipid interaction evaluation: why a 19th century solution? *Trends in Pharmacological Sciences* 31 (10), 449-454.

Sangster, J. (1989) Octanol-water partition coefficients of simple organic compounds. *Journalof Physical and Chemical Reference Data* 18 (3), 1111-1229.

Sugano, K.; Takata, N.; Machida, M.; Saitoh, K. & Terada, K. (2002) Prediction of passive intestinal absorption using bio-mimetic artificial membrane permeation assay and the paracellular pathway. *International Journal of Pharmaceutics* 241 (2), 241-251

Sugano, K.; Kato, T.; Suzuki, K.; Keiko, K.; Sajaku, T. & Mano, T. (2006) High throughput solubility measurement with automated polarized light microscopy analysis. *Journal of Pharmaceutical Sciences* 95 (10), 2115-2122.

Veith, G. D.; Austin, N. M. & Morris, R. T. (1979) A rapid method for estimating log P for organic chemicals. *Water Research* 13 (1), 43-47

Wang, J. M.; Hou, T. J. & Xu, X. J. (2009) Aqueous solubility prediction based on weighted atom type counts and solvent accessible surface areas. *Journal of Chemical Information and Modeling* 49 (3), 571–581.

Wohnsland, F. & Faller, B. (2001) High-throughput permeability pH profile and high-throughput alkane/water log P with artificial membranes. *Journal of Medicinal Chemistry* 44 (6), 923-930.

Wu, C. Y. & Benet, L. Z. (2005) Predicting drug disposition via application of BCS. Transportabsorption/elimination interplay and development of a biopharmaceutics drug disposition classification system. *Pharmaceutical Research* 22 (1), 11-23.

Zhao, Y. H.; Le, J.; Abraham, M. H.; Hersey, A.; Eddershaw, P. J.; Luscombe, C. N.; Butina, D.; Beck, G.; Sherborne, B.; Cooper, I. & Platts, J. A. (2002) Evaluation of human intestinal absorption data and subsequent derivation of a quantitative structure-activity relationship (QSAR) with the Abraham descriptors. *Journal of Pharmaceutical Sciences* 90 (6), 749-784

Zhao, Y. H.; Abraham, M. H.; Hersey, A. & Luscombe, C. N. (2003) Quantitative relationship between rat intestinal absorption and Abraham descriptors. *European Journal of Medicinal Chemistry* 38 (11-12), 939-947.

Zhao, Y. H.; Abraham, M. H.; Ibrahim, A.; Fish, P. V.; Cole, S.; Lewis, M. L.; de Groot, M. J. & Reynolds, D. P. (2007) Predicting penetration across the blood-brain barrier from simple descriptors and fragmentation schemes. *Journal of Chemical Information and Modeling* 47 (1), 170-175.

Zissimos, A. M.; Abraham, M. H.; Barker, M. C.; Box, K. J.; & Tam, K. Y. (2002a) Calculation of Abraham descriptors from solvent-water partition coefficients in four different systems; evaluation of different methods of calculation. *Journal of the Chemical Society, Perkin Transactions 2* (3), 470-477.

Zissimos, A. M.; Abraham, M. H.; Du, C. M.; Valko, K.; Bevan, C.; Reynolds, D.; Wood, J.; & Tam, K. Y. (2002b) Calculation of Abraham descriptors from experimental data from seven HPLC systems; evaluation of five different methods of calculation. *Journal of the Chemical Society, Perkin Transactions 2* (12), 2001-2010.

6

Variability of Plasma Methadone Concentration in Opiate Dependent Receiving Methadone: A Personalised Approach Towards Optimizing Dose

Nasir Mohamad[1,3], Nor Hidayah Abu Bakar[2], Tan Soo Choon[3], Sim Hann Liang[3], NIM Nazar[3], Ilya Irinaz Idrus[3] and Rusli Ismail[3]

[1]*Department of Emergency Medicine, School of Medical Sciences, Health Campus, Universiti Sains Malaysia, Kubang Kerian, Kelantan,*

[2]*Department of Pathology, Hospital Raja Perempuan Zainab II, Kota Bharu, Kelantan,*

[3]*Pharmacogenetic Research Group, Institute for Research in Molecular Medicine (INFORMM), Health Campus, Universiti Sains Malaysia, Kubang Kerian, Kelantan, Malaysia*

1. Introduction

1.1 Methadone and methadone maintenance therapy (MMT): An overview

Methadone acts on the opioid receptors and produces many of the same effects of morphine and heroin. In the treatment of opioid dependence, methadone has cross-tolerance with other opioid, including heroin and morphine and a long duration of effect. Higher doses of methadone can block the euphoric effects of heroin, morphine, and similar drugs. As a result, properly dosed methadone patients can reduce or stop altogether their use of these substances.

Methadone is a misunderstood drug and ignorance about it is common. Even professionals, physicians and pharmacists who are supposed to be the "guardians" of MMT receive very little training about the very medication that they are responsible for. To compound the issue, addiction is mostly viewed not as a disease and its care is frequently relegated to the lay public, at least until very recently. In Malaysia, addiction has solely been under the charge of "*Agensi Anti Dadah Kebangsaan*" (AADK), an agency that has mainly adopted a criminal approach to addiction. However, this has recently changed in Malaysia. Addiction is now recognized as a medical illness, under the purview of the medical professionals.

Nevertheless, many in the medical profession only have a rudimentary understanding of addiction. Most physicians, pharmacists and nurses receive very little training about addiction and much less regarding methadone. Thus, generally, both medical and other caregivers have very limited knowledge about addiction and much less about methadone. They have generally been taught to approach addiction as a character disorder and administer methadone as a substitute.

1.2 Pharmacogenetic of methadone

Methadone has variable pharmacology. It binds to the μ-opioid receptor, the NMDA ionotropic glutamate receptor to exert its effects. Its metabolism is mediated by several enzymes including CYP3A4, CYP2B6 and CYP2D6, enzymes that are polymorphic and hence exhibit great variability. It is mainly administered through the oral route and adverse effects include hypoventilation, constipation and miosis, in addition to tolerance, dependence and withdrawal difficulties.

As a full μ-opioid agonist, methadone exhibits all the opiate-like effects. Furthermore, its binding to the glutamatergic NMDA (N-methyl-D-aspartate) receptor. This makes it a receptor antagonist against glutamate which is the primary excitatory neurotransmitter in the CNS. NMDA receptors modulate long term excitation and memory formation. NMDA antagonists such as dextromethorphan (DXM), ketamine, tiletamine and ibogaine have been studied for their role in decreasing the development of tolerance to opioids and as possible for eliminating addiction /tolerance /withdrawal. Its action on the NMDA has been proposed as a mechanism by which methadone decreases craving for opioids (Xiao *et al*, 2001).

Methadone is a lipophilic drug and requires biotransformation for elimination. It has a slow metabolism and is longer lasting than morphine-based drugs. Typically its elimination half-life ranges from 15 to 60 hours with a mean of around 22 hours. Due to the polymorphic nature of its metabolism, its metabolism rates vary greatly between individuals, up to a factor of 100. This variability is apparently due to genetic variability in the production of the associated enzymes CYP3A4, CYP2B6 and CYP2D6. Several studies have been conducted to explain the intra- as well as inter-individual variability in methadone's pharmacokinetic and clinical response. Typically, methadone is a substrate for several CYP450 enzymes as well as P-glycoprotein (PGP). Many Single Nucleotide Polymorphisms (SNPs) have been reported to contribute to its variability. Furthermore, as it binds to μ-receptors, SNPs in *OPRM* gene that encodes for these receptors may contribute to the clinical response in MMT patients. Thus, SNPs in *OPRM* gene, *CYP* gene and *ABCB1 (MDR1)* gene may contribute to determine the clinical outcomes of the MMT (Lötsch *et al*, 2009).

1.3 Pharmacokinetic of methadone

The pharmacokinetic parameters of methadone were first published in 1975 (Verebely *et al*, 1975). Methadone is a lipophilic basic drug with a pKa of 9.2, which is administered orally in a racemic mixture. There is strong evidence that the enantiomers differ in their distribution and elimination, though the majority of the studies were carried out on the racemic mixture. It has been suggested that methadone undergoes adaptive changes during chronic use according to the administered doses.

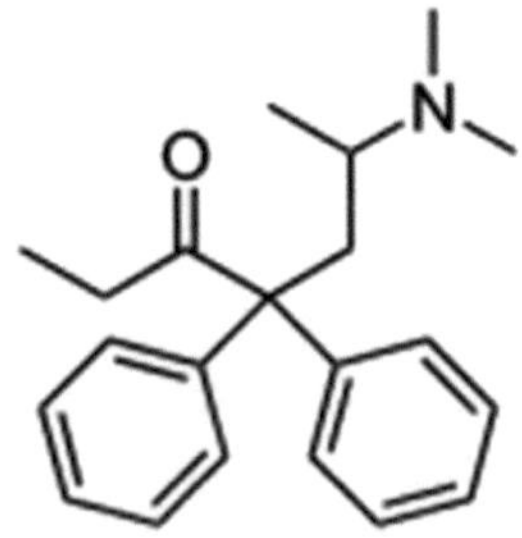

Fig. 1.1. Methadone, (*RS*)-6-(Dimethylamino)-4,4-diphenylheptan-3-one

Several attributes have been suggested such as clearance and *CYP3A4*. Accordingly, several pharmacokinetic studies have been carried out to investigate whether therapeutic drug monitoring (TDM) is effective as a clinical endpoint, on the one hand, and to study the methadone kinetic profile, on the other. There has been suggestive evidence to non-frequently monitor the kinetic of methadone to explain some unpredicted clinical response (Loimer and Schmid, 1992; Schmidt *et al*, 1993; Wolff and Hay, 1994; de Vos *et al*, 1996). It may be useful especially when all other measures have been taken adequately and a patient still cannot hold on methadone with high doses.

It should be noted that methadone Cp cannot be used directly to describe the clinical response, as a certain time is required for the drug to distribute adequately in the nervous system. Thus, some researchers have suggested the use of an effect-compartment or link-model to describe the effect appropriately (Ekblom *et al*, 1993). So far, only four studies have modeled methadone by this approach and only one among them for MMT patients (Dyer *et al*, 1999). It was noticed that there is an inverse relationship between plasma concentrations and withdrawal scores and pupil diameters. On the other hand, there was a direct relationship between plasma concentrations and pain threshold in the same patients. The area under the curve did not differ between those who reported withdrawal symptoms and those who did not. The study suggested that there is correlation between methadone clinical responses and changes in the plasma levels for methadone racemic mixture.

1.3.1 Absorption

The absorption of methadone following oral administration is fast and almost complete. The mean time to achieve peak concentration ranges from 2.5 - 30 hours depending on the formulation (Wolff *et al*, 1991). Oral bioavailability of methadone may range from as little as 45 percent up to 90 percent following a single dose (Meresaar *et al*, 1981). As methadone is a basic drug, acid secretions may contribute to such huge variability (Kukanich *et al*, 2005).

1.3.2 Distribution

Being a lipo-soluble drug, methadone distributes widely in body tissues such as: liver, lung, kidney, gut, brain, and muscle with different distribution coefficients (Sawe, 1986). In opioid addicts, the volume of distribution at a steady state (Vss) ranged from 0.2 to 9.2 L/kg. On the other hand, in patients with chronic pain, Vss ranged from 1.71 to 5.34 L/kg (Inturrisi *et al*, 1990), though higher doses are usually given in such situations.

Methadone pharmacokinetic is described as a two-compartment model. Although there are wide differences in the reported clearance, the reported terminal half-life was estimated to range from 23-26 hours. Half-life depends also on the volume of distribution, making the explanations much more complicated and inconclusive (Eap *et al*, 2002; Li *et al*, 2008)

Methadone binds to plasma protein to a high degree of 86 percent, predominantly to acute α-glycoprotein (AAG) (Romach *et al*, 1981; Eap *et al*, 1990). AAG is an acute phase protein that exhibits significant variations in its plasma levels according to the physiological and/or pathological situation of the patient (Fournier *et al*, 2000; Yang *et al*, 2006; Mestriner *et al*, 2007). AAG levels are significantly increased in stress, leading to very low concentrations in the free fraction (fu) of methadone in cancer patients compared to healthy participants (Abramson, 1982; Gómez *et al*, 1995). Therefore, some studies have measured the concentration of AAG itself to study the impact of their concentration on methadone concentration and / or clinical outcomes. Rowland and Tozer (1995) have stated that 'after a rapid input of methadone, a decrease in fu will be indicated by an increase in Cp, because Vss is proportional to fu. On the other hand, Cu levels remain unchanged. So, if the Cu is the pharmacologically active concentration, a decrease in fu will not modify the maximum response. Thus, it has been suggested that AAG is significantly higher in patients exhibiting abstinence syndrome compared to those who are stable (Garrido *et al*, 2000) and AAG may contribute to the variations in methadone plasma levels.

Other factors that may contribute to variability include age and sex. It has been suggested that these factors may explain about 33 percent of the inter-individual variations in Vss. These parameters are found to be higher in females and they are directly related to weight (Wolff *et al*, 2000).

Furthermore, it has also been suggested that a time-dependent increase in methadone clearance may result from auto-induction of its own metabolism by *CYP3A4*, and the change in Vss may be due to up or down-regulation of AAG (Rostami-Hodjegan *et al*, 1999). Therefore, a time-dependent decrease in Vss may be associated with the observed time-dependent increase in AAG.

1.3.3 Elimination

Generally, there is a huge inter-individual variability in methadone clearance that can reach up to 20 -100 folds in magnitude (Eap *et al*, 2002; Li *et al*, 2008). Methadone is eliminated by hepatic metabolism and renal excretion. It has been shown that at urinary pH of six and above, renal clearance accounts for four percent only. However, when urinary pH was lower than 6, the clearance of unchanged drug will be increased by 33 percent (Rostami-Hodjegan *et al*, 1999). It was concluded that, about 20-50 percent of the inter-individual variability can be explained by urinary excretion (KuKanich and Borum, 2008). With regard to hepatic clearance, methadone can be recognized as a drug with a low extraction ratio, 0.16 in MMT patients.

2. Objective of clinical study

2.1 General objective

To investigate factors that influence successful MMT in opiate-dependent individuals,

2.2 Specific objective

To investigate the impact of daily clinical methadone dose on plasma concentration of methadone.

3. Clinical study

The study involves opiate-dependent individuals who consented, met our study criteria and were invited to participate in the study. The study involved them taking prescribed doses of daily methadone according to Methadone Maintenance Therapy (MMT) guidelines prepared by the Malaysian Ministry of Health and be monitored regularly based on our study protocols. They were followed up for 12 months during the study period. At follow up, 5 ml of venous blood were drawn for the determination plasma methadone level using in-house methadone ELISA kit.

However, at 12th month follow up, 88 out of the 128 participants fail to meet the inclusion criteria. Thus, in order to assess the efficacy of low dose methadone on the withdrawal effect and sleeping quality, a subset of only 40 patients was further selected to participate. They were given a fixed 40 mg daily dose of methadone. Their withdrawal score and sleeping quality were assessed during the fourth week of the study.

4. Results

One hundred and twenty eight patients were enrolled for this pilot study. Their doses were titrated appropriately as tolerated. However, at 12th month follow up, 88 patients out of the 128 participants fail to meet the inclusion criteria. Thus, in order to assess the efficacy of low dose methadone on the withdrawal effect and sleeping quality, a subset of only 40 patients was further selected to participate where they were given a fixed 40 mg daily dose of methadone. Daily dose averaged 57.2 mg (SD ± 22.7) (Table 4.1) and ranged from 20 to 160 mg per day (Figure 4.1). The corresponding plasma methadone concentration averaged 281.3 ng/ml (SD ± 567.9) (Table 4.1) and ranged from 0 to 4634 ng/ml (Figure 4.2, Figure 4.3)

	Daily Dose,(mg)	Plasma Concentration, (ng/ml)
Mean	57.19828	299.842
Standard Error	2.110416	57.0856
Median	50	180.8249
Standard Deviation	22.72988	582.1612
Sample Variance	516.6473	338911.6
Kurtosis	2.263482	39.11501
Skewness	1.040586	5.905204

Table 4.1. The Summary of Statistics, Daily Methadone Dose (mg) and Plasma Methadone Concentration (ng/ml)

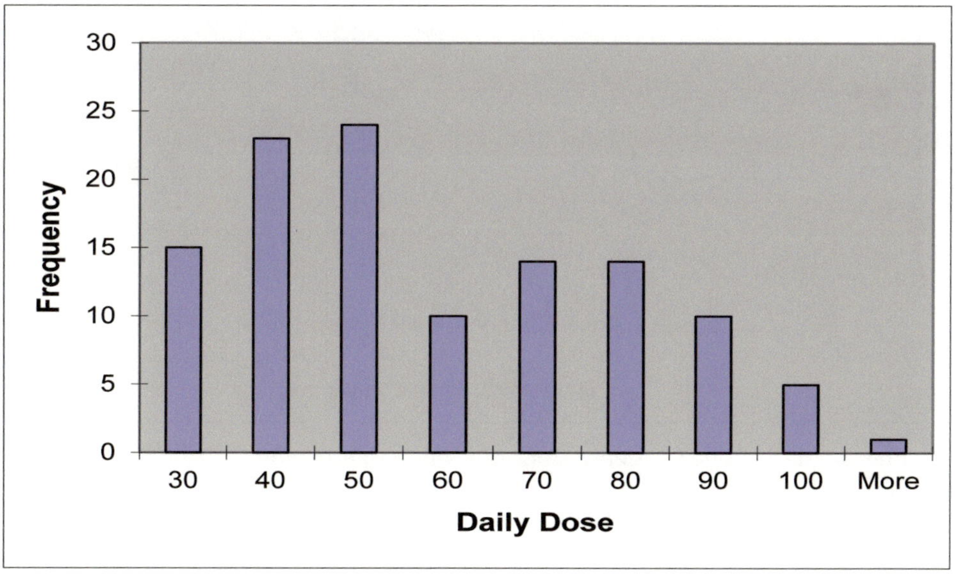

Fig. 4.1. Daily Methadone Dose in the Study Patients

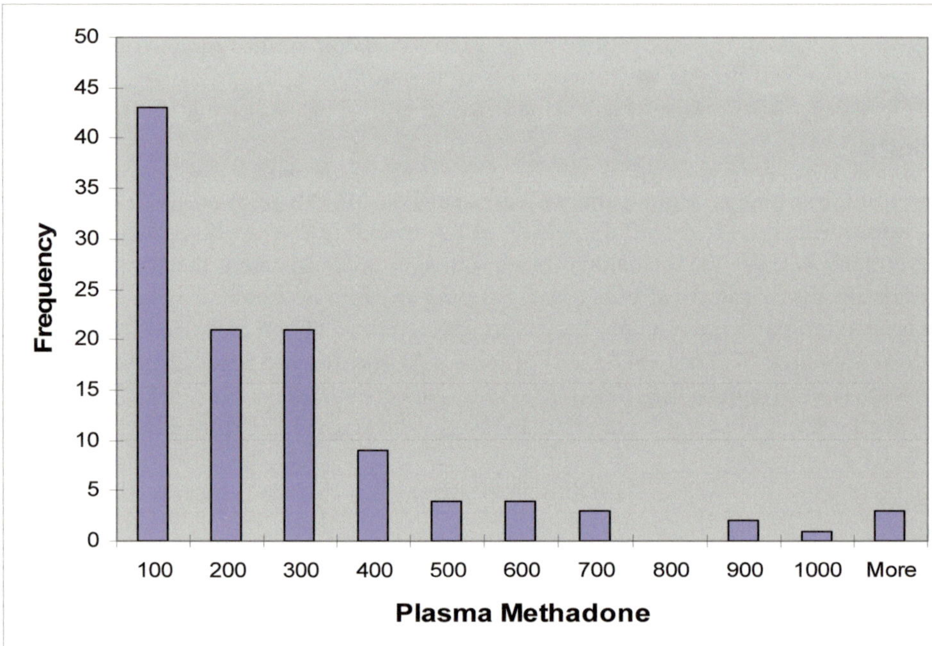

Fig. 4.2. Plasma Methadone Concentrations (ng/ml) as a function of daily methadone dose in the studied patients (outlying concentrations were removed).

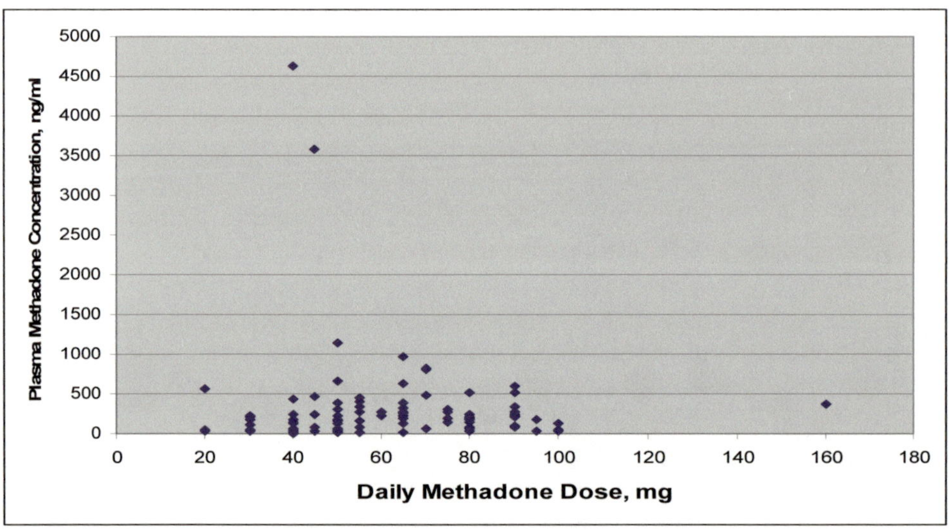

Fig. 4.3. Plasma Methadone Concentrations (ng/ml) as a Function of Daily Methadone Dose (mg) in the Studied Patients

Both the daily doses and the resulting plasma concentrations showed a non-normal distribution, more so for the plasma concentrations compared to the daily dose. Thus, although the daily dose averaged 57 mg, its median was lower at 50 mg. Similarly, although plasma concentration averaged 300 ng/ml, its median was only 181 ng/ml. A closer look revealed that 33% of patients had doses of 40 mg/day or lower, 54% received 40 - 80 mg/day dose and only 13% had doses 80 mg or more per day. In terms of plasma methadone, most, 84%, had concentrations of 400 ng/ml and 16% had 400 ng/ml and above, 400 ng/ml being the proposed minimum concentration for effectiveness. Six percent of patients on the other hand, had potentially toxic concentrations of more than 700 ng/ml. (Table 4.2 and Table 4.3)

Statistics	Day 1	Day 7	Day 14	Day 21
Mean	136.25	242.91	196.94	216.52
Standard Error	13.49	21.13	18.27	19.66
Median	135.06	194.12	162.05	190.25
Standard Deviation	80.92	126.79	109.65	117.96
Sample Variance	6548.10	16075.43	12022.56	13913.47
Skewness	0.56	1.08	2.14	2.35
Range	317.65	463.53	573.99	584.88
Minimum	14.09	92.36	60.66	81.16
Maximum	331.74	555.89	634.65	666.04

Table 4.2. Plasma Methadone Concentrations (ng/ml) on Days 1, 7, 14 and 21 While Patients Received MMT 40 mg Daily

Plasma Methadone, up to mg/ml	Day 1		Day 7		Day 14		Day 21	
	N	Cumulative %	N	Cumulative %	N	Cumulativ e %	N	Cumulativ e %
100.00	10	32.26%	2	6.06%	0	0.00%	1	3.85%
200.00	10	64.52%	16	54.55%	17	56.67%	11	46.15%
300.00	10	96.77%	7	75.76%	5	73.33%	8	76.92%
400.00	1	100.00%	3	84.85%	7	96.67%	4	92.31%
500.00	0	100.00%	1	87.88%	0	96.67%	1	96.15%
600.00	0	100.00%	4	100.00%	0	96.67%	0	96.15%
700.00	0	100.00%	0	100.00%	1	100.00%	1	100.00%
800.00	0	100.00%	0	100.00%	0	100.00%	0	100.00%

Table 4.3. Plasma Methadone Concentrations (ng/ml) on Days 1, 7, 14 and 21 While Patients Received MMT 40 mg Daily

The Subjective and Objective Withdrawal Score from patient taking MMT 40 mg daily was poorly manifested (Figure 4.4 and Figure 4.5). It showed that methadone at 40 mg a day was not adequate to suppress the withdrawal from opiate dependence.

Subjective withdrawal scores (SOW) were determined at four weeks for patients given 40 mg daily dose of methadone. Scores averaged 32 (SD ±10.4). The lowest score was 11 and the highest 51. Objective withdrawal scores (OOW) were also determined at four weeks for patients given 40 mg daily dose of methadone. Scores averaged 8.2 (SD ±1.5).

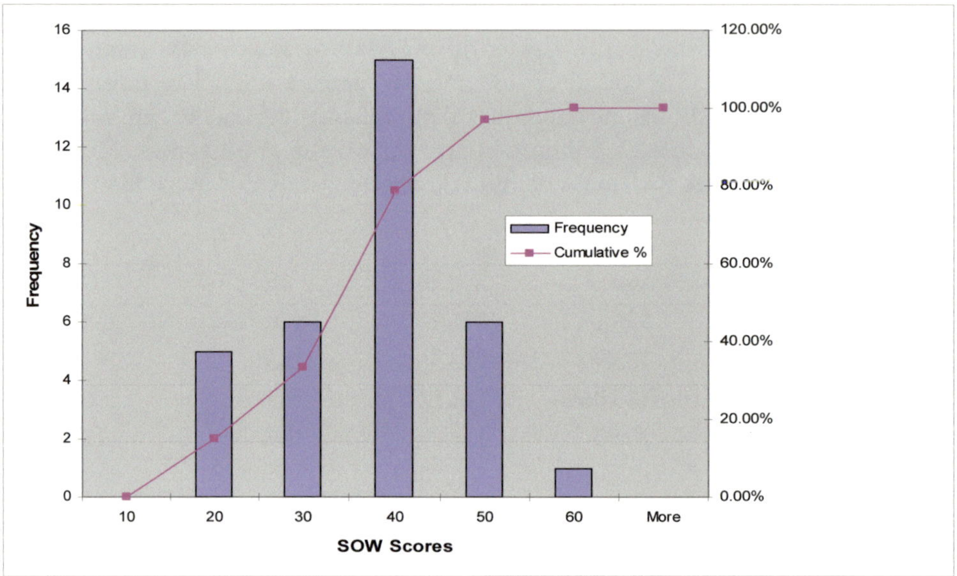

Fig. 4.4. Subjective Objective Withdrawal Scores from Patients Taking MMT 40 mg daily

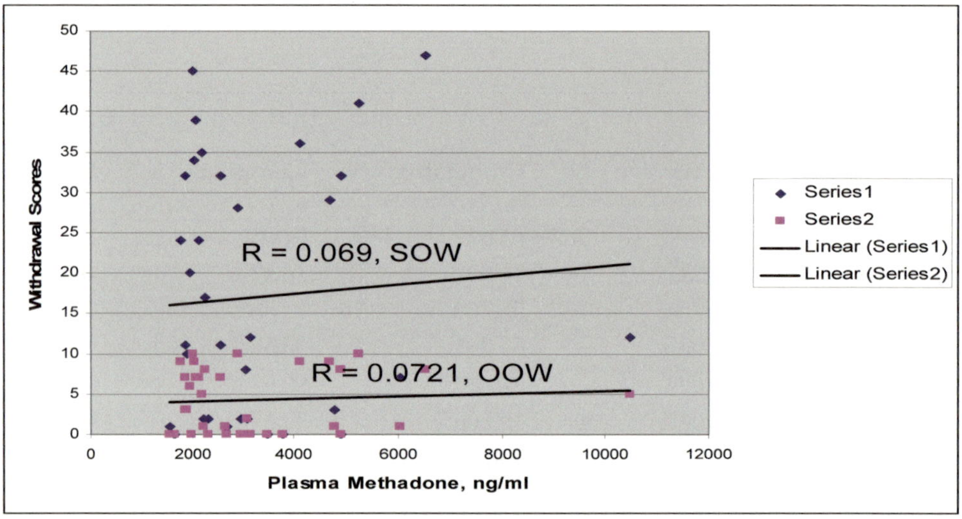

Fig. 4.5. Withdrawal Scores as a Function of Plasma Methadone Concentrations

(Series 1 = SOW; Series 2 = OOW)

5. Discussion

Methadone has a complex pharmacology. There is widespread "opiophobia" and it is frequently perceived negatively by physicians, patients and the society so much so that many just accept it as a necessary evil. The complex pharmacology and "opiophobia" present a great challenge to patients, physician and programs in terms of finding the most appropriate dose to achieve the desired results. This study was an attempt to comprehensively look at MMT. Among our notable findings included the variable ages of our patients, the male predominance, the variable daily methadone doses used and the importance of high daily maintenance dose, the variable plasma methadone obtained and its poor correlation with daily doses. Eighty eight patients were excluded from plasma concentration of methadone because they did not comply with the protocol. We investigated only 40 patients for the outcomes of MMT when the daily dose was fixed at 40 mg. We found that this daily dose was associated with high withdrawal scores implying failure of therapy.

In our clinical study, initially we enrolled 128 patients. They comprised of heroin/opiate dependent individuals receiving MMT in our clinics. As have been observed in many previous studies with MMT, patients enrolled in this study were mostly males with most in the productive age group. The youngest was 20, the oldest 56 years old. They were also mainly Malays. This fact underscores the importance of proper management of drug use disorder. These young and otherwise healthy males, if not successfully managed, are lost to the society and may lead a criminal life to feed their habits, given the difficulties, stigma and discrimination they face to be employed. Thus, instead of becoming the work force of the country needed to generate economic activity, these youngsters in turn add the burden of the country. There will be added burdens in terms of law enforcement costs, judiciary costs and other related costs. This would be over and above other costs like the society and health-care costs.

Of note was a high prevalence of HIV positivity at 36%. In most countries with good harm reduction programs for injecting drug users, the prevalence of HIV positivity is generally 1-2% (Central Intelligence Agency). The high prevalence seen in our cohort underscores the need for urgent effective measures. As there is no cure for HIV/ AIDS, this high prevalence would mean that many young Malay males in Malaysia would eventually succumb to the disease. This would reduce the pool of available males for population growth and if this is allowed to go on unabated, this will impact on the demography of the Malaysian population. Ethnic proportions can change and population growth in some communities may be halted. They may face troubles to obtain gainful employment and may resort to crimes to feed their habits, themselves and may be even their families. Co-morbid conditions like psychiatric illnesses and stigma and discrimination may make them dangerous to self, family and the society.

No age is however spared by the drug use disorder. The youngest of our patients was a 20 year-old. They began their drug habit as early as when they were 12 years. The oldest patient was 56 years of age and the oldest age a patient started with the habit was 32 years. Drug use disorder is a chronic relapsing disease. The duration of illness among our patients ranged from two years to 38 years and averaged 13 years. These have implications. For one, preventive measures for drug use disorder must begin early and should be continued through all ages. Patients afflicted with the disease should also have long follow ups as they evidently continue with their habits right through their golden years. The longer they continue on the habit, the greater is the chance for them to contract diseases like HIV, if they have not yet been infected. Being young and otherwise healthy, young addicts may find themselves constrained in various activities and this may lead them to many unhealthy practices.

Drug users do not live in isolation. They have sexual partners and families. Apart from transmission through the sharing of injection equipments, having the HIV reservoir, drug users can also transmit the disease to their sexual partners, through penetrative sex. Thus, what started as a concentrated epidemic among drug users is now showing evidence for a more generalized epidemic into the community through sexual transmission. In the beginning, less than one percent of HIV victims were females. Now it stands at about 20% and this clearly demonstrates the generalization of the HIV epidemic in Malaysia that began as a concentrated epidemic among drug users. Most of the afflicted females are also wives and spouses of drug users who are themselves HIV positive and not sex workers as many would have expected. There is however evidence for a growing epidemic among sex workers and this again has the potential to generalize into the community.

For the forty patients studied, their daily dose averaged 57.2 mg and ranged from 20 to 160 mg per day. Median dose was 50 mg per day. The corresponding plasma methadone averaged 281.3 ng/ml. It ranged from 0 to 4634 ng/ml. Daily methadone doses poorly predicted resulting plasma methadone concentrations, a hallmark for a drug metabolized by genetically polymorphic enzymes. Indeed when we measured plasma methadone concentrations in patients who received a fixed 40 mg daily methadone , they varied from 14 ng/ml to 331 ng/ml, a 23-fold difference. It is thus evident that no one dose fits all. As with many drugs used in the management of chronic diseases, methadone doses should be individualized to optimum outcomes that must be determined objectively.

It is also interesting to note that, despite claims by many physicians that relatively lower doses of methadone would be sufficient for our Malaysian patients, our observation of high withdrawal scores among patients who were maintained at 40 mg daily of methadone would imply this was not so. Severe withdrawal would discourage patients from remaining on treatment and by inference, they will not be retained. Indeed it has consistently been found that a sufficiently high dose of substitution therapy was required for improved outcome (Brady *et al*, 2005). High doses of methadone were significantly more effective in suppressing illicit heroin use and in retaining patients in the program (Family Health International; Mattick *et al*, 2003) and in producing optimum outcomes (Farré *et al*, 2002).

Inadequate doses and premature termination are the greatest threats to a successful MMT program in Malaysia. Malaysian doctors may outwardly say that they use lower methadone doses because of their fear for ethnic difference that would put their patients at higher risks for toxicity if they were to use doses as high as those recommended by the Western literature. What they may not want to admit is the fact that, inwardly, they have fears with methadone (and all opiates actually!) just for the simple reason that methadone is an opiate, just like the dreaded heroin and morphine! Indeed Malaysian doctors are not alone in this. Many doctors everywhere share the same view. Thus, despite ample evidence for the need to maintain patients at a daily dose of 80 mg to 100 mg, most patients are maintained on much less, and many are encouraged early termination.

It is probably understandable that the lay public may not understand the scientific basis for MMT and could be disparaging and become critical of it. It is however less clear why many physicians and other health care providers have the same views. Even those directly involved with MMT programs frequently fail to adhere to the basic principles of MMT. Most have actually received clear information on the pharmacologic principles underlying MMT and their claim that they want to prescribe as few medications as possible sound hollow, as they frequently easily prescribe other mood altering drugs, such as the benzodiazepines that are often prescribed with abandon and can produce psychological and physiologic dependency. Even if they claim they fear adverse effects, the adverse, physiologic effects of MMT are minimal and methadone is probably associated with the least side effects of any drug in a physician's pharmacologic armamentarium, when used appropriately. The real reason is probably more to do with the general "opiophobias" as it is known that some doctors even hesitate to use opiates even when indications are clear. Efforts should therefore be made urgently to reeducate these doctors. In their hands is the future of the nation. Their failure to prescribe adequate methadone doses will lead to therapeutic failure for MMT. This has dire consequences.

There is another problem. The expectation of the public, doctors and patients as regards treatment of addiction is to have a drug-free ending. This puts extra pressures on the doctor and patient alike and this will encourage doctors and patients to use low doses for the shortest possible time. This is despite the fact that maintenance therapy for at least two years with adequate doses is known to be associated with the maximum chance of remaining abstinent when methadone has been tapered. Many patients can thus receive less than two years of treatment with methadone with encouragements to discontinue maintenance frequently coming from health care providers working in maintenance programs. Most treating doctors also often do not try to discover reasons why patients started drug in the first place, or the existence of comorbid psychiatric illnesses. This less than holistic approach to MMT can result in increased anxiety among patients that can lead to the use of other psycho-active drugs, such as the benzodiazepines.

Notwithstanding the requirement for higher doses, as with any drugs, the dosing of methadone should be individualized (Latowsky, 2006). While low doses are associated with relapse and failure, too high a dose may lead to toxicities such as prolongation of QT interval and subsequent fatal polymorphic ventricular fibrillation (Fanoe *et al*, 2007). As regards plasma methadone concentrations, although we did not observe a clear correlation between plasma concentration and clinical effects, in the individual patients they may prove useful as illustrated in the cases we described above. Notwithstanding that, it is clear that a dose of 40 mg a day is generally inadequate. Subjective withdrawal scores (SOW) at four weeks for patients given 40 mg daily dose of methadone averaged 32 and the standard deviation was large at 10.4. The lowest score was 11 and the highest 51. Objective withdrawal scores (OOW) were also determined at four weeks for patients given 40 mg daily dose of methadone. Scores averaged 8.2 (SD ±1.5). It is evident that severe withdrawals occurred in patients maintained on 40 mg daily.

6. Conclusion

We concluded that the variable plasma methadone obtained was poorly correlated with daily doses of methadone and low dose methadone was inadequate to suppress opiate withdrawal.

A daily dose of 40 mg was associated with a high incidence of opiate withdrawal. Thus, prescription of methadone dose should be individualised to achieve a higher success of MMT.

7. Acknowledgement

I would like to thank USM (Universiti Sains Malaysia) RU grant 1001/PSSP/812056 for sponsoring this project.

8. References

Abramson, F.P. Methadone plasma protein binding: alterations in cancer and displacement from alpha 1-acid glycoprotein. *Clin Pharmaco Ther*. 1982. 32(5): 652-658.

Brady, T.M., Salvucci, S., Sverdlov, L.S., Male, A., Kyeyune, H., Sikali, E., DeSale, S. and Yu, P. Methadone dosage and retention: an examination of the 60 mg/day threshold. *Journal of Addictive Diseases.* 2005. 24(3): 23-47.

de Vos, J.W., Ufkes, J.G.R., van Brussel, G.H.A. & van den Brink, W. Craving despite extremely high methadone dosage. *Drug and Alcohol Dependence.* 1996. 40(3): 181-184.

Dyer, K.R., Foster, D.J.R., White, J.M., Somogyi, A.A., Menelaou, A. & Bochner, F. Steady-state pharmacokinetics and pharmacodynamics in methadone maintenance patients: Comparison of those who do and do not experience withdrawal and concentration-effect relationships[ast]. *Clin Pharmacol Ther.* 1999. 65(6): 685-694.

Eap, C.B., Buclin, T. & Baumann, P. Interindividual variability of the clinical pharmacokinetics of methadone: implications for the treatment of opioid dependence. . *Clin. Pharmacokinet.* 2002. 41(1153-1193.

Eap, C.B., Cuendet, C. & Baumann, P. Binding of d-methadone, l-methadone, and dl-methadone to proteins in plasma of healthy volunteers: role of the variants of alpha 1-acid glycoprotein. *Clin Pharmaco Ther.* 1990. 47(3): 338-346.

Ekblom, M., Hammarlund-Udenaes, M. & Paalzow, L. Modeling of tolerance development and rebound effect during different intravenous administrations of morphine to rats. *Journal of Pharmacology and Experimental Therapeutics.* 1993. 266(1): 244-252.

Family Health International. Managing opioid dependence: treatment and care for HIV-positive injecting drug users Disember 27,2009, from http://www.fhi.org/training/en/HIVAIDS/IDUModules/pdf/Module_04_Treatment_Care_for_HIV_positive_IDUs.pdf

Fanoe, S., Hvidt, C., Ege, P. and Jensen, G.B. Syncope and QT prolongation among patients treated with methadone for heroin dependence in the city of Copenhagen. *Heart.* 2007. 93(9): 1051-1055.

Farré, M., Mas, A., Torrens, M., Moreno, V. and CamI, J. Retention rate and illicit opioid use during methadone maintenance interventions: a meta-analysis. *Drug and Alcohol Dependence.* 2002. 65(3): 283-290.

Fournier, T., Medjoubi-N, N. & Porquet, D. Alpha-1-acid glycoprotein. *Biochimica et Biophysica Acta (BBA) - Protein Structure and Molecular Enzymology.* 2000. 1482(1-2): 157-171.

Garrido, M.J., Aguirre, C., Trocóniz, I.F., Marot, M., Valle, M., Zamacona, M.K. and Calvo, R. Alpha 1-acid glycoprotein (AAG) and serum protein binding of methadone in heroin addicts with abstinence syndrome. *Int J Clin pharmaco Ther.* 2000. 38(1): 35-40.

Gómez, E., Martinez-Jordá, R., Suárez, E., Garrido, M.J. & Calvo, R. Altered methadone analgesia due to changes in plasma protein binding: Role of the route of administration. *General Pharmacology: The Vascular System.* 1995. 26(6): 1273-1276.Xiao, Y., Smith, R.D., Caruso, F.S. & Kellar, K.J. Blockade of Rat α3β4 Nicotinic Receptor function by Methadone, its metabolites, and structural analogs. *JPET.* 2001. 299(1): 366-371.

Inturrisi, C.E., Portenoy, R.K., Max, M.B., Colburn, W.A. & Foley, K.M. Pharmacokinetic-pharmacodynamic relationships of methadone infusions in patients with cancer pain. *Clin Pharmaco Ther.* 1990. 47(5): 565-577.

KuKanich, B. & Borum, S.L. The disposition and behavioral effects of methadone in Greyhounds. *Veterinary Anaesthesia and Analgesia.* 2008. 35(3): 242-248.

Kukanich, B., Lascelles, B.D.X., Aman, A.M., Mealey, K.L. & Papich, M.G. The effects of inhibiting cytochrome P450 3A, p-glycoprotein, and gastric acid secretion on the oral bioavailability of methadone in dogs. *Journal of Veterinary Pharmacology and Therapeutics.* 2005. 28(5): 461-466.

Latowsky, M. Methadone death, dosage and torsade de pointes: risk-benefit policy implications. *J Psychoactive Drug.* 2006. 38(4): 513-519.

Liu, E., Liang, T., Shen, L., Zhong, H., Wang, B., Wu, Z. & Detels, R. Correlates of methadone client retention: a prospective cohort study in Guizhou province, China. *The International Journal on Drug Policy.* 2009. 20(4): 304-308.

Li, X. & Wei, W. Chinese materia medica: combinations and appication Hertfordshire: Donica Publishing. 2002. 75-76.

Li, Y., Kantelip, J.P., Gerritsen-van, S.P. & Davani, S. Interindividual variability of methadone response: impact of genetic polymorphism [Abstract]. *Mol Diagn Ther.* 2008. 12(2): 109-124.

Loimer, N. & Schmid, R. The use of plasma levels to optimize methadone maintenance treatment. *Drug and Alcohol Dependence.* 1992. 30(3): 241-246.

Lötsch, J., von Hentig, N., Freynhagen, R., Griessinger, N., Zimmermann, M., Doehring, A., Rohrbacher, M., Sittl, R. & Geisslinger, G. Cross-sectional analysis of the influence of currently known pharmacogenetic modulators on opioid therapy in outpatient pain centers. *Pharmacogenetics and Genomics.* 2009. 19(6):

Mattick, R.P., Breen, C. and Kimbler, J. Methadone maintenance therapy versus no opioid replacement therapy for opioid dependence. *Cochrane Database of Syst Rev.* 2003.

Meresaar, U., Nilsson, M.I., Holmstrand, J. & Änggård, E. Single dose pharmacokinetics and bioavailability of methadone in man studied with a stable isotope method. *European journal of clinical pharmacology.* 1981. 20(6): 473-478-478.

Mestriner, F.L.A.C., Spiller, F., Laure, H.J., Souto, F.O., Tavares-Murta, B.M., Rosa, J.C., Basile-Filho, A., Ferreira, S.H., Greene, L.J. & Cunha, F.Q. Acute-phase protein α-1-acid glycoprotein mediates neutrophil migration failure in sepsis by a nitric oxide-dependent mechanism. *Proceedings of the National Academy of Sciences.* 2007. 104(49): 19595-19600.

Romach, M.K., Piafsky, K.M., Abel, J.G., Khouw, V. & Sellers, E.M. Methadone binding to orosomucoid (alpha 1-acid glycoprotein): determinant of free fraction in plasma. *Clin Pharmaco Ther.* 1981. 29(2): 211-217.

Rostami-Hodjegan, A., Wolff, K., Hay, A.W.M., Raistrick, D., Calvert, R. & Tucker, G.T. Population pharmacokinetics of methadone in opiate users: characterization of time-dependent changes. *British Journal of Clinical Pharmacology.* 1999. 48(1): 43-52.

Rowland, M. & Tozer, T.N. Physiologic concepts and kinetics: distribution. In Rowland, M. and Tozer, T. N. (Eds.), *Clinical Pharmacokinetics. Concepts and Applications.* 3rd ed. Philadelphia: Lippincott Williams & Wilkins. 1995. 137–155.

Sawe, J. High-dose morphine and methadone in cancer patients. Clinical pharmacokinetic considerations of oral treatment. *Clin Pharmacokinet.* 1986. 11(2): 87-106.

Schmidt, N., Sittl, R., Brune, K. & Geisslinger, G. Rapid Determination of Methadone in Plasma, Cerebrospinal Fluid, and Urine by Gas Chromatography and Its

Application to Routine Drug Monitoring. *Pharmaceutical Research.* 1993. 10(3): 441-444-444.

Wolff, K. & Hay, A.W. Plasma methadone monitoring with methadone maintenance treatment. *Drug Alcohol Depend.* 1994. 36(1): 69-71.

Wolff, K., Rostami-Hodjegan, A., Hay, A.W.M., Raistrick, D. and Tucker, G. Population-based pharmacokinetic approach for methadone monitoring of opiate addicts: potential clinical utility. *Addiction.* 2000. 95(12): 1771-1783.

Wolff, K., Sanderson, M., Hay, A.W. and Raistrick, D. Methadone concentrations in plasma and their relationship to drug dosage. *Clinical Chemistry.* 1991. 37(2): 205-209.

Verebely, K., Volavka, J., Mulé, S. & Resnick, R. Methadone in man: pharmacokinetic and excretion studies in acute and chronic treatment. *Clinical Pharmacology and Therapeutics.* 1975. 18(2): 180-190.

Yang, Y., Wan, C., Li, H., Zhu, H., La, Y., Xi, Z., Chen, Y., Jiang, L., Feng, G. & He, L. Altered Levels of Acute Phase Proteins in the Plasma of Patients with Schizophrenia. *Analytical Chemistry.* 2006. 78(11): 3571-3576.

7

Drug Synergy – Mechanisms and Methods of Analysis

Hans-Georg Breitinger
The German University in Cairo, Egypt

1. Introduction

The term synergy is derived from the Greek *syn-ergos*, "working together". Synergies have been described in many settings and situations of life, including mechanics, technical systems, human social life, and many more. In all cases, synergy describes the fact that a system, i.e. the combination and interaction of two or more agents or forces is such that the combined effect is greater than the sum of their individual effects.
This definition implies that there are three possible ways of such an "interaction of agents or forces": these forces could simply add up, not affecting each other (no interaction), their combination could produce a greater than expected result (synergy), or the combination could lead to a result that is less than the sum of the individual effects. This "negative" summation is called antagonism.
Interactions of biologically active agents are an important aspect of pharmacology and biomedicine. In this context, interaction describes the biological activity that results from the presence of several drugs at the same time. Such situations occur in numerous clinical situations:

- combinations of cytotoxic drugs in the treatment of cancer and infections require lower doses of each drug to obtain better therapeutic effects with less side-effect toxicity.
- combinations of antibiotics likewise combine better efficiency with fewer side effects and reduced development of resistance.
- many serious clinical situations require administration of several drugs simply because of multiple therapeutic indications. Although in such a case drug combinations are not formulated to look for synergies, the interactions of these drugs need to be assessed.
- the effect of one drug may be augmented by another drug that does not produce such an effect on its own

In all these cases, multiple drugs are administered, and will show some form of interaction, synergistic, antagonistic, or none. Methods to determine and quantify drug interactions are thus an essential tool in pharmacology. Historically, extracts from plants, animals, or even soils were the first classified pharmaceuticals. These were complex mixtures rather than single agents, and some ingredients may have interacted with others. Over the years of development of pharmacy, isolation, synthesis and marketing of single drugs became the accepted standard. Whether a complex mixture or a combination of drugs is used, the biological interaction of all active substances should be known. Synergy may be observed in simple systems – two drugs that only act on one target protein can show synergism. In such a case we can study the interaction of the drugs mechanistically and determine why and how several drugs can reinforce each other (or why they do not). Synergy may also be observed in complex settings, such as patients receiving multiple medications. Usually, more than one biological target (protein, pathway, or even organ) are involved in such cases, and single mechanistic descriptions are not appropriate. Additional parameters to consider are drug absorption, tissue distribution, and clearance. It may be expected that many drugs interfere with metabolism of other drugs. Thus, a substance B that slows down clearance of an active drug A, say by blocking metabolizing enzymes or excretion, may lead to a higher effective concentration of A that remains in the body for a longer time. As a result, one would notice a greater effect of drug A when given together with B, although the two drugs have completely different modes of action. While certainly the combination of these two drugs would have a "combined effect is greater than the sum of their individual effects", their combination is synergistic in practical application, but not by the strict definition.

2. Basic models and mechanisms – Synergy on a molecular level

2.1 A simple reaction scheme for enzyme inhibition

Drug interaction and synergy has been intensively studied for more than 100 years, and some of the numerous concepts will be briefly introduced in this chapter. The simplest model cases will be presented, leading to a molecular definition of drug synergy.

Let us assume a simple enzyme following the laws of mass action and Michaelis-Menten kinetics. In the simplest case, this enzyme has an active site, where substrate is being converted into product, and possesses one or several specific binding sites for inhibitors (Fig. 1A). A competitive inhibitor by definition binds to the active site of the enzyme, displacing the substrate. Thus, a mixture of two purely competitive inhibitors will only ever target the active site. This is known as mutually exclusive binding. If only the simplest mechanistic case is considered, one would not expect a second competitive inhibitor to have any notable effect on the first one, other than raising the total amount of inhibitory molecules.

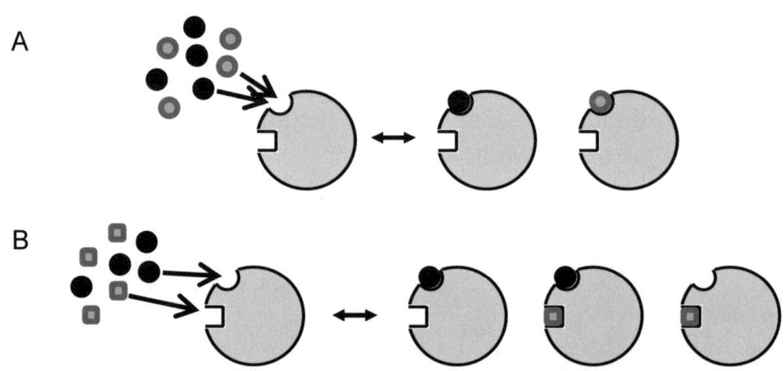

Fig. 1. Schematic representation of inhibition mechanisms (A) Competitive inhibition. Inhibitor (open circles) binds to the active site of the target protein. The agonist (solid circles) binds to the same site. By definition of competitive inhibition, all competitive inhibitors bind to the same (active) site. Thus, binding of two competitive inhibitors must be mutually exclusive, and they cannot act synergistically on the same target protein. (B) Non-competitive inhibition. Inhibitor (open squares) binds to a site different from the active site of the target molecule. In pure non-competitive inhibition agonist binding is not affected by the inhibitor. Inhibition is due to conversion of the target protein into an inactive state.

In case of non-competitive inhibition, the inhibitor binds to a location on the enzyme different from the active site. Assuming that bound inhibitor converts the enzyme into an inactive (non product-forming) state, presence of a non-competitive inhibitor simply lowers the amount of active enzyme molecules (Fig. 1B). There are states, where both substrate and inhibitor are bound to the enzyme. The effect of several non-competitive inhibitors applied together raises the question if synergy can be observed in such a simple system. If two non-competitive inhibitors bind to the same site on their target enzyme, this inhibitory site can either be occupied by inhibitor A or B, but not by both inhibitors at the same time (Fig. 2). This would be a case of mutually exclusive binding of two inhibitors. If one inhibitor is present, and the second one added, one may observe indeed a greater extend of inhibition, but this would only be due to larger amounts of inhibitory molecules being present. At all times, we could predict the total amount of inhibition by summations. In the simplest molecular case, two inhibitors targeting the same site would produce an additive effect only.

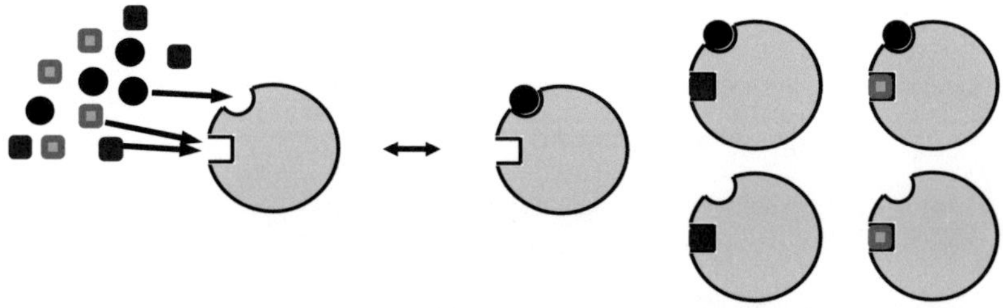

Fig. 2. Reaction scheme for two non-competitive inhibitors targeting the same site. Two non-competitive inhibitors (squares) bind to the same site on the target protein. In this case their binding is mutually exclusive. Presence of the second inhibitor increases the total amount of inhibitor causing in increased inhibitory effect. This increase is only due to simple additivity, and not synergy.

If, however, two different binding sites for non-competitive inhibitors exist on an enzyme, two inhibitors may bind simultaneously (Fig. 3). Inspection of the reaction schemes (Fig. 2, 3) shows that if two inhibitors have specific, independent sites on the enzyme, we will observe states where the enzyme indeed has two inhibitors bound (Fig. 3). These states cannot exist if both inhibitors bind to the same site (Fig. 2). Thus, if two inhibitors are able to bind simultaneously, we have a case of "mutually non-exclusive" binding. Here, presence of the second inhibitor will not only give an additive effect (increase of the number of inhibitory molecules), but will generate additional inhibited states of the enzyme. Therefore, on a molecular level we would expect a superadditive effect of two such inhibitors.

It should be noted that the considerations above are made following some basic assumptions, namely that binding of an inhibitor will convert the enzyme to an inactive state, binding of substrate and inhibitor is reversible, and binding of any compound is fully independent from all other compounds. Thus, the equilibrium binding constant for inhibitor A is the same whether A binds to the unliganded enzyme, or to the enzyme that has substrate and/or another inhibitor bound. Given these assumptions, the mechanisms for activation (Fig. 4A), and non-competitive inhibition (Fig. 4B,C) show the different states in which an enzyme exists in the presence of two non-competitive inhibitors that bind to the same site (Fig. 4B), or to different sites of the enzyme (Fig. 4B).

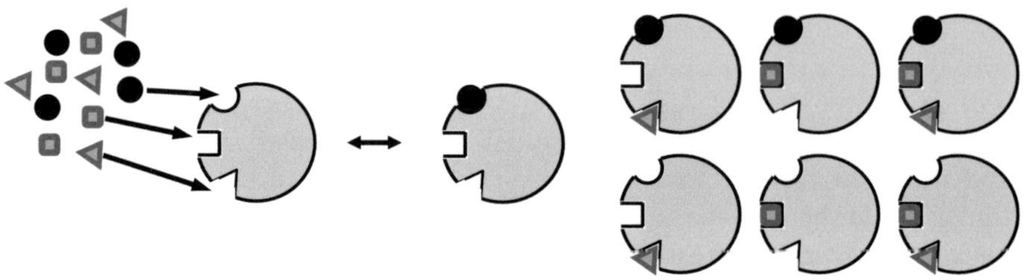

Fig. 3. Reaction scheme for two mutually non-exclusive non-competitive inhibitors. Non-competitive inhibition by two inhibitors (squares, triangles) binding to different sites on the target protein. Here, bindign of one inhibitor does not prevent binding of the other. Note that presence of the second inhibitor creates new inactive states of the target protein that are not possible if only one inhibitor is present. This applies even in the simplest theoretical case, where binding affinities of agonist and inhibitors are completely independent of each other. Thus, in the presence of two inhibitors of the same target protein that follow the rule of Bliss independence, i.e. mutually non-exclusive binding, synergy must be a necessary consequence.

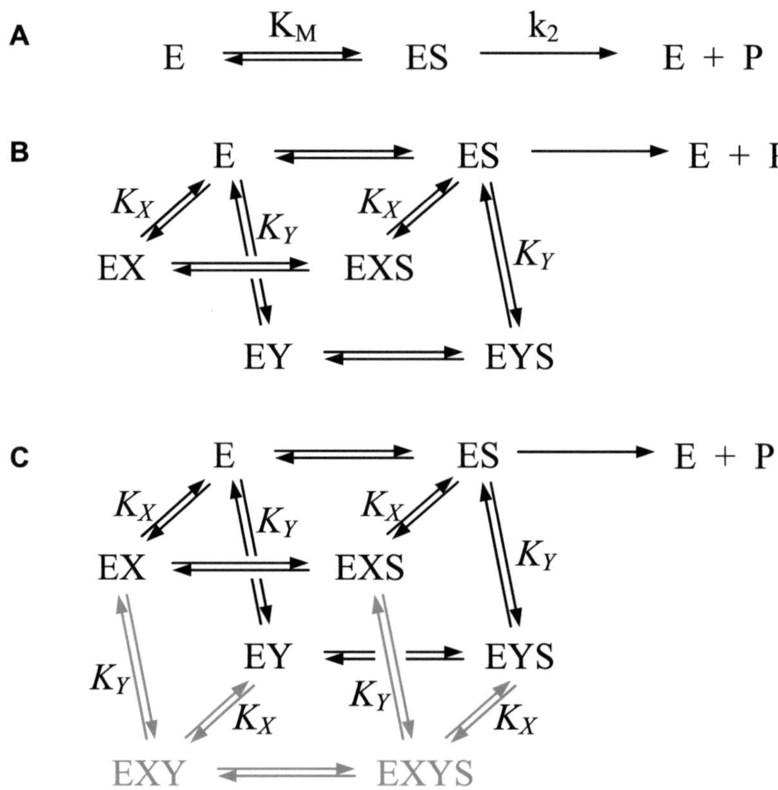

Fig. 4. Mechanism of catalysis and non-competitive inhibition of a Michaelis-Menten enzyme. (A) Mechanism for the activation of an enzyme following Michaelis-Menten kinetics. E = enzyme, S = substrate, P = product, K_M = Michaelis constant, k_2 = rate of product formation from ES. A simplified MM kinetic scheme is used, assuming no backward reaction EP → ES. (B) Inhibition of a Michaelis-Menten enzyme by two non-competitive inhibitors X and Y, which are mutually exclusive (e.g. binding to the same site). It is assumed that enzyme with

bound inhibitor is completely inactive, ie it does not form product. Either inhibitor X or Y can bind at any given time. Presence of the second inhibitor can only exert an additive effect but is not synergistic. (C) Inhibition of a Michaelis-Menten enzyme by two non-competitive inhibitors X and Y, which are mutually non-exclusive, i.e. binding to different sites on the enzyme. Here, both inhibitors may bind simultaneously, giving rise to synergistic inhibition.

2.2 Michaelis-Menten enzymes

In this section, a simple derivation of enzyme inhibition by one or two non-competitive inhibitors is given. To illustrate the consequences of mutually exclusive vs. non-exclusive binding, the simplest mechanisms are used.
From the mechanism of a Michaelis-Menten-type enzyme (Fig. 4A) and the law of mass action, we find:

$$K_M = \frac{[E][S]}{[ES]} \rightarrow [ES] = \frac{[E][S]}{K_M} \tag{1}$$

The enzyme E can only exist as free enzyme E, or enzyme-substrate-complex ES. The total enzyme concentration is $[E_{tot}]$, K_M is the Michaelis constant. Only ES can form product, the maximum rate of product formation is V_{max}.

$$[E_{tot}] = [E] + [ES] \tag{2}$$

$$V_{\max} = k_2 [E_{tot}] \tag{3}$$

V_0, the actual rate of product formation at a given concentration of substrate depends on the fraction of ES that is present in the equilibrium. Thus V_0 can be expressed in terms of "ocupancy", or f_{ES}, the fraction of enzyme present in the enzyme-substrate complex ES.

$$f_{ES} = \frac{[ES]}{[E] + [ES]} \tag{4}$$

$$V_0 = k_2 [ES] \rightarrow V_0 = V_{\max} \frac{[ES]}{[E_{tot}]}, \quad V_0 = V_{\max} \frac{[ES]}{[E] + [ES]} = V_{\max} f_{ES} \tag{5}$$

Note that this equation converts readily to the common form of the Michaelis-Menten equation, if the definition of K_M (equation 1) is substituted into equation 5.

$$V_0 = V_{\max} \frac{1}{1 + \frac{K_M}{S}} \tag{6}$$

In the presence of a single non-competitive inhibitor, additional enzyme species are possible (EX, EXS in Fig. 4B). By definition of an inhibitor, these do not lead to any product formation. Then f_{ES} becomes

$$f_{ES,X} = \frac{[ES]}{[E] + [ES] + [EX] + [EXS]} \tag{7}$$

The rate of product formation in presence of one non-competitive inhibitor is

$$V_{0,X} = V_{max} \frac{1}{\left(1+\frac{K_M}{S}\right)\left(1+\frac{X}{K_X}\right)} \quad (8)$$

For two mutually exclusive inhibitors X and Y (Fig. 4B), one obtains:

$$V_{0,X,Y} = V_{max} \frac{1}{\left(1+\frac{K_M}{S}\right)\left(1+\frac{X}{K_X}+\frac{Y}{K_Y}\right)} \quad (9)$$

And for two mutually non-exclusive inhibitors (Fig. 4C), the rate equation is

$$V_{0,X,Y} = V_{max} \frac{1}{\left(1+\frac{K_M}{S}\right)\left(1+\frac{X}{K_X}\right)\left(1+\frac{Y}{K_Y}\right)} \quad (10)$$

There is a simple technique to determine the type of enzyme inhibition by two inhibitors, and whether their action on the enzyme is synergistic. To this end, the ratio of the initial rates in the absence (control, V_0), and in the presence of inhibitor ($V_{0,X}$) is measured. S_0 is the control signal, S_X is the signal obtained in the presence of inhibitor.

$$\frac{S_0}{S_X} = \frac{V_0}{V_{0,X}} = \frac{V_{max}\frac{1}{\left(1+\frac{K_M}{S}\right)}}{V_{max}\frac{1}{\left(1+\frac{K_M}{S}\right)\left(1+\frac{X}{K_X}\right)}} = \left(1+\frac{X}{K_X}\right) \quad (11)$$

Thus, a straight-line curve is obtained when S_0/S_X is plotted against [X], the (varied) concentration of inhibitor X. The slope of this line (Fig. 6) gives the inhibition constant K_X. This plot is linear over the entire range of inhibitor concentration.
In the case of two mutually exclusive inhibitors, the ratio becomes

$$\frac{S_0}{S_{X,Y}} = \frac{V_0}{V_{0,X,Y}} = \frac{V_{max}\frac{1}{\left(1+\frac{K_M}{S}\right)}}{V_{max}\frac{1}{\left(1+\frac{K_M}{S}\right)\left(1+\frac{X}{K_X}+\frac{Y}{K_Y}\right)}} = \left(1+\frac{X}{K_X}+\frac{Y}{K_Y}\right) \quad (12)$$

Presence of the second inhibitor only results in an additional term (Y/K_Y) that shifts the $S_0/S_{X,Y}$ curve upwards. This term indicates additivity of the two inhibitors, but inhibitory potency (slope of the curve) is not altered.
For two mutually non-exclusive inhibitors, the ratio is

$$\frac{S_0}{S_{X,Y}} = \frac{V_0}{V_{0,X,Y}} = \frac{V_{\max}\dfrac{1}{\left(1+\dfrac{K_M}{S}\right)}}{V_{\max}\dfrac{1}{\left(1+\dfrac{K_M}{S}\right)\left(1+\dfrac{X}{K_X}\right)\left(1+\dfrac{Y}{K_Y}\right)}} = \left(1+\frac{X}{K_X}\right)\left(1+\frac{Y}{K_Y}\right) \tag{13}$$

The difference between mutually exclusive and non-exclusive inhibitors can directly be seen from an experiment where the concentration of inhibitor X is held constant, and only [Y] is varied. Equation 13 can be rearranged to:

$$\frac{S_0}{S_{X,Y}} = 1+\frac{X}{K_X}+\frac{Y}{K_Y}\left(1+\frac{X}{K_X}\right) \tag{14}$$

Compared to the case of mutually exclusive inhibitors, the curve of $S_0/S_{X,Y}$. Y is shifted upwards by a constant concentration of X, and the slope of the curve also increases by a factor of $(1+X/K_X)$.

The ratio method shown here applies to the simplest case of synergistic action of drugs, two substances binding to the same target. It requires some basic kinetic data to be collected and gives a simple linear graph that can be quickly inspected for a qualitative result whether two substances act on the same or on different sites on an enzyme, and thus whether these two substances can be synergistic on their target or not. It should be noted that by taking the ratios, the control signal (uninhibited case, i.e. the largest signal) is divided by a signal that becomes progressively smaller and thus carries a higher error. It is needed to detect whether two curves have the same slope (mutually exclusive binding, additive effect), or different slopes (mutually non-exclusive binding, synergy). This difference has to be clearly demonstrated from experiment and data analysis, requiring data of sufficient quality to make this distinction.

The technique provides two important pieces of information:

1. The value of K_X, the inhibition constant, is unchanged if two inhibitors are only additive, and is decreased (~ higher inhibitory potency) in the presence of the second inhibitor. Therefore, we have a clear, mechanism-derived definition of synergy on the molecular level.
2. Conversely, the method allows to determine whether two inhibitors bind to the same, or to different sites on an enzyme. This may be an important result for drug development, and is obtained without need of structural data. (Note: strictly speaking, the result only tells whether binding of two inhibitors is mutually exclusive or non-exclusive)

The method has originally been presented for ligand-gated ion channels by Karpen and Hess (Karpen, Aoshima et al. 1982; Karpen and Hess 1986), and subsequently been used for the study of action of multiple inhibitors on ion channels (Karpen, Aoshima et al. 1982; Karpen and Hess 1986; Breitinger, Geetha et al. 2001; Raafat, Breitinger et al. 2010).

The basic mechanism presented here is by far not sufficient to describe multimeric enzymes, enzynmes requiring cofactors, and various modes of inhibition. Enzymes may form multimers, binding of one inhibitor may affect binding of other others, and binding sites my overlap. More complex mechanisms of inhibition of Michaelis-Menten enzymes have been discussed, including those of several inhibitors acting on a single enzyme (Palatini 1983). Action of several inhibitors as well as antagonistic interaction of enzyme inhibitors have been studied (Asante-Appiah and Chan 1996; Schenker and Baici 2009), and a major development in drug interaction analysis was the detailed mathematical treatment of enzyme kinetics and inhibition by Chou and Talalay (Chou 1976; Chou and Talalay 1977; Chou and Talalay 1981; Chou 2006; Chou 2010), covering the mechanistic Michaelis-Menten approach as well as logistic approaches.

2.3 Ligand-gated ion channel receptors

Ligand-gated ion channels are principal mediators of rapid synaptic transmission between nerve cells and in the neuromuscular junction. Compared to Michaelis-Menten type enzymes, their mechanism of activation is more complex, requiring an additional transition (Hess 1993; Colquhoun 1998). First step of ion channel activation is binding of the activating ligand (a neurotransmitter), which is governed by the principle of mass action (Hess 1993; Colquhoun 1998). Usually, more than one ligand molecule is required; depending on receptor type, models with two or three ligands binding prior to efficient channel opening have been discussed. Ligand binding induces an conformational change, where the receptor protein converts from the closed to an open ion-conducting state (Fig. 5A) (Hess 1993; Colquhoun 1998). Only the passing ions generate an electric signal and this signal can be recorded using patch-clamp techniques. Similar to the ES complex in enzymes, only the liganded receptor can undergo the opening transition. The mechanisms of non-competitive inhibition by two inhibitors binding to the same (Fig. 5B), or different (Fig. 5C) sites have been given. A similar derivation to the one for MM-enzymes can then be made.

The signal in this case is not a rate of product formation, but an ionic current, namely the rate of ion translocation through the open channel. Assuming a constant transmembrane voltage, and only one conducting state (ie only one channel size, in reality several conductance levels have been observed for each ion channel receptor).

The observed signal S_L would then be:

$$S_L = I_L = n_{Ch} J_{ion} \tag{15}$$

where I_L is the observd current, n_{Ch} is the number of open channels, and J_{ion} is the ion translocation rate. The maximum current signal would be observed if all ion channel were open at the same time. F_{open}, the fraction of open channels, would then be equal to 1 (a theoretical value only).

$$S_{\max} = I_{\max} F_{open} \tag{16}$$

Assuming that only receptors with two bound ligands can undergo the opening transition (Fig. 5A), we can define the fraction of open channels as

$$F_{open} = \frac{\overline{[RL_2(open)]}}{[R]+2[RL]+[RL_2]+\overline{[RL_2(open)]}} \tag{17}$$

Using the law of mass action, we can define

$$K_D = 2\frac{[R][L]}{[RL]} \tag{18}$$

$$K_D = \frac{[RL][L]}{[RL_2]} \tag{19}$$

$$\phi = \frac{[RL_2]}{[RL_2(open)]} \tag{20}$$

we can then obtain

$$S_0 = I_{\max} F_{open} = I_{\max} \frac{1}{\left(\frac{K_D}{L}+1\right)^2 \phi + 1} \tag{21}$$

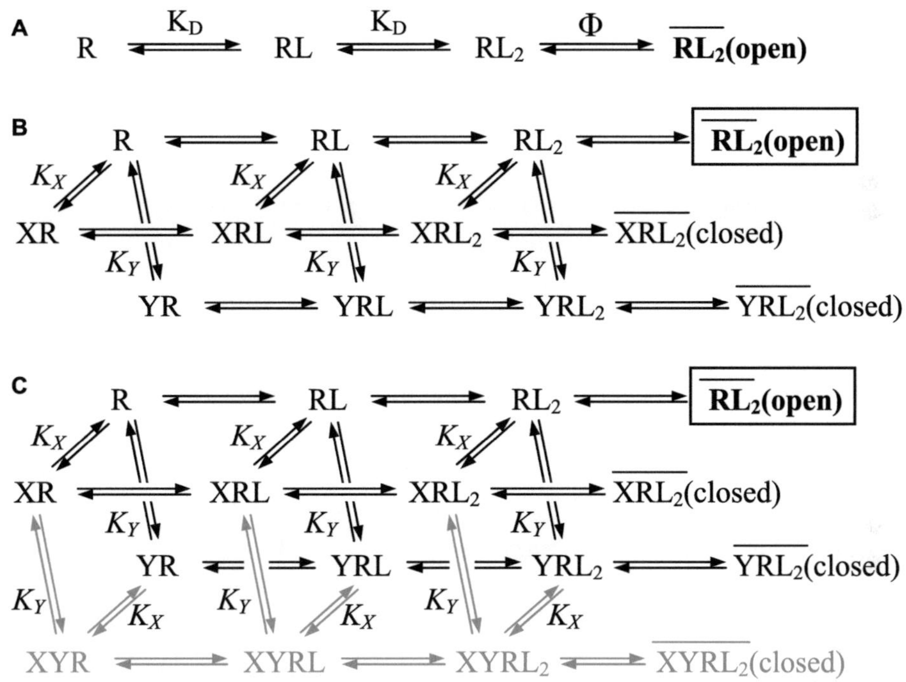

Fig. 5. Mechanisms of activation and non-competitive inhibition of ion channel receptors (A) Minimum mechanism for the activation of a ligand-gated ion channel. Note that the channel-opening reaction comprises two elementary steps, ligand binding (dissociation constant K_D) and conformational change to the open state (open-close equilibrium Φ). R = receptor, L = activating ligand. In this example binding of two ligand molecules is needed prior to channel opening. (B) Inhibition of an ion channel receptor by two non-competitive inhibitors X and Y, which are mutually exclusive (e.g. binding to the same site). Either inhibitor X or Y can bind at any given time. Presence of the second inhibitor can only exert an additive effect but is not synergistic. (C) Inhibition of an ion channel receptor by two non-competitive inhibitors X and Y, which are mutually non-exclusive, targeting different sites on the receptor. Synergism is then observed as a necessary consequence of two mutually non-exclusive inhibitors.

In the presence of one non-competitive inhibitor X, we obtain the following equation for the signal S_X:

$$S_X = I_{\max} \frac{1}{\left[\left(\frac{K_D}{L}+1\right)^2 \phi + 1\right]\left(1+\frac{X}{K_X}\right)} \tag{22}$$

where K_X is the inhibition constant, L is the concentration of activating ligand, and X the concentration of inhibitor. One can now readily compute the ratios of control current signal to signal in presence of inhibitor:

$$\frac{S_0}{S_X} = \frac{I_{\max} \frac{1}{\left[\left(\frac{K_D}{L}+1\right)^2 \phi + 1\right]}}{I_{\max} \frac{1}{\left[\left(\frac{K_D}{L}+1\right)^2 \phi + 1\right]\left(1+\frac{X}{K_X}\right)}} = 1 + \frac{X}{K_X} \tag{23}$$

In case of two inhibitors binding to the same site (mutually exclusive), the ratio again becomes

$$\frac{S_0}{S_{X,Y}} = 1 + \frac{X}{K_X} + \frac{Y}{K_Y} \tag{24}$$

For two non-exclusive inhibitors, targeting different sites on the recpetor, this ratio then is

$$\frac{S_0}{S_{X,Y}} = 1 + \frac{X}{K_X} + \frac{Y}{K_Y}\left(1+\frac{X}{K_X}\right) \tag{25}$$

Equations 23 – 25 are identical to equations 11-14.
Similar to the treatment of Michaelis-Menten enzymes, we obtain again a system of linear equations that describes the action of one or two inhibitors of ion channel receptors. If the concentration of inhibitor X is held constant, and the concentration of the second inhibitor, Y, is varied, the ratio S_0 / $S_{X,Y}$ is shifted up by a constant amount X/K_X but the slope ($1/K_Y$) is unchanged. The slope of the ratio curve represents the inhibitory potency, and the constant upward shift is due to the additive effect of two mutually exclusive inhibitors.
In the presence of two mutually non-exclusive inhibitors, the slope (ie inhibitory potency) is increased by a factor of ($1 + X/K_X$). Thus, if the mechanism underlying this analysis were followed, the "amount of synergy" could be calculated as $1 + X/K_X$. Often, quality of the data does not permit this quantitation, although the qualitative demonstration of synergy (increased inhibitory potency of drug A in the presence of drug B) is statistically safe. Thus, by taking the ratios of control and inhibited signals, we arrive at an equation that becomes mechanism-independent and corresponds to the principal equations used to describe drug interactions. The ratio method results in a simple graph that describes the type of joint action of two inhibitors on a common enzyme, neurotransmitter receptor, or general target protein (Fig. 6).

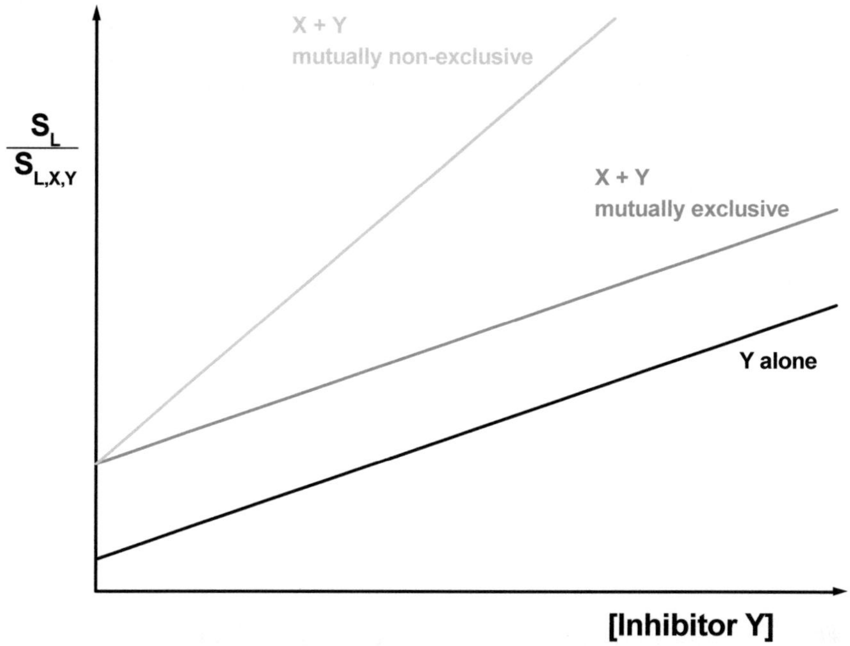

Fig. 6. Ratio method graph. Graph of signal ratio $S_0/S_{X,Y}$ vs inhibitor concentration for the case of one inhibitor (black curve), two mutually exclusive inhibitors (gray curve), and two mutually non-exclusive inhibitors (light gray curve). In case of mutually non-exclusive binding the inhibitory potency of inhibitor Y is increased in the presence of inhibitor X, as indicated by the lower value of K_Y computed from the slope of the inhibition ratio curve. Note that the formalism described here becomes mechanism-independent and applies to Michaelis-Menten type enzymes as well as to more complex mechanisms of ion channel receptor inhibition.

So far, a simple description of the action of two inhibitors on a common target has been derived. The mechanisms were based upon (i) a common binding site for two inhibitors, leading to mutually exclusive binding (Fig. 2), or (ii) two independent binding sites, leading to mutually non-exclusive binding (Fig. 3), Indeed, these simple models underlie (i) the principle of Loewe additivity (Loewe 1953; Berenbaum 1989), also referred to "similar", or "homodynamic" action of drugs. Here, the expectation value for zero interaction is just additivity. Independent inhibitor sites (Fig. 3), in contrast, correspond to Bliss independence, "dissimilar", "heterodynamic", or "independent" action of drugs (Bliss 1939; Berenbaum 1989). The combined effect of two such drugs will be more than additive, fulfilling the basic criterion of synergy. It has been recognized that these are the two limiting mechanisms for drug interaction (Bliss 1939; Finney 1942; Plackett and Hewlett 1948), and indeed both models are being used in the literature as zero interaction reference (Greco, Bravo et al. 1995).
It is intuitive, and favoured by this author to view the concept of Loewe additivity as the zero interaction reference, and noting the superadditive response from Bliss independence as synergism. This definition is widely accepted (Segel 1975; Chou and Talalay 1977; Berenbaum 1989). Furthermore, it allows for a very intuitive definition of zero interaction, proposed by Loewe: if drug A and B are the same, B being a dilution of A. Naturally, action of "both" drugs would be similar, and thus we have a perfect model of additivity.

However, what happens if we already know that drug A and B have completely different modes of action? Two drugs could be targeting different enzymes in a biochemical pathway. Of such a combination of drugs - having dissimilar action - we would expect superadditive behaviour. Can we call this synergy, or is it just expected from the mechanism and is now our zero reference? Arguments can be found for either view, and both models (and many more) are thus used and debated in the literature.

Once we move to more complicated systems, mechanism-based analysis is no longer feasible, and more general descriptions of drug interaction are needed. However, they all relate to the basic models of additivity and independence that were described above.

Equation 25 can be rearranged into the form

$$\frac{S_0}{S_{X,Y}} = 1 + \frac{X}{K_X} + \frac{Y}{K_Y} + \frac{X}{K_X}\frac{Y}{K_Y} \tag{26}$$

This equation is similar to a general equation that describes describing the joint action of two drugs on a specific target or biochemical process, presented by Greco et al. (Greco, Bravo et al. 1995).

$$1 = \frac{D_1}{ID_{X,1}} + \frac{D_2}{ID_{X,2}} + f\left(\frac{D_1}{ID_{X,1}}, \frac{D_2}{ID_{X,2}}, \alpha, p\right) \tag{27}$$

Here, D_1 and D_2 are concentrations of drug 1 and 2 in a mixture; $ID_{X,1}$ and $ID_{X,2}$ are the concentrations that produce a certain effect (corresponding to EC_{50}, or IC_{50} values); α is the synergism/antagonism parameter and p represents additional parameter(s) describing the "interaction" (joint action) of the two drugs.

The models and derivations given above are indeed the simplest approach to synergism between drugs. At this time, we do not even have a complete description of the action of every drug. It has been pointed out that under physiological conditions, it is expected that indeed presence of a drug will always result in an altered state of metabolism and thereby affect other drugs (Gessner 1974). In many patients multiple drug regimes have to be given, and the metabolism of a critically ill person may differ from a healthy "control" volunteer. Taken together, medical reality is not sufficiently described by simplified models. However, as shown above, even from simple model cases we can understand mechanisms of synergy and can derive mechanism-independent formalisms to determine the type of joint action of drug combinations.

In biomedical modelling, an alternative approach is the use of a mechanism-free description of activity, such as enzyme activity, ion channel function, the throughput of an entire biochemical pathway, or even cell survival in toxicity assays. The most common approach is the use of logistic equations that simply connect concentration of an effector (agonist or inhibitor) to the measured effect (enzyme activity, product formation, cell survival). The most comonly used formalism is that of the Hill equation.

$$E_0 = E_{\max} \frac{1}{1 + \left(\frac{EC_{50}}{L}\right)^n} \tag{28}$$

Here, E_0 is the observed effect, E_{max} is the maximum signal, EC_{50} is the concentration of ligand L that produces 50 % of the maximum response, and n is a coefficient defining the steepness of the dose-response curve. The similarity to Michaelis-Menten type enzyme kinetics is obvious, yet the logistic formalism is not based on any mechanism. Indeed, complex clinical situations require use of mechanism-free models to analyze drug interactions (Chou 1976; Berenbaum 1978; Berenbaum 1980; Chou and Talalay 1981; Berenbaum 1989; Tallarida 1992; Greco, Bravo et al. 1995).
In the following section some principles and formalisms for the analysis of drug synergism are briefly reviewed. An exhaustive review of all concepts is outside the scope of this text, readers are directed to several excellent, comprehensive reviews (Berenbaum 1989; Greco, Bravo et al. 1995; Tallarida 2001; Chou 2002; Toews and Bylund 2005; Chou 2006; Tallarida 2006; Bijnsdorp, Giovannetti et al. 2011).

3. Mechanisms and techniques of synergy testing in complex biomedical settings

An example, modified from Berenbaum (Berenbaum 1989) is that of a woodcutter, able to cut 10 trees in a day. He is joined by a second woodcutter, also able to cut down 10 trees in a day. Together, they manage to cut 15 trees in one day. How do we describe this situation?
One approach is that cutter A achieves 10 trees per day, our expectation value. Addition of cutter B results in 15 trees being cut, so there is synergy. Such an approach has been proposed e.g. by Gaddum, who only considered the effect of one agent and whether it was affected by another one being added (Gaddum 1940). This formalism is not used widely, as it obviously assigns synergism to the effects of several drugs too readily.
Conversely, one would say that with two cutters, each able to cut 10 trees per day, the expectation value is 20 trees/day. If only 15 are achieved, they are antagonising each other. This is the application of additivity, and clearly, the combined effect is sub-additive, 20 trees would be just additive, and more than 20 would mean synergy.
Mechanistically, one might argue that if cutter A works on a tree, then cutter B would not work on the same tree. Their action would be mutually exclusive, and the additive result would be expected. If, however, they are willing to work at the same tree together, they will be able to cut this tree in a much shorter time. In this case, they would be able to cut more than 20 trees in a day and their action would be mutually non-exclusive, leading to synergy.
As stated above, pure mechanistic analysis is not sufficient (and not possible) for most clinical cases, so a general, mechanism-free analysis of drug interaction is needed. Berenbaum (Berenbaum 1989) has pointed out the similarity to non-parametric statistical tests that do not require information about the meaning of the values, or the distribution of populations from where the values originate. The equivalent in dose-response analysis is a logistic equation, that just describes a dose-response curve without any requirement of a mechanism. In such a setting, one would just define the desired outcome (enzyme inhibition, cell death, reduction of virus titer, ...), and then measure the effect achieved by varying doses of each drug alone, and in combination.
The mechanisms shown above illustrate just the simplest mechanistic model. In real life, the situation is more complicated, as mechanisms of enzyme or receptor acitivity are more complex. Furthermore medical intervention is not only directed at single proteins, but at entire pathways or controlling structures, such as transcription factors, that initiate or control biochemical processes. Some therapies, such as cancer chemotherapy even aim at

cell destruction, i.e. they interfere with a complete living organism. In most of these situations, mechanisms of action are not known, or are too complex to work with. The additional problem is that with increasing complexity of the biological system, one finds an increasing paucity of experimental data. Even a simple dose-response curve, traditionally recorded with seven sensibly spaced concentration points, carries a significant error. By the rule of parsimony, one has to choose the simplest possible mechanism to describe experimental data. Thus, research is confronted with the dilemma of either oversimplification, or overinterpretation of results – a working compromise between these two extremes is needed. The pertinent models and methods have been extensively analyzed and reviewed in two excellent papers by Berenbaum (Berenbaum 1989), and Greco et al. (Greco, Bravo et al. 1995).

Some of the main concepts are just briefly described:

- Median effect analysis
- Interaction index, isobole method and combination index
- Response surface analysis

3.1 Median effect analysis

Chou et al. derived the median effect equation which follows from a detailed derivation of MM enzyme mechanisms (Chou 1976; Chou and Talalay 1977; Chou and Talalay 1981; Chou 2006).

$$\frac{d}{M} = \frac{E_d}{1 - E_d} \tag{29}$$

where d is the dose of a drug, E_d the effect caused by this amount of drug, M the median (dose causing 50 % effect, i.e. EC_{50} or IC_{50}). Indeed, such an equation can be derived by rearrangement of the Michaelis-Menten equation (6):

$$\frac{[S]}{K_M} = \frac{\frac{V_0}{V_{\max}}}{1 - \frac{V_0}{V_{\max}}} \tag{30}$$

Here, [S] is the substrate concentration that gives the observed V_0, K_M is the Michaelis constant, and V_0/V_{max} is the effect caused by [S], expressed here as the fractional velocity. The median effect equation has been proposed as a central, unified equation from which the basic equation sets of Henderson-Hasselbalch, Scatchard, Hill, and Michaelis-Menten can be derived (Chou 2006; Chou 2010). The median effect equation has been derived from MM-type enzymes from mathematical analysis. It can be extended to multiple-site systems in the form (Chou 2006)

$$\frac{E_d}{1 - E_d} = \left(\frac{d}{M}\right)^n \tag{31}$$

where n is the constant giving the slope of the dose-response curve. Note that n has often been equated with the number of binding sites, but this is an oversimplification that should be avoided since it is not valid in most cases. The value of n may be a measure of the degree of cooperativity between binding sites, but nothing more.

The equation can also be expressed in the form

$$\frac{f_A}{f_{UA}} = \left(\frac{d}{M}\right)^n \tag{32}$$

where f_A and f_{UA} are the fractions of affected and unaffected enzyme, respectively. The importance of the median effect equation is that it is composed of ratios of effects (E_d, $(1-E_d)$, or f_A and f_{UA}) and of the dose ratio (actual dose d, median dose M). Although derived from mechanistic analysis, the median effect equation cancels out mechanism-specific constants, and just links dose and effect in dimensionless ratios. This makes it a very versatile tool for the analysis of complex systems. The median effect equation can be linearized by taking logarithms on either side, giving the Hill plot (see Berenbaum 1989) which is a straight line for the plot of $\log(f_A/f_{UA})$ vs. log d.

$$\log\left[\frac{f_A}{f_{UA}}\right] = n(\log d - \log M) \tag{33}$$

Thus the median effect equations can be seen as an extremely useful rearranged form of dose-response curves, linking ratios of drug doses to ratios of observed effects. The median equation will work with both, mechanism-based (eg Michaelis-Menten), and effect-based (eg logistic) equations, and provides a dimensionless measure for drug effects. The technique has been extensively tested and derived from mechanistic as well as purely mathematical considerations. The group of T.C. Chou have pioneered this field and developed software packages (CompuSyn ands CalcuSyn) that allow reliable testing of drug interaction parameters (Chou 2002; Chou 2006; Chou 2010). Well-founded in theory, the technique has found widespread use (Chou 2002; Chou 2006; Chou 2010; Bijnsdorp, Giovannetti et al. 2011), and the initital paper by Chou and Talalay (Chou and Talalay 1984) has been intensely cited and discussed.

3.2 Interaction index, isobole method and combination index

The interaction of two or more drugs to produce a combined effect can be described by the interaction index I (Berenbaum 1977).

$$I = \frac{D_1}{ID_{X,1}} + \frac{D_2}{ID_{X,2}} \tag{34}$$

or written in terms of the median equations above

$$I = \frac{d_1}{M_1} + \frac{d_2}{M_2} \tag{35}$$

where, D_1 , D_2 d_1 and d_2 are concentrations of drug 1 and 2 that produce a certain effect if applied together; $ID_{X,1}$, $ID_{X,2}$, M_1 and M_2 are the concentrations that produce the same effect when given alone. For instance, if we want 50 % inhibition, then equation 34 would be:

$$I = \frac{D_1}{IC_{50,1}} + \frac{D_2}{IC_{50,2}} \tag{36}$$

Here, $IC_{50,1}$ and $IC_{50,2}$ are the IC_{50} values of drug 1 and drug 2 alone. D_1 and D_2 are the doses of drug 1 and 2, respectively, that also produce 50 % inhibition when given together. The interaction index, proposed by Berenbaum (Berenbaum 1977), should be constant in case of zero interaction. The method has been extended by Berenbaum (Berenbaum 1985) and developed into a general method based on analysis of each drug alone and then simulating the combined action of both drugs based on Loewe additivity (see also Greco, Bravo et al. 1995).
The interaction index underlies one of the most widely used graphical representations of drug synergism and antagonism, the isobologram. Isoboles were first used by Fraser in 1870 (Fraser 1870; Fraser 1872) as simple, intuitive illustration without mathematical derivation. Here, the doses of drugs A and B give abscissa and ordinate, respectively, and the effect of drug combinations is plotted as graph (Fig. 7). In the example (Fig. 7), the effect plotted is for 50 % inhibition of an enzyme. The effects of each drug alone (i.e. IC_{50}) can be read from the axes. The isobologram shows an effect, such as IC_{50} (IC_{10} or IC_{80}, whatever effect is of interest) and which drug concentration is needed to achieve this effect.

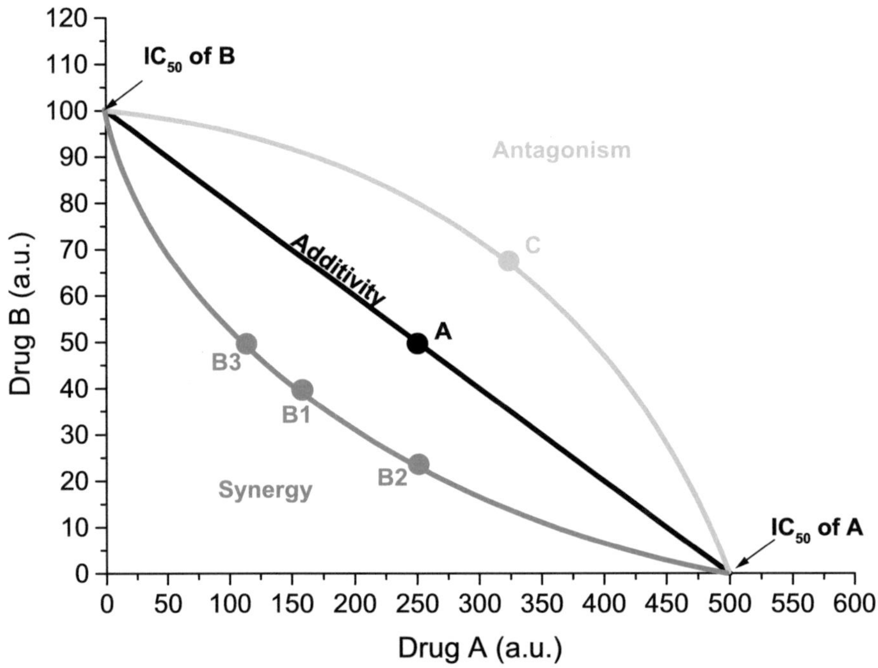

Fig. 7. Isobologram. Abscissa and ordinate units are the concentrations of drugs A and B. The solid black line connects concentrations that produce the same effect on the target protein, enzyme, or system. In this example, the IC_{50} line is given. In the simulation, drug A has an IC_{50} (concentration giving 50 % inhibition) of 500 a.u. (arbitrary units), IC_{50} of drug B is 100 a.u. From additivity (black line), the combination of 250 a.u. of A with 50 a.u. of B should also give 50 % inhibition (point A). If, 50 % inhibition are achieved at lower concentrations of the two drugs (e.g. 150 a.u. of A and 40 a.u. of B, point B1), the drugs would show synergism. If the observed inhibition by the combination was less than 50 %, drug A and B would interact in an antagonistic way (point C). Model lines of synergism (gray line) and antagonism (light gray line) are drawn. Note that in case of synergy between two drugs, the IC_{50} curve would not be a straight line but an upward concave (gray line), in case of antagonism a downward concave (light gray line). In practical application, one

would determine IC_{50} of one drug in the presence of a constant concentration of the other. IC_{50} would be found with the combination of 250 a.u. of A and 24 a.u. of B (point B2), or 110 a.u. of A and 50 a.u. of B (point B3).

Equations 34 - 36 define straight lines for two drugs that do not show any interaction (synergism or antagonism). Two drugs showing aditivity wold be expected to fall on the additivity line (Fig. 7). If the two drugs act synergistically, lower concentrations would be needed in the mixture to achieve the same effect. Their combination graph would be an upward concave (gray line in Fig. 7), following the unequality

$$\frac{D_1}{ID_{X,1}} + \frac{D_2}{ID_{X,2}} < 1 \tag{37}$$

Conversely, two antagonistic drugs would require higher doses in combination to achieve the same effect, and the resulting isobole would be an upward convex line (red line in Fig. 7), of the general (un)equation

$$\frac{D_1}{ID_{X,1}} + \frac{D_2}{ID_{X,2}} > 1 \tag{38}$$

Representing a form of median effect equationry, isoboles have become a useful tool to present complex modes of drug interaction. An excellent review by Greco et al (Greco, Bravo et al. 1995) derives isoboles as 2-D sections through three-dimensional plots of drug action data. Depending on the shapes of the dose-response curves of both drugs, isoboles do not need to be linear (Greco, Bravo et al. 1995). Also, drug combinations may be biphasic, showing concentration ranges of synergy and ranges of antagonism (Berenbaum 1989).
Equations 34 and 35 apply to the case of Loewe additivity, where the two drugs do not show synergy or antagonism. For drugs showing any type of interaction, equation 34 was extended to define a combination index (CI), indicating type and amount of interaction between two (or more) drugs with respect to the experimantal parameter being studied (Chou and Talalay 1983).

$$CI = \frac{D_1}{ID_{X,1}} + \frac{D_2}{ID_{X,2}} \begin{array}{l} > 1 \text{ for antagonism} \\ = 1 \text{ for additivity} \\ < 1 \text{ for synergy} \end{array} \tag{39}$$

The CI can take values between 1 and infinity for antagonism, and runs between 0 and 1 for synergy. Chou and Chou (1988) have introduced the dose reduction index DRI (Chou and Chou 1988), which is based on the interpretation of the Combination index equation (39). Assuming that two drugs show synergy, one expects that a lower dose of each is needed to achieve the same effect. This lower concentration (D_1 and D_2 in equations 34-39) can be related to the median (IC_{50} in equation 36), to give the dose reduction index DRI.

$$CI = \frac{1}{(DRI)_1} + \frac{1}{(DRI)_2} \tag{40}$$

Both, combination index CI and DRI can be used to plot drug combination data for visualization of synergy or antagonism (Fig. 8, see (Chou 2006)).

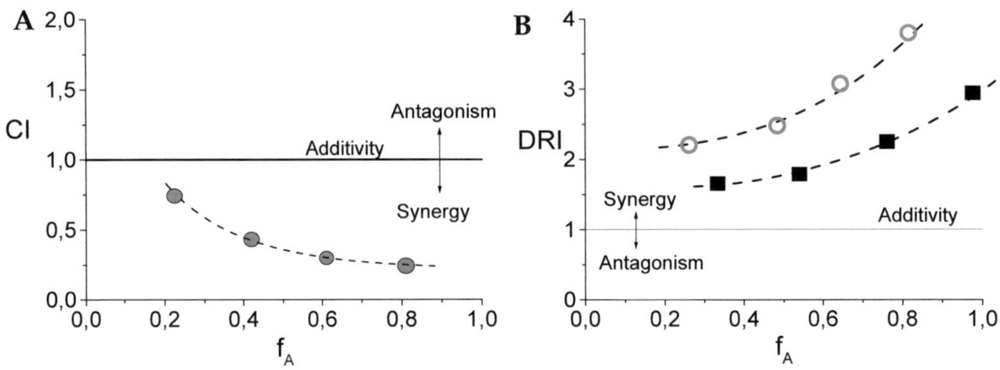

Fig. 8. Visualization of drug interaction data. (A) CI-f_A plot: The combination index CI is plotted versus f_A, the fraction of affected enzyme or biological function. (B) DRI plot: the dose reduction index DRI is plotted against f_A. See text for definitions of terms.

3.3 Response surface analysis

Response surfaces can be calculated and are a way to represent effects of drug combinations as a contour plot where drug concentrations are plotted as a horizontal x-y- plane, and the effect is plotted on the z axis. Isoboles can be seen as 2D sections through response surfaces, and the method allows graphical analysis of drug interaction data, albeit at requirement of quite some mathematical and computational effort. From the dose-response data of each drug alone, the expected response surface based on the zero interaction reference of choice, is plotted. Then actual drug combination data are entered into the plot, and similar to isobole analysis, deviations from the reference surface indicate synergism or antagonism. The technique has been applied to synergism studies (Tallarida, Stone et al. 1999), and its general use reviewed and commented in great detail (Berenbaum 1989; Greco, Bravo et al. 1995; Tallarida 2001).

3.4 Practical limitations

There is a need for a definition of synergy, antagonism, and the zero case (neither one nor the other). Sometimes, specific problems are discussed and authors feel compelled to use a unique treatment of the data. Pharmacologists, stasticians, clinicians, and representatives from other fields have different views and concepts. In various major reviews, 13 models to treat drug combination data have been proposed. The author would not encourage decisions as to right or wrong. Each model may be appropriate for a given situation, and not applicable to others. However, all models discussing synergy can be traced back to only two types of the "zero" (no interaction) case as discussed before

- Loewe Additivity

  Both drugs exert an effect but are mutually exclusive, either one or the other can be active at a given time. This corresponds to a common site of interaction in the simplest mechanistic case (Fig. 2).
- Bliss Independence

  Both drugs are mutually non-exclusive, both can be active at the same time. In the simplest case, each drug has a specific, independent interaction site (Fig. 3).

Indeed all models refer to these two basic cases. Obviously, both have a different expecation of joint action of two drugs. Loewe additivity is best described by equation 34, and any deviation from this may be considered as synergy. In case of Bliss independencs, one would expect both drugs to act independently, and therefore the zero case already includes a more than additive effect of both drugs. The author sees two problems with this definition: (i) two purely additive drugs would have to be called antagonistic, including the sham combination of a drug with itself. (ii) If two mutually non-exclusive drugs already produce a superadditive effect, and we do not yet call this synergy, how do we define "true" synergy? In terms of isoboles, the baseline (no synergy, no antagonism) is already curved, in the ratio method (Fig. 6), the slope of the inhibition curve is increased already for the zero case, and one calculates a CI of less than one. Thus, to identify synergy, one has to select a gradual increase. It may be fairly easy to identify a deviation from a straight line (isobole), but for the CI a deviation from <1 to <<1 is expected. In the ration method, the steepness of th slope may be hard to compute, as the ratio $S_X/S_{control}$ is toe be calculated from small numerical values and thus carries a large error.

Thus the definition of Loewe additivity is preferred by this author as the definition of no synergy. As shown in Fig.s 2 and 3, it can clearly be defined in mechanistic term. Dose-response analysis also follows the definition. Addtivity correctly describes the purest control experiment, sham mixtures of the same drug, and it follows the general definition of synergy, where a combination produces more thant the sum of the individual components.

It should be noted, however, that in many clinical applications, drug combinations are used that target two completely different target proteins, or pathways. In radiotherapy, the combination of radiation and drugs work together, and in combination lower doses of either are required compared to a single treatment. No baseline of Loewe additivity can be proposed for such a combination. Likewise, combinations of drugs that target completely different cellular pathways may work synergistically towards cell killing even though the two drugs are not mutually exclusive in their activity. Obviously, there is no single methodology that is appropriate for all biomedical situations.

An additional problem in interpreting drug combination data is the quality of the measured data. Biological systems invariably carry experimental error, and thus borderline cases are almost impossible to assign. For example, a combination index is calculated to be 0.9 – is this a real deviation from unity (and thus synergy), or is it experimental error?

Even with the best data, however, analysis of joint action of two drugs has another inherent problem. Two different drugs may have different dose-response characteristics. In this case, changes in effective concentrations may suggest synergy where there is none. A principal illustration of this problem is given in Fig. 9 (adapted from Chou (Chou 2006; Chou 2010)), showing that the same relative concentration change can produce quite different effects (Fig. 9 A,B). Even for a single compound, there is a marked difference whether one investigates concentrations below or around EC_{50}, or near saturation. Addition of the same drug in the concentration range around EC_{50} (ie the steepest part of the dose-response curve) gives rise to a strong increase in signal which may be misinterpreted as synergy. The shapes of isobolograms for drugs with different dose-response characteristics, and the complications resulting from this fact have been extensively studied (Berenbaum 1989; Greco, Bravo et al. 1995; Tallarida 2001; Chou 2006).

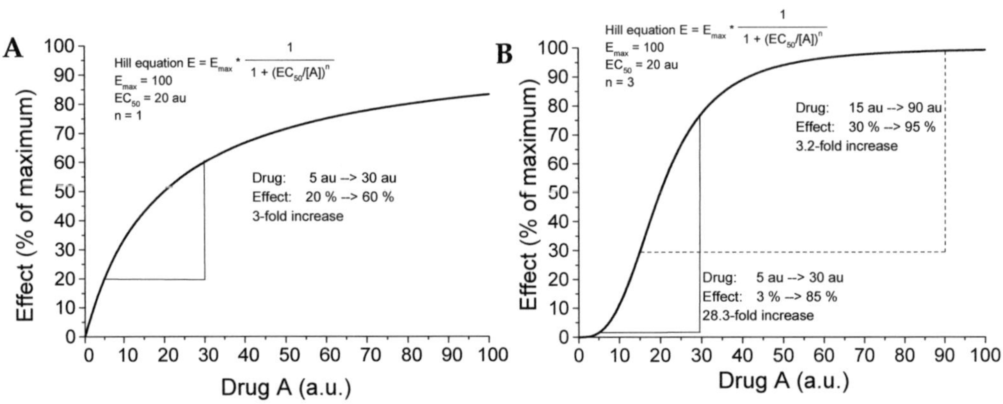

Fig. 9. Dose-effect curves of different shape. Both curves were simulated using the Hill equation and the parameters E_{max} = 100 % , EC_{50} = 20 au (arbitrary units). (A) Curve simulated for n =1 (hyperbolic curve). (B) Simulated for n = 3 (sigmoidal curve). Note the difference in curve shape, and the different effect of a change of concentration of agonist A from 5 to 30 au. In the hyperbolic case, the effect increases 3-fold, in the sigmoidal case, the increase is 28.3-fold. Effects of changes in agonist concentration are different depending on the response range where they happen. Sigmoidal dose-response curves are steepest around the median (panel B). In the example, a 6-fold raise in concentration (from 5 to 30 au) will cause a 28.3-fold increase in the observed effect. Raising the concentration from 15 to 90 au, the effect only increases 3.2-fold. Thus, if presence of a second drug B increases cooperativity of drug A, or if drug B shifts the relevant dose-response range of A towards the median by purely additive (non-synergistic) means, one would observe a higher increase in effect than expected from addition and wrongly interpret this as synergy.

4. Borderlines of synergism – Potentiation, coalism, inertism, metabolic interference

From the simplest models presented here to advanced discussions, the situations of synergy could be traced back to the simple principles of additivity vs. independence. In all those cases, both drugs were having the same effect alone or in combination. The only difference was the magnitude of the effects. Synergism can also occur with combinations of drugs or methods that have completely different modes of action. In cancer therapy a combination of radiation and cytotostatica is often used. Combination of substances and environmental conditions (heat, pH, radiation) have indeed been analyzed for synergy (Johnson, Eyring et al. 1945). There are cases of one drug having no activity, but augmenting the activity of another, as observed for antinociception by acetaminophen in combination with phentolamine (Raffa, Stone et al. 2001). The extreme case would be the combination of two drugs that have no effect alone, but are effective in combination. On the othe hand, self-synergy of paracetamol has been described by Tallarida et al., who showed that the drug binds to targets in different locations and thus facilitates its own activity (Raffa, Stone et al. 2000). An interesting approach is an attempt to predict drug synergism from gene microarray data (Jin, Zhao et al. 2011).

Effect of drug combination	Both drugs have same effect individually	Only one drug is effective individually	None of the two drugs has an effect individually
Greater than zero reference	Synergy, Synergism	Synergism (potentiation)	Coalism
Equal to zero reference	Additiviy / Independence	Inertism	Inertism
Smaller than zero reference	Antagonism	Antagonism	

Table 1. The terminology of the combined action of drugs (after Greco, Bravo et al. 1995)

Another effect leading to apparent synergy or antagonism is the effect some drug may have on uptake, metabolism and clearance of other drugs. Depending on the route of administration, metabolism by first liver pass must be considered, including one of the most critical steps of drug biotransformation, namely oxygenation (thus hydrophilization) by cytochrome P450, an oxygenase that catalyzes oxygenations of substrates using NADPH and oxygen (O_2). This oxygenation R-H → R-OH is a crucial step in metabolism and eventual clearance of drugs and pharmaceuticals from the body. To date, 56 subtypes of cytochrome P450 are found in humans, some of which are critical in metabolism of endogenous substances such as medical drugs. Substances interfering with cytochrome P450 may, therefore, have an impact on drug clearance and thus on the actual concentration of a certain drug in the body (Flockhart 1995; Flockhart and Oesterheld 2000; Shin, Park et al. 2002; Takada, Arefayene et al. 2004).

Resource	Internet address	Comment
Drug interactions checker	http://www.drugs.com/drug_interactions.html	Tool to query compounds that interact with a given drug
Medscape drug interaction checker	http://reference.medscape.com/drug-interactionchecker	Tool to report on interactions between two drugs
Cytochrome P450 drug interaction table	http://medicine.iupui.edu/clinpharm/ddis/	List of drugs metabolized by cyt P450 isoforms (Flockhart 2007)
Grapefruit juice/citrus fruit juice interactions	http://www.mayoclinic.com/health/food-and-nutrition/AN00413	Short list of drugs that interact with dietary citrus fruits
Private resources	http://www.environmentaldiseases.com/article-drug-interactions.html	Website discussing case individual studies of interfering drugs

Table 2. Internet tools for drug interactions in clinical settings

There are numerous internet tools that list known drug interactions. A brief list of some such resources is given in table 2. Thus, some practical aspects have been covered, although synergisms and other interactions of drugs are not yet given enough weight in approval or recommendations of drug use. This is particularly relevant for the less well-defined field of herbal remedies. Their interaction with anticancer agents has been studied (Sparreboom, Cox et al. 2004), but our knowledge in this area is still far from comprehensive.

To date, the study of drug interaction in the biomedical field is widespread and must include the following aspects:

- mechanism of action of a single drug
- mechanisms of action of two (or more) drugs acting on the same physiological target
- interaction of two drugs through side effects, secondary targets, etc
- effects on metabolism of the primary drug
- top-down observations of the performance of drug combinations in patients

Going down this list it becomes clear that pure mechanistic studies - although essential - are not sufficient to cover all aspects of drug interaction. Clinical observation is the - equally essential - other end of the spectrum and the gap between these two positions is indeed narrowing.

5. References

Asante-Appiah, E. & W. W. Chan (1996). Analysis of the interactions between an enzyme and multiple inhibitors using combination plots. *Biochem J* Vol. 320 (Pt 1), pp. 17-26.

Berenbaum, M. C. (1977). Synergy, additivism and antagonism in immunosuppression. A critical review. *Clin Exp Immunol* Vol. 28, No. 1, pp. 1-18.

Berenbaum, M. C. (1978). A method for testing for synergy with any number of agents. *J Infect Dis* Vol. 137, No. 2, pp. 122-130.

Berenbaum, M. C. (1980). Correlations between methods for measurement of synergy. *J Infect Dis* Vol. 142, No. 3, pp. 476-480.

Berenbaum, M. C. (1985). The expected effect of a combination of agents: the general solution. *J Theor Biol* Vol. 114, No. 3, pp. 413-431.

Berenbaum, M. C. (1989). What is synergy? *Pharmacol Rev* Vol. 41, No. 2, pp. 93-141.

Bijnsdorp, I. V., E. Giovannetti & G. J. Peters (2011). Analysis of drug interactions. *Methods Mol Biol* Vol. 731, No., pp. 421-34.

Bliss, C. I. (1939). The toxicity of poisons applied jointly. *Ann Appl Biol* Vol. 26, pp. 585-615.

Breitinger, H.-G., N. Geetha & G. P. Hess (2001). Inhibition of the serotonin 5-HT3 receptor by nicotine, cocaine, and fluoxetine investigated by rapid chemical kinetic techniques. *Biochemistry* Vol. 40, No. 28, pp. 8419-8429.

Chou, T. C. (1976). Derivation and properties of Michaelis-Menten type and Hill type equations for reference ligands. *J Theor Biol* Vol. 59, No. 2, pp. 253-276.

Chou, T. C. (2002). Synergy determination issues. *J Virol* Vol. 76, No. 20, pp. 10577; author reply 10578

Chou, T. C. (2006). Theoretical basis, experimental design, and computerized simulation of synergism and antagonism in drug combination studies. *Pharmacol Rev* Vol. 58, No. 3, pp. 621-681.

Chou, T. C. (2010). Drug combination studies and their synergy quantification using the Chou-Talalay method. *Cancer Res* Vol. 70, No. 2, pp. 440-446.

Chou, T. C. & J. H. Chou (1988). Distinction between multiple ligand exclusivity and competitiveness in receptor binding topology. *FASEB J.* Vol. 2, pp. A1778.

Chou, T. C. & P. Talalay (1977). A simple generalized equation for the analysis of multiple inhibitions of Michaelis-Menten kinetic systems. *J Biol Chem* Vol. 252, No. 18, pp. 6438-6442.

Chou, T. C. & P. Talalay (1981). Generalized equations for the analysis of inhibitions of Michaelis-Menten and higher-order kinetic systems with two or more mutually exclusive and nonexclusive inhibitors. *Eur J Biochem* Vol. 115, No. 1, pp. 207-216.

Chou, T. C. & P. Talalay (1983). Analysis of combined drug effects: a new look at a very old problem. *Trends Pharmacol Sci* Vol. 4, No., pp. 450–454.

Chou, T. C. & P. Talalay (1984). Quantitative analysis of dose-effect relationships: the combined effects of multiple drugs or enzyme inhibitors. *Adv Enzyme Regul* Vol. 22, No., pp. 27-55.

Colquhoun, D. (1998). Binding, gating, affinity and efficacy: the interpretation of structure-activity relationships for agonists and of the effects of mutating receptors. *Br J Pharmacol* Vol. 125, No. 5, pp. 924-947.

Finney, D. J. (1942). The analysis of toxicity tests on mixtures of poisons. *Ann. App!. Biol.* Vol. 29, No., pp. 82-94.

Flockhart, D. A. (1995). Drug interactions and the cytochrome P450 system. The role of cytochrome P450 2C19. *Clin Pharmacokinet* Vol. 29 Suppl 1, No., pp. 45-52.

Flockhart, D. A. (2007). Drug Interactions: Cytochrome P450 Drug Interaction Table. *Indiana University School of Medicine* . http://medicine.iupui.edu/clinpharm/ddis/

Flockhart, D. A. & J. R. Oesterheld (2000). Cytochrome P450-mediated drug interactions. *Child Adolesc Psychiatr Clin N Am* Vol. 9, No. 1, pp. 43-76.

Fraser, T. R. (1870). An experimental research on the antagonism between the actions of physostigma and atropia. *Proc. Roy. Soc. Edin.* Vol. 7, No., pp. 506-511.

Fraser, T. R. (1872). The antagonism between the actions of active substances. *Br. Med. J.* Vol. 2, No., pp. 485-487.

Gaddum, J. H. (1940). *Pharmacology*. Oxford University Press, London.

Gessner, P. K. (1974). *The isobolographic method applied to drug interactions*. In: Drug Interactions. P. L. Morselli, S. Garattini & S. N. Cohen (Eds), pp. 349-362, Raven Press, New York.

Greco, W. R., G. Bravo & J. C. Parsons (1995). The search for synergy: a critical review from a response surface perspective. *Pharmacol Rev* Vol. 47, No. 2, pp. 331-385.

Hess, G. P. (1993). Determination of the chemical mechanism of neurotransmitter receptor-mediated reactions by rapid chemical kinetic techniques. *Biochemistry* Vol. 32, No. 4, pp. 989-1000.

Jin, G., H. Zhao, X. Zhou & S. T. Wong (2011). An enhanced Petri-net model to predict synergistic effects of pairwise drug combinations from gene microarray data. *Bioinformatics* Vol. 27, No. 13, pp. i310-316.

Johnson, F. H., H. Eyring, R. Steblay, H. Chaplin, C. Huber & G. Gherardi (1945). The Nature and Control of Reactions in Bioluminescence : With Special Reference to the Mechanism of Reversible and Irreversible Inhibitions by Hydrogen and Hydroxyl Ions, Temperature, Pressure, Alcohol, Urethane, and Sulfanilamide in Bacteria. *J Gen Physiol* Vol. 28, No. 5, pp. 463-537.

Karpen, J. W., H. Aoshima, L. G. Abood & G. P. Hess (1982). Cocaine and phencyclidine inhibition of the acetylcholine receptor: analysis of the mechanisms of action based on measurements of ion flux in the millisecond-to-minute time region. *Proc Natl Acad Sci U S A* Vol. 79, No. 8, pp. 2509-2513.

Karpen, J. W. & G. P. Hess (1986). Cocaine, phencyclidine, and procaine inhibition of the acetylcholine receptor: characterization of the binding site by stopped-flow measurements of receptor-controlled ion flux in membrane vesicles. *Biochemistry* Vol. 25, No. 7, pp. 1777-1785.

Loewe, S. (1953). The problem of synergism and antagonism of combined drugs. *Arzneimittelforschung* Vol. 3, No. 6, pp. 285-290.

Palatini, P. (1983). The interaction between full and partial inhibitors acting on a single enzyme. A theoretical analysis. *Mol Pharmacol* Vol. 24, No. 1, pp. 30-41.

Plackett, R. L. & P. S. Hewlett (1948). Statistical aspects of the independent joint action of poisons, particularly insecticides; the toxicity of a mixture of poisons. *Ann Appl Biol* Vol. 35, No. 3, pp. 347-358.

Raafat, K., U. Breitinger, L. Mahran, N. Ayoub & H. G. Breitinger (2010). Synergistic inhibition of glycinergic transmission in vitro and in vivo by flavonoids and strychnine. *Toxicol Sci* Vol. 118, No. 1, pp. 171-182.

Raffa, R. B., D. J. Stone, Jr. & R. J. Tallarida (2000). Discovery of "self-synergistic" spinal/supraspinal antinociception produced by acetaminophen (paracetamol). *J Pharmacol Exp Ther* Vol. 295, No. 1, pp. 291-294.

Raffa, R. B., D. J. Stone, Jr. & R. J. Tallarida (2001). Unexpected and pronounced antinociceptive synergy between spinal acetaminophen (paracetamol) and phentolamine. *Eur J Pharmacol* Vol. 412, No. 2, pp. R1-2.

Schenker, P. & A. Baici (2009). Simultaneous interaction of enzymes with two modifiers: reappraisal of kinetic models and new paradigms. *J Theor Biol* Vol. 261, No. 2, pp. 318-329.

Segel, I. H. (1975). *Enzyme Kinetics*. John Wiley, New York.

Shin, J. G., J. Y. Park, M. J. Kim, J. H. Shon, Y. R. Yoon, I. J. Cha, S. S. Lee, S. W. Oh, S. W. Kim & D. A. Flockhart (2002). Inhibitory effects of tricyclic antidepressants (TCAs) on human cytochrome P450 enzymes in vitro: mechanism of drug interaction between TCAs and phenytoin. *Drug Metab Dispos* Vol. 30, No. 10, pp. 1102-1107.

Sparreboom, A., M. C. Cox, M. R. Acharya & W. D. Figg (2004). Herbal remedies in the United States: potential adverse interactions with anticancer agents. *J Clin Oncol* Vol. 22, No. 12, pp. 2489-2503.

Takada, K., M. Arefayene, Z. Desta, C. H. Yarboro, D. T. Boumpas, J. E. Balow, D. A. Flockhart & G. G. Illei (2004). Cytochrome P450 pharmacogenetics as a predictor of toxicity and clinical response to pulse cyclophosphamide in lupus nephritis. *Arthritis Rheum* Vol. 50, No. 7, pp. 2202-2210.

Tallarida, R. J. (1992). Statistical analysis of drug combinations for synergism. *Pain* Vol. 49, No. 1, pp. 93-97.

Tallarida, R. J. (2001). Drug synergism: its detection and applications. *J Pharmacol Exp Ther* Vol. 298, No. 3, pp. 865-872.

Tallarida, R. J. (2006). An overview of drug combination analysis with isobolograms. *J Pharmacol Exp Ther* Vol. 319, No. 1, pp. 1-7.

Tallarida, R. J., D. J. Stone, Jr., J. D. McCary & R. B. Raffa (1999). Response surface analysis of synergism between morphine and clonidine. *J Pharmacol Exp Ther* Vol. 289, No. 1, pp. 8-13.

Toews, M. L. & D. B. Bylund (2005). Pharmacologic principles for combination therapy. *Proc Am Thorac Soc* Vol. 2, No. 4, pp. 282-289; discussion 290-291.

8

Herbal Medicine in the Treatment of Malaria: *Vernonia amygdalina*: An Overview of Evidence and Pharmacology

Anoka A. Njan
Department of Pharmacology and Toxicology, Faculty of Pharmaceutical Scinces, Usmanu Danfodiyo University, Sokoto, Nigeria

1. Introduction

Traditional medicines occupy a central place among rural communities of developing countries for the provision of health care in the absence of an efficient public health care system (WHO, 2003).

The use of traditional remedies is common in sub-Saharan Africa, and visits to traditional healers remain a mainstay of care for many people because of preference, affordability, and limited access to hospitals and modern health practitioners (Homsy et al., 1999).

It is an important part of medical care in Uganda and throughout Africa, representing first line therapy for 70% of the population, (Homsy et al., 2004). For many, traditional herbal medicines may be the only source of treatment available. The main reasons to explain this are: traditional medicines are often more accessible compared with licensed drugs; there are no records attesting the resistance to whole-plant extracts possibly due to the synergistic action of their constituents; phytotherapy, possibly produces fewer adverse effect than chemotherapy (Willcox and Bodeker, 2000).

In Africa more than 2,000 plants have been identified and use as herbal medicines. However, very few of these plants have been screened for safety in resource-constrained countries including Uganda. It is time to ask in a systematic and scientific manner how these local treatments work, what are the best means to establish their safety and can they be used as traditionally prepared? The source of antimalarial drugs such as artemisinin derivatives and quinolines currently in use today were isolated from medicinal plants. Renewed interest in traditional pharmacopoeias has meant that researchers are concerned not only with determining the scientific rationale for plants usage, but also with the discovering of novel compounds of pharmaceutical value for the treatment of malaria.

Herbals are as old as human civilization and they have provided a complete storehouse of remedies to cure acute and chronic diseases. Numerous nutraceuticals are present in medicinal herbs as key components. Scientific evaluation of herbal products has been limited, yet herbal products are the most commonly consumed health care products. Because of known pharmacological effects and potential interaction of many of these compounds with therapeutic drugs, a history of herbal intake should be considered as part of routine medical history and should be evaluated before any change in prescription drugs and before medical procedures (Schwartz et al 2000)

At present, work conducted on traditional medicine in Africa has mainly concentrated on the collection, identification, and classification of herbal products for treatment of different ailments. However, research in the areas of safety and toxicology is lacking.
Traditional medicines, like modern pharmaceuticals can do harm, but because humans have been using herbal drugs for long time, they are considered safe and non-toxic so the toxicological actions of these agents have been mostly ignored, even while the effectiveness is either already known or under study (O'Hara et al., 1998). Willcox (1999), carried out a clinical study on 'AM' (coded to protect the intellectual property right of the traditional healers), a popular antimalarial herb that has a long history of use among the people of south-western Uganda. In her result, 'AM' significantly reduced parasite count between day 1 and day 7, patients showed symptomatic improvement, but 50% of them experienced some side effects including vomiting, nausea and stomach upset. These were partly attributed to malaria itself as well as to 'AM' ingestion (Willcox, 1999).
If the origin of herbs' toxicity is not identified, the adverse effects may be wrongly associated with other environmental exposures or some traditional belief. Failure to establish the true cause of exposure also means that the patient continues taking the toxic herb. Thus, the screening of traditional remedies for safety and toxicity is recommended to protect public health. On the other hand, several plants used in Uganda traditional medicine can cause damage to genetic material and therefore have potential to cause long-term damage in patients when administered as medicinal preparations (Steenkamp, 2005).

1.1 The main groups of active principle or constituents obtained from medicinal herbs

The therapeutic effects of plant species are determined by their constituents. These affect the condition and function of the various human body organs, clear up residual symptoms or destroy the cause of the disease in most cases infectious micro-organisms. They help increase the body's resistance to disease, retard or delay the processes of natural aging or facilitate the adaptation of the organism to certain conditions (Forantisek, 2001). Over the centuries, man used medicinal plants even though he was unable to find a rational explanation for their effects. It was not until the 19th century and after the rapid development of organic chemistry and pharmacology, that man determined which active or group of principles are responsible for a given therapeutic effect. Knowledge of these substances frequently served as a model for the synthetic preparation of new medicines, enabling the drug to be modified and made more effective. It was soon discovered that a better therapeutic effect was often obtained by the particular combination of active principle naturally present in each plant that by a single, isolated substance. The most important constituents are the secondary metabolism in plants, which includes alkaloids, glycosides, essential oils, tannins and the bitter principles. Products of secondary metabolism of plants are responsible for the plants' therapeutics effects. Of greater importance for the plants themselves of course are the products of primary metabolism which are necessary for the proper function of the basic life processes in plants. Primary metabolism products are also used by man. This group includes sugars, fatty oils, organic acids, vitamins and protein. These products of primary metabolism themselves may have no therapeutic effect but may possibly increase the efficiency of the therapeutically important principles (70)

1.2 *Vernonia amygdalina*

(Aseraceae), also called bitter leaf is a popular African vegetable that grows as a shrub or small tree indigenous to Central and East Africa including Uganda (Huffman et al, 1996). It produces large mass of forage and is drought tolerant (Hutchioson and Dalziel, 1963), it is 2 - 5 m with petiolate leaf of about 6 mm diameter and elliptic shape. The leaves are green with a characteristic odour and a bitter taste. No seeds are produced and the tree has therefore to be distributed through cutting. It is known locally as Omubirizi in south-western Uganda and used traditionally for pain relief and malaria attack. Patients are instructed to soak the plant leave in hot water about (80°C). They should then drink half a glass (about 0.25l) two times daily for 4-7 days. Smaller doses are prescribed for children according to their weight.They are used as vegetable and stimulate the digestive system in some other countries in the continent.

This plant has ethnomedical use in treating veneral diseases, gastrointestinal problems and malaria (Kambizi et al, 2001; Huffman et al, 2003; Hamill et al, 1992). Furthermore, they are used as local medicine against leech, which are transmitting bilharzias. Free living chimpanzees eat the leaves, if they have attacked by parasites (Huffman, M.A. 2003). There are reports concerning the hypoglycaemic, antineoplastic antibacterial and antioxidant properties of the plant. (Akah et al, 1992; Izevbigie et al, 2004; Taiwo et al, 1999; Iwalewa et al, 2005). Despite the varied uses of the plant, there are no information on its analgesic properties and exact toxicology on sub-chronic exposure, although some reports describe its antiplasmodial effects (Abosi et al 2005; Masaba et al 2000; Tona et al, 2004; Wilcox et al, 1999). Previous phytochemical reports have shown the presence of steroid, saponins, flavonoids.

2. Methods

2.1 Research design

Ninety traditional healers were identified through community and healers association leaders. Once identified, study staff members approached the individuals to determine eligibility. Eligibility criteria included 30 years of age and older, recognition as a traditional healer by the local community council, and having established an active practice in the community. Three districts (Kanungu/Bwindi area, Bushenyi and Mbarara) south-western Uganda were identified. With consent a taxonomist samples of antimalarial herb were obtained for this research study.

To evaluate consistency, interviews were conducted by a person specially trained in interview administration and who is fluent in the language of the participants.

The ethnographic interview included questions about common plant names, sources of products, method of preparation, purpose of use, quantity of herbs use and perceived benefit of herbs in ameliorating malaria symptoms and improving overall health. Ethical forms were used in order to assure them of the defense of their knowledge and intellectual property right was applied. Traditional healer's name, age, gender, and ethnicity tribe, were asked. We relied on the knowledge of healers and the taxonomist to select the products of greatest importance. This enabled us target products that have a high likelihood of possessing significant pharmacological activity.

A strategy was developed that respected the healers' rights to maintain propriety of unique blends of herbal medicine. Also, a memorandum of understanding was developed that disclosed our study objective, which is to characterize the pharmacologic activity and to elucidate the toxicity of these remedies in order to determine any potential adverse effect. We emphasized that we were interested in general knowledge about the remedy and not in specific formulation, and that it was not our intention to use the knowledge gained from this study for commercial profit. Rather we would report back to them in a workshop the remedy's indication and contraindication after completion of the study. We requested that all parties sign the agreement and copies were kept in a secure file. The result of the study was used to determine the most common botanical/herbal products used by the healers to treat malaria. Among the herbal products, *Vernonia amygdalina* which appeared in 80% in the interview was chosen for studies.

Fidelity level: The fidelity level (Fl) (Alexiades et al, 2000) among the healers from the same district was calculated according to the following formula:

$$Fl (\%) = (Np/N) \times 100$$

Np is the number of healers from one given district that claim a use of a plant species to treat a particular disease, and N is the number of healers from the same district that use the plants as a medicine to treat any given disease. The formula was applied in order to compare data from different district where the survey was performed.

2.2 Extract preparation

Leaves of *V. amygdalina* were collected from the botanical garden of the Rukararwe Traditional Medicine Health Center, a division of Rukararwe Partnership Workshop for Rural Development (RPWRD) in Bushenyi district. The plant was authenticated by Dominic Byarugaba, a botanist with the Department of Plant Biology, Mbarara University of Science and Technology (MUST), Uganda. A voucher specimen is kept in the department. The plant material was air-dried and grounded into a coarse powder. About (350g) of this powder were macerated in 2 L of distilled water for 24 h with occasional shaking (GFL 3017 Germany) and then extracted using a soxhlet extractor (Gallemkamp, England). The resultant extract was evaporated in a water bath, under controlled temperature not exceeding the one used by the healers in their plant preparation (80°C) to yield a 32.3 g of semi solid residue.

2.3 Animals

Adult Wistar rats (130 – 150g) and Swiss albino mice (18 – 26g) of either sex, maintained at Animal Facility Centre were used for the acute toxicity and 14 days sub-chronic experiments. The animals were kept in plastic cages at room temperature and moisture, under a naturally illuminated environment of 12:12 h dark/light cycle. Animals were fed the standard diet and had access to tap water *ad libitum*.

Male Wistar rats were used for the 6 week exposure studies.. At dosing, animals were 8 to 12 weeks old. All animals were clinically monitored at the time of delivery and during acclimation period, and were maintained at the Animal Facility Centre. Animals found unsuitable were excluded from the experiment. Animals were housed in plastic cages under same conditions described above; they were fed with standard diet (Mice pallet), and had access to tap water *ad libitum*. The animal experiments were conducted according to the NIH Guide on Laboratory Animals for Biomedical Research (NIH, 1978) and ethical guidelines for investigation of experimental pain in conscious animals (Zimmermann et al, 1983).

2.4 Antiplasmodial activity

The test was conducted according to the curative procedure described earlier (Saidu et al, 2000; Adzu et al, 2003). A donor mouse infected with rodent malaria (*Plasmodium berghei*) was anaesthetized with chloroform and the abdomen opened. Blood was collected through cardiac puncture with a sterile needle and syringes in such a way that 0.2 ml of the blood containing about 1 x 10^7 infected red cells. Twenty-five mice were inoculated i.p. with 0.2 mL each. The mice were then randomized and grouped into five (n = 5) and treated as follows on day 3 (D_3). Group 1 received normal saline, group 2 received chloroquine (CQ, 5mg/kg, i.p.); while groups 3-5 received (50, 100, and 200 mg/kg, i.p.). The treatment continued daily until day 7. Thick and thin blood smear were collected daily from tail blood, fixed with methanol, stained with 4% Giemsa at pH 7.2 for 45 min and examined microscopically (Nikon YS2-H Japan). The increase/decrease in parasitaemia, defined as the number of infected and uninfected red blood cell RBCs, were counted on five different fields, and mean survival time (within 30 days) was recorded.

2.5 Evaluate the antinociceptive activity of the selected antimalarial

2.5.1 Acetic acid-induced writhing in mice

Analgesia was assessed according to the method of Siegmund et al. (1957), as was modified by Koster et al, 1959). The mice were divided into different groups (of five mice each). They were differently pre-treated with the extract (50, 100, 200mg/kg i.p), aspirin (100mg/kg i.p) and normal saline (10ml/kg i.p). 30, 60, 90 and 120min after the treatment, 0.7% acetylsalicylic acid (ASA) (Sigma Chemicals Co) 10ml/kg i.p was administered to the mice. They were placed in a transparent cage, 5mins after administration of acetic acid, the number of abdominal constrictions (writhes) made within 10min of every mouse was counted. The results of the treatment groups were compared with those of normal saline pre-treated control. The percentage of the writhes was calculated as (test mean/control mean) × 100.

2.5.2 Formalin test

For the formalin studies, rats were injected with 0.05 ml of formalin (2.5% formaldehyde) into the sub-plantar surface of the left hind paw 30min after treatment with saline, extract or ASA. Severity of pain (for both control and test groups (n = 5)) were simultaneously observed and rated as scores using (Dubuisson et al, 1977) pain measurements. This was rated as follows: (0) rat can bear weight on injected paw; (1) light resting of the paw on floor; (2) partial elevation of the injected paw, and (3) total elevation, licking and biting of paw. These observation were recorded every minute for the first 10 min (early phase) and at every 5 min for the period between 15 and 60min (late phase).

2.5.3 Tail-flick test

This test as first described [28], and subsequently modified (Janssen et al, 1969; Asongalem et al 2004a) was used. Briefly, before treatment, the terminal (2 cm) of each rat tail was immersed in hot water contained in a 500ml beaker and maintained at 55 ± 1°C using a thermo-regulated hot plate (Ugo Basile, Socrel DS-35) and the time (in seconds) between the onset of stimulation and tail withdrawal was measured as the tail-flick latency. Twenty five rats that shows response within 0 – 4 s were selected and grouped into five (n = 5) for the study. Immediately after basal latency assessment, normal saline, reference drug (Pethidine hydrochloride; Bayer, England) or the plant extract were administered and the reaction time again recorded at 30 and 60min. after administration the extract. (50 – 200 mg/kg p.o) (Sanchez-Mateo et al, 2006).

2.6 Acute and sub-chronic toxicity of the herbs

2.6.1 Acute – toxicity test

The intraperitoneal (i.p) acute toxicity of the extract was evaluated in Swiss albino mice using a slightly modified Lorke's method (Lorke, 1998). Briefly, this method involved the determination of LD_{50} value in biphasic manner. The animals were starved of feed but allowed access to water 24 h prior to the study. In the initial investigatory step (phase 1), a range of doses of the extract producing the toxic effects was established. This was done by intraperitoneal administration of geometric doses of the extract (10, 100, 1000, 1500 mg/kg) to four groups of mice (n = 4). Based on the results obtained, a phase 2 investigatory step was done by giving more specific doses (200, 400, 600, 800 mg/kg i.p) to four other groups of mice.

The mice were observed for 24 h for such behavioral signs as, excitement, dullness, ataxia or death. The LD_{50} was estimated from the geometric mean of the dose that caused 100% mortality and the dose which caused no lethality.

The same procedure was used in rats which received (1000, 2000, 3000, 5000 mg/kg oral) in phase 1 and (1500, 3000, 4000, 5000 mg/kg oral) in the second phase.

2.6.2 Two weeks sub-chronic toxicity test

Twenty eight Wistar rats divided into four weight-matched groups, of seven rats each, (both sexes) were used for the study. Three test groups received 500, 1000, 2000 mg/kg *V. amygdalina* by gavage with biomedical needle (G 16, Length 76.2mm, diameter 3mm, Straight Harvard Apparatus) for 14 days. The control group received normal saline.

Food and water intake were measured daily while the animal's body weights were taken every other day. All animals were observed at least once daily for clinical signs (behavior such as lethargy, hyperactivity, depression and diarrhea). On day 14, immediately prior to euthanasia, all animals were anesthetized with chloroform and bled via the descending aorta for hematology and clinical chemistry determination. Organs were dissected and weighed to determine absolute and relative weight. The blood for clinical chemistry was allowed to clot in microtainer separator tubes, centrifuged and sera collected and stored at -20^{0}C till ready for biochemical analyses. Commercial kits for Biosystem BTS-310, (Biosystem S.A Costa Brava 30, Barcelona, Spain) and Vitrous DT systems, Orthoclinical Diagnostics Johnson Company (US17) were used to analyze liver function, renal function and the electrolyte test.

The hematological tests were carried out in an ethylene diamine tetra-acetic acid (EDTA) – anticoagulated blood. Hemoglobin (Hb) concentration was analysed by the cyanmethaemoglobin method, packed cell volume (PCV) by the micro-method, and white blood cell (WBC, total and differential) and platelet counts by visual methods Dacia et al, 1991). The mean cell hemoglobin concentration (MCHC) was calculated by dividing Hb by PCV (Dioka et al, 2002).

2.6.3 Six weeks sub-chronic toxicity test

For the six-week exposure studies, twenty eight male Wistar rats were divided into four weight-matched groups of seven rats each. Three of the four test groups received 750 1500, 3000 mg/kg *V. amygdalina* by gavage with biomedical needle (G 16, Length 76.2mm, diameter 3mm, Straight Harvard Apparatus) consecutively for 43 days. The control group received distilled water vehicle only, via gavage.

Food and water intake were measured daily while the animal's body weights were taken preexposure and weekly during exposure. All animals were observed at least once daily for clinical signs (behavior such as lethargy, hyperactivity, depression and diarrhea), and once/week clinical observations were performed on each rat by removing it from its cage and examining it for changes in general health. On day 44, immediately prior to euthanasia, all animals were anesthetized with chloroform and bled via the descending aorta for hematology and clinical chemistry determination. Organs were dissected and weighed to determine absolute and relative weight. The blood for clinical chemistry was allowed to clot in microtainer separator tubes, centrifuged and sera collected and stored at -70 ^{0}C until performing the biochemical analyses. The biochemical and hematological parameter were analyzed in the (New Italian Laboratory). Mbarara University of Science and Technology (MUST).

The collected plasma samples were analyzed using a (HumanStar 180 and Humalyze 2000, Germany) autoanalyzer. Sixteen biochemical parameters were studied; plasma sodium, potassium and chloride were also assayed with (Humalyzer 17410, Germany) autoanalyzer with appropriate Human Kits.

Hematological parameters were analyzed using (Beckman and Coulter, USA) with the appropriate kit (Coulter ACT 5 diff Diluent's).

3. Results

In the study, a total of 90 healers from - sub-county from the three districts were interviewed. Most of them were members of traditional healers association in their district. Men dominate the practices of traditional medicine.

Most of the traditional healers interviewed (81 out of 90), indicated to have passed through a several routes to become healers. All of the 81 were raised in families with traditional healers, who had involved them in the healing process and they were familiar with the profession. After some time they started to practice on their own. All reported on the importance of the family environment of a traditional healer in the context of acquiring knowledge and experience by members of the family. Furthermore it was reported that, the entrance into practice through these routes is facilitated through training by an experienced healer or a family member, who decides when the apprentice is ready to become an independent healer or to take up the practice. Eight out of 81 of the traditional healers indicated to have been instructed through dreams by their ancestral spirits to take up the traditional healing practice. They were required to learn and observe traditional healing procedures as dictated by the spirits. Indeed, the ancestral spirits are considered to be supernaturally powerful and ignoring them is to invite punishment to an individual and or her family. Of the 90 healers interviewed, two indicated to be self-taught healers.

The leaves are the most frequently used plant part (56.3%), the root and fruits are used about 30% and 8.5% respectively, and the less used plant part is the bark (5.3%). The majority of the remedies are prepared in the form of decoction of fresh leaves. In our study area people do usually not store remedies for prolonged period of time. When needed they go out and collect the plant and prepare the remedy from fresh or sun dried material. Powders are prepared by pounding the fresh plant part or the crushed plant material after sun drying,

Decoction is the most frequent method way of remedy preparation (65%) followed by infusion (13%), which is used for the powders; the maceration (11%) is mostly used for the

root preparation. Some remedies are prepared from a single plant species; however, in a few cases mixtures of plants or other substances are added as noted in Table 2
Most of the remedies are taken orally and by external application as body bath, steam bath, and as ointment. Fumigation is mainly used in the treatment of headache and chest pain.
For most of the remedies, the administered dose depends on the patient's age, physical and health condition, and the duration of the illness. The doses vary from a teacup (70 ml) for adults to a handful (25 ml) for a child; a lack of agreement among the healers on doses of remedies was sometimes noted. The variation of the doses from one healer to another may show that the plants have a low degree of toxicity. For pharmacological investigation the active doses of these plants may not be high since they appear to treat the patients with low doses. The duration of treatment is not given for all remedies. According to the healers duration of treatment is difficult to determine and depends on how long the patient has been ill. The patient is supposed to take the remedy until healed. The only person able to determine the end of a treatment is the patient himself since the remedy is taken at home in the absence of the healers.
The reported adverse effects for the use of these medicinal plants are vomiting and dizziness. According to the healers these effects are generally due to an overdose of the remedy. The adverse effects are generally moderate, and disappear at the end of the treatment. Also, patients are advice to drink a lot of milk, meat soup or porridge made from sorghum to help alleviate serious side effects.

Districts	Sub-County	Numbers of healers	Sex		Age range
			Males	Females	
Kanungu		5	4	1	28–76
		5	3	2	30–79
		5	5	0	42–85
		5	5	0	35–55
		5	4	1	65–85
Bushenyi	kyangyenyi	5	5	0	47–70
	Kigarama	5	5	0	38–80
		5	5	1	27–70
		5	5	0	49–104
		5	5	0	56–80
Mbarara	Nyakayojo	10	8	2	45–73
	Kinoni	10	10	0	55–62
	Rugando	10	9	1	50–61
	Bugamba	10	9	1	50-59

Table 1. An overview of the traditional healers interviewed.

3.1 Acute toxicity test

The median lethal dose LD_{50} was established to be 560 ± 1.21 mg/kg i.p. in mice and 3.32 ± 0.15 g/kg oral in rats. Adverse signs of gaiting, reduction in stereotypic activities and deaths were however seen in high doses.

3.2 Acetic acid-induced writhing in mice

The aqueous extract of *V. amygdalina* (50, 100, 200mg/kg i.p) exhibited a significant (P<0.05) antinocicetive activity against acetic acid-induced writhing in mice. 50 and 100 mg/kg oral doses exhibited a dose-dependent anti-nociception that progressively reduced over a period of 90 min post-treatment. However, at 120min the reduced anti-nociceptive activity increases again at these doses. The dose of 200 mg/kg on the other hand caused a total anti-nociception up to 120min. These results compared favorably with those of aspirin (100mg/kg i.p; Fig 1).

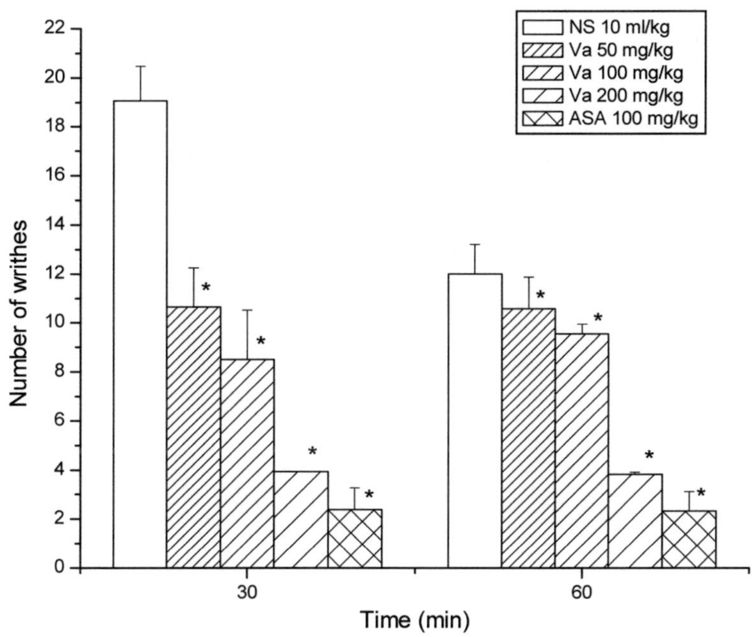

Fig. 1. Effect of aqueous extract of *V.amygdalina* leaves on acetic acid-induced writhing in mice for 5 min (NS, normal saline; Va, *V. Amygdalina*; ASA acetysalicylic acid). All data are presented as means ± S.E.M., n=5. The asterisk (*) denotes, significance (p<0.05) between treated group and NS control

3.3 Formalin and tail-flick tests

The extract at doses of 100 and 200 mg/kg induced significant (p<0.05) reduction in pain response in both phases (aphasic and tonic) of pain induced by formalin in comparison with control (Fig 2).

In all cases ASA, a positive analgesic agent demonstrated significant anti-nociceptive action with a slightly stronger pharmacological intensity than *V. amygdalina* at 200 mg/kg in the late phase. The extract exerted no significant effect on nociception in tail-flick as values obtained correspond with those with saline. However pethidine the reference agent markedly prolonged the tail-flick reaction time in rats (Fig 3)

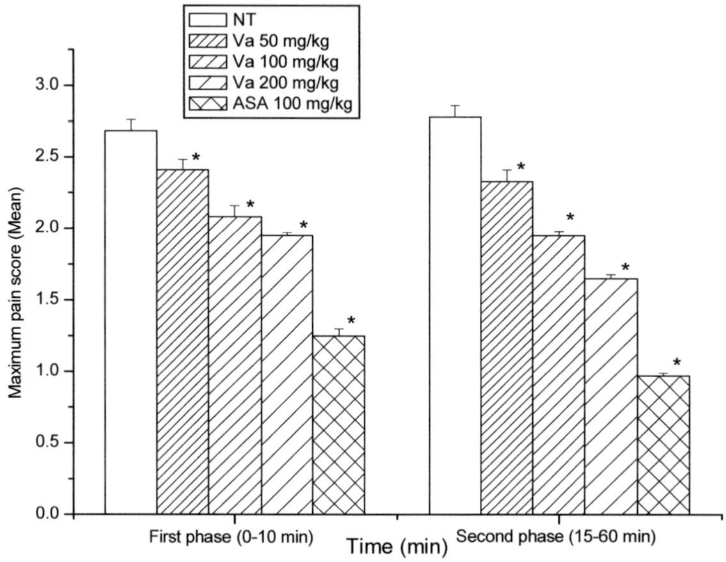

Fig. 2. Effect of aqueous extract of *V.amygdalina* leaves on formalin test in rats (NT, non treated animals; Va, *V. Amygdalina*; ASA acetyl salicilic acid). All data are presented as means ± S.E.M., n=5. The asterisk (*) denotes significance ($p<0.05$) between treated group and NT control

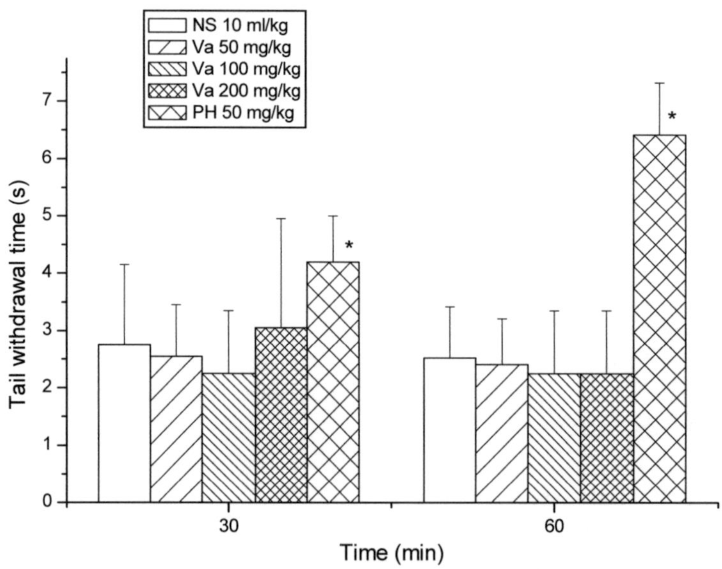

Fig. 3. Effect of aqueous extract of *V.amygdalina* leaves on thermal stimulus-induced tail-flick test in rats (NS, normal saline; Va, *V. Amygdalina*; PH, penthidine hydrochloride). All data are presented as means ± S.E.M., n=5. The asterisk (*) denotes significance difference ($p<0.05$).

3.4 Antiplasmodial activity

The extract caused a significant ($P < 0.05$) and dose-dependent reduction in mean parasitaemia in mice infected with Plasmodium berghei in comparison to CQ (5 mg/kg). The extract caused a parasitaemia reduction of 52% in 50 mg/kg, 64% and 73% in 100 and 200 mg/kg respectively (Table 2). One animal death was recorded in the 200 mg/kg extract groups throughout the 30 days observation period of the experiment while the remaining mice recovered fully. All mice in the saline group were lost within 15 days of the study.

Treatment	Dose (mg/kg, p.o.)	Mean prasitaemia (D_2 –D_6)	Inhibition (%)
NS (10ml/kg)	-	14.2 ± 0.25	-
V. amygdalina	50	6.7 ± 0.17*	52.8
	100	5.0 ± 0.22*	64.8
	200	3.7 ± 0.17*	73.9
CQ	5	3.1 ± 0.25*	78.2

Values are mean count S.E.M. (for n = 5)
*Significantly (p<0.05) different from saline control group
N.S., Normal saline

Table 2. Curative activity of the aqueous extract of *V. amygdalina* and CQ against *Plasmodium berghei* in mice.

3.5 Sub-chronic toxicity (14 days exposure)

No treatment deaths occurred and no treatment related clinical signs were noted during the study. The extract did not exert significant changes on mean body and organ weight, fluid and food intake (Table 3). All animals demonstrated a progressive increase in body weight during the exposure. The organ weights were expressed as a percentage of the body weight (% relative organ weight), rather than as absolute weights, so as to take into consideration differences in the organ weight that may solely be attributable to differences in the body weights of the respective rats. The hematology result showed a significant decrease ($p<0.05$) in red blood count at the dose of 2000mg/kg compared to control (Table 4). The result of the clinical chemistry parameter showed a dose-dependent increase in direct and total bilirubin, there was also an increase in uric acid at the doses of 500 and 1000mg/kg compared to control (Table 5).

3.6 Six weeks exposure

Clinical observation, Body and organ weight

At the end of the 43-day-period of drug administration, No overt signs of toxicity were seen in any of the animals during the course of the study. No statistical difference was observed between the body and organ weight of the control group and the assay group in the male rats receiving the three doses, all animals exhibited a gain in body weight. Organ weights (% relative organ weights) were similar to those of the corresponding organs from the control. (Fig 5 and 6).

Treatment (mg/kg)	Food Intake (g SEM)	Fluid Intake (mL SEM)	Weight (g SEM)												
			Initial Body	Final Body	Liver		Heart		Kidney		Lungs		Spleen	
					Absol.	Relat.	Absol.	Relat.	Absol.	Relat.	Absol.	Relat.	Absol.	Relat.
0(Control)	131.82 7.04	155.63 11.64	147.92 7.35	178.92 6.51	7.03 0.18	3.96 0.19	0.65 0.02	0.35 0.01	1.43 .49	0.79 .02	1.42 0.12	0.80 0.07	0.84 0.05	0.48 .04
500	131.82 10.52	148.33 19.22	161.38 14.77	181.11 14.11	6.78 0.42	3.72 0.47	0.83 0.09	0.46 0.08	1.34 0.09	0.76 .06	1.66 0.23	0.97 .20	0.76 0.62	0.43 .03
1000	113.49 10.14	120.16 6.51	137.62 14.32	158.17 17.93	5.37 0.58	3.64 0.52	0.64 0.08	0.44 0.07	1.26 .10	0.85 .11	1.50 .10	0.99 0.11	0.63 .05	0.46 .05
2000	129.82 12.20	147.16 12.18	134.58 9.72	156.94 6.85	6.43 0.11	4.17 0.41	0.74 0.06	0.48 0.06	1.36 .09	0.88 .07	1.33 .09	0.87 0.07	0.74 0.42	0.48 .05

Values are expressed as mean ± S.E.M. for n = 7
Relative organs weight = Absolute Organ Weight X 100
Final Organ Weight

Table 3. Effect of *V. Amygdalina* on daily food and fluid intake, body weights and organs weight of rats. (14days exposure)

Parameter	Control	500mg/kg	1000mg/kg	2000mg/kg
Hb (g/dl)	12.17± 0.27	9.97± 0.73	11.88± 0.78	10.54±0.47
PCV (%)	36.14±0.79	29.71±2.20	35.42± 2.34	31.42± 1.41
MCHC (g/dl)	32.14±0.34	30.28±0.60	32.00±0.65	30.85±0.40
RBC (x 10^{12}/L)	4.64±0.13	3.84±0.25#	4.30±0.35#	3.58±0.14#
Platelet (x 10^9)	156.42±3.77	139.85±4.38	153.28±6.95	136.71±3.82#
WBS (x 10^9/L)	6.57±0.43	5.57±0.87	6.68±0.51	3.47±0.89#
Neutrophil (%)	20.57±2.42	25.57±1.95*	24.00±1.77*	21.00±1.67
Lymphocyte (%)	79.28±2.53	74.42±1.95	77.4±2.47	83.28±3.48*

Values are expressed as means ± S.E.M for n = 7
* Significantly increased (P≤0.05) compared to control.
# Significantly reduced (P≤0.05) compared to control.

Table 4. Effect of *V. amygdalina* on selected hematological parameter in rats (14days Exposure)

Parameters	Control	500 mg/kg	1000 mg/kg	2000 mg/kg
AKL.Phos (iu/L)	212.1±2.21	215.5±3.77	218.8±8.11	218.7±3.45
Total Protein (g/L)	71.5± 1.11	74.3±2.69	77.0± 0.54	73.7± 2.21
Albumin (g/L)	38.3± 1.25	39.7± 1.04	40.0± 0.94	39.6± 0.76
Direct Biliru (μMol/L)	1.8± 0.82	2.5± 1.01*	3.2± 1.51*	4.0± 1.78*
Total Biliru (μMol/L)	4.2±2.65	6.28±2.63*	5.71±2.53*	6.57± 3.19*
ALT (iu/L)	32.7±5.80	34.60±10.18	35.10±11.04	33.70± 6.23
AST (iu/L)	42.28±10.27	40.43±10.68	41.29±12.32	41.14± 5.52
Chol (μMol/L)	1.23±0.32	0.92±0.33	1.25±0.34	1.10± 0.28
Trig (μMol/L)	0.51±0.04	0.86± 0.18	0.60±0.60	0.47± 0.06
HDL (iu/l)	0.44±0.39	0.44± 0.31	0.36±0.07	0.42± 0.44
LDL (μMol/L)	0.37±0.20	0.53± 0.19	0.69±0.20	0.64± 0.16
VLDL (μMol/L)	0.23±0.02	0.39±0.08	0.27±0.02	0.21± 0.03
CHO/HDL (μMol/L)	2.80±0.84	1.95±0.73	2.60±0.69	2.72± 0.80
K^+ (mMol/L)	6.92±028	8.04±0.50	7.02±0.52	7.35± 0.48
Na^+ (mMol/L)	139.14± 3.34	140.71± 5.84	147.43 ±2.79*	145.57 ± 1.06*
Cl^- (mMol/L)	107.57 ± 2.72	110.70 ± 5.32	117.40 ±4.37*	114.00 ± 1.46*
HCO_2^- (mMol/L)	23.71±0.91	22.28±1.32	21.14±0.39	21.14± 0.40
Uric Acid (μMol/L)	106.6± 6.74	164.6± 19.18	168.6±8.21	134.8±9.50
Urea (mMol/L)	6.80±0.44	7.31±0.39	6.82±0.72	4.60± 0.41#
Creat (mMol/L)	76.57±2.80	73.71± 8.4	70.14±2.52	76.85± 4.06

Values are expressed as means ± S.E.M. for n = 7
* Significantly increased (P≤0.05) compared to control.
# Significantly reduced (P≤0.05) compared to control.
ALT, Alanin Amino transferase
AST. Aspartate amino transferase
ALK. Phos, Alkaline Phosphatase.

Table 5. Effects of *V.Amygdalina* on Clinical Chemistry Parameter in rats. (14days exposure)

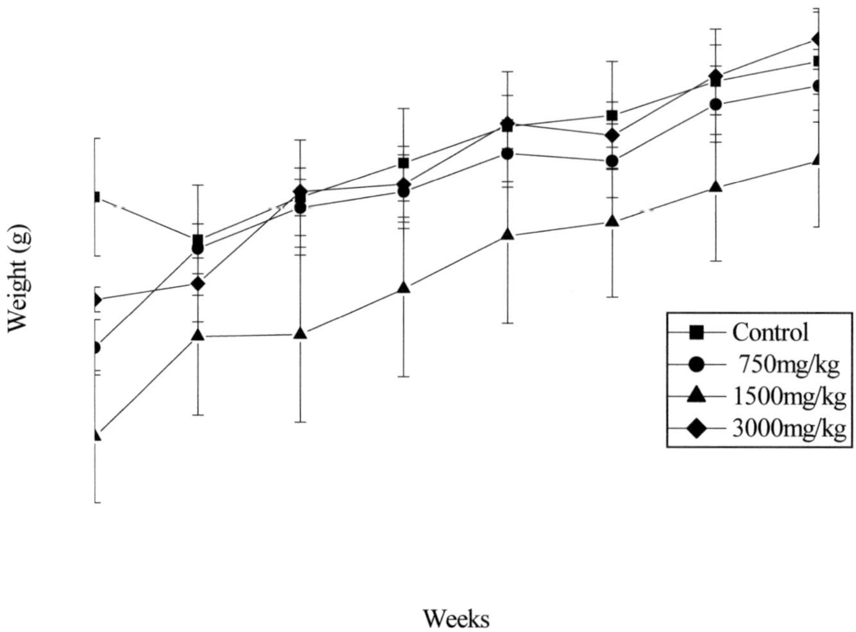

Fig. 5. Evolution of the mean ±SE of rat body weight during the subchronic toxicity of *Vernonia amygdalina* extract.

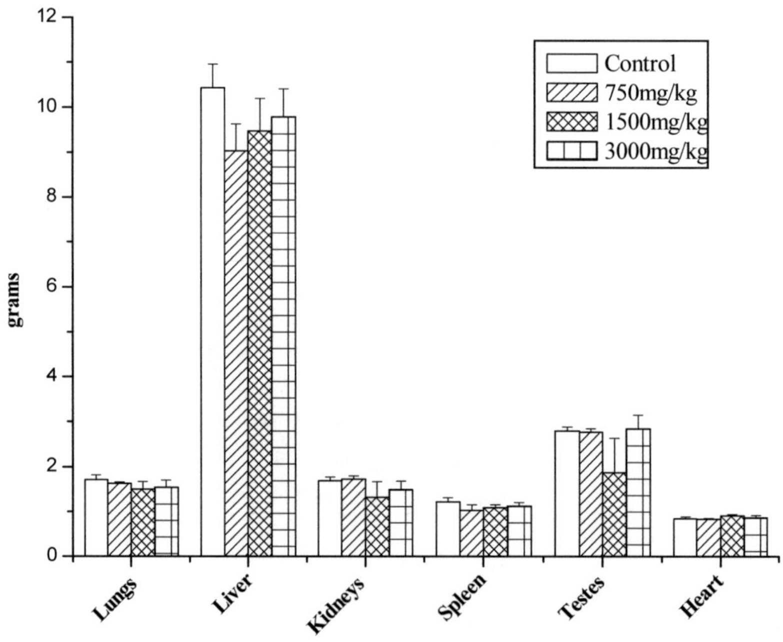

Fig. 6. Plots of the mean SE. Of the harvested organ weights during the sub-chronic toxicity study of *V.amygdalina* extract.

3.7 Hematological analysis

The mean values of the nine haematological parameters are reported in (Table 6)

Doses mg/kg	WBC (10^9/ l)	RBC (10^{12}/l)	HGB (g/dl)	HCT (%)	MCV (fL)	MCH (pg)	MCHC (g/dl)	PLT (10^9/µ/)	MPV (fL)	NE (%)	LY (%)
Control	4.8±0.8	8.4±1.2	16.9±2	44±6	53±4	20±2	38±2	429±50	6.7±0.1	0.5±0.01	4.1±0.7
750mg/kg	6.6±1.0	8.7±1.1	17.2±3	45±1	52±4	19±1	38±4	464±18	6.5±1.0	1.0±0.4*	5.4±0.8
1500mg/kg	8.0±0.7*	8.2±0.6	16.7±1	43±3	53±2	20±0.3	38±3	555±43	6.5±0.1	0.7±0.1	6.9±0.6*
3000mg/kg	8.5±0.3*	8.4±0.2	17.1±0.2	44±8	52±3	20±0.3	38±3	436±161	6.7±0.3	0.7±0.1	7.3±0.3*

Values presented as mean ± standard deviation.
n = 7
WBC = White blood cell; RBC = Red blood cell; HGB = Hemoglobin; HCT = Hematocrit; MCV = Mean corpuscular volume; MCH = Mean corpuscular hemoglobin; MCHC = Mean corpuscular hemoglobin concentration; PLT = Platelets; NE = Neutrophil; LY = Lymphocyte
Statistical analysis: ANOVA, then Dunnett's test
*Mean value of group is significantly different from control at $p<0.05$

Table 6. Mean hematology values of rats after repeated (6 weeks) oral dosing with extract leave of *V.amygdalina.*

The WBC count presented a significant increase in the two high doses (8.47 ± 0.3 in 3000 mg/kg/d) and (8.02 ± 0.7 in 1500 mg/kg/d) versus control (4.80 ± 0.8).
There was a significant increase in the lymphocyte values in high doses (7.33 ± 0.2 in 3000 mg/kg/d) and (6.94 ± 0.6 in 1500 mg/kg/d) as compared to control (4.13 ± 0.7)

There was also a significant increase in the values of Neutrophil count (1.08 ± 0.7 in 750 mg/kg/d) versus control (0.53 ± 0.02). However, no major difference was noted between the control and assayed groups.

3.8 Biochemical analysis

Clinical chemistry analysis of the rats indicate increased ASAT and ALAT ratios in the 1500 mg/kg/d dose, compared to control values (Table 7). In addition, significant increased in HDL levels were noted in the same dose level when compared to controls.

Dose Mg/kg/d	ASAT (U/L)	ALAT (U/L)	ALB (g/dl)	TRIG (mg/dl)	UREA (mg/dl)	CALC (mg/dl)	T.PROT (g/L)	PHOS (mg/dl)	CREAT (mg/dl)	T.BIL (mg/dl)	URICAC (μmol/l)	D.BIL (mg/dl)	T.CHO (mg/dl)	HDL mg/dl)	LDL (mg/dl)	K (mmol/l)	NA (mmol/l)	AMY (U/L)
Control	132	93	3.4	120	52	12	33	24	0.5	0.38	80	0.20	88	4.1	68	5.9	152	1196
	±26	±4	±0.1	±15	±3	±3	±10	±6	±0.3	±0.1	±30	±.02	±10	±0.7	±9	±0.2	±3	±49
750	202	94	3.5	115	56	14	39	40	0.6	0.42	81	0.12	69	3.4	55	5.7	146	1301
	±29	±9	±0.2	±13	±2	±4	±15	±11	±0.2	±0.1	±40	±.03	±10	±0.5	±7	±0.3	±5	±36
1500	373*	186*	3.7	112	56	6.4	24	28	0.6	0.80	70	0.18	83	6.7*	59	5.9	147	1219
	±77	±26	±0.2	±17	±3	±1.8	±5	±5.9	±0.2	±0.2	±25	±.02	±19	±0.7	±15	±0.4	±4	±94
3000	313	140	3.3	104	57	3.9	24	16	0.5	0.58	148	0.10	76	4.8	56	5.9	151	1267
	±63	±23	±0.1	±15	±3	±1.2	±4	±3.0	±0.02	±0.1	±19	±.02	±7	±0.6	±6	±0.4	±2.4	±63

n = 7, Values presented as mean ± standard deviation
ASAT = Aspartate aminotransferase; ALAT = Alanine aminotransferase; ALB = Albumin; TRIG = Triglyceride; CAL = Calcium; T.PROT = Total protein; PHOS = Phosphate; CREAT = Creatine; T. BILI = Total bilirubin ; D. BILI = Direct bilirubin; T.CHO = Total Cholesterol; HDL = High density lipoprotein; LDL = Low density lipoprotein; K = Potassium; NA = Sodium; AMY = Amylase
Statistcal analysis: ANOVA, Dunnett's test
*Mean values of groups is significantly different from control at $p<0.05$.

Table 7. Mean clinical chemistru values of rats after repeated (6 weeks) orad dosing with aqueous extract leave of *V.amygdalina*.

4. Discussion

As herbal medicine become more popular especially in rural areas, pharmacological evidences to understand the action of these medicine and the underlying mechanisms, to support the proper and safe use of these medicine are indispensable

Our ethnopharmacology survey showed that medicinal plants are still widely used by the population in the area where the study was conducted. Several types of preparations of plants were used. The plants grow over an extended area and are used by healers separated by long distances.

In the current study, the analgesic effect of the leave extract of *Vernonia amygdalina* was assessed using three nociceptive animal models. In the writhing response model, acetic acid is injected into the peritoneal cavity of mice. The acid causes nociception in the abdomen due to the release of various substances that excite pain nerve ending (Raj, 1996). According to previous reports this assay is commonly used in mice to detect both central and peripheral analgesic efficacy of agents (Dewey, 1970; Fukawa et al 1980), *V amygdalina* showed an ability to diminish the numbers of the writhing episode in a dose-dependent manner. The results of the writhing test alone did not ascertain whether antinociceptive effects are central or peripheral.

The formalin test is considered a model for chronic pain (Duduisson and Dennis, 1977). In this test, animals present two distinct nociceptive behavior phases, which probably involve different stimuli. The first phase initiates immediately after formalin injection and lasts 3 to 5 mins, resulting from chemical stimulations of nociceptor. The second phase initiates 15 to 20 mins after formalin injection, lasts 20 to 40 mins and seems to depend on a peripheral mechanism as well as a central one. While substance P and bradykinins are involved in the first phase, histamine, 5HT, prostaglandins and bradykinin are involved in the second phase. The effect of extract was significant in both phases. Since the mechanism of the analgesic effect of *V. amygdalina* is apparent in these two models, it can however be speculated that this effect may be linked to processes in the prevention of sensitization of the nociceptor, down-regulation of the sensitized nociceptor and/or blockade of the nociceptor at peripheral and/or central levels.(Ferreira, 1990). Another possible mechanism may be that the extract blocks effect or the release of endogenous substances, including prostaglandin E_2 (PG_{E2}) and $PGF_{2\alpha}$ that excites pain nerve ending which is found in writhing response test model of mice (Deraedt, et al, 1980).

The extract fails to exhibit antinociceptive effect in the tail-flick test, as values obtain were not significantly different from control animals. Pethidine (50mg/kg p.o.) the reference drug used exhibited significant antinociceptive effect in rats. It is known that the tail-flick (thermal nociceptive) response appears to be a spinal reflex sensitive to opioid $_{\mu}$-agonists and non-thermal tests to opioid $_{\kappa}$-agonists (Abbott, 1988; Furst et al, 1988), furthermore thermally-induced pain is also mediated by Aδ and C fibers. The data in the present study suggest the involvement of $_{\kappa}$ opioid receptors in the analgesic activity and a decrease activity of Aδ and C fibers against inflammatory-induced activation but not thermally-induced activation (Puig and Sorkin, 1980).

Aqueous extracts of *V. amygdalina* were found to have *in vivo* activities against *P. berghei* in mice. At 200 mg/kg the antiplasmodial activity were comparable to CQ treated mice. Empirically, this plant is used in decoction alone, other plants may be added to reduce the side effect of nausea that result from the herb's bitter taste (15).

The acute oral toxicity results from the *V. amygdalina* extract (3.32 ± 0.15 g/kg p.o) indicate that the extract may be safe based on the chemical labeling and classification of acute systemic toxicity on oral LD_{50} values, recommended by the organization for Economic Cooperation and Development (Walum et al,1986). It has, however, been reported, that the median lethal dose is not an absolute value but is an inherently variable biologic parameter that cannot be compared to constants such as molecular weight or melting point (Oliver, 1986). The adverse signs of gaiting, reduction in stereotypic activities and deaths were however seen in high doses.

In the sub-chronic study, the hematologic parameter shows a decrease in the RBC counts and an increased neutrophil in the treated groups. The serum chemistry parameter shows an increase in the direct and total bilirubin value. In several organs, mainly heart and liver, cell damage is followed by increased levels of a number of cytoplasmic enzymes in the blood, a phenomenon that provides the basis for clinical diagnosis of heart and liver diseases . For example, liver enzymes are usually raised in acute hepatotoxicity but tend to decreased with prolonged intoxication due to damage to the liver cells (Orisakwe et al, 2004). In this study, the extract did not exert significant effects on the serum chemistry parameters, the increased in bilirubin levels were probably due to the decrease RBC values.

Since the traditional healers reported use of the drug as prophylactics against malaria, male rats were exposed to the extract for 6 weeks. No extract-related deaths occurred, the clinical condition of the animals, body weight gain, and food consumption were unaffected. Clinical pathology parameters (hematology, serum chemistry) exhibited no treatment-related effect. Organ weight changes can be sensitive indicators of target organ toxicity, and significant changes in organ weights may occur in the absence in changes in other pathology parameters (Bailey,S.A., 2004), for example, increased liver weight associated with hepatic cytochrome P450 induction is a common finding in toxicology studies. Liver weight increases of up to 20% relative to control without microscopic evidence of hepatocellular hypertrophy or changes in serum chemistries (Amacher, et al., 2000). Similarly modest dose-related changes in kidney weight commonly occur in toxicology studies without histopathologic evidence of cellular alteration (Greaves, P. 2000).

In conclusion, the results of this study showed analgesic activity of the extract with clear and significant antiplasmodial effects in mice, no indication of toxicity in rats, incidental findings below or above standard reference levels were all within control values based on historical reference ranges. This might explain the pharmacological basis for the successes in pain and malaria treatment claimed by traditional healers who use *V. amygdalina.*

5. Acknowledgments

This study received financial support from Innovation at Makerere Committee (I@mak.com) grant. The authors are grateful to Prof. F.I.B. Kayanja (Mbarara University of Science and Technology) for his valuable input. We also thank The Rukararwe Traditional Medicine Health Center in Bushenyi District for providing plant material for the study.

6. References

Abosi AO, Raseroka BH: In vivo antimalarial activity of *Vernonia amygdalina. Br J Biomed Sci* 2003;60:89–91.

Adzu B, Abbah J, Vongtau H, Gamaniel K: Study on the used of *Cassia singueana* in malaria ethnopharmacy. *J Ethnopharmacol* 2003;88:261–267.

Akah PA, Okafor CI: Hypoglycaemia effect of *Vernonia amygdalina* Del in experimental rabbits. *Plant Med Res* 1992;1:6–10.

Amacher,D.E. et al (1998) The relationship among microsomal enzyme induction, liver weight and histological change in rat toxicology studies, *Food Chem.Toxicol.* 36, 831,

Asongalem, E.A., Foyet, H.S., Ngogang, J., Folefoc, G.N., Dimo, T., Kamchouing, P. Analgesic and anti-inflammatory activities of *Ergeron floribundus*. *J Ethnopharmacol* 2004a, 91: 301-308.

Bailey, S. A., Zidell, R. H., and Perry R. W., (2004) Relationships between organ weight and body/brain weight in the rat: what is the best analytical endpoint? *Toxicl. Pathol.*, 32, 448.

Deraedt R, Jougney S, Falhout M: Release of prostaglandin E and F in an algogenic reaction and its inhibition. *Eur J Pharmacol* 1980;51:17–24.

Dewey, W.L., Harris, L.S., Howes, J.F., Nuite, J.A. The effect of various neurohumoral modulators on the activity of morphine and the narcotic antagonists in the tail-flick and phenylquinous tests. *J Pharmacol.Exp.Ther* 1970, 175: 435 - 442

Dioka C, Orisakwe OE, Afonne OJ, *et al.*: Investigation into the haematologic and hepatotoxic effects of rinbacin in rats. *J Health Sci* 2002;48:393–398.

Dubuisson, D, Dennis SG: The formalin test: a qualitative study of analgesic effects of morphine, meperidine and brain stem stimulation in rats and cats. *Pain* 1977;4:161–174.

Dubuisson, D., Dennis, S.G. The formalin test: a qualitative study of analgesic effects of morphine, meperidine and brain stem stimulation in rats and cats. *Pain* 1977, 4:161-174.

Ferreira SH: A classification of peripheral analgesics based upon their mode of action. In: *Migraine: A Spectrum of Ideas* (Sandler M, Collins GM, eds.). Oxford University Press, Oxford, 1990, pp.59–72.

Fukawa K, Kawano O, Hibi M, Misaki M, Ohba S, Hatanaka Y: A method for evaluating analgesic agents in rats. *J Pharmacol Methods* 1980;4:251–259.

Greaves,P., (2000) *Histopathology of Preclinical Toxicity studies,* 2nd ed., Elsevier, Amsterdam, chap 9

Guide for the Care and Use of Laboratory Animals, revised. NIH publication No. 83-23. National Institutes of Health, Bethesda, MD, 1978.

Hamill FA, Apio A, Mubiro NK, Mosango M, *et al.*: Traditional herbal drugs of Southern Uganda 1. *J Ethnopharmacol* 2000;70: 281–300.

Homsy J.K.E., Kabatesi D., Mubiru F., Kwamya L., Tusuba C., Kasolo S., Mwebe D., Ssentamu L., Okello M., King R., Evaluating herbal medicine for the management of

Homsy J.K.E., King R., Balaba D., Kabatesi D. Traditional health practitioners are key to scaling up comprehensive care for HIV/AIDS in sub-Saharan Africa. AIDS, 2004 18(12)1723-1725.

Huffman MA, Koshimizu K, Ohigashi H: Ethnobotany and zoopharmacognosy of *Vernonia amygdalina*, a medicinal plant used by humans and chimpanzees. In: *Compositae: Biology Utilization. Proceedings of the International Compositae Conference* (Caligary PDS, Hind DJN, eds.). The Royal Botanical Garden, Kew, UK, 1996, pp. 351–360.

Huffman MA: Animal self-medication and ethno-medicine exploration and exploitation of the medicinal properties of plant. *Proc Nutr Soc* 2003;62:371–381.

Iwalewa EO, Adewunmi CO, Omisote NO, *et al.*: Pro-and antioxidant effects and cytoprotective potentials of nine edible vegetables in southwest Nigeria. *J Med Food* 2005;4:539–544.

Izevbigie EB, Bryant JL, Walker A: A novel natural inhibitor of extracellular signal-regulated kinases and human breast cancer cell growth. *Exp Biol Med* 2004;229:163–169.

Janssen, P.A.J., Niemegeers, C.J.E., Dony, J.G.H. The inhibitory effect of fentanyl and other morphine-like analgesic on the warm water induced tail withdrawal reflex in rats. Arzneim-Forsch *Drug Res* 1963, 6: 502-507

K.Saidu, J. Onah, A. Orisadipe, A.Olusola, C. Wambebe, Kgamaniel, (2000) Antiplasmodial, analgesic, and anti-inflammatory activities of the aqueous extract of the stem bark of Erythrina senegalensis. Journal of Ethnopharmacology 71,275 - 280.

Kambizi L, Afolayan AJ: An ethnobotanical study of plants used for the treatment of sexually transmitted disease. *J Ethnopharmacol* 2001;77:5–9.

Koster, R., Anderson, N., De Beer, E. J. Acetic acid for analgesic screening. Federation Proceedings 1959, 18: 412.

Lorke D: A new approach to practical acute toxicity testing. *Arch Toxicol* 1998;5:275–289.

Masaba SC: The antimalarial activity of *Vernonia amygdalina* Del. (Compositae). *Trans R Soc Trop Med Hyg* 2000;94:694–695.

O'Hara, M; Kiefer D; Farrel K and Kemper K (1998) A review of 12 commonly used medicinal herbs. *Arch. Fam. Med.* 7: 523-536.

Oliver JA: Opportunities for using fewer animals in acute toxicity studies. In: *Chemical Testing and Animal Welfare*. The National Chemicals Inspectorate, Solna, Sweden, 1986, pp. 119–143.

Orisakwe OE, Njan AA, Afonne OJ, Akumka DD, Orish VN, Udemezue OO: Investigation into the nephrotoxicity of Nigerian bonny light crude oil in albino rats. *Int J Environ Res Public Health* 2004;2:91–95.

Raj PP: Pain mechanisms. In: *Pain Medicine, A Comprehensive Review*. Mosby-Year Book, St. Louis, 1996, pp. 12–24.

Sanchez-Mateo CC, Bonkanka CX, Hernandez-Perez M, Rabanal RM: Evaluation of analgesic and topical anti-inflammatory effects of *Hypericum reflexum* L. fil. *J Ethnopharmacol* 2006;107:1–6.

Sanchez-Mateo, C.C., Bonkanka, C.X., Hernandez-Perez, M., Rabanal, R.M. Evaluation of analgesic and topical anti-inflammatory effects of *Hypericum reflexum* L. fil. *J Ethnopharmacol* 2006, 107: 1-6.

Siegmund EA, Cadmus RA, Lu G: Screening of analgesic including aspirin-type compound based upon the antagonism of chemically induced writhing in mice. *J Pharmacol Exp Ther* 1957;119:184–186.

Taiwo O, Xu HX, Lee SF: Antibacterial activites of extracts from Nigerian chewing sticks. *Phytother Res* 1999;8:675–679.

Tona L, Cimanga RK, Mesia K, *et al.*: Antiplasmodial activity of extracts and fractions from seven medicinal plants. *J Ethnopharmacol* 2004;93:27–32.

WHO, (2003). Assessment and monitoring of antimalarial drug efficacy for the treatment of uncomplicated faciparum malaria. Geneva.

Wilcox ML: A clinical trial of 'AM', a Uganda herbal remedy for malaria. *J Public Health Med* 1999;21:318–324.

Willcox, M.L, G. Bodeker (2000). Plant-based malaria Control: research initiative on traditional antimalaria methods. *Parasitology Today* 16: 220 - 221.

Zimmermann M: Ethical guidelines for investigations of experimental pain in conscious animals. *Pain* 1983;16:109–110.

9

Experimental and Computational Methods Pertaining to Drug Solubility

Abolghasem Jouyban[1] and Mohammad A. A. Fakhree[2]
[1]Drug Applied Research Center and Faculty of Pharmacy,
[2]Liver and Gastrointestinal Diseases Research Center,
Tabriz University of Medical Sciences, Tabriz,
Iran

1. Introduction

Solubility of a drug is one of its important physico-chemical properties. More attention has been paid to the aqueous solubility since water is the unique solvent of biological systems. It is obvious that a drug should be reached to its receptors in the body through the aqueous and non-aqueous media. The chance of a low water soluble drug to be appeared in the market place is very low and nearly 40 % of the drug candidates fail to reach higher phases of the drug trials simply because of their low water solubility. The solubility in non-aqueous solvents is not too important from clinical viewpoint however these solubilities play curious roles in drug discovery and development investigations. Most of drugs are synthesized in non-aqueous media and/or extracted from natural sources using non-aqueous extracting solvents. Different polymorphs of some drugs could be produced from their crystallization using organic solvents.

There are various methods for solubility determination of drugs which is discussed in this chapter. The experimental determination is tedious and time-consuming process and sometimes there is restrictions in the availability of enough amount of a drug candidate to be used in the solubility measurements, especially in the early stages of drug discovery investigations in which only small amount of a drug is synthesized/extracted and large number of preliminary biological tests should be carried out. To cover this limitation, and in order to provide a faster and easier tool, mathematical models have been developed to correlate/predict the solubility of drugs. These models are discussed in this chapter to provide an overall view for a pharmaceutical scientist who is working in the research and development department of a company and/or a research laboratory within academia. In addition to the accurate calculations which are expected from these models, the simplicity of the required computations is another parameter which should be taken into account, since more complex computations did not attract more attention in the pharmaceutical industry.

1.1 Solubility and dissolution

When talking about solubility, there are two concepts which might be confused with each other: solubility and dissolution. The term solution (i.e. thermodynamic solution) is used to define the state which is thermodynamically stable and shows the neat result of an equilibrium between a solute (the compound which is going to be dispersed molecularly in another medium which is called solvent) and its dissolved form in the medium. The dissolving process is the migration of the molecules of the solute to the solvent medium and makes the solution which after reaching a steady state is called homogenous solution and can be represented by the following equilibrium:

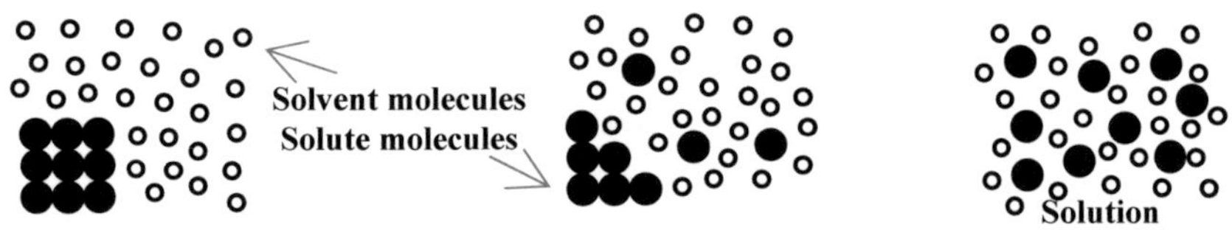

$$X_{Solid} + Y_{Liquid} \longleftrightarrow [Concenteration]$$

How much a solute is molecularly dispersed in the solvent is called solubility and the rate of dissolving is called dissolution. Hence, the solubility value is a thermodynamic property while the dissolution rate is a kinetic one. In other words, time has no effect on solubility value and is not important in its related subjects, but it is important in dissolution related subjects.

The solubility is important in stable forms including liquid formulations and dissolution is important in transient states including the release of the drug from its formulation to biological fluids and permeability (Sinko and Martin, 2006). In pharmaceutical sciences, especially in formulation, designing a stable liquid formulation requires the knowledge on the solubility value and an effective drug delivery to the body mostly depends on the dissolution rate which is affected by the solubility (Allen et al., 2006). However, they both affect each other based on Noyes-Whitney equation (Sinko and Martin, 2006):

$$\frac{dW}{dt} = \frac{DA(C_S - C)}{L} \tag{1}$$

where *dW/dt* is the rate of dissolution, *A* is the surface area of the solid which is in direct contact with the molecules of the solvents, *C* is the concentration of the solute in the medium (dissolved amount), C_S is the concentration of the solute in the diffusion layer, *D* is the diffusion coefficient, and *L* is the thickness of the diffusion layer.

Based on the discussed topics, solubility and dissolution are in relation with each other, but not the same. So, they must not be used in place of each other as the consequences can be awful! For example, a drug substance might be highly soluble, but dissolves slowly (or vice versa). So, in the formulation of such compounds, the difference between solubility and dissolution must be considered.

1.2 Solubility of base form of drugs

The apparent solubility (S_{App}) of a weak electrolyte is expressed by:

$$S_{App} = S_M + S_I \tag{2}$$

in which S_M is the molecular form of the drug and S_I is the ionized form of the drug in the solution. For strong electrolytes, S_I is predominant whereas for nonelectrolytes S_M is the only form of the solubilized drug in the solution. S_M is also called intrinsic solubility or S_0. In early stages of drug discovery, only small amount of the new drug is available and its purity is not assured. In this stage, the solubility determination in acidic and/or basic solutions could be used in practice. Increased apparent solubility in acidic or basic medium reveals that the new drug is a basic or an acidic solute. No increase in the solubility means that the drug is a nonelectrolyte. Increased solubility in both acidic and basic media indicates either zwitterionic or amphoteric behaviour. The intrinsic solubility of a drug could be determined from apparent solubility data at various pH values. When the purity of a drug candidate is not assured, a phase-solubility diagram, i.e. the solubility at different solute:solvent ratios, is recommended. In this diagram, the co-solute effect (self association, complexation, solubilization) increases the solubility and the common ion effect decreases the solubility and no change in the solubility might mean that drug is pure and no interaction exists.

1.3 Solubility of salt form of drugs

Salt formation of weak acidic or basic drugs is one of their solubility increasing methods since the ionized species have greater solubility in water and other polar solvents and a number of drugs are marketed as their salt forms. The most common salts used for salt formation of acidic drugs are sodium, potassium, calcium and zinc and those for basic drugs are hydrochloride, sulphate, mesylate, maleate, phosphate, tartrate, citrate and besylate (Wells, 1988). Different slats of a given drug possess various solubilities. As an example, the solubility of lamotrigine with the counterions of tartrate, saccharinate, succinate and fumarate are 2.63, 1.37, 0.61 and 0.43 millimole per liter (Galcera and Molins, 2009). The selection of the salt of a drug is mainly carried out by trial and error basis considering practical issues such as cost of raw materials, ease of crystallization, percent yield, thermal stability and hygroscopicity of the resulting salt. Black et al. (2007) investigated the salt formation of 17 salt forms of ephedrine and reported their physicochemical properties and tried to develop a relationship between these properties which was not successful. Any model representing the properties of salt forms of drugs is a highly in demand subject in the pharmaceutical industry. As an example, the relation between the dielectric constant of the solvent and the solubility of drugs in their salt form, can be mentioned (Fakhree et al., 2010).

1.4 Solubility of pharmaceutical macromolecules

Polymers and macromolecules are important parts of drug design and development. The emerging technology of proteins, peptides, DNA and RNA sequences as pharmaceutical active ingredients makes it necessary for consideration of their physicochemical properties in pharmaceutical sciences, including solubility. For the beginning, in terms of macromolecules, it is better to use dispersion versus solubility in a medium and this makes a difference between their solubility in comparison with small organic molecules. The dispersion of the macromolecules in the solution results in formation of new properties for the solution such as increase in viscosity, light scattering, molecular network formation (e.g. gel) etc (Sinko and Martin, 2006). Another important note about macromolecules, is the fact that they have been produced in an aqueous medium and have philia to watery media (not always, but in most of the cases). Hence, they are sensitive to presence of organic solvents and might be precipitated by addition of the organic solvents (unlike small organic nonelectrolyte molecules which dissolve in organic media more than aqueous solutions).

The solubility of proteins is influenced by the ratio of the hydrophobic and hydrophilic residues of amino acids and their arrangement in the final structure of the protein (Bolen, 2004). For example, globular proteins have hydrophobic residues in their core and hydrophilic residues in their surface. It is also affected by the pH and ionic strength of the water, presence of organic solvents and other polymers (Burgess, 2009). When talking about the solubility of proteins, there are different kinds of low solubility for the proteins:

1. in-vitro low solubility due to structural properties of the protein (hydrophobic residues),
2. in-vivo low solubility due to over expression of the protein in an organism (*E. coli*),
3. amyloid formation which results in aggregation of the proteins because of their hydrophobic, residue charge, and β-sheets in the structure, and
4. low solubility due to conformational changes (Trevino et al., 2008).

For increasing a protein's aqueous solubility, one of the strategies is addition of additives such as L-arginine and L-glutamic acids. Fusion of peptides and proteins is another method which is addition of a solubilizing sequence of amino acids or protein to the structure of the low soluble protein. Mutation in the hydrophobic amino acids sequences to hydrophilic ones is another strategy. However, this might not work in all of the cases (Trevino et al., 2008). Another approach is screening to find a more soluble homologue of that protein in other organisms (Waldo, 2003).

1.5 Solubility of drugs in biological fluids

For understanding the dissolution of a drug in the human body fluids, it is crucial to focus on the solubility of drugs in more realistic environment and to acquire larger amount of experimental data for simulating the solubility at different pHs, in the presence of bile salts etc which exists in the real solubilization media within human body. Solubility data of drugs in biorelevant media are increasingly required in early phases of drug discovery to predict the bioavailability of a drug after oral administration.

1.6 Solubility modifications

Solubility modification of drugs is required in separation, purification, analysis and formulation investigations and different methods are used to achieve the increased/decreased solubility values.

1.6.1 Solubility increasing

Several methods have been used to enhance the aqueous solubility of drugs including cosolvency, hydrotropism, complexation, ionisation, use of the surface active agents, crystal structure modifications and addition of ionic liquids. These methods have been discussed in details in the literature (Myrdal and Yalkowsky, 1998). Mixing a permissible non-toxic organic solvent with water, i.e. cosolvency, is the most common and feasible technique to enhance the aqueous solubility of drugs. The common cosolvents which, are used in the pharmaceutical industry are ethanol, propylene glycol, glycerine, glycofural, polyethylene glycols (mainly 200, 300 and 400), N,N-dimethyl acetamide, dimethyl sulfoxide, 2-propanol, dimethyl isosorbide, N-methyl 2-pyrrolidone (NMP) and room temperature ionic liquids (Rubino, 1990; Mizucci et al., 2008; Jouyban et al., 2010a). Their applications and possible side effects have been discussed in the literature (Spiegel and Noseworthy, 1963; Tsai et al., 1986; Patel et al., 1986; Golightly et al., 1988; Rubino, 1990). Hydrotropes are a class of amphiphilic molecules that cannot form organized structures, such as micelles, in water but they increase the aqueous solubility of drugs. Often strong synergistic effects are observed when hydrotropes are added to aqueous surfactant or polymer solutions. Caffeine and nicotinamide are well known hydrotropic agents and their ability to solubilize a wide variety of therapeutic drugs including riboflavin (Lim and Go, 2000) has been demonstrated. Complexation of drugs is another solubilization technique and there are a number of reports on complexation of drugs by cyclodextrins. Ionization is applicable for weak electrolytes and the solubility of some drugs could be increased by changing pH of the solution.

1.6.2 Solubility decreasing

In precipitation and crystallization processes as a part of extraction and purification of the pharmaceutically related compounds, lowering the solubility is desirable. Lowering the solubility for pharmaceutical compounds might include using of temperature alteration, addition of antisolvent, using of a low soluble salt or ester of the drug, and producing low soluble polymorphs (Blagden et al., 2007; Widenski et al., 2009).

Precipitation or crystallization both can be used in this regard depending on the rate of solubility decreasing. If it is happened quickly, then the solid state might be in amorphous form and the process called precipitation. If the lowering of solubility takes place in a controlled way that crystal growth can happen, then the process called crystallization. Precipitation of proteins and macromolecules such as DNA and RNA are other examples for this kind of solubility modification. In protein biosynthesis and extraction, different methods of desolubilization are used which include: salting out, isoelectric point precipitation, precipitation with organic solvents, addition of non-ionic hydrophilic polymers, flocculation by polyelectrolytes, and addition of polyvalent metallic ions (Burgess, 2009). Another reason making it desirable to precipitate macromolecules such as proteins, DNA, and RNA is pre-treatment of biological analytes before starting analyses.

Recrystallization is another process which is used in pharmaceutical sciences and means to dissolve a compound in a medium, and by modifying the physicochemical conditions made the dissolved compound to crystallize again. This technique is widely used in crystal engineering technology which can produce amorphous, different polymorphs, and psudopolymorphs of a drug (Blagden et al., 2007). This is important in modification of pharmaceutically interested physicochemical properties such as compressibility in formulation process, size of particles, dissolution rate, as well as solubility (Allen et al., 2006; Gibaldi et al., 2007).

The above mentioned processes are related to preformulation processes. In formulation of pharmaceutical active ingredients the desire for lowering solubility can be seen in designing of sustained release and depot dosage forms or drug delivery systems (Allen et al., 2006; Gibaldi et al., 2007). For making a sustained release dosage form of a drug, different formulation techniques such as use of polymeric matrix, osmotic pumps, and crystallization of a poorly water soluble compound are used. For designing a depot drug delivery system, possible solutions include: use of low soluble salts or esters of a drug (e.g. methylprednisolone acetate), addition of additives (e.g. zinc and insulin), very concentrated non-aqueous solutions of drug (e.g. Leuprolide and NMP), and depot dosage forms (e.g. implants of low soluble compounds such as sex hormones) (Strickley, 2004; Allen et al., 2006; Gibaldi et al., 2007).

Also low solubility is useful when stability of a pharmaceutical compound is low in its solubilized form (Sinko and Martin, 2006). Hence, suspension formulations (i.e. ready to use and lyophilized powder for suspension preparation) might be a useful strategy.
In the recent decade, emerging technologies such as micro-formulation, micro-encapsulation, nano-formulation, and nano-encapsulation are using solubility decreasing principals as a part of their processes. This is usually done by addition of antisolvent and fine particle stabilizers to gain a suspension with micro/nano-sized particles.

2. Experimental methods for determination of solubility

The solubility of a drug could be measured experimentally using two procedures, namely the thermodynamic and kinetic solubility methods. The thermodynamic solubility determination methods are not feasible at the early discovery stage because of the large sample requirement, low throughput and laborious sample preparation. The kinetic solubility determinations could be used as an alternative method at this stage.

2.1 Determination of thermodynamic solubility

Solubility determination of drugs in a liquid could be classified as analytical and synthetic methods. The main advantage of the analytical (shake flask) method is the possibility of measuring a large number of samples simultaneously however this method is tedious and time-consuming.

2.1.1 Shake flask method

The shake-flask method of Higuchi and Connors (1965) is the most reliable method for low soluble compounds and widely used solubility measurement method. In this method, an excess amount of drug is added to the solubility medium. The added amount should be enough to make a saturated solution in equilibrium with the solid phase. In case of acidic or basic drugs dissolved in an un-buffered solubility medium, further addition of the solid could change pH of the solution and consequently the solubility of the drug (Wang et al., 2002; Kawakami et al., 2005; Jouyban and Soltanpour, 2010). Depending on the dissolution rate and type of agitation used, the equilibration time between the dissolved drug and the excess solid could be varied. Equilibration is often achieved within 24 hours. To ensure the equilibration condition, the dissolution profile of drug should be investigated. The shortest time needed for reaching the plateau of drug concentration against time could be considered as a suitable equilibration time. Any significant variation on dissolution profile after reaching the equilibration should be inspected, since there are a number of possibilities including degradation of the drug and also its polymorphic transformation. Both these affect the solubility values of a drug dissolved in the dissolution media. Heating, vortexing or sonicating the sample prior to equilibration could shorten the equilibration time. To overcome the poor wettability of low soluble drugs, one may use small glass microspheres or sonication. Then the two phases, solid and solution phases, are separated using two common methods of filtration and/or centrifugation. Filteration is the easiest method, however, the possible sorption of the solute on the filter should be considered as a source of error in solubility determination, especially for very low soluble drugs. Pre-rinsing the filter with the saturated solution could reduce the sorption of the solute on the filter by saturating the adsorption sites. Centrifugation or ultra-centrifugation is preferred in some cases, and the higher viscosity of the saturated solutions, e.g. in mixed solvents, should be kept in mind as a limitation. A combination of filtration and centrifugation is also could be used. The UV spectrophotometric analysis is the most common and the easiest analytical method. The next is the HPLC methods both in isocratic and gradient elution modes. The HPLC analysis could also detect the possible impurities or degradation products if a highly selective method was used. X-ray diffraction (XRD) and differential scanning calorimetry (DSC) of the residual solid separated from the saturated solution confirm the possible solid phase transformations during equilibration.

2.1.2 Synthetic method

The synthetic method (Hankinson and Thompson, 1965; Ren et al., 2005; Yang et al., 2008; Yu et al., 2009) which is so called laser monitoring technique (Li et al., 2006), last crystal disappearance method (Hao et al., 2005) and dynamic method (Peisheng and Qing, 2001; Weiwei et al., 2007; Wang et al., 2008) is based on disappearance of the solid drug (from the mixture of solvent and drug) monitored by a laser beam. The history of this method backs to 1886 and first introduced by Alexejew and then modified by other research groups (Ward, 1926). The disappearance of drugs could be achieved either by changing the temperature or by addition of a known amount of the solvent. It is claimed that the synthetic method is much faster and more reliable than analytical method (Yang et al., 2008). Figure 1 illustrates a schematic representation of the most completed set up used in the synthetic method.

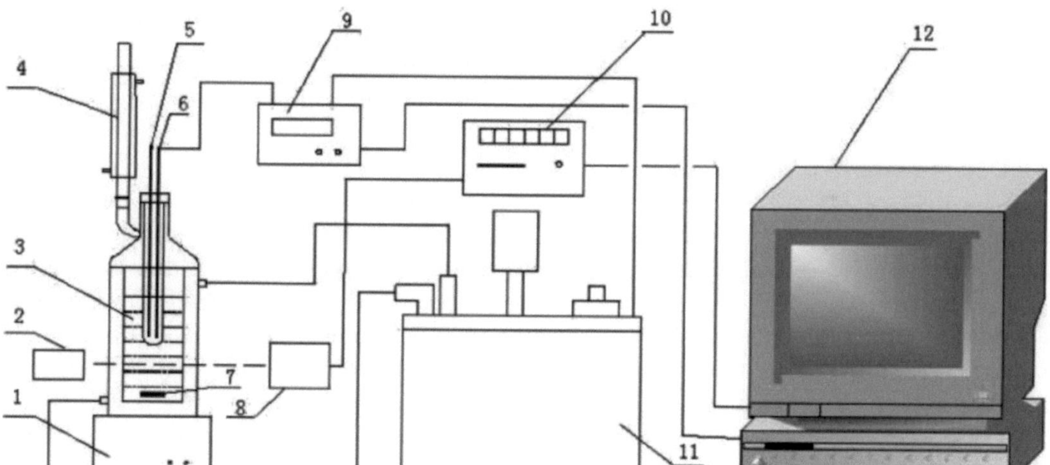

Fig. 1. Schematic representation of the synthetic method for determination of solubility of drugs; 1, magnetic stirrer; 2, laser generator; 3, jacketed glass vessel; 4, condenser pipe; 5, thermometer; 6, thermocouple; 7, rotor; 8, photoelectric transducer; 9, controller; 10, laser strength display; 11, constant temperature bath; 12, workstation. (Figure is reproduced from Ren et al., 2005).

The solubility apparatus consisted of a jacketed glass vessel (varying from 60 to 250 mL) maintained at the desired temperature by circulating water that was provided by a constant-temperature bath. The water temperature was controlled by a workstation with a temperature accuracy of (0.1 K) achieved continuous stirring, and a condenser (or a perforated rubber cover) was fitted to reduce the solvent's evaporation. A thermometer with an uncertainty of 0.01 K was used to determine the temperature of the system. A laser beam was used as a tool to observe dissolving the solid in liquid. The signal transmitted through the vessel was collected by a detector that decided the rate of temperature rise and estimated the equilibrium point of the given system on the basis of the signal change. The solute and the solvent were prepared using an electronic balance with the estimated uncertainty in the mole fraction of less than 0.001. A predetermined quantity of drug and solvent was placed into the jacketed vessel. The system was slowly heated (heating rate increase is 0.5 to 2 $K \cdot hr^{-1}$) with continuous stirring. When the solute particles disappeared thoroughly, the signal approached a maximum value. The workstation judged the signal difference at 10-min intervals; if the interval was less than 10, then the workstation gave an order to stop heating and record the temperature. The temperature recorded was the liquid temperature of a given composition upon the complete dissolution of the drug (Ren et al., 2005). In another version of this set up, predetermined masses of drug and solvent were placed in the vessel and the contents were stirred continuously at a constant temperature. As the particles of the drug are dissolved, the intensity of the laser beam increased gradually and reaches to the maximum value when the drug is dissolved completely. Then an additional known mass of the drug is introduced to the vessel and the procedure is repeated until the laser beam could not return to the maximum value which means the last addition could not be dissolved. The total amount of the added drug is recorded and used to calculate the solubility value (Yang et al., 2008). The synthetic method is preferred over shake flask method for solubility determination of drugs in viscous solvents where separation of the excess solids from saturated solutions is not achievable (Grant and Abougela, 1983).

2.2 Determination of kinetic solubility

In drug discovery and development, one of the rationalized methods is high-throughput screening (HTS) which includes the design and synthesis of a large set(s) of chemicals to find hit compounds based on specific physicochemical properties (PCPs) and to develop lead compound. One of the important PCPs in determination of hit and lead compounds is aqueous solubility (Pan et al., 2001; Alsenz and Kansy, 2007; Hoelke et al. 2009). However, in practice it is not possible to experimentally determine thermodynamic solubility value in HTS approaches. This is because of large number of compounds which might be more than 1000 compounds in each HTS experiment or little amount of synthesized compounds which is around a few milligrams and is another limiting factor (Pan et al., 2001; Alsenz and Kansy, 2007; Hoelke et al. 2009).

Kinetic solubility determination methods were used for covering this problem. The advantages of the kinetics solubility determination in comparison with thermodynamic solubility determination methods are capability to being easily automated, accuracy, rapidity and requiring less amount of the solute (Pan et al., 2001; Alsenz and Kansy, 2007; Hoelke et al. 2009). Its disadvantages might include not assessing the crystal effect on the solubility, the cosolvent action of the dimethyl sulfoxide (DMSO), and its applicability is good for compounds which have solubility more than 10^{-6} molar. Some of the well established approaches include: nephelometric, UV-Spectroscopic, and HPLC methods which are discussed in the following.

2.2.1 Nephelometric method

The nephelometry is based on turbidimetry. Figure 2 shows a schematic view of the mechanism of turbidimetry. For sample preparation in this method, a 10 millimolar concentration of a solute was prepared by dissolving suitable amounts of the solute in DMSO. Then, this stock solution is used to prepare sample solutions in the range of 5×10^{-7} to 5×10^{-4} molar. For concentrations above the 10^{-4} molar, the solutions prepared by direct dilution of the stock solution and for the lower concentrations, serial dilutions were used where the dilutant is a buffer. These dilutions are directly take place in a 96-well plate with the total 5% concentration of DMSO and the final volume of ≈200 µL (Pan et al., 2001; Hoelke et al. 2009). This optimum volume is based on the fact that light scattering (for a specific condition) is nearly constant for a range of particle sizes (Pan et al., 2001) which make the process reproducible and accurate.

For sample analyzing after the preparation section, the 96-well plate is placed in a nephelometer apparatus for measurement of the light scattering. It uses a laser beam (with a fixed wavelength in the range of 550-750 nm) as the light source, and a detector which is placed with a specific angle to the light source. Based on plotting turbidity against prepared concentrations, and drawing its asymptotes and finding their meeting point x coordination, gives the kinetic solubility (see Figure 3) (Pan et al., 2001; Hoelke et al. 2009).

With this method, the kinetic solubility for a plate of 96 samples can be measured in a few minutes.

2.2.2 UV/Vis-spectroscopic method

There are two methods using UV/Vis-spectroscopy for kinetic solubility determination: Method 1 is based on turbidimetry and the other is based on light absorbance intensity as a function of concentration (Pan et al., 2001).

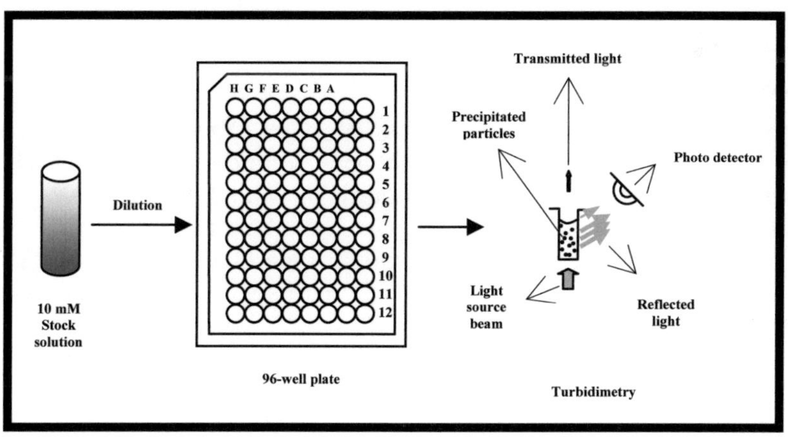

Fig. 2. Schematic representation of turbidimetry.

2.2.2.1 UV/Vis-spectroscopic method 1

The sample preparation is like nephelometry method, but the analyzing is with a 96-well plate UV/Vis-spectroscopy apparatus. This provides a wider range of wavelength to choose for reading the samples turbidity (190-1000 nm) (Pan et al., 2001). The lower the wavelength, the smaller particle is detected. However, in practice, wavelengths greater than 500 nm is used. This is because of the fact that most of organic compounds which have UV absorbance (e.g. contain a benzene ring) also have fluorescence property and might interfere with turbidimetry which reads the amount of reflected light (or fluorescence emission light) (Pan et al., 2001). An example of this is phenol red which has light absorption in 430 and 560 nm and is exited by these wavelengths which results in fluorescence emission (Pan et al., 2001). Another limitation is the UV absorbance of the most plates which are made of plastics (Pan et al., 2001).

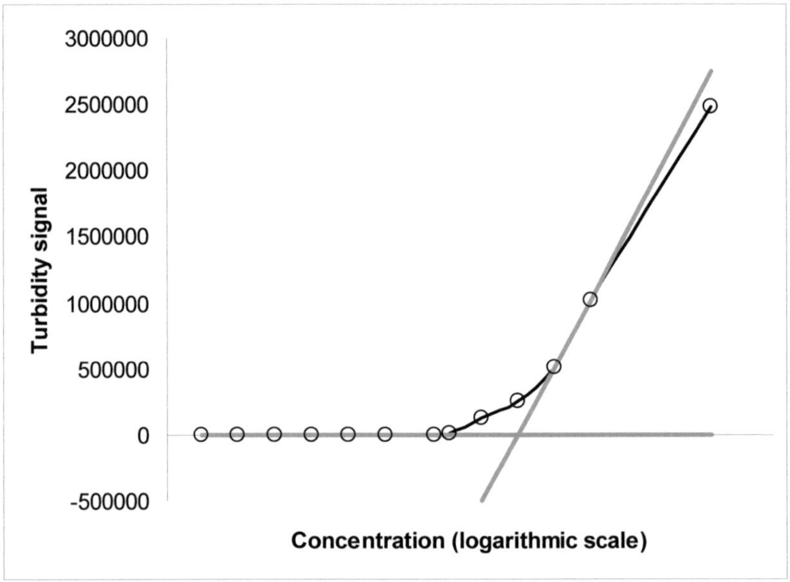

Fig. 3. The method for finding kinetic solubility.

2.2.2.2 UV/Vis-spectroscopic method 2

In this method, sample dilution in range of 7×10^{-9} to 5×10^{-4} molar is performed. But after precipitation of the stock solution by the aqueous solution, the samples are filtered to another plate. And in this part, 20% acetonitrile is added to the filtered samples for prevention of solute precipitation during analysis. Then the plate is read with a 96-well plate UV/Vis-spectroscopy apparatus and the recorded data changed to molar concentration (determined by calibration curve obtained by standard solutions using another plate) (Pan et al., 2001; Hoelke et al. 2009).

2.2.3 HPLC method

The sample preparation for this method is the same as UV/Vis-spectroscopic method 2 and the transferring of samples to the 96-well plate is not required. However, filtration of samples is done prior to injection to the HPLC or online filtration is applied. A calibration curve is required for the determination of the concentrations of the prepared samples. This method is the most accurate one in comparison with other mentioned methods (limit of detection < 10^{-8} molar). But it must be considered that it consumes much more time (around 6 hours for 96 samples) (Pan et al., 2001; Hoelke et al. 2009). A comparison between the mentioned methods is given in Table 1.

Method	Calibration	Specificity	Easy	Cut off	LOD	Rapidity
Nephelometric	Not required	Low	Yes	No	Low	High
UV/Vis 1	Not required	Low	Yes	<500 nm	Low	High
UV/Vis 2	Required	Medium	No	<250 nm	Medium	Medium
HPLC	Required	High	No	No	High	Low

Table 1. The comparison between four kinetic solubility determination methods

Kinetic solubility values are valuable source in early stage of drug discovery in place of thermodynamic solubility values where there is good correlation between trends of these two values for a set of compounds (Hoelke et al. 2009). However, because of the amorphic nature of the solutes, in most of the cases the kinetic solubility is higher than thermodynamic solubility values. The effect of 5% DMSO as a cosolvent on the solubility value in kinetic solubility determination methods also should be considered. This is very important where most of the drugs have very low aqueous solubility and very small amounts of solubilizing agents such as cosolvents (e.g. DMSO) enhance their solubility largely.

Also the effect of time after dilution is important, especially in turbidimetry methods. Hoelke et al. have shown that by increasing the time after dilution and precipitation, the determined solubility become smaller (Hoelke et al. 2009).

2.3 Data validation

The collected data could be compared with the previously reported data in order to ensure the accuracy of the experimental procedure employed. Any mistake in the dilution steps, and miscalculations, or using un-calibrated instruments, such as un-calibrated balances, temperature variation and some other factors could be resulted in different solubility values for a given drug dissolved in a solvent at a fixed temperature.

3. Computational methods for solubility prediction

Computational methods in recent decades have become an important part of drug design and discovery. They are classified as theoretical, semi empirical and empirical equations. Most of models used in pharmaceutical sciences are semi-empirical (which is theoretical correlation of experimentally determined values) or empirical equations (which is mathematical correlation of experimentally determined values). Examples for semi-empirical models are those correlations which use physicochemical parameters in their relationships. In other word, it is needed for them to be calculated based on experimental determinations at least for one time. For example in Noyes-Whitney equation, the diffusion coefficient must be determined at least for one time for a solute. So the Noyes-Whitney equation is a semi-empirical model. The quantitative structure property relationships (QSPR) and quantitative structure activity relationships (QSAR) are examples for empirical modelling. The pioneer for this type of equations in pharmaceutical sciences is Prof. Crowin H. Hansch. He has developed a QSPR model for solubility prediction of liquids, based on their partition coefficient (Hansch et al., 1968):

$$-\log S = 1.339 \log P - 0.978 \quad (3)$$

where log$P$ is the logarithm of the partition coefficient between octanol and water for a specific liquid.
In another grouping, the correlation could be developed using linear modelling or non-linear modelling. Linear modelling is the simple linear regression (or multiple linear regression) and non-linear modelling is artificial neural network, as examples. There are advantages and disadvantages for each type of modelling which is listed in the Table 2:

Modelling type	Advantages	Disadvantages
Linear	- Simple to perform - Fast - Robust - Reproducible - Easy to use - The resulted model can be analyzed theoretically - Performable with small number of cases	- It cannot analyze non-linear and complex behaviour - Most of the time the results have low accuracy
Non-linear	- Can analyze non-linear and complex behaviour - The results have high accuracy	- Easily over fitting occurs - Many iterations are required - Need almost large number of cases - Reproducibility is hard - You must have the trained model to be able to predict new cases - It gives a black box instead of a model

Table 2. Advantages and disadvantages of linear and non-linear modelling in QSPR studies

In QSPR modelling, the variables used for correlation of physicochemical properties are called descriptors. These descriptors include simple structure derived parameters (e.g. number of carbon atoms, number of single bonds), overall structural parameters (e.g. molecular weight, and molecular volume), structure residues parameters (e.g. distance between two atoms, total charge on oxygen atoms), or physicochemical properties (e.g. melting point, partition coefficient). In solubility correlation almost all kinds of descriptors have been used. Around half of the models use log$P$ as one of descriptors in modelling (Dearden, 2006). The following categories of descriptors have been used in solubility correlation:

1. PCPs (such as melting point, molecular weight, molar refraction, …),
2. structure related descriptors (such as molecular volume, solvent accessible surface area, number of rotatable/rigid bonds, number of hydrogen bond donor/acceptor atoms, …),
3. quantum chemical descriptors (such as optimized total energy, HOMO and LUMO energies, …),
4. topological parameters,
5. molecular connectivity indices,
6. electrostatic state (E-state) descriptors,

7. group contribution method or fragment based approach (different fragments derived rom structure, SMILIES/InChI codes),
8. solvatochromic parameters (Dearden, 2006; Katritzky et al., 2010; Jouyban et al., 2010b).

Other descriptors have been used as well, and a number of mixtures of the mentioned parameters are used, too. In the next section, the easiest and the most accurate models for solubility prediction are discussed. Also approaches like mobile order theory and differential equations of activity coefficient for the calculation of solubility have been used as semi-empirical methods (Dearden, 2006; Katritzky et al., 2010).

For modelling, multiple linear regression (MLR), partial least square (PLS), support vector machine (SVM), artificial neural network (ANN), random forest (RF), Monte Carlo simulation (MCS), and other methods are used. Mostly, correlation coefficients of the non-linear methods are better than linear methods and the related errors are smaller (Dearden, 2006; Katritzky et al., 2010). This might suggest a nature of non-linear behaviour for solubility.

3.1 Aqueous solubility

Available models and software to predict the aqueous solubility of drugs were reviewed in a recent work (Jouyban et al., 2008). Solubility of drugs in water could be predicted using different models presented in the literature. The general single equation of Yalkowsky is the simplest and the most common method in the pharmaceutical area. The model requires experimental melting point (*mp*) and logarithm of partition coefficient (log*P*) as input data and is expressed as:

$$\log S_W = 0.5 - 0.01(mp - 25) - \log P \tag{4}$$

where S_w is the molar aqueous solubility of a drug at 25 °C. If the solute has a melting point less than 25 °C, the (mp-25) term is set to zero (Ran et al., 2001). The two parameters, log*P* and *mp* are good representatives of effects of hydrophobicity and crystal packing on the solubility of a certain solute. Jain et al. (2008) provided some theoretical background for general single equation from thermodynamic principles. The simplicity of the model is its main advantage and a possible disadvantage is the melting point as an experimental parameter which may not be available for some of the compounds in early stages of drug discovery. An attempt has been made to predict the melting points from chemical structure was not successful (Jain and Yalkowsky, 2010) and it is recommended to use experimental values of melting point in the computations using general single equation (Chu and Yalkowsky, 2009). Also drugs with high melting points which decompose before melting are not suitable to be predicted by this model. The log*P* is measured using experimental methods such as HPLC, and/or calculated by some computational methods, then applied to solubility prediction.

The linear solvation energy relationship is another model developed by Abraham and his co-workers (Stovall et al., 2005a) and is presented as:

$$\log S_W = 0.395 - 0.955E + 0.320S + 1.155A + 3.255B - 0.785A \cdot B - 3.330V \tag{5}$$

in which E is excess molar refraction of the compound, S is dipolarity/polarizability, A and B are hydrogen bond acidity and basicity, respectively, which these later three parameter (S,

A and B) determined from solubility data of a compound in water and different organic solvents, the $A \cdot B$ term is a representative of hydrogen-bond interactions between acidic and basic functional groups of the drug in its pure solid or liquid, V is one percent of the McGowan volume and simply is calculated using group contribution method (Stovall et al., 2005).

In a recent work from our group, a simple equation was proposed to predict the aqueous solubility of drugs trained by the solubility data of pharmaceuticals (220 drugs) and was validated using various validation methods (Shayanfar et al, 2010). The proposed model is:

$$\log S_W = -1.120E - 0.599C\log P \quad (6)$$

Both parameters (E and Clog*P* or computed log*P*) employed in equation 6 are computed using Pharma-Algorithms (Pharma Algorithms, 2008), therefore, the model is an *in silico* model and no experimental data is required in the prediction procedure. In the pharmaceutical literature, an external prediction set consisting of aqueous solubility of 21 pharmaceutical and non-pharmaceutical compounds (Ran et al., 2001) usually were used to test the prediction capability of the proposed models. This data could not well represent the aqueous solubility data of pharmaceutical compounds, and another data set has been proposed consisting of the solubility of 75 official drugs collected from the literature. A list of the proposed test set and the experimental and predicted aqueous solubilities using equations 1-3 are listed in Table 3.

Drug	Experimental	Equation 4	Equation 5	Equation 6
Acetaminophen	-1.06	-1.18	-0.63	-1.39
Acetazolamide	-2.49	-1.18	0.06	-1.43
Acyclovir	-2.24	-0.37	0.91	-1.26
Allopurinol	-2.26	-2.19	0.38	-1.30
Amiloride	-3.36	-1.96	-0.07	-2.74
Amoxicilin	-2.17	-0.11	-1.90	-2.38
Antipyrine	0.39	-0.9	-1.16	-1.91
Atenolol	-1.30	-0.98	-1.85	-1.81
Atropine	-2.12	-1.77	-3.77	-2.43
Azathioprine	-3.21	-1.98	-1.95	-3.16
Baclofen	-1.67	-0.53	-1.84	-0.76
Benzocaine	-2.33	-1.98	-1.82	-2.14
Celecoxib	-3.74	-3.73	-5.38	-4.55
Chloramphenicol	-2.11	-1.57	-2.16	-2.55
Chlorpromazine	-5.27	-4.82	-5.97	-5.72
Ciprofloxacin	-3.73	-1.11	-2.78	-2.04
Colchicine	-0.96	-1.76	-3.93	-3.00
Cortisone	-3.00	-2.72	-4.43	-2.88
Dapsone	-3.19	-2.43	-2.05	-2.94
Diazepam	-3.76	-3.34	-4.58	-4.06

Diethylstilbestrol	-4.57	-5.805	-4.94	-4.82
Digoxin	-4.16	-3.12	-10.31	-4.94
Diltiazem	-2.95	-4.39	-4.64	-4.41
Ephedrine	-0.47	-0.52	-1.28	-1.65
Estradiol	-4.84	-4.95	-4.53	-4.43
Famotidine	-2.48	-0.09	-1.18	-2.53
Fluorouracil	-1.03	-1.24	0.55	-0.38
Gemfibrozil	-3.16	-4.26	-4.44	-3.54
Griseofulvin	-4.61	-3.45	-3.47	-3.28
Guaifenesin	-0.60	-0.36	-1.10	-1.45
Haloperidol	-4.43	-4.08	-5.44	-4.22
Halothane	-1.71	-1.68	-1.99	-1.56
Hydrochlorothiazide	-2.63	-1.61	-1.04	-2.18
Hydroquinone	-0.18	-1.66	-0.23	-1.56
Isoniazid	0.01	-0.154	0.97	-0.85
Ketoprofen	-3.25	-2.73	-3.95	-3.27
Labetalol	-3.45	-3.44	-4.32	-3.75
Lamotrigine	-3.14	-4.05	-3.48	-4.26
Levodopa	-1.72	-0.02	-0.35	-0.29
Lindane	-4.60	-4.08	-4.53	-3.76
Lovastatin	-6.01	-5.40	-6.42	-4.18
Manitol	0.06	1.08	0.89	-0.18
Maprotiline	-4.69	-5.28	-5.91	-5.03
Meprobamate	-1.82	-1.36	-1.62	-1.44
Mercaptopurine	-3.09	-1.84	-0.70	-1.66
Metoclopramide	-3.18	-2.99	-2.85	-3.04
Metronidazole	-1.22	-0.585	-1.14	-1.09
Minoxidil	-1.98	-2.97	-2.19	-2.46
Mitomycin C	-2.56	-2.53	-0.12	-2.46
Mycophenolic acid	-4.39	-3.30	-4.99	-3.19
Nifedipine	-4.78	-2.10	-3.71	-2.42
Nitrofurantoin	-3.24	-2.19	-0.98	-2.03
Nitroglycerin	-2.26	-1.19	-2.22	-1.66
Omeprazole	-3.62	-3.21	-3.00	-4.43
Oxytetracycline	-3.09	0.07	-4.04	-3.30
p-Aminobenzoic acid	-1.37	-1.93	-0.65	-1.65
Papaverine	-3.87	-4.43	-4.66	-4.67
Phenobarbital	-2.29	-2.39	-1.90	-2.59
Phenytoin	-3.99	-4.07	-3.20	-3.35
Progesterone	-4.40	-4.35	-5.64	-4.08
Propofol	-3.05	-3.38	-3.82	-3.28
Propoxyphene	-5.01	-4.38	-6.45	-4.14
Prostaglandin-E_2	-2.47	-2.73	-5.22	-3.16

Quinine	-2.82	-2.11	-4.01	-4.06
Riboflavin	-3.65	-0.43	-2.77	-2.21
Salicylic acid	-1.93	-2.87	-1.53	-2.24
Sertraline	-4.94	-6.59	-6.17	-4.98
Sulfacetamide	-1.23	-0.99	-0.83	-1.64
Terfenadine	-6.69	-6.63	-9.05	-6.39
Testosterone	-4.06	-4.02	-4.89	-3.66
Theophylline	-1.38	-2.09	-0.18	-1.71
Thiabendazole	-3.48	-4.68	-3.21	-3.94
Tolbutamide	-3.46	-2.93	-3.13	-2.93
Trimethoprim	-2.95	-2.22	-6.11	-2.61
Warfarin	-3.89	-3.19	-7.40	-3.61

Table 3. List of the test data set for evaluating the capability of the models for aqueous solubility prediction, the experimental ($\log S_W$) and predicted values by equations 4-6

The solubility value of a drug is affected by pH which is largely depends on whether the compound has acid/base ionizable functional groups. Most of the pharmaceutical compounds are weak acids or bases which could be dissociated according to the following equlibria:

$$Acidic\ Drug:\quad HA + H_2O \xleftrightarrow{pKa} A^- + H_3O^+ \quad , \quad pK_a = \frac{\left[A^-\right]\cdot\left[H_3O^+\right]}{\left[HA\right]}$$

$$Basic\ Drug:\quad B + H_2O \xleftrightarrow{pKb} BH^+ + OH^- \quad , \quad pK_b = \frac{\left[BH^+\right]\cdot\left[OH^-\right]}{\left[B\right]}$$

where HA and B are acidic and basic drugs, respectively, pK_a is the acid dissociation constant, and pK_b is basic dissociation constant. The solubility of a weak acid or base in solutions with different pH is calculated by Henderson–Hasselbalch equation:

$$Acidic\ Drug:\quad \log S_T = \log S_0 + \log\left(10^{pH-pKa} + 1\right) \tag{7a}$$

$$Basic\ Drug:\quad \log S_T = \log S_0 + \log\left(10^{pKa-pH} + 1\right) \tag{7b}$$

where S_T and S_0 are total and intrinsic solubility, respectively. So for solubility prediction of a drug at different pH values we need to have intrinsic solubility and pK_a value for the drug (Sinko and Martin, 2006).

However, having a specific pK_a value for a compound does not mean it will have complete activity in every pH values which is the case for most of the drugs which do not have complete activity in aqueous solutions.

There are some mathematical models for calculation of the solubility and pK_a of the compounds (Dearden, 2006; Jouyban, 2009; Katritzky et al., 2010). However, complete activity will be gained in two conditions: 1- infinite dilution and 2- strong acidic condition for basic compounds (or strong basic condition for acidic compounds).

3.2 Solubility in organic solvents

Few models were presented to calculate the solubility of drugs in organic solvents. Yalkowsky et al. (1983) calculated the mole fraction solubility of weak electrolytes and non-electrolytes in n-octanol at 30 °C as:

$$\log X_{Oct} = -0.011mp + 0.15 \tag{8}$$

$$\log X_{Oct} = -0.013mp + 0.44 \tag{9}$$

Dearden and O'Sullivan (1988) proposed the following equation for calculating the molar solubility of drugs in cyclohexane (S_{Cyc}):

$$\log S_{Cyc} = -0.0423mp + 1.45 \tag{10}$$

which was tested on the solubility of 12 pharmaceuticals and the mean percentage deviation was 85.1 (± 21.6) % (Jouyban, 2009).
Sepassi and Yalkowsky (2006) proposed another version of equation 8 to compute the molar solubility of drugs in octanol as:

$$\log S_{Oct} = -0.01(mp - 25) + 0.5 \tag{11}$$

The mean percentage value of equation 11 was 147 (± 247) % (Jouyban, 2009).
The Abraham solvation model provides a more comprehensive solubility prediction method for organic solvents (Abraham et al., 2010). The Abraham model written in terms of solubility is:

$$\log\left(\frac{S_S}{S_W}\right) = c + e \cdot E + s \cdot S + a \cdot A + b \cdot B + v \cdot V \tag{12}$$

where S_S and S_W are the solute solubility in the organic solvent and water (in mole/L), respectively. In equation 12, the coefficients c, e, s, a, b and v are the model constants (i.e. solvent's coefficients), which depend upon the solvent system under consideration. These coefficients were computed by regression analysis of measured $\log\left(\frac{S_S}{S_W}\right)$ values, infinite dilution activity coefficients and partition coefficients of various solutes against the corresponding solute parameters (Abraham and Acree, 2005). The Abraham solvent coefficients (c, e, s, a, b and v) and Abraham solute parameters (E, S, A, B and V) represent the extent of all known interactions between solute and solvents in the solution (Stovall et al., 2005b).

3.3 Solubility at different temperatures

Solubility of a solute in an ideal solution could be mathematically represented by van't Hoff equation:

$$\log S = \frac{a}{T} + b \tag{13}$$

where a is the slope of the linear plot of $\ln S$ against $\frac{1}{T}$ and b is the intercept. The a term is equal to $\frac{-\Delta H_f}{2.303R}$ and b is equal to $\frac{\Delta H_f}{2.303RT_m}$ for ideal solutions in which R is the molar gas constant and T_m is the melting point expressed as K. Equation 13 provides good relationship in the narrow range of temperature. For ideal solutions, the enthalpy of mixing is zero, therefore the enthalpy of solution (ΔH_s) is equal to the enthalpy of fusion (ΔH_f). The ΔH_s is always endothermic for ideal solutions, and the solute solubility will be increased by increasing the temperature. The pattern is different for gases, liquids and solids as shown in Figure 4 where the solubility of gases decreases with increased temperature. The Hildebrand equation is an alternative model and expressed as:

$$\log S = a \ln T + b \tag{14}$$

in which a and b are the adjustable parameters. Equations 13 and 14 fail to represent the solubility-temperature relationship of most of pharmaceutical compounds in water and other pharmaceutically interested solvents especially at a wide temperature range. There are some physico-chemical reasons for this deviation from linear relationships, e.g. formation of polymorphs or solvate forms of the drug, which was discussed in details by Grant et al. (1984). To represent such data, a combined version of the van't Hoff and Hildebrand equations could be used. The equation is:

$$\log S = \frac{a}{T} + b \ln T + c \tag{15}$$

in which a, b and c are the adjustable parameters calculated by a least square analysis (Grant et al., 1984).

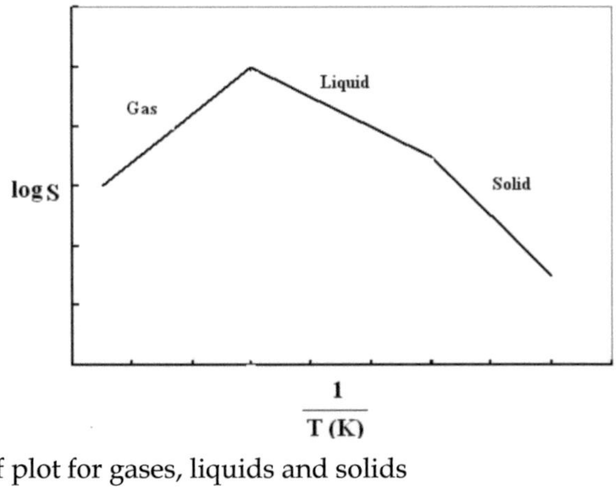

Fig. 4. The van't Hoff plot for gases, liquids and solids

3.4 Solubility in mixed solvents

The log-linear model of Yalkowsky is the simplest and famous model to calculate the solubility of pharmaceuticals in mixed solvent systems and is expressed by:

$$\log S_m = \log S_2 + \sigma \cdot f_1 \tag{16}$$

where S_m is the solubility of the solute in the mixed solvent system, S_2 denote the aqueous solubility of drug, σ is the solubilization power of the cosolvent and theoretically is equal to $(\log(S_1 / S_2))$ in which S_1 is the solubility in the neat cosolvent (Yalkowsky and Roseman, 1981). The general form of the log-linear model for multi-component solvent systems could be written as:

$$\log S_m = \log S_2 + \sum \sigma_i f_i \tag{17}$$

where σ_i and f_i are the solubilization power and the fractions of cosolvent i *(*Li, 2001*)*. Valvani *et al.* (1981) reported a linear relationship between σ and logarithm of drug's partition coefficient ($\log P$) which is a key relationship and could improve the prediction capability of the log-linear model. The relationship was expressed as:

$$\sigma = M \cdot \log P + N \tag{18}$$

where *M* and *N* are the cosolvent constants and are not dependent on the solute's nature. The numerical values of *M* and *N* were reported for most of the common cosolvents earlier (Li and Yalkowsky, 1998) and listed in Table 4. This version of the log-linear model could be considered as a predictive model and provided the simplest solubility estimation method and requires the aqueous solubility of the drug and its experimental/calculated log*P* value as input data. The log-linear model was developed to predict the solubility of drugs at room temperature (22 – 27 °C) however the solubility at other temperatures are also required in the pharmaceutical industry.

Solvent system	M	N
Acetone - water	1.14	-0.10
Acetonitrile – water	1.16	-0.49
Butylamine – water	0.64	1.86
Dimethylacetamide – water	0.96	0.75
Dimethylformamide – water	0.83	0.92
Dimethylsulphoxide – water	0.79	0.95
Dioxane – water	1.08	0.40
Ethanol – water	0.93	0.40
Ethylene glycol – water	0.68	0.37
Glycerol – water	0.35	0.26
Methanol – water	0.89	0.36
Polyethylene glycol 400 – water	0.74	1.26
1-Propanol – water	1.09	0.01
2-Propanol – water	1.11	-0.50
Propylene glycol - water	0.77	0.58

Table 4. Updated Table from (Li and Yalkowsky, 1998; Millard et al., 2002.)

The Jouyban-Acree model was adopted from the combined nearly ideal binary solvent/Redlich-Kister equation proposed by Prof. Acree (1992) which was derived from a thermodynamic mixing model that includes contributions from both two-body and three-body interactions (Hwang et al., 1991). The model was presented for solubility calculations in binary solvents at a fixed temperature and expressed as:

$$\log S_m = f_1 \log S_1 + f_2 \log S_2 + f_1 f_2 \sum_{i=0}^{2} A_i (f_1 - f_2)^i \tag{19}$$

where A_i stands for the model constants. The A_i values are calculated by regressing $(\log S_m - f_1 \log S_1 - f_2 \log S_2)$ against $f_1 f_2$, $f_1 f_2 (f_1 - f_2)$ and $f_1 f_2 (f_1 - f_2)^2$ by a no intercept least squares analysis (Jouyban-Gharamaleki and Hanaee, 1997). The applicability of the model was extended to other physico-chemical properties in mixed solvents at various temperatures as:

$$\log S_{m,T} = f_1 \log S_{1,T} + f_2 \log S_{2,T} + \frac{f_1 f_2}{T} \sum_{i=0}^{2} J_i (f_1 - f_2)^i \tag{20}$$

where $S_{m,T}$, $S_{1,T}$ and $S_{2,T}$ are the solubility in solvent mixture, mono-solvents 1 and 2 at temperature T (K) and J_i is the model constants. The main limitations of the Jouyban-Acree model for predicting drug solubilities in solvent mixtures are: a) it requires two data points of solubilities in mono-solvent systems, and b) numerical values of the model constants. To overcome the first limitation, the solubility prediction methods in mono-solvent system should be improved. To address the second limitation, the following solutions were examined during last couple of years:

i. the J_i terms are obtained using solubility of structurally related drugs in a given mixed solvent system, and then predict the un-measured solubility of the related drugs where the expected mean percentage deviation was ~ 17 % (Jouyban-Gharamaleki et al., 1998).
ii. the model constants could be calculated using a minimum number of experimental data points, i.e. three data points, and then predict the solubilities at the rest of solvent compositions where the expected prediction mean percentage deviation was < 15 % (Jouyban-Gharamaleki et al., 2001).
iii. the trained versions of the Jouyban-Acree models could be employed for solubility prediction of drugs in the aqueous mixtures of a number of organic solvents were reported. Using this version of the model, only the solubility data in mono-solvents are required. Table 5 listed the numerical values of the Jouyban-Acree model constants for the 5 cosolvents studied.

Solvent system	J_0	J_1	J_2	Prediction % error
Dioxane - water	958.44	509.45	867.44	27
Ethanol – water	724.21	485.17	194.41	48
Polyethylene glycol 400 – water	394.82	-355.28	388.89	40
Propylene glycol - water	37.03	319.49	-	24
Ethanol – ethyl acetate	382.987	125.663	214.579	13

Table 5. The constants of the Jouyban-Acree model for a number of solvent systems, data taken from (Jouyban and Acree, 2007; Jouyban, 2008)

iv. in the trained versions of the Jouyban-Acree model, we assumed the extent of the solute-solvent interactions are the same, however, it is not the case since various solutes possess different functional groups leading to various extent of the solute-solvent interactions. To cover this point, the deviated solubilities from the trained versions of the Jouyban-Acree model were correlated using available solubility data sets in ethanol - water and dioxane - water mixtures at various temperatures and the following equations are obtained:

$$\begin{aligned}\log S_{m,T} &= f_1 \log S_{1,T} + f_2 \log S_{2,T} \\ &+ \left(\frac{f_1 f_2}{T}\right)\{558.45 + 358.60E + 22.01S - 352.97A + 130.48B - 297.10V\} \\ &+ \left(\frac{f_1 f_2 (f_1 - f_2)}{T}\right)\{45.67 - 165.77E - 321.55S + 479.48A - 409.51B + 827.63V\} \\ &+ \left(\frac{f_1 f_2 (f_1 - f_2)^2}{T}\right)\{-493.81 - 341.32E + 866.22S - 36.17A + 173.41B - 555.48V\}\end{aligned} \quad (21)$$

and

$$\begin{aligned}\log S_{m,T} &= f_1 \log S_{1,T} + f_2 \log S_{2,T} \\ &+ \left(\frac{f_1 f_2}{T}\right)\{648.01 - 404.99E + 428.69 + S340.99A - 59.03B - 56.94V\} \\ &+ \left(\frac{f_1 f_2 (f_1 - f_2)}{T}\right)\{-135.95 - 41.11E - 192.19S + 237.81A + 363.87B + 310.30V\} \\ &+ \left(\frac{f_1 f_2 (f_1 - f_2)^2}{T}\right)\{-1102.49 - 667.02E + 2070.16S + 421.15A - 924.73B - 271.54V\}\end{aligned} \quad (22)$$

The mean percentage deviation values for ethanol and dioxane were 34 and 22 %, respectively (Jouyban et al., 2009).

v. a generalized version of the Jouyban-Acree model was proposed using its combination with the Abraham solvation parameters where the model constants of the Jouyban-Acree model were correlated with the functions of the Abraham solvent coefficients and the solute parameters as:

The mean percentage deviation of this model was 42 % for 152 data sets which was significantly less than that of the log-linear model (78 %). Figure 5 shows the relative frequency of the individual percentage deviations of the predicted solubilities using equations 23 and 16 (log-linear) in which the error distribution of equation 23 is better than that of the log-linear model. It should be noted that the Jouyban-Acree model requires two experimental data points, i.e. $S_{1,T}$ and $S_{2,T}$, whereas the log-linear model needs just aqueous solubility of the drug as input data. The main advantage of equation 23 is that it could be used to predict the solubility in mixed solvents where the Abraham solvent parameters (i.e. c, e, s, a, b and v) are available. Table 6 listed these parameters for a number of more common solvents in the pharmaceutical industry. Unfortunately these parameters are not available for a number of more common pharmaceutical cosolvents, such as propylene glycol and polyethylene glycols, and this is a disadvantage for this model.

$$\begin{aligned}\log S_{m,T} &= f_1 \log S_{1,T} + f_2 \log S_{2,T} \\ &+ \left(\frac{f_1 f_2}{T}\right)\begin{Bmatrix}1639.07 - 561.01\left[(c_1 - c_2)^2\right] - 1344.81\left[E(e_1 - e_2)^2\right] - 18.22\left[S(s_1 - s_2)^2\right] \\ -3.65\left[A(a_1 - a_2)^2\right] + 0.86\left[B(b_1 - b_2)^2\right] + 4.40\left[V(v_1 - v_2)^2\right]\end{Bmatrix} \\ &+ \left(\frac{f_1 f_2 (f_1 - f_2)}{T}\right)\begin{Bmatrix}-1054.03 + 1043.54\left[(c_1 - c_2)^2\right] + 359.47\left[E(e_1 - e_2)^2\right] - 1.20\left[S(s_1 - s_2)^2\right] \\ +30.26\left[A(a_1 - a_2)^2\right] - 2.66\left[B(b_1 - b_2)^2\right] - 0.16\left[V(v_1 - v_2)^2\right]\end{Bmatrix} \\ &+ \left(\frac{f_1 f_2 (f_1 - f_2)^2}{T}\right)\begin{Bmatrix}2895.07 - 1913.07\left[(c_1 - c_2)^2\right] - 901.29\left[E(e_1 - e_2)^2\right] - 10.87\left[S(s_1 - s_2)^2\right] \\ +24.62\left[A(a_1 - a_2)^2\right] + 9.79\left[B(b_1 - b_2)^2\right] - 24.38\left[V(v_1 - v_2)^2\right]\end{Bmatrix}\end{aligned} \quad (23)$$

In addition to the above discussed models to predict the solubility of drugs in solvent mixtures, there are some models derived from molecular thermodynamic approaches. These models require relatively complex computations and did not attract more attention in the pharmaceutical area. These models provide comparable prediction accuracies with the above discussed models. As an example, the prediction error of a method based on statistical mechanical fluctuation solution theory varied 0.3-58 % (Ellegaard et al., 2010) whereas the corresponding value for the common models in the pharmaceutical area varied between 8 to 19 % (Jouyban-Gharamaleki et al., 1999).

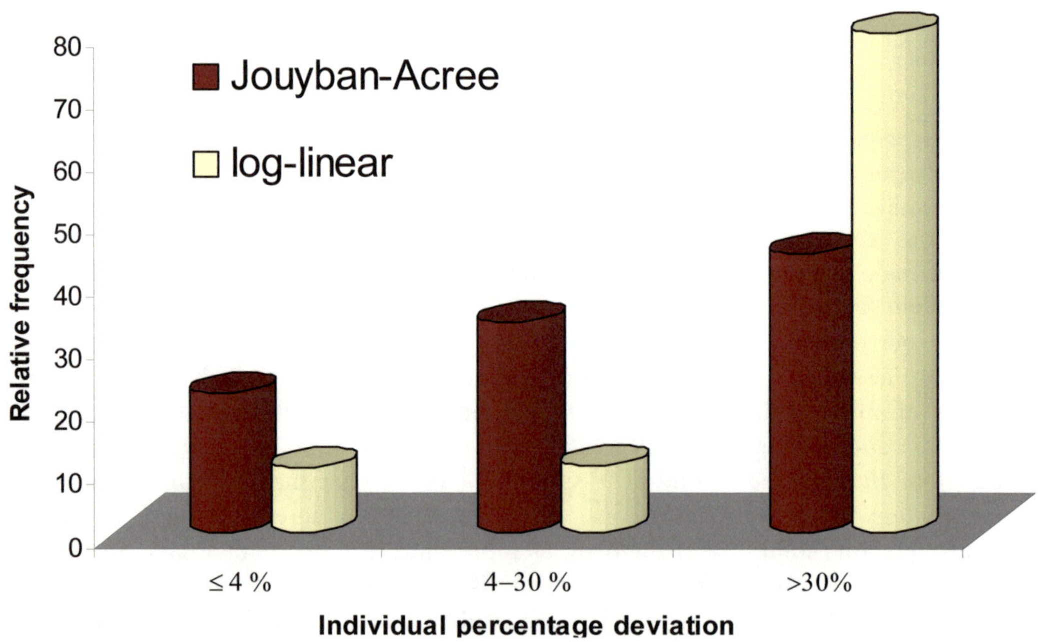

Fig. 5. The relative frequencies of the predicted solubilities in binary solvent mixtures using Jouyban-Acree and log-linear models

Solvent	c	e	s	a	b	v
Acetone	0.335	0.349	-0.231	-0.411	-4.793	3.963
Acetonitrile	0.413	0.077	0.326	-1.566	-4.391	3.364
Dimethyl formamide	-0.438	-0.099	0.670	0.878	-4.970	4.552
Dioxane	0.098	0.350	-0.083	-0.556	-4.826	4.172
Ethanol	0.208	0.409	-0.959	0.186	-3.645	3.928
Ethylene glycol	0.243	0.695	-0.670	0.726	-2.399	2.670
Methanol	0.329	0.299	-0.671	0.080	-3.389	3.512
2-Propanol	0.063	0.320	-1.024	0.445	-3.824	4.067
Water	-0.994	0.577	2.549	3.813	4.841	-0.869

Table 6. The Abraham solvent parameters of a number of common solvents (data taken from Stovall et al., 2005a; 2005b)

3.5 Solubility in the presence of surfactants

Equation 24 is one of the equations used for the solubility calculation in presence of surfactant (Rangel-Yagui et al., 2005):

$$\chi = \frac{(S_T - S_W)}{(C_{Surfactant} - cmc)} \tag{24}$$

where χ is the ratio of the concentration of the drug in micelles to the concentration of the micellar surfactant molecules, S_T is the total drug solubility in the solution, S_W is the aqueous solubility of the drug, $C_{Surfactant}$ is the molar concentration of the surfactant in the solution, and *cmc* is the critical micelle concentration. Another equation is (Rangel-Yagui et al., 2005):

$$K = \frac{S_T - S_W}{S_W} \tag{25}$$

where K is the micelle-water partition coefficient of the drug.

However, these equations require at least two other experimental data as input for total solubility prediction of the drug in micellar solutions.

Abraham et al. (1995) have proposed two models for prediction of K for different solutes in the presence of sodium dodecylsulfate (SDS) as:

$$\begin{aligned} &\log K_x = 1.201 + 0.542E - 0.400S - 0.133A - 1.580B + 2.793V \\ &R = 0.9849 \quad , \quad N = 132 \quad , \quad \text{standard deviation} = 0.171 \end{aligned} \tag{26}$$

and

$$\log K_x = 1.129 + 0.504 \log P + 1.216V$$
$$R = 0.9755 \quad , \quad N = 132 \quad , \quad \text{standard deviation} = 0.215 \tag{27}$$

where K_x is the definition of K of equation 25 in mole fraction unit (Abraham et al., 1995).
Ghasemi and coworkers have developed a MLR model for micellar solubility prediction in the presence of SDS for a diverse set of compounds:

$$\log K_S = -0.638 + 0.001E_b + 0.384MR - 0.112LUMO + 0.570C\log P - 0.001\mathrm{Re}\,pE$$
$$R^2 = 0.9679 \quad , \quad N = 62 \quad , \quad RMSEP = 0.124 \tag{28}$$

where K_S is the micellar solubility, E_b is bending energy, *MR* is molar refractivity, LUMO is the lowest unoccupied molecular orbital, Clog*P* is logarithm of calculated partition coefficient and *RepE* is the repulsion energy (Ghasemi et al., 2008). In other work, they have proposed a QSPR model for micellar solubility prediction for a diverse set of compounds in presence of cetyltrimethylammonium bromide (CTAB) as:

$$\log K_S = -1.1522 + 0.0070MP + 0.8089 \log P - 0.1262DPLL$$
$$R^2 = 0.9624 \quad , \quad N = 40 \quad , \quad RMSEP = 0.169 \tag{29}$$

where *MP* is melting point of the solute, and *DPLL* is the dipole length of the solute (Ghasemi et al., 2009).
However, as mentioned above, at least intrinsic solubility is required for total solubility prediction in the presence of a surfactant and they cannot be used as *ab initio* QSPR models for solubility prediction.

3.6 Solubility in the presence of complexing agents

In most of the cases, by adding complexing agents (e.g. cyclodextrins) to the solution, the solubility of a specific ligand (i.e. drug) is enhanced. But this enhancement could have different types as illustrated in Figure 6.
As has been seen, different kinds of drugs show different behaviours. But except for one condition, in the smaller amounts of complexing agent, the solubility changes are the same for other types. This common part of the curves is considered as a straight line with a slope of:

$$Slope = \frac{K_{1:1}S_0}{1 + K_{1:1}S_0}$$
$$K_{1:1} = \frac{[Host.Ligand]}{[Host]\cdot[Ligand]} \tag{30}$$

where $K_{1:1}$ is the complex formation coefficient, [*Host.Ligand*] is the concentration of the formed complex between drug and complexing agent, [*Host*] is the concentration of the complexing agent, and [*Ligand*] is the concentration of the drug (Sinko and Martin, 2006; Brewster and Loftsson, 2007). To correlate solubility value in presence of a complexing agent in this part of the solubility curve, one can use the following equation:

$$S_{Total}^{Complex} = S_0 + Slope \cdot C_{Host} \tag{31}$$

where $S_{Total}^{Complex}$ is the total solubility amount in the presence of a complexing agent, S_0 is the intrinsic solubility, *Slope* is the slope of the first part of solubility curve versus complexing agent concentrations, and C_{Host} is the concentration of the complexing agent (Sinko and Martin, 2006; Brewster and Loftsson, 2007).

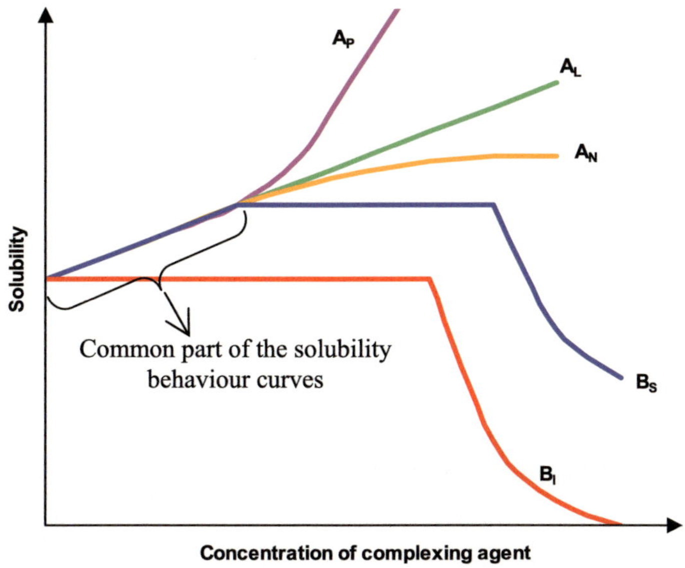

Fig. 6. Possible different solubility behaviours in the presence of complexing agent.

Again, like the pH and surfactant effects, one must have intrinsic solubility and *Slope* (or $K_{1:1}$) for solubility prediction in presence of complexing agents. However some QSPR models have been developed for prediction of *Slope* (or $K_{1:1}$). But most of them only considered the effect of complexing agent on the solubility enhancement (i.e. *Slope*). Demian (2000) has proposed equation 32 for the correlation of the *Slope* of the above mentioned equation for aromatics and terpenes with hydroxypropyl-β-cyclodextrin:

$$\begin{aligned} &Slope = 2.86 - 0.11 \times SterimolL - 0.34 \times \log P \\ &R = 0.788 \quad , \quad N = 19 \quad , \quad \text{standard error} = 0.336 \end{aligned} \tag{32}$$

where *SterimolL* is a steric parameter which is calculated by ChemOffice software (Demian, 2000). Choi et al. (2006) have developed a QSPR model for the correlation of the *Slope* for A_L type solubility curves between drugs and α/β/γ-cyclodextrines as following:

$$\begin{aligned} &Slope = -0.012E_{h-g} + 0.102E_{np\_h-g} + 0.328E_{np\_g-g} + 0.305 \\ &R^2 = 0.913 \quad , \quad N = 63 \quad , \quad \text{standard error} = 0.028 \end{aligned} \tag{33}$$

where E_{h-g} is the interaction energy between host and guest, E_{np_h-g} is the difference between nonpolar components of free energy of solvation of the host–guest complex and those of individual host and guest molecules, E_{np_g-g} is the difference between nonpolar components of free energy of solvation of the guest–guest dimer and those of individual guest molecule (Choi et al., 2006). These energy values are calculated after a Monte Carlo docking simulation between each drug and related complexing agent. Trapani et al. (2005) have developed a QSPR model for the correlation of the ratio of the total versus intrinsic solubilities of 25 drugs in the presence of 2-hydroxypropyl-β-cyclodextrin as following:

$$\log \frac{S_{Total}^{Complex}}{S_0} = 3.766 + 0.182CMR - 0.150C\log P - 0.00683TPSA - 0.0844\delta_{tot} \tag{34}$$
$$R^2 = 0.793 \quad , \quad N = 25 \quad , \quad Q^2 = 0.711$$

and

$$\log \frac{S_{Total}^{Complex}}{S_0} = 1.827 - 0.00508MW + 0.0122MV - 0.179C\log P - 0.00547TPSA \tag{35}$$
$$R^2 = 0.763 \quad , \quad N = 25 \quad , \quad Q^2 = 0.605$$

where *CMR* is calculated molecular refractivity, *TPSA* is total polar surface area, δ_{tot} total solubility parameter, *MW* is molecular weight, and *MV* is molecular volume. Equation 34 was derived using a MLR method and equation 35 was derived using a PLS method (Trapani et al., 2005).
However, as mentioned earlier, none of these models can be applied directly for solubility prediction in the presence of complexing agents and intrinsic solubility is required for all of them.

3.7 Available software

There is almost a large number of software for solubility prediction. A thorough review of these software was provided in an article (Jouyban et al., 2008). In this chapter, more useful solubility prediction applications and those which are newly developed or related with drug design and development is discussed.
ACD/Solubility DB predicts aqueous solubility at different pH with an accuracy of average error of 0.47±0.67 (in decimal logarithm) for solubility prediction of 1125 compounds (ACD/Labs).
ACD/DMSO Solubility predicts whether a compound is soluble (a result of 1) or insoluble (a result of 0) in DMSO. Using a hybrid model of logistic regression with PLS method, its predictive model was trained with solubility related physicochemical parameters, and considering the effects of charged groups, atom chains, and ring scaffolds. It provides 30% high reliability, 70% moderate reliability and <1% low reliability in prediction, with an overall accuracy of 82% in correct prediction (Japertas et al.).
Simulations plus' ADMET predictor™, predicts aqueous solubility using 2D and 3D descriptors as input data with average error of 0.432 and 0.423 in logarithm scale for 2817 and 711 number of compounds in train and test sets, respectively (ADMET Predictor™). It can also predict the solubility in biorelevant medium of the fasted state simulated gastric fluid (FaSSGF), the fasted state simulated intestinal fluid (FaSSIF), and the fed state simulated intestinal fluid (FeSSIF). Its average errors in logarithm scale for FaSSGF are 0.510 and 0.470 for 137 and 20 compounds, respectively. Its average errors in logarithm scale for FaSSIF are 0.469 and 0.417 for 141 and 16 compounds, respectively. Its average errors in logarithm scale for FeSSIF are 0.424 and 0.409 for 136 and 21 compounds, respectively. These predictive tools are designed using 2D descriptors as inputs and ADMET Modeler's ANNE

methodology for modelling (ADMET Predictor™). This package also can predict possibility of supersaturation in water. It calculates ratio of kinetic solubility versus intrinsic solubility and if the result is higher than 1.3, then the answer to possibility of supersaturation is true. It classified 95 and 23 out of 97 and 24 compounds correctly as train and test sets (ADMET Predictor™).

Finally, Solvomix is a recently developed free software available via Handbook of Solubility Data for Pharmaceuticals as a tool for prediction of solubility in monosolvents and mixtures of solvents. It uses GSE and Abraham models for the prediction of solubility in monosolvents and trained versions of log-linear model of Yalkowsky and Jouyban-Acree model for solubility prediction in mixtures of solvents (Jouyban, 2009).

4. Conclusion

Although preparation of a drug solution is a simple procedure, the associated problems are still a challenging subject in the pharmaceutical area. Brief review of its importance, various experimental and computational methods to determine the solubility and a number of more common methods to alter the solubility are discussed in this chapter. A comprehensive compilation of aqueous solubility data of chemical/pharmaceutical compounds is available from a reference work of Yalkowsky et al. 2010. The solubility data of pharmaceuticals in organic mono-solvents and also aqueous and non-aqueous solvent mixtures are compiled in a recent work (Jouyban, 2009).

5. Acknowledgment

This work is dedicated to Professor S.A. Mahboob, Tabriz University of Medical Sciences, Tabriz, Iran, for his life long efforts in training pharmacy students in Tabriz.

6. References

Abraham, M.H.; Chadha, H.S.; Dixon, J.P.; Rafols, C. & Treiner, C. (1995). Hydrogen Bonding. Part 40. Factors That Influence the Distribution of Solutes between Water and Sodium Dodecylsulfate Micelles. *Journal of the Chemical Society, Perkin Transactions 2*, pp. 887-894, ISSN *0300-9580*

Abraham, M.H. & Acree Jr., W.E. (2005). Characterisation of the Water-Isopropyl Myristate System. *International Journal of Pharmaceutics*, Vol. 294, pp. 121-128, ISSN *0378-5173*

Abraham, M.H.; Smith, R.E.; Luchtefeld, R.; Boorem, A.J.; Luo, R. & Acree Jr., W.E. (2010). Prediction of Solubility of Drugs and Other Compounds in Organic Solvents. *Journal of Pharmaceutical Sciences*, Vol. 99, pp. 1500-1515, ISSN *0378-5173*

ACD/Labs. Advanced Chemistry Development. Available from http://207.176.233.196/products/phys_chem_lab/aqsol/

ADMET Predictor™. Simulations plus inc. available from http://www.simulations-plus.com/Products.aspx?grpID=1&cID=11&pID=13

Acree Jr., W.E. (1992). Mathematical Representation of Thermodynamic Properties. Part II. Derivation of the Combined Nearly Ideal Binary Solvent (NIBS)/Redlich-Kister Mathematical Representation from a Two-Body and Three-Body Interactional Mixing Model. *Thermochimica Acta*, Vol. 198, pp. 71-79, ISSN *0040-6031*

Allen, L.V.; Popovich, N.G. & Ansel, H.C. (2006). *Ansel's Pharmaceutical Dosage Forms and Drug Delivery Systems*, Lippincott Williams & Wilkins, ISBN 978-078-1770-17-0, Philadelphia, US

Alsenz, J. & Kansy, M. (2007). High Throughput Solubility Measurement in Drug Discovery and Development. *Advanced Drug Delivery Reviews*, Vol. 59, pp. 546-567, ISSN *0169-409X*

Black, S.N.; Collier, E.A.; Davey, R.J. & Roberts, R.J. (2007). Structure, Solubility, Screening, and Synthesis of Molecular Salts. *Journal of Pharmaceutical Sciences*, Vol. 96, pp. 1053-1068, ISSN *0022-3549*

Blagden, N.; de Matas, M.; Gavan, P.T. & York, P. (2007). Crystal Engineering of Active Pharmaceutical Ingredients to Improve Solubility and Dissolution Rates. *Advanced Drug Delivery Reviews*, Vol. 59, pp. 617-630, ISSN *0169-409X*

Bolen, D.W. (2004). Effects of Naturally Occurring Osmolytes on Protein Stability and Solubility: Issues Important in Protein Crystallization. *Methods*, Vol. 34, pp. 312-322, ISSN *1046-2023*

Brewster, M.E. & Loftsson, T. (2007). Cyclodextrins as Pharmaceutical Solubilizers. *Advanced Drug Delivery Reviews*, Vol. 59, pp. 645-666, ISSN *0169-409X*

Burgess, R.R. (2009). Chapter 20 Protein Precipitation Techniques. *Methods in Enzymology*, Vol. 463, pp. 331-342, ISSN *0076-6879*

Choi, Y.; Cho, K.W.; Jeong, K.; Paik, S.R. & Jung, S. (2006). Computational Prediction for the Slopes of A_L-Type Phase Solubility Curves of Organic Compounds Complexed with α-, β-, or γ-Cyclodextrins Based on Monte Carlo Docking Simulations. *Journal of Inclusion Phenomena*, Vol. 55, pp. 103-108, ISSN *1388-3127*

Chu, K.A. & Yalkowsky, S.H. (2009). Predicting Aqueous Solubility: The Role of Crystalinity. *Current Drug Metabolism*, Vol. 10, pp. 1184-1191, ISSN *1389-2002*

Dearden, J.C. & O'Sullivan, J.G. (1988). Solubility of Pharmaceuticals in Cyclohexane. *Journal of Pharmacy and Pharmacology*, Vol. 40, p. 77P, ISSN *0022-3573*

Dearden, J.C. (2006). In Silico Prediction of Aqueous Solubility. *Expert Opinion on Drug Discovery*, Vol. 1, pp. 31-52, ISSN *1746-0441*

Demian, B.A. (2000). Correlation of the Solubility of Several Aromatics and Terpenes in Aqueous Hydroxypropyl-β-cyclodextrin with Steric and Hydrophobicity Parameters. *Carbohydrate Research*, Vol. 328, pp. 635-639, ISSN *0008-6215*

Ellegaard, C.; Abidsko, J. & O'Connell, P.O. (2010). Molecular Thermodynamic Modelling of Mixed Solvent Solubility. *Industrial and Engineering Chemistry Research*, Vol. 49, pp. 11620-11632, ISSN *0888-5885*

Fakhree, M.A.A.; Delgado, D.R.; Martínez, F. & Jouyban, A. (2010). The Importance of Dielectric Constant for Drug Solubility Prediction in Binary Solvent Mixtures: Electrolytes and Zwitterions in Water+Ethanol. *AAPS PharmSciTech*, Vol. 11, pp. 1726-1729, ISSN *1530-9932*

Galcera, J. & Molins, E. (2009). Effects of the Counterion on the Solubility of Isostructural Pharmaceutical Lamotrigine Salts. *Crystal Growth and Design*, Vol. 9, pp. 327-334, ISSN *1528-7483*

Ghasemi, J.; Abdolmaleki, A.; Asadpour, S. & Shiri, F. (2008). Prediction of Solubility of Nonionic Solutes in Anionic Micelle (SDS) Using a QSPR Model. *QSAR and Combinatorial Science*, Vol. 27, pp. 338-346, ISSN *1611-020X*

Ghasemi, J.B.; Abdolmaleki, A. & Mandoumi, N. (2009). A Quantitative Structure Property Relationship for Prediction of Solubilization of Hazardous Compounds Using GA-

Based MLR in CTAB Micellar Media. *Journal of Hazardous Materials*, Vol. 161, pp. 74-80, ISSN *0304-3894*

Gibaldi, M.; Lee, M. & Desai, A. (2007). *Gibaldi's Drug Delivery Systems in Pharmaceutical Care*, Lea & Febiger, ISBN 978-158-5281-36-7, Philadelphia, US

Golightly, L.K.; Smolinkse, S.S.; Bennett, M.L.; Sunderland III, E.W. & Rumack, B.H. (1988). Pharmaceutical Excipients Adverse Effects Associated with Inactive Ingredients in Drug Products (Part I). *Medical Toxicology and Adverse Drug Experience*, Vol. 3, p. 128-165, ISSN *0113-5244*

Grant, D.J.W. & Abougela, I.K.A (1983). A Synthetic Method for Determining the Solubility of Solids in Viscous Liquids. *International Journal of Pharmaceutics*, Vol. 16, pp. 11-21, ISSN *0378-5173*

Grant, D.J.W.; Mehdizadeh, M.; Chow, A.H.L. & Fairbrother, J.E. (1984). Non-Linear van 't Hoff Solubility - Temperature Plots and Their Pharmaceutical Interpretation. *International Journal of Pharmaceutics*, Vol. 18, pp. 25-38, ISSN *0378-5173*

Hankinson, R.W. & Thompson, D. (1965). Equilibria and Solubility Data for Methanol - Water -1-Nitropropane Ternary Liquid System. *Journal of Chemical and Engineering Data*, Vol. 10, pp. 18-19, ISSN *1520-5134*

Hansch, C.; Quinlan, J.E. & Lawrence, G.L. (1968). The Linear Free-Energy Relationship Between Partition Coefficients and the Aqueous Solubility of Organic Liquids. *Journal of Organic Chemistry*, Vol. 33, pp. 347-350, ISSN *0022-3263*

Hao, H.X.; Hou, B.H.; Wang, J.K. & Zhang, M.J. (2005). Solubility of Erythriol in Different Solvents. *Journal of Chemical and Engineering Data*, Vol. 50, pp. 1454-1456, ISSN *1520-5134*

Higuchi, T. & Connors, K.A. (1965). Phase-solubility techniques. *Advances in Analytical Chemistry and Instrumentation*. Vol. 4, pp. 117-212

Hoelke, B.; Gieringer, S.; Arlt, M. & Saal, C. (2009). Comparison of Nephelometric, UV-Spectroscopic, and HPLC Methods for High-Throughput Determination of Aqueous Drug Solubility in Microtiter Plates. *Analytical Chemistry*, Vol. 81, pp. 3165-3172, ISSN *0003-2700*

Hwang, C.A.; Holste, J.C.; Hall, K.R. & Mansoori, G.A. (1991). A Simple Relation to Predict or to Correlate the Excess Functions of Multicomponent Mixtures. *Fluid Phase Equilibria*, Vol. 62, pp. 173-189, ISSN *0378-3812*

Jain, P.; Sepassi, K. & Yalkowsky, S.H. (2008). Comparison of Aqueous Solubility Estimation from AQUAFAC and GSE. *International Journal of Pharmaceutics*, Vol. 360, pp. 122-147, ISSN *0378-5173*

Jain, P. & Yalkowsky, S.H. (2010). Prediction of Aqueous Solubility from SCRATCH. *International Journal of Pharmaceutics*, Vol. 385, pp. 1-5, ISSN *0378-5173*

Japertas, P.; Maas, P. & Petrauskas, A. DMSO Solubility Prediction. Available from http://www.acdlabs.com/products/pc_admet/physchem/dmso/

Jouyban-Gharamaleki, A. & Hanaee, J. (1997). A Novel Method for Improvement of Predictability of the CNIBS/R-K Equation. *International Journal of Pharmaceutics*, Vol. 154, pp. 245-247, ISSN *0378-5173*

Jouyban-Gharamaleki, A.; Barzegar-Jalali, M. & Acree Jr., W.E. (1998). Solubility correlation of structurally related drugs in binary solvent mixtures. *International Journal of Pharmaceutics*, Vol. 166, pp. 205-209, ISSN *0378-5173*

Jouyban-Gharamaleki, A.; Valaee, L.; Barzegar-Jalali, M.; Clark, B.J. & Acree Jr., W.E. (1999). Comparison of Various Cosolvency Models for Calculating Solute Solubility in

Water-Cosolvent Mixtures. *International Journal of Pharmaceutics,* Vol. 177, pp. 93-101, ISSN *0378-5173*

Jouyban-Gharamaleki, A.; York, P.; Hanna, M. & Clark, B.J. (2001) Solubility Prediction of Salmeterol Xinafoate in Water-Dioxane Mixtures. *International Journal of Pharmaceutics,* Vol. 216, pp. 33-41, ISSN *0378-5173*

Jouyban, A. & Acree Jr., W.E. (2007). Prediction of Drug Solubility in Ethanol-Ethyl Acetate Mixtures at Various Temperatures Using the Jouyban-Acree Model. *Journal of Drug Delivery Science and Technology,* Vol. 17, pp. 159-160, ISSN *1773-2247*

Jouyban, A.; Fakhree, M.A.A. & Shayanfar, A. (2008). Solubility prediction methods for drug/drug like molecules. *Recent Patent on Chemical Engineering,* Vol. 1, pp. 220-231, ISSN *1874-4788*

Jouyban, A.; Soltanpour, Sh.; Soltani, S.; Tamizi, E.; Fakhree, M.A.A. & Acree Jr., W.E. (2009). Prediction of Drug Solubility in Mixed Solvents Using Computed Abraham Parameters. *Journal of Molecular Liquids,* Vol. 146, 82-88, ISSN *0167-7322*

Jouyban, A. (2009) *Handbook of Solubility Data for Pharmaceuticals,* CRC Press, ISBN 978-143-9804-85-8, Boca Raton, USA.

Jouyban, A. & Soltanpour, Sh. (2010). Solubility of Pioglitazone Hydrochloride in Binary and Ternary Mixtures of Water, Propylene Glycol, and Polyethylene Glycols 200, 400 and 600 at 298.2 K. *AAPS PharmSciTech, Vol.* 11, pp. 1713-1717, ISSN *1530-9932*

Jouyban, A.; Fakhree, M.A.A. & Shayanfar, A. (2010a). Review of Pharmaceutical Applications of N-Methyl-2-Pyrrolidone. *Journal of Pharmacy and Pharmaceutical Sciences,* Vol. 13, pp. 524-535, ISSN *1482-1826*

Jouyban, A.; Fakhree, M.A.A.; Shayanfar, A. & Ghafourian, T. (2010b). QSPR Modelling Using Catalan Solvent and Solute Parameters. *Journal of Brazilian Chemical Society,* In press, ISSN *0103-5053*

Katritzky, A.R.; Kuanar, M.; Slavov, S.; Hall, C.D.; Karelson, M.; Kahn, I. & Dobchev, D.A. (2010). Quantitative Correlation of Physical and Chemical Properties with Chemical Structure: Utility for Prediction. *Chemical Reviews,* Vol. 110, pp. 5714-5789, ISSN *0009-2665*

Kawakami, A.; Miyoshi, K. & Ida, Y. (2005). Impact of the Amount of Excess Solids on Apparent Solubility. *Pharmaceutical Research,* Vol. 22, pp. 1537-1543, ISSN *0724-8741*

Li, A. & Yalkowsky, S.H. (1998) .Predicting Cosolvency. 1. Solubility Ratio and Solute logKow. *Industrial and Engineering Chemistry Research,* Vol. 37, pp. 4470-4475, ISSN *0888-5885*

Li, A. (2001). Predicting Cosolvency. 3. Evaluation of the Extended Log-Linear. *Industrial and Engineering Chemistry Research,* Vol. 40, pp. 5029-5035, ISSN *0888-5885*

Li, X.; Yin, Q.; Chen, W. & Wang, J. (2006). Solubility of Hydroquinone in Different Solvents from 276.65 to 345.10 K. *Journal of Chemical and Engineering Data,* Vol. 51, pp. 127-129, ISSN *1520-5134*

Lim, L.-Y. & Go, M.-L. (2000). Caffeine and Nicotinamide Enhances the Aqueous Solubility of the Antimalarial Agent Halofantrine. *European Journal of Pharmaceutical Sciences,* Vol. 10, pp. 17–28, ISSN *0928-0987*

Millard, J.F.; Alvarez-Nunez, F.A. & Yalkowsky, S.H. (2002). Solubilization by Cosolvents. Establishment Useful Constants for the Log-Linear Model. *International Journal of Pharmaceutics,* Vol. 245, 153-166, ISSN *0378-5173*

Mizuuchi, H.; Jaitely, V.; Murdan, S. & Florence, A.T. (2008). Room Temperature Ionic Liquids and Their Mixtures: Potential Pharmaceutical Solvents. *European Journal of Pharmaceutical Sciences*, Vol. 33, pp. 326-331, ISSN *0928-0987*

Myrdal, P.B. & Yalkowsky, S.H. (1998). Solubilization of Drugs, In: *Encyclopedia of Pharmaceutical Technology*, Swarbrick, J. & Boylan, J.C. (Eds.), 161-217, Marcel Dekker, ISBN 978-082-4728-19-9, New York, US

Pan, L.; Ho, Q.; Tsutsui, K. & Takahashi, L. (2001). Comparison of Chromatographic and Spectroscopic Methods Used to Rank Compounds for Aqueous Solubility. *Journal of Pharmaceutical Sciences*, Vol. 90, pp. 521-529, ISSN *0022-3549*

Patel, D.M.; Bernardo, P.; Cooper, J. & Forrester, R.B. (1986). Glycerine. In: *Handbook of Pharmaceutical Excipients*, 203-213, America and Great Britain Pharmaceutical Societies, London, UK

Peisheng, M.A. & Qing, X. (2001). Determination and Correlation for Solubility of Aromatic Acids in Solvents. *Chinese Journal of Chemical Engineering*, Vol. 9, pp. 39-44, ISSN *1004-9541*

Pharma-Algorithms (2008). ADME Boxes, Version 4.0, PharmaAlgorithms Inc., Toronto, Canada

Ran, Y.; Jain, N. & Yalkowsky S.H. (2001). Prediction of Aqueous Solubility of Organic Compounds by the General Solubility Equation (GSE). *Journal of Chemical Information and Computer Science, Vol.* 41, pp. 1208-1217, ISSN *0095-2338*

Rangel-Yagui, C.deO.; Pessoa Jr., A. & Tavares, L.C. (2005). Micellar Solubilization of Drugs. *Journal of Pharmacy and Pharmaceutical Sciences*, Vol. 8, pp. 147-163, ISSN *1482-1826*

Ren, B.Z.; Chong, H.G.; Li, W.R. & Wang F.A. (2005). Solubility of Potassium p-Chlorophenoxyacetate in Ethanol + Water from (295.61 to 358.16) K. *Journal of Chemical and Engineering Data*, Vol. 50, pp. 907-909, ISSN *1520-5134*

Rubino, J.T. (1990). Cosolvents and Cosolvency, In: *Encyclopedia of Pharmaceutical Technology*, Swarbrick, J. & Boylan, J.C. (Eds.), 375-398, Marcel Dekker, ISBN 978-082-4728-19-9, New York, US

Sepassi, K. & Yalkowsky, S.H. (2006). Solubility Prediction in Octanol: A Technical Note. *AAPS PharmSciTechnol*, Vol. 7: p. E1-E8, ISSN *1530-9932*

Shayanfar, A.; Fakhree, M.A.A. & Jouyban, A. (2010). A Simple QSPR Model to Predict Aqueous Solubility of Drugs. *Journal of Drug Delivery Science and Technology*, Vol. 20, pp. 467-476, ISSN *1773-2247*

Sinko, P.J. & Martin, A.N. (2006). *Martin's Physical Pharmacy and Pharmaceutical Sciences*, Lippincott Williams & Wilkins, ISBN 978-078-1750-27-1, Philadelphia, US

Spiegel, A.J. & Noseworthy, M.M. (1963). Use of Nonaqueous Solvents in Parenteral Products. *Journal of Pharmaceutical Sciences*, Vol. 52 pp. 917-927, ISSN *0022 -3549*

Stovall, D.M.; Acree Jr., W.E. & Abraham M.H. (2005a) Solubility of 9-Fluorenone, Thianthrene and Xanthene in Organic Solvents. *Fluid Phase Equilibria*, Vol. 232, pp. 113-121, ISSN *0378-3812*

Stovall, D.M.; Givens, C.; Keown, S.; Hoover, K.R.; Barnes, R.; Harris, C.; Lozano, J.; Nguyen, M.; Rodriguez, E.; Acree Jr., W.E. & Abraham, M.H. (2005b). Solubility of Crystalline Nonelectrolyte Solutes in Organic Solvents: Mathematical Correlation of 4-Chloro-3-Nitrobenzoic Acid and 2-Chloro-5-Nitrobenzoic Acid Solubilities with the Abraham Solvation Parameter Model. *Physics and Chemistry of Liquids*, Vol. 43, pp. 351-360, ISSN *0031-9104*

Strickley, R.G. (2004). Solubilizing Excipients in Oral and Injectable Formulations. *Pharmaceutical Research*, Vol. 21, pp. 201-230, ISSN *0724-8741*

Trapani, A.; Lopedota, A.; Denora, N.; Laquintana, V.; Franco, M.; Latrofa, A.; Trapani, G. & Liso, G. (2005). A Rapid Screening Tool for Estimating the Potential of 2-Hydroxypropyl-β-Cyclodextrin Complexation for Solubilization Purposes. *International Journal of Pharmaceutics*, Vol. 295, pp. 163-175, ISSN *0378-5173*

Trevino, S.R.; Scholtz, J.M. & Pace, C.N. (2008). Measuring and Increasing Protein Solubility. *Journal of Pharmaceutical Sciences*, Vol. 97, pp. 4155-4166, ISSN *0022-3549*

Tsai, P.S.; Lipper, R.A. & Worthington, H.C. (1986). Propylene Glycol, In: *Handbook of Pharmaceutical Excipients*, 241-242, America and Great Britain Pharmaceutical Societies, London, UK

Valvani, S.C.; Yalkowsky, S.H. & Roseman, T.J. (1981). Solubility and Partitioning IV: Aqueous Solubility and Octanol-Water Partition Coefficients of Liquid Nonelectrolytes. *Journal of Pharmaceutical Sciences*, Vol. 70, pp. 502-507, ISSN *0022-3549*

Waldo, G.S. (2003). Genetic Screens and Directed Evolution for Protein Solubility. *Current Opinion in Chemical Biology*, Vol. 7, pp. 33-38, ISSN *1367-5931*

Wang, L.C.; Ding, H.; Zhao, J.H.; Song C.Y. & Wang J.S. (2008). Solubility of Isonicotinic Acid in 4-Methylpyridine + Water from (287.65 to 361.15) K. *Journal of Chemical and Engineering Data,* Vol. 53, pp. 2544-2546, ISSN *1520-5134*

Wang, Z.; Burrell, L.S. & Lambert, W.J. (2002). Solubility of E2050 at Various pH: A Case in Which Apparent Solubility Is Affected by the Amount of Excess Solid. *Journal of Pharmaceutical Sciences, Vol.* 91, pp. 1445-1455, ISSN *0022-3549*

Ward, H.L. (1926). The Solubility Relations of Naphthalene. *Journal of Physical Chemistry,* Vol. 30, pp. 1316-1333, ISSN *0022-3654*

Weiwei, S.; Peisheng, M.A.; Lihua, F. & Zhengle X. (2007). Solubility of Glutamic Acid in Cyclohexane, Cyclohexanol, Their Five Mixtures and Acetic Acid. *Chinese Journal of Chemical Engineering,* Vol. 15, pp. 228-232, ISSN *1004-9541*

Wells, J.I. (1988). *Pharmaceutical Preformulation,* ISBN 978-074-5802-76-3, Ellis Harwood Ltd., Chiester, England.

Widenski, D.J.; Abbas, A. & Romagnoli, J.A. (2009). Effect of the Solubility Model on Antisolvent Crystallization Predicted Volume Mean Size. *Chemical Engineering Transactions*, Vol. 17, pp. 639–44

Yalkowsky, S.H. & Roseman, T. (1981) Solubilization of Drugs by Cosolvents In: *Techniques of Solubilization of Drugs*, Yalkowsky, S.H. (Ed.), 91-134, Marcel Dekker, ISBN 978-082-4715-66-3, New York, US

Yalkowsky, S.H.; Valvani, S.C. & Roseman, T.J. (1983). Solubility and Partitioning. VI: Octanol Solubility and Octanol-Water Partition Coefficients. *Journal of Pharmaceutical Sciences*, Vol. 72, pp. 866-870, ISSN *0022-3549*

Yalkowsky, S.H.; He, Y. & Jain, P. (2010) *Handbook of Aqueous Solubility Data,* CRC Press, ISBN 978-143-9802-46-5, Boca Raton, USA.

Yang, Z.S.; Zeng, Z.X.; Xue W.L. & Zhang Y. (2008). Solubility of Bis(benzoxaolyl-2-methyl) Sulfide in Different Pure Solvents and Ethanol + Water Binary Mixtures between (273.25 and 325.25) K. *Journal of Chemical and Engineering Data,* Vol. 53, pp. 2692-2695, ISSN *1520-5134*

Yu, Q.; Black, S. & Wei H. (2009). Solubility of Butanedioic Acid in Different Solvents at Temperatures between 283 K and 333 K. *Journal of Chemical and Engineering Data,* Vol. 54, pp. 2123-2125, ISSN *1520-5134*

Part 2

Toxicity

10

Toxic Effects of Cadmium on Crabs and Shrimps

Xianjiang Kang[1], Shumei Mu[1], Wenyan Li[2] and Na Zhao[1]
[1]*College of Life Sciences, Hebei University,*
[2]*College of Basic Medicine, Hebei University,*
China

1. Introduction

Cadmium (Cd) is one of the most toxic heavy metals for humans; the main source of nonoccupational exposure to Cd includes smoking, air, and food and water contaminated by Cd (Nagata et al., 2005). In addition, herbal medicine is another source of Cd. The World Health Organization (WHO) estimates that 4 billion people or 80 percent of the world population, presently use herbal medicine (Naithani et al., 2010). Several articles have reported of adverse effects of these herbal preparations due to the presence of high level of heavy metals such as Cd, lead, chromium, nickel, etc. (Naithani et al., 2010). Saeed et al. (2010) investigated twenty five herbal products. The results revealed that the concentrations of some heavy metals, including Cd, were far greater than the permissible limits proposed by the International Regulatory Authorities for herbal drugs. Acute or chronic exposure of Cd causes respiratory distress, lung, breast and endometrial cancers, cardiovascular disorders and endocrine dysfunction (Åkesson et al., 2008; Chang et al., 2009; Messner et al., 2009; Nagata et al., 2005; Naithani et al., 2010; Navas-Acien et al., 2004).

In addition, Cd is a common inorganic contaminant of coastal sediments and waters due to anthropogenic pollution and natural sources (Ivanina et al., 2008, 2010; Sokolova et al., 2004). It can be accumulated in aquatic animals (e.g. crabs, shrimps, oysters and mussels) after entering through different way such as respiratory tract, digestive tract, surface penetration etc. (Dailianis & Kaloyianni, 2004; Dailianis et al., 2009; Ivanina et al., 2008, 2010; Li et al., 2008b; Sokolova, 2004; Sokolova et al., 2004; Wang L. et al., 2001, 2002a,b, 2008; Wang Q. et al., 2003; Zhao et al., 1995). It is seriously harmful to the growth of aquatic life and survival, resulting in decline of their populations. At the same time, as aquatic food products, these animals exposed to Cd might threaten human health.

1.1 Cd accumulation and distribution in crabs and shrimps

Cd in waters can be absorbed by aquatic organisms via respiratory system, digestive system and body surface without significant excretion (Rainbow & White, 1989; van Hatton et al., 1989). And we can get valuable information for evaluating the level of Cd pollution in waters and sediments by assaying Cd concentration in crabs and shrimps.

1.1.1 The difference of Cd accumulation and distribution in different tissues

Experiments have confirmed that Cd absorption and accumulation by crabs and shrimps had obvious differences among the various body segments. Accumulated Cd was distributed to all organs with the highest proportions of body content being found in the exoskeleton, gills, hepatopancreas, and so on.

The first organ in which Cd accumulates is the exoskeleton. Cd has similar chemical properties to calcium (Ca), the main component of the exoskeleton, such as the same charge number, the similar ion diameter and electronic number. Therefore, the Cd in waters can replace the Ca entering the body via exoskeletons (Jennings & Rainbow, 1979). The gill is a respiratory organ for crabs or shrimps. It plays an important role in the absorption and transport of heavy metals (Silvestre et al., 2004; Silvestre et al., 2005a) and is the target organ of Cd in waters. The hepatopancreas are detoxicating organs in crabs and shrimps which can change the toxic heavy metal into non-toxic compounds and reduce the toxicity of the heavy metal in the body. Thus the Cd concentration is higher in the hepatopancreas.

1.1.2 Factors influencing Cd accumulation and distribution

Due to the different treatment methods, the accumulation and distribution of Cd are different in different organs. When *Carcinus maenas* was exposed to seawater at Cd dose of 10 ppm, the midgut gland contained absorbed 10% of the total Cd, while the exoskeleton contained. When Cd was absorbed from a food source, the midgut gland contained 16.9% of the absorbed Cd whereas the exoskeleton contained only 22.2% (Jennings & Rainbow, 1979). It can be inferred that in bath experiments, the exoskeleton was in direct contact with Cd and accumulated the most Cd; in feeding regimes, the exoskeleton had the lower proportion accumulation. This result was consistent with those in unpolluted areas (Bjerregaard & Depledge, 2002; Davies et al., 1981; Falconer et al., 1986). American lobster, *Homarus americanus* were fed with three kinds of diets containing Cd (based on crab muscle; based on crab muscle adding ascorbic acid; based on casein for protein source). The result showed that Cd accumulated in hepatopancreas was higher in the lobsters fed with the first two diets than in ones fed with casein (Chou et al., 1987). In addition, *Sinopotamon yangtsekiense* had the highest concentration of Cd in the exoskeleton after acute exposure (Silvestre et al, 2005b), while *Eriocheir sinensis* had highest Cd concentration in the gills after chronic exposure for 30 d adding the acute exposure for 3 d (Wang Q. et al., 2003).

The environment can also affect the absorption and accumulation of Cd. An increase in the Cd concentration in the environment will result in increased Cd accumulation. Namely, the accumulation of Cd has obvious dose-dependent relationship (Wang L. et al., 2001; Wang Q. et al., 2003).

Ca in the water environment will prevent the absorption and accumulation of Cd because it can form the competitive relationship with Cd. Therefore, accumulated Cd in the body will be less whenever the Ca concentration in water increases (Wright, 1977).

Beltrame et al. (2010) reported that sex, habitat, and seasonality could influence heavy-metal concentrations in the burrowing crab (*Neohelice granulata*) from a coastal lagoon in Argentina.

The accumulation of Cd in all tissues were markedly higher in postmoult (A1–2 and B1–2) compared to intermoult (C1, C3 and C4) and premoult (D0–3) in male shore crab *C. maenas* (Nørum et al., 2005). This shows that accumulation and distribution of Cd in crabs and shrimps can also be related to the status of the organisms.

1.2 The influence of Cd on the enzyme activity in crabs and shrimps

Small amounts of Cd can be detoxicified into non-toxic substance by metallothionein in the organism (van Hatton et al., 1989). Excessive Cd will damage the body, however, as it will combine with protein molecules having sulphur, hydroxyl and amino group, and restrain some enzyme system activity. In addition, because the affinity of Cd with sulfhydryl groups is stronger than zinc (Zn), it can replace the enzyme-bond Zn and cause the enzyme to lose its function (Müller & Ohnesorge, 1982).

1.2.1 The influence of Cd on antioxidant enzymes system in crabs and shrimps

One of the mechanisms for Cd toxicity to animals is the oxidative damage. On one hand, Cd can cause the body to produce excessive active oxygen. On other hand, it can change the expression and vitality of antioxidant enzymes. Antioxidant enzymes mainly include the superoxide dismutase (SOD), catalase (CAT), glutathione peroxidase (GPX), glutathione enzyme turn sulfur (GST), etc. They can effectively scavenge active oxygen in the body and avoid oxidative damage to the body (Wang L. et al., 2007). Numerous studies have been published on the influence of Cd on antioxidant enzymes in terrestrial creatures, while reports about shrimps and crabs are rare. In one study the Cd concentration was 0.025 mg/L and 0.05 mg/L in water, and SOD, CAT and GPX activities in *Charybdis japonica* could be stimulated after 0.5 d, and then reduced during the experimental period (Pan & Zhang, 2006). When crabs (*S. yangtsekiense*) were exposed to the reagent with a dose range of 7.25-116.00 mg/L for 24, 48, 72 and 96 h, the activities of SOD, CAT and GPX increased initially and decreased subsequently (Li et al. 2008; Wang L. et al., 2008; Yan et al., 2007). After Immersing the juvenile crab *E. sinensis* in 2.0 mg/L water, the activities of SOD, CAT and GPX in hepatopancreas were all initially decreased, and then recovered to some degree during the duration of the study (Liu et al., 2003). This showed that low concentration of Cd stimulated antioxidant enzymes activity while high concentration inhibited antioxidant enzymes activity.

1.2.2 The influence of Cd on metabolic enzymes in crabs and shrimps

Glutamic-pyruvic transaminase (GPT) and glutamic-oxalacetic transaminease (GOT) are the important aminotransferase in the protein metabolism. Low concentration of Cd stimulated the activity of GPT and GOT in *Scylla serrata* while high Cd concentrations showed apparent inhibition. The results showed the obvious dose-effect relations (Tang et al., 2000). Effects of Cd on GOT and GPT activity are also tissue-specific. GPT and GOT activity decreased significantly in the heart, gills and hepatopancreas after *Macrobrachium rosenbergii* was poisoned by Cd, but increased in the green glands. This may be because green gland is excretory organ with strong detoxicification (Zhao et al., 1995). GPT activity in serum of *E. sinensis* increased with increasing Cd concentration after poisoning. That might be because tissues were damaged and the enzyme released into serum (Lu et al., 1989).

Lactic dehydrogenase (LDH) plays an important role in the carbohydrate metabolism. The crab *Uca pugilator* were immersed in 2.0 mg/L water for 24 h, 48 h, LDH activity reduced in hepatopancreas and that is opposite in the abdominal muscles (Devi et al.,1994).

Alkaline phosphatase is a kind of low-specific phosphomonoesterase which plays an important role in nucleinic acid, protein and lipid metabolic. The influence of Cd on enzymatic activity in *S. serrata* also exhibited dose-effect relationship that was similar to that observed above (Tang et al., 2000).

1.2.3 The influence of Cd on Na^+-K^+-ATPase in crabs and shrimps

Na^+-K^+-ATPase are ubiquitous in organism. It is the most important enzyme during the process of osmotic regulation and ion exchange in crustaceans. It is involved in cellular transmembrane transport of Na^+ and K^+ and sustains the ion gradient and membrane potential inside and outside cells. Cd can be directly combined with ATPase to execute function. In low concentration, the change rule of the enzyme is more complicated. In high concentration, enzyme activity will be loss. When *S. serrata* was exposed to 0.3 µg/L Cd, Na^+-K^+-ATPase activity in hepatopancreas and gills showed temporary activation in 10 d, followed by inhibition at longer exposure times (Daksna, 1988). Crabs *E. sinensis* were submitted to acute (0.5 mg/L for 1, 2 or 3 d), chronic (10 or 50 µg/L for 30 d) or chronic (immediately followed by acute) exposure. After 3 d of acute exposure, the respiratory anterior gill ultrastructure and Na^+/K^+-ATPase activities were significantly impaired. In contrast to acute exposure, chronic exposure did not induce any observable effects. Moreover, crabs submitted to chronic immediately followed by acute exposure showed normal hyper-osmoregulatory capacity with no change in gill Na^+/K^+-ATPase activity. These results demonstrated that a chronic Cd exposure could induce acclimation mechanisms related to osmoregulation in this euryhaline decapod crustacean (Silvestre et al., 2005a).

1.3 The influence of Cd on the ultrastructure of crabs and shrimps

Studies concerning the influence of Cd on the ultrastructure of crabs and shrimps have appeared in the past few years. The published studies have focused on the destruction of membrane systems and morphologic changes of cells. Cd can accelerate cellar lipid peroxidation and cause the accumulation of lipid peroxides. These free radicals and their reaction products, peroxides, can often cause various biological macromolecules, including DNA, to change structures and properties through chemical reactions, such as hydrogen abstraction, oxidation sulfhydryl and carbon chain destruction. Cd can also decompose the unsaturated fatty acid into malondialdehyde (MAD) by peroxiding and cause biological macromolecules to crosslink into abnormal macromolecules which degrade membrane structure and alter the membrane permeability (Shukla et al., 1989).

After the crabs *E. sinensis* were exposed to Cd, many changes appeared in the R-cell in hepatopancreas, such as organells decrease, mitochondria damage, endoplasmic reticulum expansion, and thinning of the cytoplasm matrix (Wang L. et al., 2001). Cd can partly disintegrate the mitochondrial cristae of neurosecretory cells in *E. sinensis* (Li et al., 2008). Whenever injected into the crab *S. yangtsekiense*, Cd resulted in damage to the organells with membrane structure, and the mitochondria was damaged first, which suggested that mitochondria was a sensitive organelle to Cd that could be used to show the amount of damage caused by Cd (Wang L. et al., 2002a,b). Cd could cause the morpha of female ovaries to change markedly in *S. henanese*, such as the increase of fragmentations and adherences. The oval prosenchyma of egg cells became significantly larger. Egg membrane were much thicker. At the same time, the particulate protuterances on the surface of eggs cells decreased. The boundary between egg cells became more and more unclear. These morphological changes may be a form of self-preservation in eggs which can reduce the damage through self-adjustment, whereas with the increase of Cd dosage, the irreconcilable morpha damage would become much larger (Meng, 2006).

1.4 The influence of Cd on ovarian development in crabs and shrimps

1.4.1 The influence of Cd on ovarian development

Studies regarding the effects of Cd on ovarian development in crabs and shrimps have been conducted since the 1990s. The majority of experiments showed that Cd inhibited ovarian growth, reduced hatch rates of the fertilized eggs and led to embryonic deformity.

Reddy et al. (1997) found Cd could inhibit 5-HT-induced ovarian maturation in the red swamp crayfish, *Procambarus clarkia*. Lee et al. (1996) documented that Cd deformed eyespots, reduced hatching success, and inhibited growth of oocytes of *Callinectes sapidus*. Naqvi et al. (1993) reported that *P. clarkia* treated with Cd hatched 48 eggs with a hatching rate of only 17%. In comparison, untreated individuals hatched 203 eggs with a hatching rate of 95%. Some results were not consistent with the above observations. For exemple, red swamp crayfish fed with duckweeds containing Cd for 14 d had significantly bigger ovary index and total fat content than the respective groups fed with unpolluted duckweeds (Devi et al., 1996).

1.4.2 The mechanism for the iInfluence of Cd on ovarian development

There are different views regarding the mechanism of how Cd affects ovary development. Reddy et al. (1997) suggested that the inhibition of Cd on ovarian maturation in P. clarkii was due to the metal inhibiting 5- Hydroxytryptamine (5-HT)-stimulated gonad-stimulating hormone (GSH) release, and preventing the ovaries from responding to this hormone. Rodriguez et al. (2000) studied the effect of Cd on oocyte growth of the fiddler crab *U. pugilator* during the slow vitellogenesis phase of ovarian maturation of this crab. Only when eyestalks were present (intact crabs in vivo experiments or in the incubation media in vitro experiments) , the oocyte growth was inhibited by Cd. So the authors suggested that Cd could act to increase the secretion of the gonad-inhibiting hormone (GIH) from the sinus gland in the eyestalks, and then GIH inhibited the oocytes directly or indirectly. On the contrary, no significant (P >0.05) change of the gonadosomatic index was observed with intact female crab *Chasmagnathus granulata* exposed to 0.5 mg/L Cd, whereas eyestalk-ablated exposed females showed significantly (P<0.05) lower gonadosomatic index values than their respective controls. This indicated that Cd interfered with extra-eyestalk hormones. The experimental results shows a possible interference of Cd with the transduction pathway of methyl farnesoate or 17-hydroxyprogesterone.On the other hand, Cd has an inhibitory effect on GIH secretion from the eyestalk.

2. The reproductive toxicity of the Cd to the Chinese crab *E. sinensis*

The ovarian growth in the Chinese crab is a process with oogonium multiplication, oocyte enlargement and yolk protein synthesis. It is the basis for the development of follow-up individual and is regulated by their own complex endocrine system. In the condition of internal hormone imbalance or external hormonal stimulation, the process of yolk synthesis will be affected. The gonad-inhibiting hormone (GIH), gonad-stimulating hormone (GSH), methyl ester (MF), progesterone and estradiol in the body can adjust ovarian development together. The existence of heavy metals in water as environment endocrine disruptors will cause certain damage for the shrimps and crabs. In this section, ovarian index (OI), oocyte diameter and yolk protein accumulation, GIH, progesterone and estradiol levels in hemolymph were meassured and ovarian ultrastructural changes were observed after *E. sinensis* was treated with Cd. The influence of Cd on ovarian development and its mechanism are discussed. The discussion provides information regarding the effects of environmental endocrinal disrupter such as heavy metal on the health of animals and human.

Juvenile female crabs for this experiment were obtained from Baiyangdian Lake, Hebei province, China. In the laboratory, the crabs were maintained for at least 2 weeks prior to the start of an experiment in fresh water, prepared to have a temperature of 25 °C and were fed uncooked potatoes daily. During the experiment, crabs were distributed into 3 groups of 15 crabs per group. The first group served as the control. Other animals were exposed to Cd concentrations of 0.25 and 0.50 mg/L (Cd added as $CdCl_2 \cdot 2.5H_2O$). The duration of exposure was 12 d. After exposure, the OI, oocyte diameter, yolk protein, GIH, progesterone and estradiol levels in hemolymph were meassured and ovarian ultrastructural changes were observed.

The results showed crabs exposed to 0.50 mg Cd/L had significiantly smaller ovarian index than controls. The difference between crabs exposed to 0.25 mg/L and controls were not significiant. The influence of Cd on OI presented the dose-effect relations.

The influence of Cd on oocyte diameter had the similar regularity.

	OI (%)	oocyte diameter (μm)
controls	0.503±0.162	50.729±2.254
0.25mg/L Cd	0.293±0.149	45.792±1.599
0.50mg/L Cd	0.241±0.026*	40.771±2.097*

* Significant difference to control group (P < 0.05)

Table 1. The effect of Cd on ovarian index and oocyte diameter

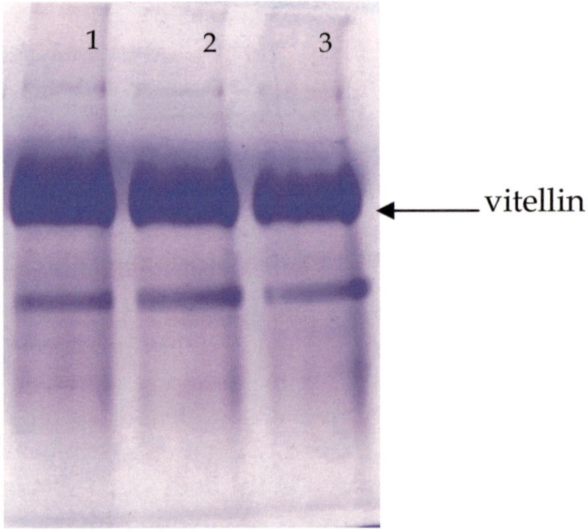

Fig. 1. Native PAGE maps of vitellin

1. map of native PAGE with CBB staining of ovary crude extracts in controls; 2. map of native PAGE with CBB staining of ovary crude extracts exposed to 0.25 mg/L Cd; and 3. map of native PAGE with CBB staining of ovary crude extracts exposed to 0.50 mg/L Cd

Through native PAGE with ovarian coarse extraction fluid of different groups and gray scan with Bandscan 5.0, the control group had the highest vitellin level, the group in 0.25 mg/L Cd had the second highest level, and the group in 0. 50 mg/L Cd had the lowest level. The percentage of ovary total protein charged for livetin had the above regularity. These results documented the accumulation of vitellin and the percentage of ovary total protein charged for livetin decreased with the increase of Cd concentration.

Semi-quantitative analysis of GIH in hemolymph was achieved by enzyme-linked immune sorbent assay (ELISA) method. GIH relative concentration in the crabs exposed to Cd is higher than those in controls. The relative concentration of GIH increased with increasing Cd concentration (see Table 2). These results suggest that Cd might stimulate secretion of GIH.

Progesterone and estradiol levels in hemolymphand measured by radioimmunoassay (RIA) are given in table 2. Compared with control group, groups exposed to Cd had higher progesterone level and lower estradiol level. There were no significant difference between 0.25 mg/L Cd group and control group while there were significant difference between 0.50 mg/L Cd group and control group.

	GIH absorbance	Progesterone level (ng/mL)	Estradiol level (pg/mL)
controls	0.138±0.019	0.91±0.16	180.28±24.01
0.25mg/L Cd	0.168±0.014	1.16±0.17	157.45±24.53
0.50mg/L Cd	0.432±0.021	1.49±0.32*	150.65±26.57*

* Significant difference to control group ($P < 0.05$)

Table 2. GIH absorbance, estradiol and progesterone levels in the hemolymph of each treatment

Observed by transmission electron microscope, normal nuclear appeared round and nuclear matrix was uniformly distributed. The surface of inner nuclear membrane was smooth and perinuclear cisternae was relatively small (Fig.2). In 0.25 mg/L group, outer nuclear membrane appeared folding deformation and swelled slightly. Nuclear material concentrated slightly and the electronic density was not uniform. Perinuclear cisternae became larger (Fig.3). In 0.50 mg/L group, the most notable changes were observed in nuclei. Outer nuclear membrane showed obvious folding deformation and the nuclear material more highly concentrated. The inner nuclear membrane nearly disappeared. Perinuclear cisternae became larger (Fig.4).

In the primary vitellogenesis phase, normal oocyte nuclei exhibit regular roundness. Nuclear membrane looked like moniliform and the moniliform particles distribute uniformly (Fig.5). Most of the vesicles of the endoplamic reticulum in the cytoplasm also showed regular roundness which is attached on by ribosomes (Fig.6). After being exposed to 0.50 mg/L Cd, nuclear membrane were crimpy and distorted, and moniliform particles of nuclear membrane appeared pile and damage (Fig.7). The vesicles of the endoplamic reticulum became swelled and dissolved. Electronic density in vesicles decreased, even vacuolization. Ribosomes on the endoplamic reticulum gradually fell off (Fig.8).

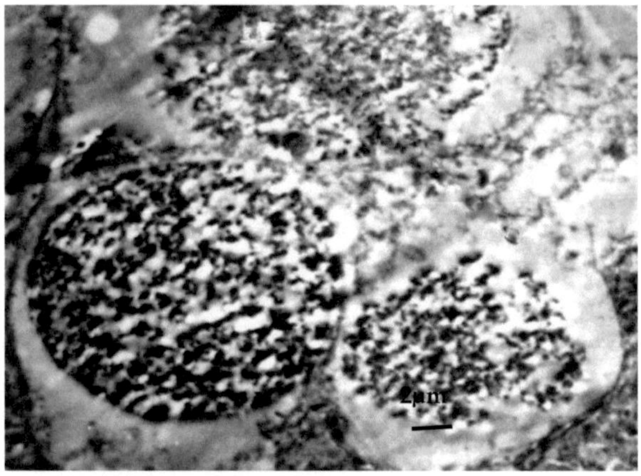

Fig. 2. Normal nuclear of reproductiving

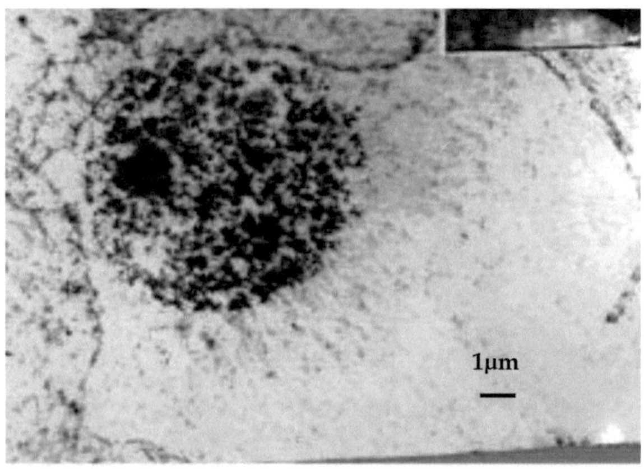

Fig. 3. Nuclear of reproductiving oogonia oogonia exposed to 0.25 mg/L Cd

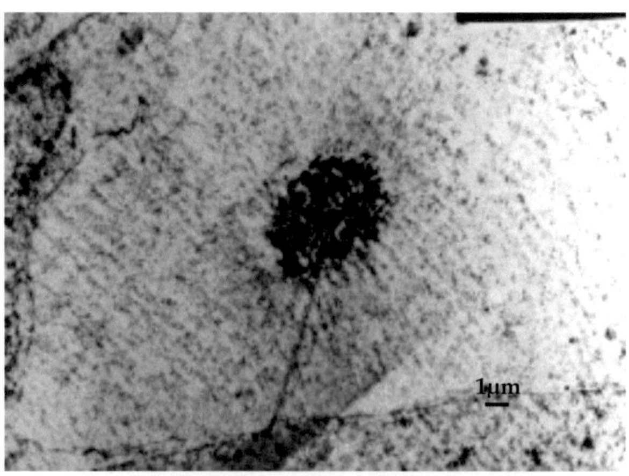

Fig. 4. Nuclear of reproductiving oogonia

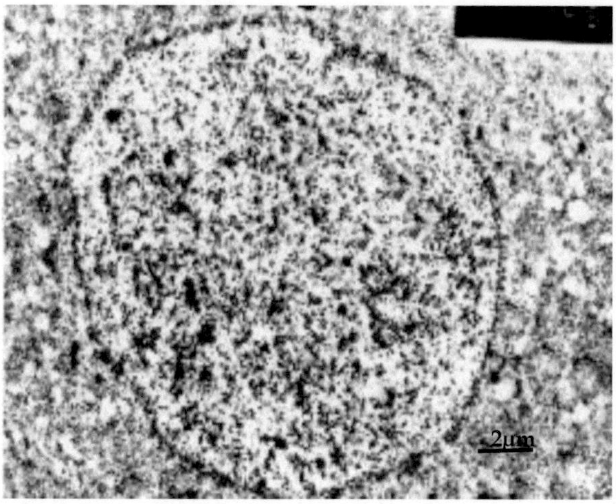

Fig. 5. Normal nuclear of the oocytes in exposed to 0.50 mg/L Cd primary vitellogenesis phase

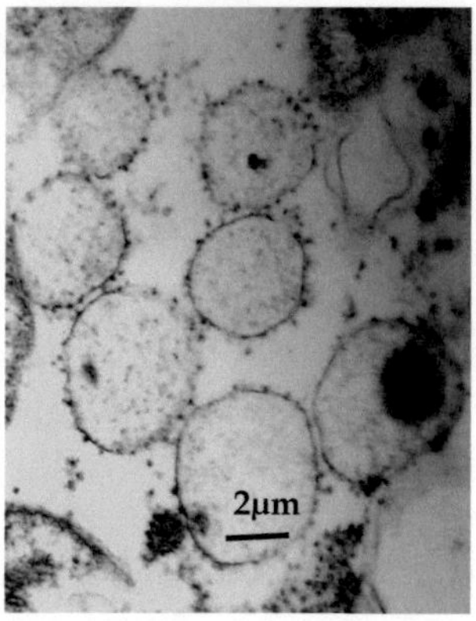

Fig. 6. Normal endoplamic reticulum vesicle

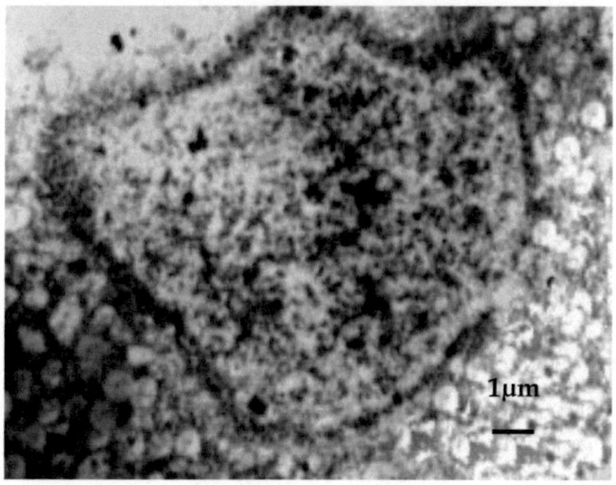

Fig. 7. Nuclear of the oocytes in primary vitellogenesis phase exposed to 0.50 mg/L Cd

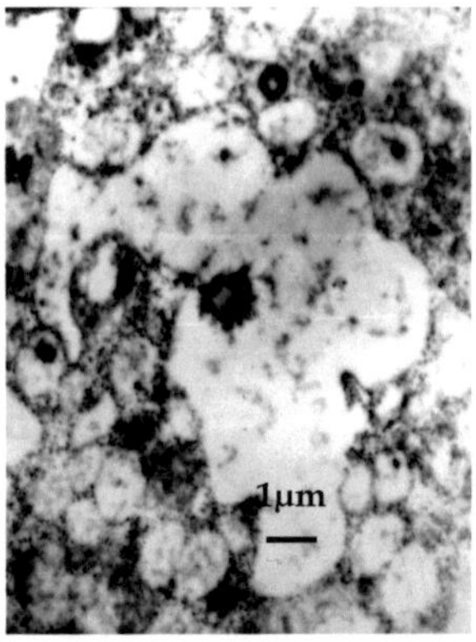

Fig. 8. Endoplamic reticulum vesicles exposed to 0.50 mg/L Cd

3. Effects of Cd on proliferation of spermatogenic cells from *M. nipponense in vitro*

The toxic effects of Cd on male reproductive system is obvious, it can significantly damage the testicles and the testicular parenchyma cells, leading to pathological testicular alterations and morphological abnormalities of spermatozoa, directly affected the reproductive capacity (Luo et al., 1993; Mohan et al., 1992; Saygi et al., 1991).

Culture of spermatogenic cells *in vitro* is important in development. Establishing the model of culture of spermatogenic cells in vitro is helpful for studying the regulate mechanism of spermatogenesis. In addition, the environment factor and presence of a poisonous substance can have grave effect on idioplasm, and thus restrict the development of marine species. Studying the effects of poisonous substances on reproduction and differentiation of spermatogenic cells has theoretical significance on clarifying the mechanism of poisonous substance, and has practical significance on idioplasm profect and health breed aquatics.

Juvenile male *M. nipponense* (20 to 25 mm body length) for the experiments were purchased from Baiyangdian Lake, Hebei Province, China. Spermatogenic cells of *M. nipponense* were isolated and sublimated with the method of trypsinization and differential speed adherence. Cell suspensions were seeded into M199 medium (pH 7.2, supplemented with 10% fetal bovine serum (FBS), 1 g/L glucose, 0.3 g/L glutamine, 0.11 g/L sodium pyruvate, 0.01% 2-mercaptoethanol, 100 IU/mL penicillin, 100 IU/mL streptomycin, 20 μg/mL gentamicin) and kept under 5% CO_2 at 26°C for 12 h before being incubated with various concentrations of Cd (5, 50, 500, 1 000 ng/mL). Equal volumes of culture medium containing no Cd were added to the control groups. Subsequently, MTT [3-(4, 5-dimethylthia- zole-2-yl)-2,5-diphenyl-tetrazoliumbromide] assay (Mosmann, 1983) was used to evaluate the proliferation of spermatogenic cells after 0 h, 24 h, 48 h, 72 h, 96 h exposure.

MTT assay is widespread method to assess cell viability. In living cells, MTT is deoxidized by mitochondrial dehydrogenases to a blue formazan product. The results can be read on a multi-well scanning spectrophotometer (ELISA reader) and the absorption of dissolved formazan correlates with the number of alive cells (Mosmann, 1983). Cytotoxic compounds (e.g. heavy metals) are able to damage and destroy cells, and thus decrease the reduction of MTT to formazan, the absorbance value therefore will decline.

A concentration-response curve for Cd obtained with the MTT assay is shown in Fig. 9. Before 24 h, the absorbance curve of each group showed no regularity; downward trend of the curve was not obvious. 24 h later, the absorbance of groups exposed to Cd at dose of 50 ng/mL, 500 ng/mL, 1 000 ng/mL, but not 5 ng/mL, were significantly lower than those of the controls ($P < 0.01$). The cell proliferation rate was found to decrease with increasing Cd concentration, and after 24 h exposure the absorbance of each concentration was significantly different from the absorbance at the start of the experiment ($P < 0.01$). In brief, rate of cell proliferation showed negative correlation with dose and exposure time at 50 ng/mL, 500 ng/mL, 1 000 ng/mL after 24 h.

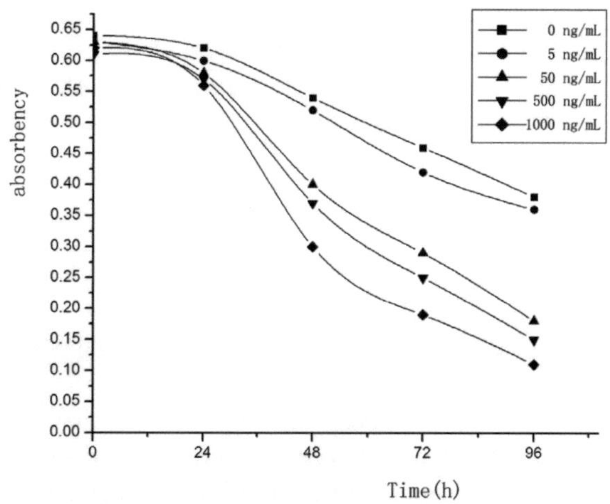

Fig. 9. Absorbency of spermatogenic cells disposed with Cd

There is growing evidence that suggests the mechanism of cytotoxicity of Cd may be mitochondrial dysfunction (Sokolova, 2004; Sokolova et al., 2004; Ivanina et al., 2010). In terrestrial plants and mammals, Cd is known as a powerful modulator of mitochondrial function, inhibiting electron transport chain, increasing generation of reactive oxygen species (Sokolova, 2004, as cited in Miccadei & Floridi, 1993 and Wallace & Starkov, 2000), and stimulating proton leak through the inner mitochondrial membrane (Sokolova, 2004, as cited in Belyaeva et al., 2001). In marine mollusks, such as oysters, Cd also affects mitochondrial function (Sokolova, 2004; Sokolova et al., 2004; Ivanina et al., 2010). These data strongly suggest that mitochondria are key intracellular targets for Cd (Sokolova, 2004). Heavy metals, such as Cd, are known to induce apoptosis and necrosis in invertebrates and vertebrates and result in increased cellular mortality (Benoff et al., 2004; Sokolova et al., 2004, as cited in Li et al., 2000 and Sung et al., 2003). In vertebrates, undergoing Cd stress, cells activate the classical intrinsic death pathway, in which mitochondria have a central role (Sokolova et al., 2004, as cited in Shih et al., 2004 and Hüttenbrenner et al., 2003). Cd exposure induces apoptosis in oyster immune cells and does so through a mitochondria/caspase-independent pathway (Sokolova et al., 2004). These results suggest that the mechanism of apoptosis induced by Cd exposure is very complex.

In our study, the results of MTT assay showed that Cd restrained the proliferation of isolated spermatogenic cells from *M. nipponense*. According to other investigations, it is due to cells apoptosis or necrosis induced by Cd exposure. The cause is unclear and further research will be needed.

4. Conclusion

As noted above, Cd exhibits biochemical and physiological toxicity for crabs and shrimps, affecting on activity of antioxidant enzymes, affecting metabolic enzymes, affecting Na+-K+-ATPase, etc. In some cases, Cd had a stimulating action at low concentration and inhibiting activity at high concentration.

Cd showed noticeable effects on the reproduction of crabs and shrimps. 1. Female crabs exposed to 0.50 mg/L Cd showed significantly ($P < 0.05$) lower the gonadal somatic index, oocyte diameter values and the ovary vitellin than controls. These proved certain concentration of Cd inhibited ovary development in *E. sinensis*. 2. Cd stimulated the secretion of GIH, increased progesterone level and decreased estradiol level in haemolymp. 3. The vesicles of the endoplamic reticulum became swelled and dissolved; ribosomes on the endoplamic reticulum gradually fell off by Cd toxicity. 4. Cd restrained the proliferation of isolated spermatogenic cells from *M. nipponense* at dose of 50, 500, 1 000 ng/mL after 24 h exposure.

5. Acknowledgment

This project was supported by the Hebei Province Natural Science Fund (C2011201028).

6. References

Åkesson, A., Julin, B., Wolk, A. (2008). Long-term Dietary Cadmium Intake and Postmenopausal Endometrial Cancer Incidence: A Population-Based Prospective Cohort Study. *Cancer Research*, Vol.68, No.15, (August 2008), pp. 6435–6441, ISSN 0008-5472

Beltrame, M. O., De Marco, S. G., Marcovecchio, J. E. (2010). Influences of sex, habitat, and seasonality on heavy-metal concentrations in the burrowing crab (*Neohelice granulata*) from a coastal lagoon in Argentina. *Archives of Environmental Contamination and Toxicology*, Vol.58, No.3, (April 2010), pp.746-56, ISSN 0090-4341

Benoff, S. H., Millan, C., Hurley, I. R., et al. (2004). Bilateral increased apoptosis and bilateral accumulation of cadmium in infertile men with left varicocele. *Human Reproduction*, Vol.19, No.3, (January 2004), pp.616-627, ISSN 0268-1161

Bjerregaard, P., Depledge, M. H. (2002). Trace metal concentrations and contents in the tissues of the shore crab *Carcinus maenas*: effects of size and tissue hydration. *Marine Biology*, Vol.141, No.3, pp.741–752, ISSN 0025-3162

Chang, X. L., Jin T. Y., Chen L., et al. (2009). Metallothionein I Isoform mRNA Expression in Peripheral Lymphocytes as a Biomarke for Occupational Cadmium Exposure. *Experimental Biology and Medicine*, Vol.234, pp.666–672, ISSN 1535-3702

Chou, C. L., Uthe, J. F., Castell, J. D., et al. (1987). Effect of dietary cadmium on growth, survival, and tissue concentrations of cadmium, zinc, copper, and silver in juvenile American lobster (*Homarus americanus*). *Canadian Journal of Fisheries and Aquatic Sciences*, Vol.44, No.8, (August 1988), pp.1443–1450, ISSN 0706-652X

Dailianis, S., Kaloyianni, M. (2004). Cadmium induces both pyruvate kinase and Na^+/H^+ exchanger activity through protein kinase C mediated signal transduction, in isolated digestive gland cells of *Mytilus galloprovincialis* (L.). *The Journal of Experimental Biology*, Vol.207, pp.1665-1674, ISSN 0022-0949

Dailianis, S., Patetsini, E., Kaloyianni M. (2009). The role of signalling molecules on actin glutathionylation and protein carbonylation induced by cadmium in haemocytes of mussel *Mytilus galloprovincialis* (Lmk). *The Journal of Experimental Biology*, Vol.212, pp.3612-3620, ISSN 0022-0949

Dhavale, D. M., Masurekar, V. B., Giridhar, B. A. (1988). Cadmium induced inhibition of Na^{+}-K^{+}-ATPase activity in tissues of crab *Scylla serrata* (Forskal). *Bulletin of Environmental Contamination and Toxicology*, Vol.40, No.5, (May 1988), pp.759-763, ISSN 0007-4861

Davies, I. M., Topping, G., Graham, W. C., et al. (1981). Field and experimental studies on cadmium in the edible crab *Cancer pagurus*. *Marine Biology*, Vol.64, No.3, pp.291–297, ISSN 0025-3162

Devi, M., Reddy, P. S., Fingerman, M. (1993). Effect of cadmium exposure on lactate dyhydrogenase activity in the hepatopancreas and abdominal muscle of the fiddler Crab, *Uca pugilator*. *Comparative biochemistry and physiology C. pharmacology and toxicology*, Vol.106, No.3, (November 1993), pp.739-742, ISSN 1532-0456

Devi, M., Thomas, D. A., Barber, J. T., et al. (1996). Accumulation and physiological and biochemical effects of cadmium in a simple aquatic food chain. *Ecotoxicology and environmental safety*, Vol.33, No.1, (Febrary 1996), pp.38-43, ISSN 0147-6513

Falconer, C. R., Davies, I. M., Topping, G. (1986). Cadmium in edible crabs (*Cancer pagurus* L.) from Scottish coastal waters. *Science of the Total Environment*, Vol.54, No.2, (October 1986), pp.173–183, ISSN 0048-9697

Ivanina, A. V., Cherkasov, A. S., Sokolova, I. M. (2008). Effects of cadmium on cellular protein and glutathione synthesis and expression of stress proteins in eastern oysters, *Crassostrea virginica* Gmelin. *The Journal of Experimental Biology*, Vol.211, pp. 577-586, ISSN 0022-0949

Ivanina, A. V., Eilers, S., Kurochkin I. O., et al. (2010). Effects of cadmium exposure and intermittent anoxia on nitric oxide metabolism in eastern oysters, *Crassostrea virginica*. *The Journal of Experimental Biology*, Vol.213, pp. 433-444, ISSN 0022-0949

Jennings, J. R., Rainbow, P. S. (1979). Studies on the uptake of cadmium by the crab *Carcinus maenas* in the laboratory: I Accumulation from seawater and a food source. *Marine Biology*, Vol.50, No.2, pp.131–139, ISSN 0025-3162

Lee, R. F., O'Malley, K., Oshima, Y. (1996). Effects of toxicants on developing oocytes and embryos of the blue Crab, *Callinectes sapidus*. *Marine Environmental Research*, Vol.42, No.1-4, pp.125-128, ISSN 0141-1136

Li, W. Y., Kang, X. J., Guo, M.S., et al. (2008a). Acute toxicity of Cd2+ to the the Chinese Mitten Crab (*Eriocheir sinensis*). *Hebei Fisheries*, No.2, pp.12-15,39, ISSN 1004-6755

Li, W. Y., Kang, X. J., Mu, S. M., et al. (2008b). Research Advance of Toxicological Effects of Cadmium on Shrimps and Crabs. *Fisheries Science*, Vol.27, No.1, (January 2008), pp.47-50, ISSN 1003-1111

Li, Y. Q., Wang,L. ,Liu, N., et al. (2008). Effects of cadmium on enzyme activity and lipid peroxidation in freshwater crab *Sinopotamon yangtsekiense*. *Acta Hydrobiologica Sinica*, Vol.32, No.3, (May 2008), pp. 373-379, ISSN 1000-3207

Liu, X. L., Zhou, Z. L.,Chen, L. Q. (2003). Effect of cadmium on antioxidant enzyme of the juvenile *Eriocheir sinensis*. *Marine Science*, Vol.27, No.8, (August 2003), pp.59-62, ISSN 1000-3096

Lu, J. R., Lai, W., Du, N. S. (1989). Effects of cadmium on ultrastructure of R-cell in hepatopancreas and serum glutamic-pyruvic transaminase (SGPT) activity of *Eriocheir sinensis. Journal of Ocean University of Qingdao*, Vol.19, No.2, pp.62-68, ISSN 1672-5174

Luo, G. Z., Zou, M. J., Wu, Y. X., et al.(1993). Toxic Effect of Trace Element Cadmium on the Mouse Testes. *Journl of Guiyang Medical College*, No.4, pp.251-255, ISSN 1000-2707

Medesani, D. A., López Greco, L. S., Rodríguez, E. M. (2004). Interference of cadmium and copper with the endocrine control of ovarian growth, in the estuarine crab *Chasmagnathus granulata. Aquatic Toxicology*, Vol.69, No.2, (August 2004), pp.165–174, ISSN 0166-445X

Meng, Fan. (2006). The effects of plumbum and cadmium on the cytoarchitecture of fresh crab (*Sinopotamon henanense*), 18.06. 2008, Available from http://10.186.5.116/kns50/detail.aspx?filename=2006101999.nh&dbname=CMFD2006

Messner, B., Knoflach, M., Seubert, A., et al. (2009). Cadmium Is a Novel and Independent Risk Factor for Early Atherosclerosis. *Arteriosclerosis Thrombosis and Vascular Biology*, Vol.29, (September 2009), pp.1392-1398, ISSN 1079-5642

Mohan, J., Moudgal, R. P., Panda, J. N. (1992). Effects of cadmium salt on phosphomonoesterases activity and fertilizing ability of fowl spermatozoa. *Indian Journal of Experimental Biology*, Vol.30, No.3, (March 1992), pp.241-243, ISSN 0019-5189

Mosmann, T. (1983). Rapid colorimetric assay for cellular growth and survival: Application to proliferation and cytotoxicity assays. *Journal of Immunological Methods*, Vol.65, No.1-2, (December 1983), pp. 55-63, ISSN 0022-1759

Müller, L., Ohnesorge, F. K. (1982). Different response of liver parenchymal cells from starved and fed rats to cadmium. *Toxicology*, Vol.25, No.2-3, pp.141-150, ISSN 0300-483X

Nagata, C., Nagao, Y., Shibuya, C., et al. (2005). Urinary Cadmium and Serum Levels of Estrogens and Androgens in Postmenopausal Japanese Women. *Cancer Epidemiology, Biomarkers & Prevention*, Vol.14, (March 2005), pp.705-708, ISSN 1055-9965

Naithani, V., Pathak, N., Chaudhary, M. (2010). Evaluation of Heavy Metals in Two Major Ingredients of Ampucare. *International Journal of Pharmaceutical Sciences and Drug Research*, Vol.2, No.2, (April-June, 2010), pp.137-141, ISSN 0975-248X

Naqvi, S. M., Howell, R. D. (1993). Toxicity of cadmium and lead to juvenile red swamp crayfish, *Procambarus clarkii,* and effects on fecundity of adults. *Bulletin of Environmental Contamination and Toxicology*, Vol.51, No.2, pp.303–308, ISSN 0007-4861

Navas-Acien, A., Selvin, E., Sharrett, A. R., et al. (2004). Lead, Cadmium, Smoking, and Increased Risk of Peripheral Arterial Disease. *Circulation*, Vol.109, (June 2004), pp.3196-3201, ISSN 0009-7322

Navas-Acien, A., Tellez-Plaza, M., Guallar E., et al. (2009). Blood Cadmium and Lead and Chronic Kidney Disease in US Adults: A Joint Analysis. *American Journal of Epidemiology*, Vol.170, No.9, (August 2009), pp.1156–1164, ISSN 0002-9262

Nørum, U., Bondgaard, M., Pedersen, T. V., et al. (2005). In vivo and in vitro cadmium accumulation during the moult cycle of the male shore crab *Carcinus maenas*—

interaction with calcium metabolism. *Aquatic toxicology Amsterdam Netherlands*, Vol.72, No.1-2, pp.29–44, ISSN 1879-1514

Pan, L. Q., Zhang, H. X. (2006). Metallothionein, antioxidant enzymes and DNA strand breaks as biomarkers of Cd exposure in a marine crab, *Charybdis japonica*. *Comparative Biochemistry and Physiology Part C: Toxicology & Pharmacology*, Vol.144, No.1, (September 2006), pp.67-75, ISSN 1532-0456

Rainbow, P. S., White, S. L. (1989). Comparative strategies of heavy metal accumulation by crustaceans: zinc, copper and cadmium in a decapod, an amphipod and a barnacle. *Hydrobiologia*, Vol. 174, No.3, pp. 245–262, ISSN 0018-8158

Reddy, P. S., Tuberty, S. R., Fingerman, M. (1997). Effects of Cadmium and Mercury on Ovarian Maturation in the Red Swamp Crayfish, *Procambarus clarkii*. *Ecotoxicology and environmental safety*, Vol.37, No.1, (June 1997), pp.62-65, ISSN 0147-6513

Rodríguez, E. M., López Greco, L. S., Fingerman M. (2000). Inhibition of ovarian growth by cadmium in the fiddler Crab, *Uca pugilator* (Decapoda, Ocypodidae). *Ecotoxicology and Environmental Safety*, Vol.46, No.2, (June 2000), pp. 202-206, ISSN 0147-6513

Saeed, M., Muhammad, N., Khan, H., et al. (2010). Analysis of toxic heavy metals in branded Pakistani herbal products. *Journal of the Chemical Society of Pakistan*, Vol.32, No.4, pp. 471-475, ISSN 0253-5106

Saygi, S., Deniz, G., Kutsal, O., et al. (1991). Chronic effects of cadmium on kedney, liver, testis, and fertility of male rats. *Biological Trace Element Research*, Vol.31, No.3, pp.209-214, ISSN 0163-4984

Shukla, G. S., Hussain, T., Srivastava, R. S., et al. (1989). Glutathione peroxidase and catalase in liver, kidney, testis and brain regions of rats following cadmium exposure and subsequent withdrawal. *Industrial Health*, Vol. 27, No.2, pp.59-69, ISSN 0019-8366

Silvestre, F., Trausch, G., Péqueux, A., et al. (2004). Uptake of cadmium through isolated perfused gills of the Chinese mitten crab, *Eriocheir sinensis*. *Comparative Biochemistry and Physiology - Part A: Molecular & Integrative Physiology*, Vol.137, No.1, (January 2004), pp.189-196, ISSN 1095-6433

Silvestre, F., Trausch, G., Devos, P. (2005a). Hyper-osmoregulatory capacity of the Chinese mitten crab (Eriocheir sinensis) exposed to cadmium; acclimation during chronic exposure. *Comparative Biochemistry and Physiology Part C: Toxicology & Pharmacology*, Vol.140, No.1, (January 2005), pp.29–37, ISSN 1532-0456

Silvestre F., Duchêne, C., Trausch G., et al. (2005b). Tissue-specific cadmium accumulation and metallothionein-like protein levels during acclimation process in the Chinese crab *Eriocheir sinensis*. *Comparative Biochemistry and Physiology Part C: Toxicology & Pharmacology*, Vol.140, No.1, (January 2005), pp.39-45, ISSN 1532-0456

Sokolova, I. M. (2004). Cadmium effects on mitochondrial function are enhanced by elevated temperatures in a marine poikilotherm, *Crassostrea virginica* Gmelin (Bivalvia: Ostreidae). *The Journal of Experimental Biology*, Vol.207, pp. 2639-2648, ISSN 0022-0949

Sokolova, I. M., Evans, S., Hughes, F. M. (2004). Cadmium-induced apoptosis in oyster hemocytes involves disturbance of cellular energy balance but no mitochondrial permeability transition. *The Journal of Experimental Biology*, Vol.207, (June 2004), pp.3369-3380, ISSN 0022-0949

Tang, H., Li, S. J., Wang, G. Z., et al. (2000). Effects of Cu^{2+}, Zn^{2+}, Cd^{2+} on three metabolic enzymes of the larval crab of *Scylla serrata*. *Journal of Xiamen University (Natural Science Edition)*, Vol.39, No.4, pp.521-525, ISSN 0438-0479

van Hatton, B., de Voogt, P., van den Bosch, L., et al. (1989). Bioaccumulation of cadmium by the freshwater isopod *Asellus aquaticus* (L.) from aqueous and dietary sources. *Environmental Pollution*, Vol.62, No.2-3, pp.129-151, ISSN 0269-7491

Wang, L., Yang, X. Q., Wang, Q., et al. (2001). The accumulation of Cd^{2+} and the effect on EST in five tissues and organs of *Eriocheir sinensis*. *Acta Zoologica Sinica*, Vol.47, No.S1, pp.96-100, ISSN 0001-7302

Wang, L., Sun, H. F., Li, C. Y. (2002a). Effects of cadmium on spermatogenesis in freshwater crab (*Sinopotamon yangtsekiense*). *Acta Zoologica Sinica*, Vol.48, No.5, pp.677-684, ISSN 0001-7302

Wang, L., Sun, H. F. (2002b). Effect of cadmium on ultrastructure of myocardial cell of freshwater crab, *Sinopotamon yangtsekiense*. *Acta Hydrobiologica Sinica*, Vol.26, No.1, (January 2002), pp. 9-13, ISSN 1000-3207

Wang, L., Yan, B., Liu, N., et al. (2008). Effects of cadmium on glutathione synthesis in hepatopancreas of freshwater crab, *Sinopotamon yangtsekiense*. *Chemosphere*, Vol.74, No.1, (December 2008), pp.51-56, ISSN: 0045-6535

Wang, L., Li, Y. Q., Yan, B., et al. (2007). Effect of Cadm ium on SOD and POD Isozyme in Tissues of Freshwater Crab (*Sinopotamon henanense*). *Chinese Journal of Applied & Environmental Biology*, Vol.13, No.6, (December 2007), pp.823-829, ISSN 1006-687X

Wang, Q., Wang, L., Xi, Y.Y. (2003). The Acute toxcity and accumulated of Cd^{2+} in freshwater crab *Sinopotamon yangtsekiense*. *Journal of Shanxi University (Natural Science Edition)*, Vol.26, No.2, pp.176-178, ISSN 0253-2395

Wright, D. A. (1977). The effect of calcium on cadmium uptake by the shore crab *Carcinus maenas*. *Journal of Experimental Biology*, Vol.67, No.2, pp.163–173, ISSN 0022-0949

Yan, B., Wang, L., Li, Y. Q., et al. (2007). Effects of cadmium on hepatopancreatic antioxidant enzyme activity in a freshwater crab *Sinopotamon yangtsekiense*. *Acta Zoologica Sinica*, Vol. 53, No.6, pp. 1121-1128, ISSN 0001-7302

Zhao, W. X., Wei, H., Jia, J., et al. (1995). Effects of cadmium on transaminase and structures of tissues in freshwater giant prawn (*Macrobrachium rosenbergii*). *Journal of fisheries of China*, Vol.19, No.1, pp.21-27, ISSN 1000-0615

11

Paraquat, Between Apoptosis and Autophagy

Rosa A. González-Polo, José M. Bravo-San Pedro, Rubén Gómez-Sánchez, Elisa Pizarro-Estrella, Mireia Niso-Santano and José M. Fuentes
Centro de Investigación Biomédica en Red Sobre Enfermedades Neurodegenerativas (CIBERNED),
Departamento de Bioquímica y Biología Molecular y Genética, E. Enfermería y TO, Universidad de Extremadura, Cáceres
Spain

1. Introduction

Paraquat (PQ, methyl viologen), 1,1'-dimethyl-4,4'-bipyridinium (Figure 1), is a commonly used, potent herbicide. It was first synthesised in 1882 by Weidel and Russo, as recorded by Hadley in his review of 1979 (Haley, 1979), and its redox properties were discovered by Michaelis and Hill in 1933 (Haley, 1979). Initially, PQ was used as an indicator of oxidation-reduction because in the absence of molecular oxygen, donating an electron to paraquat (PQ^{2+}) generated a monocationically stable violet or blue form that is commonly known as methyl viologen (Dinis-Oliveira *et al.*, 2008). However, its properties as an herbicide were not discovered until 1955, and in 1962, it was introduced into global markets.
The PQ is registered and used in approximately 100 countries worldwide and is the second most commonly used herbicide in the world after gliphosate. Despite this, its use is currently banned in the European Union (EU), but the import of products from outside the EU for patients who have been treated with PQ has not.
In its recommended rating of "pesticides by risk," WHO (World Health Organization) considers composite PQ to be moderately toxic (Category II) (World Health Organization 2004). The ECB (European Chemicals Bureau) classifies PQ as being very toxic (R26) by inhalation, toxic (R25) orally and moderately toxic (R24) dermally.
PQ is included in the family of herbicides called bipyridines. It is an herbicide that is non-selective and functions systemically through contact without acting on the leaves of green plants. Among its advantages, it is rapidly absorbed by the leaves of plants that have been sprayed, but clay soil causes it to be biologically inactive.
Its action on plants has been shown to occur on chloroplasts and is based on its redox cycle. PQ interferes with photosynthesis at the level of photosystem I. At this point, PQ blocks the flow of electrons from ferredoxin and $NADP^+$ so that electrons from photosystem I would reduce PQ, which transfers divalent cations (normal state) to monovalent cations (reduced state). The monovalent cation reduces oxygen to the superoxide radical (O_2^-), which is produced by the loss of activity of the chloroplasts and the subsequent cell damage that leads to plant death. There is controversy about the use of PQ in agriculture because herbicides are toxic to humans and the environment, especially when not taking the proper precautions. Specifically, in addition to the adverse effects on humans, one of the greatest

risks occurs in the absorption of the herbicide when being applied to crops. When rats ingested toxic amounts of PQ (either accidentally or voluntary), the initial absorption occurred in the small intestine where the amount absorbed by the stomach was negligible, especially if there was parallel food intake, and the majority was excreted in the urine and feces (Daniel & Gage, 1966). It can also be absorbed and causes damage when it contacts with the skin, especially when there was a previously damaged area that would cause an abrasion contact zone (J. G. Smith, 1988). When applied with a nasal spray, droplets can penetrate the lungs through inhalation. When used in the absence of any physical barrier protection (goggles, masks, gloves, etc.), PQ can be highly toxic. Once absorbed into the body, PQ could affect different organs, with the liver and kidneys being more sensitive to oral ingestion and the lungs being more sensitive to inhalation. In autopsies of dead patients that suffered from voluntary PQ poisoning, different organs were damaged. The brain damage consisted of widespread edema, subepidermal and subarachnoid haemorrhage (which had an uneven distribution in different patients) and inflammation of the meninges, which could be a secondary consequence that resulted from lung damage and hypoxia based on its characteristics (Grant *et al.*, 1980).

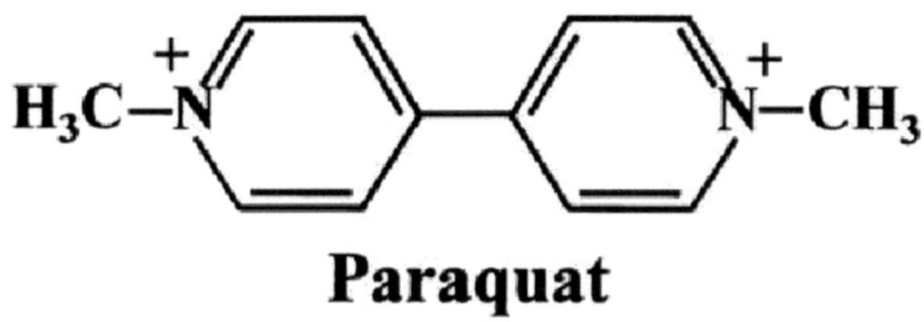

Fig. 1. Chemical structure of paraquat

Together with the correlations observed in epidemiological studies between the use of PQ and the development of Parkinson's disease (PD) (Tanner *et al.*, 2011), the structural similarity between PQ and the active metabolite (MPP^+) of the neurotoxin called MPTP, widely accepted as a model of parkinsonism, led us to postulate the existence of a relationship between the pesticide and the origin of the disease (Costello *et al.*, 2009; Di Monte *et al.*, 1986; Hertzman *et al.*, 1990; Liou *et al.*, 1997). Both neurotoxic effects that generated oxidative stress activated different pathways (Richardson *et al.*, 2005). Currently, PQ is a valid model for studying neurotoxicity based on oxidative stress, such as for MPP^+. Further, studies have examined the relationship between the application and exposure of this pesticide and the development of PD, which is widely accepted for MPP^+, and increasing studies have found a role of PQ in oxidative stress and cell death. The toxicity induced by PQ as an herbicide makes it toxic to mammalian cells. The redox cycling of PQ (Figure 2) in biological systems has two important implications: one is the generation of reactive oxygen species (ROS), and the other is the depletion of reducing agents (NADH and NADPH) necessary for proper function, affecting different cellular processes, such as the synthesis of fatty acids. Similar to inside the plant cell, PQ requires an electron donor to be reduced in neurons. The potential standard reduction (E) of a compound indicates the affinity of the compound to accept electrons. PQ has an E of -0.45 V. The potential E of the redox couples, NAD^+/ NADH and $NADP^+$/ NADPH, is -0.32V and -0.324V, respectively, where PQ, under physiological conditions and with the aid of diaphorase within the cell, could accept electrons from either reducing agent. The MPP^+ E is - 1.18 V, and this indicates that PQ has a greater ability to accept electrons than MPP^+ (Drechsel & Patel, 2008). Among the cellular enzymes that could donate electrons to PQ (PQ-enzymes with diaphorase), it has been examined mitochondrial complex I (NADH-ubiquinone reductase complex) (Fukushima *et al.*, 1993), thioredoxin reductase (Gray *et al.*, 2007), NADPH, ferredoxin oxidoreductase (Liochev *et al.*, 1994), NADPH oxidase (Bonneh-Barkay *et al.*, 2005) and NOS (nitric oxide synthase) (Patel *et al.*, 1996) in addition to other enzymes. The mitochondria have been shown to be a major source of ROS generation within the PQ-induced mechanism, which may induce PQ-diaphorase activity during breathing (Drechsel & Patel, 2008). Once PQ has been reduced, it could be oxidised by oxygen and generate superoxide molecules, which occurs in the cell during oxidative stress. This could be activated by different pathways to initiate cell damage through different components and the activation of different cellular mechanisms, such as autophagy (R. A. Gonzalez-Polo *et al.*, 2007b), dysfunction of the proteasome (Yang & Tiffany-Castiglioni, 2007) and cell death by apoptosis (Dinis-Oliveira *et al.*, 2008; R. A. Gonzalez-Polo *et al.*, 2007a; R. A. Gonzalez-Polo *et al.*, 2004; McCarthy *et al.*, 2004; Niso-Santano *et al.*, 2011; Niso-Santano *et al.*, 2010; Richardson *et al.*, 2005). It is commonly accepted that the key mechanism in PQ-mediated toxicity was due to the oxidative stress-derived superoxide anion produced in the redox cycle (Drechsel & Patel, 2008; Patel *et al.*, 1996). The fact that the key element in PQ-mediated toxicity was the generation of superoxide anions was demonstrated by the overexpression or silencing of superoxide dismutase (SOD), which led to an alteration of the toxic effects generated by PQ (Patel *et al.*, 1996). The superoxide anion generated in the redox cycling of PQ could be transformed by various reactions and ROS (Bus & Gibson, 1984) primarily generated by the hydroxyl radical (HO^-) and hydrogen peroxide (H_2O_2). These reactive oxygen species have been shown to be responsible for the oxidative stress that initiates different cascades inside the cell and causes apoptosis. Moreover, both cell death and changes in its regulation have been implicated in various diseases, including cancer and neurodegenerative diseases (Leist & Jaattela, 2001). More specifically, various studies have linked apoptosis induced following the exposure to various toxic compounds with the loss of neurons that occur during the development of various neurodegenerative diseases, such as Alzheimer's disease (AD) (Loo et al., 1993) and PD (Andersen, 2001; Fall & Bennett, 1999; Hartmann *et al.*, 2000). In addition, previous studies have shown that PQ induced apoptosis in the primary cultures of rat cerebellar granule cells (R. A. Gonzalez-Polo *et al.*, 2004) and an increase in the expression of genes related to apoptosis in SH-SY5Y cells (Moran *et al.*, 2008). Therefore, we examined PQ as a model for studying the neurotoxicity based on the generation of oxidative stress, such as in PD, to determine the fundamental role of superoxide anions in the redox cycling of the herbicide.

2. Paraquat induces apoptosis

The first time that the term apoptosis appeared was in a paper from John Kerr, Andrew Wyllie and Alastair Currie, in 1972 (Kerr *et al.*, 1972). The name was derived from the 'dropping off' or 'falling off' of petals from flowers or leaves from trees.

Apoptosis, or programmed cell death, is characterised by several morphological features, such as DNA degradation into oligonucleosomal fragments, chromatin condensation, reduction in nuclear and cellular fractions, phosphatidylserine exposure on the outward-facing side of the plasma membrane and preservation of organelle structure and plasma membrane integrity, which leads to the generation of apoptotic bodies, or vesicles in the cytoplasm containing tightly packed organelles with or without nuclear fragments. This type of cell death contrasts with necrosis, which is uncontrolled, accidental and pathological cell death. However, these two cell death pathways have been shown to crosstalk, which has been described as the "apoptosis-necrosis continuum" (Zeiss, 2003).

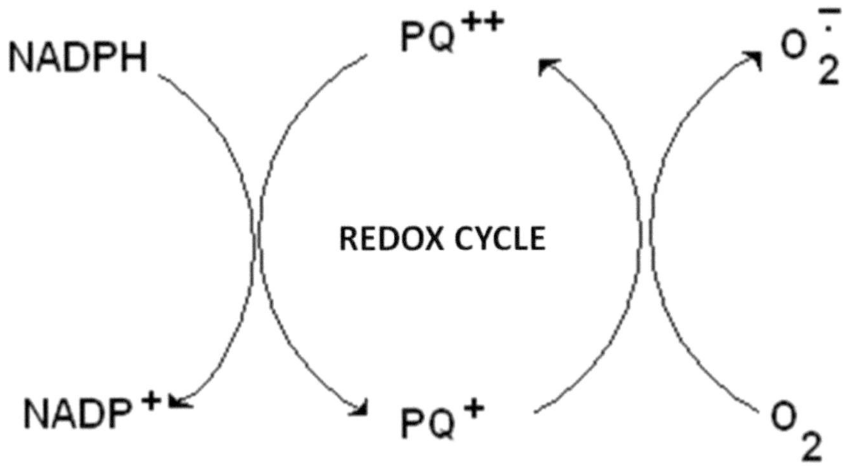

Fig. 2. Redox cycle of paraquat

Previous studies demonstrating the regulation of apoptosis came from *Caenorhabditis elegans* where 131 of the 1090 somatic cells in *C. elegans* were under the control of programmed cell death. In 1985, the Horvitz's lab discovered four important genes (*Ced-3, Ced-4, Ced-9, Egl-1*) that are involved in the regulation of cell death (Fixsen *et al.*, 1985). Previous studies have shown that apoptosis was necessary to define whether cells should live or die. However, there are other forms of programmed cell death and other possible mechanisms that have not yet been discovered (Debnath *et al.*, 2005; Formigli *et al.*, 2000; Sperandio *et al.*, 2000). Several mechanisms of cell death have already been shown to be involved in maintaining the balance between life and death (Boya *et al.*, 2005; Lum *et al.*, 2005; Ravikumar *et al.*, 2006). Apoptosis most commonly occurs during development and aging as a homeostatic mechanism. Although it has been shown to be used as a defence mechanism, such as when cells become damaged, during an immune response (Norbury & Hickson, 2001), or as a pathological process in cancer and autoimmune lymphoproliferative syndrome in which apoptosis was suppressed and led to the development and progression of tumours (Kerr *et al.*, 1994; Worth *et al.*, 2006), neurodegenerative diseases, autoimmune diseases and ischaemia-associated injury where there is excessive apoptosis (Ethell & Buhler, 2003; Freude *et al.*, 2000; C. J. Li *et al.*, 1995). Traditionally, apoptosis has been considered to be an irreversible process; however, several reports have demonstrated that these apoptotic cells could be rescued from programmed cell death (Geske *et al.*, 2001; Hoeppner *et al.*, 2001; Reddien *et al.*, 2001).

The mechanisms of apoptosis are highly complex and involve an energy-dependent cascade of molecular events. Apoptosis can be initiated by a variety of stimuli, but previous studies have shown that there are two main apoptotic pathways: the death receptor or extrinsic pathway and the mitochondrial or intrinsic pathway. However, these two pathways are connected, and some molecules of one pathway have been shown to influence the other pathway (Igney & Krammer, 2002). Further, a third pathway was found in T cells and had been shown to occur through cytotoxicity and perforin-granzyme-dependent cell death (via granzyme A or granzyme B). Basically, the extrinsic pathway is activated by the death receptors (DR), which are localised on the cell surface, through the recognition of their specific ligands. In comparison, the intrinsic pathway is initiated after several intracellular triggers, called "stress signals", such as cytoskeleton disruption, hypoxia, DNA damage, macromolecular synthesis inhibition and endoplasmic reticulum stress, which induce the mitochondria to release pro-apoptotic factors into the cytosol. However, both pathways and the granzyme B pathway terminate in the execution pathway that activates caspases (cysteine-aspartic acid proteases), and they have been shown to be responsible for developing the well-known features of apoptosis (Amarante-Mendes & Green, 1999). In contrast, the granzyme A pathway is a caspase-independent cell death pathway, which has been shown to act in parallel (Martinvalet *et al.*, 2005). The cell's decision has been shown to be determined by the Bcl-2 protein family. The regulation of the Bcl-2 family of proteins is important (Gross *et al.*, 1999).

It is well known that the toxicity of PQ was due to the production of ROS (Bus & Gibson, 1984; Mollace *et al.*, 2003), which has been partially generated by xanthine oxidase (Kitazawa *et al.*, 1991; Sakai *et al.*, 1995). Therefore, it has been shown that PQ could induce apoptotic cell death in cerebellar granule cells using this xanthine oxidase system (R. A. Gonzalez-Polo *et al.*, 2004). In addition, it has been reported that PQ induced apoptosis in other animal models, such as human lung epithelial cells (Cappelletti *et al.*, 1998), PC12 cells (X. Li & Sun, 1999), mouse 32D cells (Fabisiak *et al.*, 1997), primary mesencephalic cells and dopaminergic neuronal cells (Gomez-Sanchez *et al.*, 2010; Peng *et al.*, 2004).

PQ has structural homology to MPP^+, which has been linked to PD in epidemiological studies (Hertzman *et al.*, 1990; Liou *et al.*, 1997). In this vein, *PINK1*-silenced neuroblastoma cells were more sensitive and exhibited increased apoptosis compared with control cells following PQ treatment (Gegg *et al.*, 2009). Silencing *DJ-1* in neuroblastoma cells induced apoptotic cell death, and the treatment with PQ increased apoptosis (R. Gonzalez-Polo *et al.*, 2009).

The cytotoxic actions of PQ have been shown to involve oxidative stress by producing superoxide anions through the mitochondrial electron transport chain (Dinis-Oliveira *et al.*, 2006; McCormack *et al.*, 2002). PQ has been shown to be reduced by mitochondrial complex I and, thus, impair the respiration complex that led to the generation of ROS to induce selective neurodegeneration in dopaminergic neurons in the substantia nigra pars compacta (Fei *et al.*, 2008) and apoptosis by activating different intracellular pathways. PQ has been shown to induce apoptosis through the mitochondrial intrinsic pathway associated with p53 (Yang & Tiffany-Castiglioni, 2008). JNK proteins have been implicated in dopaminergic neuronal death induced by rotenone, PQ and 6-hydroxydopamine (6-OHDA) (Choi *et al.*, 1999; Klintworth *et al.*, 2007; Newhouse *et al.*, 2004; Niso-Santano *et al.*, 2006). PQ activates cell death through JNK and its downstream target c-Jun (Peng et al. 2004) and induces high levels of pro-apoptotic Bcl-2 family members (Bak, Bid, BNip3 and Noxa) in conjunction with cytochrome c release and caspase-3 activation (Fei *et al.*, 2008).

Another mechanism by which PQ has been shown to activate cell death involves chronic endoplasmic reticulum (ER) stress (Chinta *et al.*, 2008; Holtz & O'Malley, 2003; Ryu *et al.*, 2002). The increase in the expression of GRP family proteins, the increased phosphorylation of eIF2a and the induction of GADD153 expression was reported following PQ treatment in dopaminergic N27 cells (Chinta *et al.*, 2008) . These results were consistent with previous studies that demonstrated the transcriptional upregulation of ER stress and unfolded protein response (UPR)-specific proapoptotic genes following exposure to MPP^+ and 6-OHDA (Holtz & O'Malley, 2003; Ryu *et al.*, 2002). Several neurodegenerative diseases feature the accumulation of abnormal proteins as a result of the inhibition of the cellular proteasome activity and ER stress. Paraquat treatment led to a significant decrease in 20S proteasome activity (Chinta *et al.*, 2008). The inhibition of proteasome activity initiated the formation and accumulation of ubiquitinated protein aggregates (Lam *et al.*, 2002).

PQ was shown to induce IRE1/ASK1/JNK activation (Niso-Santano *et al.*, 2010; Yang *et al.*, 2009). IRE1 is an ER-resident transmembrane protein that is activated in response to ER stress. IRE1 phosphorylates ASK1, which has been shown to play a key role in the activation of p38/JNK signalling in neurotoxin-induced cell culture models of PD, such as MPTP and paraquat-induced apoptosis in dopaminergic neuronal cells (Niso-Santano *et al.*, 2010).

Recent studies have shown that paraquat induced acetylation of core histones in cell culture models of PD and that the inhibition of HAT activity by anacardic acid significantly attenuated paraquat-induced caspase-3 enzyme activity, indicating that histone acetylation played a role in paraquat-induced apoptosis (Song *et al.*).

3. PQ induces autophagy

Autophagy is an intracellular lysosome-mediated catabolic mechanism that is responsible for the bulk degradation and recycling of damaged or dysfunctional cytoplasmic components and intracellular organelles (Klionsky & Emr, 2000). Autophagy is an evolutionarily conserved cellular response to both extracellular stress conditions (nutrient deprivation and hypoxia) and intracellular stress conditions (accumulation of damaged organelles and cytoplasmic components). Autophagy is a physiological degradative process employed during embryonic growth and development, cellular remodelling and the biogenesis of some subcellular organelles, such as multi-lamellar bodies (Filonova *et al.*, 2000; Hariri *et al.*, 2000; Sattler & Mayer, 2000). Autophagic cell death has been shown to involve the accumulation of autophagic vacuoles in the cytoplasm of dying cells and in mitochondrial dilation and the enlargement of the ER and the Golgi apparatus.

Different types of autophagy are classified depending on the mechanism driving the degradation of the substrate in the lysosomal lumen (Klionsky *et al.*, 2007). We could distinguish three types of autophagy:

1. Macroautophagy: is often referred to as "autophagy". In this process, the material to be degraded becomes trapped in double-membrane vesicles to form a structure known as the autophagosome (Baba *et al.*, 1994; Fengsrud *et al.*, 1995). Macroautophagy has been shown to involve a number of genes called *ATGs* (autophagy-related genes), which have been shown to encode more than 30 proteins. Autophagosome membranes are derived from a structure called the pre-autophagosome, phagophore or early autophagosome (Fengsrud *et al.*, 1995; Mizushima *et al.*, 2001; Suzuki *et al.*, 2001). The first step towards the formation of the late autophagosome is the expansion of the phagophore (pre-autophagosome) membrane. Therefore, the carbon terminus of the protein LC3 (encoded by the gene *ATG8*) is attached to

a residue of phosphatidyl-ethanolamine (PE) in the membrane of the phagophore and with two other proteins encoded by *ATG12* and *ATG5* that also bind to the inner membrane, leading to the formation of the autophagosome. This autophagosome then fuses with lysosomes, forming the autophagolysosome where the degradation of the material occurs due to the action of lysosomal enzymes.

2. Microautophagy: In this process, the material to be degraded becomes trapped by the lysosomes through the invagination of its membrane. Once introduced into the lysosome, the material becomes degraded by lysosomal enzymes similar to macroautophagy.

3. Chaperone-mediated autophagy (CMA): In this autophagy, the material to be degraded is damaged or misfolded protein that has been translocated into the lysosomal lumen through the lysosomal membrane. This translocation is mediated by cytosolic and lysosomal chaperones, involving the carrier LAMP-2A (lysosome-associated membrane protein 2A).

Dysfunctions in autophagy have been implicated in various diseases, such as cancer (Kondo & Kondo, 2006), cardiomyopathy (Nakai *et al.*, 2007) or neurodegenerative processes (Martinez-Vicente & Cuervo, 2007; Ravikumar & Rubinsztein, 2004). In neurodegenerative diseases, an increase in the formation of autophagic vacuoles in the *substantia nigra* of patients with PD (Anglade *et al.*, 1997), Huntington's disease (Kegel *et al.*, 2000; Sapp *et al.*, 1997) and AD (Butler & Bahr, 2006; Nixon *et al.*, 2005; Zheng *et al.*, 2006) has been shown. This raises questions about the role of autophagy in these neurodegenerative processes. Previous studies have suggested that the increased number of autophagic vacuoles was responsible for neuronal death; however, in contrast, other studies have suggested a protective role for autophagy, contributing to the increased degradation of damaged proteins, which could induce apoptosis (U. Bandyopadhyay & Cuervo, 2007).

Changes have been described in the ubiquitin-proteasome system associated with PD. Several studies have suggested that once the ubiquitin-proteasome system has been damaged, autophagy becomes over-regulated, increasing the number of protein aggregates degraded by this mechanism (Iwata *et al.*, 2005; Massey *et al.*, 2006), which has been considered to be the default pathway when protein aggregates could not be eliminated by the proteasome (Olanow, 2007; Rideout *et al.*, 2004). However, if the pathogenic insult was maintained, this compensatory mechanism was unable to maintain cellular balance, leading to neuronal death (Trojanowski & Lee, 2000).

Recently, converging evidence suggests that the impairment of homeostatic mechanisms processing unwanted and misfolded proteins plays a central role in the pathogenesis in PD (Olanow, 2007). Impairment of the autophagy-lysosomal pathway has been shown to be related to the development of PD (Pan *et al.*, 2008). Activation of autophagy was also identified within peripheral blood mononuclear cells from PD patients (Prigione *et al.*, 2010). This self-regulatory concept of autophagy supports the hypothesis that increased signalling of autophagy occurred in mice with a malfunctioning lysosome that was accompanied by the aggregation of the protein α-synuclein (Meredith *et al.*, 2002). Increased levels of α-synuclein were reported in both the frontal cortex and the ventral midbrain, and α-synuclein positive inclusions in the substantia nigra neurons of mice treated with PQ were found (Manning-Bog *et al.*, 2002). The association of dopaminergic neuronal death with α-synuclein upregulation and aggregation following PQ toxicity is relevant as a PD model.

Because PQ induced the accumulation of autophagic vacuoles and increased the degradation of proteins in the cytoplasm of SH-SY5Y cells (R. A. Gonzalez-Polo *et al.*, 2007a), this indicates that the increased oxidative stress could activate autophagy in the initial stages of mitochondrial dysfunction to have a protective role in paraquat-induced cell death

(R. A. Gonzalez-Polo *et al.*, 2007a, 2007b). Moreover, our group has shown that PQ exposure induced an early reticulum stress response that was correlated with the adaptive activation of autophagy, characterised by the accumulation of autophagic vacuoles, activation of beclin-1, accumulation of LC3-II, p62 degradation, and mammalian target of rapamycin dephosphorylation (R. A. Gonzalez-Polo *et al.*, 2007a, 2007b; Niso-Santano *et al.*, 2011). This response was increased in cells that overexpressed wild-type (WT) ASK1 (apoptosis signal kinase 1) protein. In this model, the inhibition of autophagy caused an exacerbation of the apoptosis induced by ASK1 WT overexpression with or without PQ. These results suggest that autophagy has an important role in the cell death/survival events produced by PQ and ASK1 that contribute to neuronal degeneration.

Therefore, increased autophagy might be a new strategy for the treatment of neurodegenerative diseases (Menzies *et al.*, 2006). It is encouraging to consider enhancing the autophagic capacity as a therapeutic strategy in the prevention of neurodegeneration because studies have shown that the abnormal regulation of autophagic pathways may lead to apoptosis and cell death (Walls *et al.*, 2010).

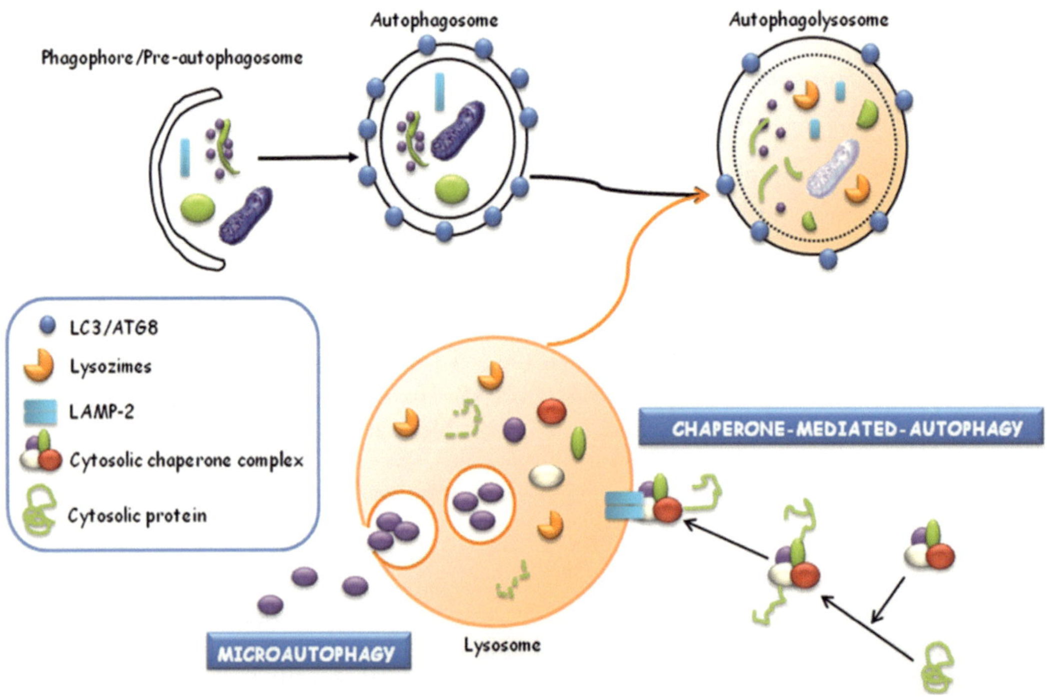

Fig. 3. Schematic representation of the different types of autophagy

4. Paraquat and Parkinson´s disease-related proteins

As previously described, PD is characterised by the selective degeneration of dopaminergic neurons. The aetiology of PD is unknown but has a multifactorial origin that involves both genetic and environmental factors. The interaction of both factors was, in part, involved in the selective death of dopaminergic neurons observed in PD. Apart from the studies that have identified human mutations as a basis for disease, the high number of individuals with sporadic PD have an unknown aetiology. These individuals have multifactorial disease in which the environment plays important roles. PQ is an environmental agent that has been associated with PD. A recent study by Caroline Tanner concluded that people using PQ and rotenone were 2.5 times more likely to develop PD than those who were not in contact with them (Tanner *et al.*, 2011). Therefore, there is a relationship between the toxicity of PQ and PD. This interaction is not known; however, several studies directly indicate the interaction of PQ with PARK genes.

The development of PD was attributed to different events, such as mitochondrial dysfunction, oxidative stress or the aggregation of proteins. These events could be important to understanding the relationship between PQ and PARK genes (Table 1).

Gene	Locus	Protein name	Inheritance	Function
PARK 1/4	4q21.3-q22	α-synuclein	AD	Lewy`s body component
PARK 2	6q25-27	Parkin	AR	E3 ubiquitin ligase
PARK 3	2p13	¿?	AD	¿?
PARK 5	4p14	UCHL-1	AD	Ubiquitin C-terminal hydrolase
PARK 6	1p35-36	PINK1	AR	Mitochondrial kinase
PARK 7	1p36	DJ-1	AR	Antioxidant agent
PARK 8	12q12	LRRK2	AD	Kinase, GTPase
PARK 9	1p36	ATP13A2	AR	ATPase, cationic transport
PARK 10	1p32	¿?	AD	¿?
PARK 11	2q36-q37	GIGYF2	AD	Receptor tyrosine kinase signaling
PARK 12	Xq21-q25	¿?	X-linked	¿?
PARK 13	2p13	HTRA2/OMI	AD	Serine protease
PARK 14	22q13.1	PLA2G6	AR	Fosfolipase A2
PARK 15	22q11.2	FBXO7	AR	E3 ubiquitin ligase
PARK 16	1q32	RAB7L1	¿?	¿?
PARK 17	4p	GAK/DGKQ	¿?	¿?
PARK 18	6p	HLA-DRA	¿?	¿?

Table 1. Some characteristics of PARK genes

The increase in oxidative stress has been observed in the substantia nigra of PD brains, as demonstrated by the increased lipid, protein, and DNA oxidation or increased total iron content (Bagchi *et al.*, 1995; Mattson, 2006). This alteration of cellular redox balance may be produced by different mechanisms because of the enzymatic conversion to secondary reactive products and/or ROS by the depletion of antioxidant defences or the impairment of antioxidant enzyme function (Abdollahi *et al.*, 2004). Autosomal recessive PD-associated genes such as parkin, DJ-1 and PTEN-induced putative kinase 1 (PINK), have been shown to be involved in mitochondrial function, which suggests that mitochondrial dysfunction and the generation of ROS were central events in the pathogenesis of PD. Therefore, further study of the implication of these proteins in PQ toxicity would be of interest.

In contrast, the misfolding and aggregation of proteins is another pathway of cell toxicity in PD. The failure of α-synuclein (PD-related protein) clearance by the ubiquitin-proteasome system UPS (ubiquitin proteosome system) led to its accumulation over time and to the formation of fibrillar aggregates and Lewy bodies. In this vein, there is a relationship between PQ toxicity and PD because exposure to PQ has been shown to induce proteasome dysfunction and α-synuclein aggregation (Ding & Keller, 2001; Fei *et al.*, 2008; Goers *et al.*, 2003; Manning-Bog *et al.*, 2002; Yang & Tiffany-Castiglioni, 2007).
Therefore, there is a relationship between the toxicity exerted by PQ and different *PARK* genes.

4.1 α-synuclein (PARK1, PARK4) and paraquat

Lewy bodies (LBs) are abnormal aggregates of protein that develop inside the nerve cells in PD. The presence of α-synuclein in these aggregates has been shown to play an important role in the formation of LBs (Masliah *et al.*, 2000; Spillantini *et al.*, 1997). The mechanisms that promote intraneuronal α-synuclein assembly remain poorly understood. Missense mutations (A53T, A30P and E46K) or multiplications (duplications and triplications) in the *α-synuclein* gene (*PARK1/4*) caused autosomal-dominant parkinsonism (Polymeropoulos *et al.*, 1997), but it is still unclear whether fibrils of aggregated α-synuclein, as found in LBs, have a causative role in the more common forms of PD or could be a marker for the underlying pathogenetic process. α-synuclein has three common forms, monomers, dimers, and protofibrils, and it is thought that an excess of the protofibril forms inhibited UPS *in vitro* (McNaught *et al.*, 2001) and *in vivo* (Dyllick-Brenzinger *et al.*, 2010). α-synuclein protofibrils have been shown to directly lead to oxidative stress that could further impair UPS by reducing ATP levels, inhibiting the proteasome and by the oxidation of parkin.
Studies have indicated that the interaction of environmental factors with alterations in α-synuclein might be involved in the aetiology of PD. The interaction of α-synuclein with PQ toxicity has been extensively examined. PQ has been shown to potentiate α-synuclein-induced toxicity (Norris *et al.*, 2007). PQ preferentially binds to the partially folded α-synuclein intermediate because PQ has been shown to induce a conformational change in α-synuclein and significantly increase the rate of the formation of α-synuclein fibrils *in vitro* (Uversky *et al.*, 2001). *In vivo*, rodent studies have shown that the administration of PQ induced an increase in α-synuclein levels in the brain. These results suggest that the upregulation of α-synuclein as a result of toxic insult and the direct interactions between the protein and environmental agents are potential mechanisms leading to α-synuclein pathology in neurodegenerative disorders (Manning-Bog *et al.*, 2002).

4.2 PINK1/PARKIN (PARK6/PARK2) and paraquat

Another hallmark PD characteristic is mitochondrial dysfunction. In *post-mortem* analysis in the substantia nigra, some patients with PD showed complex I deficiency (Schapira *et al.*, 1989). In addition, the oxidative stress was higher in patients with parkinsonism (Jenner, 2003). In this sense, *PINK1* (*PARK6*) and *Parkin* (*PARK2)* are 2 genes related to PD that may be involved in the regulation of mitochondrial homeostasis.
Parkin mutations were first linked to an autosomal recessive juvenile-onset form of PD in Japanese families (Kitada *et al.*, 1998; Matsumine *et al.*, 1997). Numerous parkin mutations have been described, including deletions, multiplications and missense mutations (Hattori & Mizuno, 2004). Parkin protein acts as an E3 ubiquitin protein ligase in the UPS (Shimura *et al.*, 2000). Ubiquitination of proteins is essential to start to proteasomal protein degradation.

Therefore, parkin mutations should lead to an incorrect ubiquitination, blocking the degradation of the protein and leading to protein accumulation. Mutant parkin has been shown to impair mitochondrial function and morphology in human fibroblasts and to sensitise the cells to an insult with PQ, producing higher levels of oxidised proteins in the *Parkin*-mutant samples than in controls (Grunewald *et al.*, 2010). PQ has also been demonstrated to induce alterations in parkin solubility and result in its intracellular aggregation (C. Wang *et al.*, 2005).

PINK1 is a serine/threonine kinase capable of autophosphorylation. This protein has an N-terminal mitochondrial targeting signal (MTS), is synthesised as a full-length version (FL) and is processed into at least two cleaved forms (Δ1 and Δ2) (W. Lin & Kang, 2008). PINK1 is considered to be a mitochondrial protein with a role in protecting against oxidative stress and apoptosis in *in vitro* models (Valente *et al.*, 2004). Mutations in *PINK1* have been associated with autosomal recessive PD (Valente *et al.*, 2004) and with *PINK1* KO flies with motor deficits and disorganised mitochondrial morphology (Clark *et al.*, 2006). For the link between PINK1 and the toxicity of PQ, studies using silencer PINK1 have shown an increase in oxidative stress and ATP depletion and a higher sensitivity to PQ (Gegg *et al.*, 2009). Similar results have been observed in studies that examined PINK1 nonsense and missense mutations (Grunewald *et al.*, 2009).

4.3 DJ-1 (PARK7) and paraquat

DJ-1 is a small protein that belongs to the ThiJ/PfpI protein superfamily (S. Bandyopadhyay & Cookson, 2004) that was initially identified as an oncogene that interacted with H-Ras (Nagakubo *et al.*, 1997). The involvement of DJ-1 in neurodegeneration was found when it was discovered that the DJ-1 gene (*PARK7*) was the cause of autosomal recessive PD in a Dutch family (Bonifati *et al.*, 2003). Different pathogenic mutations have been identified in the *PARK7* gene, including truncation, exonic deletions and homozygous and heterozygous missense mutations (Hague *et al.*, 2003). L166P is the most dramatic point mutation, whereas other mutations, such as A104T and M26I, have a weaker destabilising effect on the protein structure. The L166P mutation is located in the centre of α-helix 7, which is a major part of the hydrophobic patch. This mutation has been shown to destabilise the dimeric structure of DJ-1 by promoting the unfolding of its C-terminal region, resulting in rapid degradation (Miller *et al.*, 2003; Moore *et al.*, 2003). However, the frequency of DJ-1 mutations was low, with it being estimated at approximately 1-2 % in early onset PD. The physiological function of DJ-1 is unclear, but it may have a role in protecting against mitochondrial damage in response to oxidative stress (Canet-Aviles *et al.*, 2004).

The link between DJ-1 and PQ exposure has been correlated with autophagy and the apoptotic process. An active role for DJ-1 in the autophagic response produced by PQ has been suggested. In a study using transfected cells exposed to PQ and DJ-1-specific siRNA, an inhibition of the autophagic events induced by the herbicide, the increased sensitisation during PQ-induced apoptotic cell death and the exacerbation of apoptosis in the presence of the autophagy inhibitor 3-methyladenine (R. A. Gonzalez-Polo *et al.*, 2009) had been shown. Interestingly, PQ-induced toxicity and proteasome dysfunction was potentiated in a DJ-1 deficiency (Lavara-Culebras & Paricio, 2007; Menzies *et al.*, 2005). In another study using DJ-1 null cells from the DJ-1(-/-) mouse embryos, DJ-1 null cells showed a resistance to PQ-induced apoptosis, including reduced poly (ADP-ribose) polymerase and procaspase-3. Therefore, DJ-1 could be important to maintain mitochondrial complex I, and complex I could be a key target in the interaction of PQ toxicity and DJ-1 in PD (Kwon *et al.*, 2011). In

DJ-1-deficient mice treated with PQ, decreased proteasome activities and increased ubiquitinated protein levels were found, and these pathologies were not observed in brain regions of normal mice treated with PQ (Yang *et al.*, 2007). In another mouse study, the loss of DJ-1 increased the sensitivity to oxidative insults but did not produce neurodegeneration. Similar results have been found when analysing *Drosophila melanogaster* mutants for the DJ-1 orthologous genes, DJ-1alpha and DJ-1beta, that resulted in increased sensitivity to PQ insults, reduced lifespan and motor impairments. However, these mutations did not lead to dopaminergic neuronal loss (Lavara-Culebras & Paricio, 2007)

4.4 LRRK2 (PARK8) and paraquat

In 2002, *PARK8* gene mutations were discovered as a major genetic cause associated with hereditary parkinsonism (Paisan-Ruiz *et al.*, 2004). The *PARK8* gene was associated with PD in studies of a Japanese Sagamihara family who responded positively to treatment with L-DOPA, which had parkinsonism that presented with an unknown aetiology of the disease (Funayama *et al.*, 2002). Other studies examined two additional families (German and Canadian) who also had an autosomal dominant, late-onset parkinsonism (Zimprich *et al.*, 2004).

In the LRRK2 structure, two functional domains, kinase and GTPase domains, were shown to be present. The G2019S mutation was present in the kinase domain specific to the binding site for Mg^{2+} (Kachergus *et al.*, 2005). This mutation facilitates the access of the kinase domain to its substrates, which increases autophosphorylation 2.5-fold the phosphorylation of other substrates, such as myelin basic protein (MBP), 3-fold for the LRRK2 autophosphorylation without the presence of this mutation (Jaleel *et al.*, 2007; West *et al.*, 2005), which is responsible for the increased toxicity of this molecule (Greggio *et al.*, 2006). In the GTPase domain, the R1441C has been the most studied mutation, and there is controversy as to the influence of GTPase mutations on the kinase activity that was observed in some studies in which the increase was similar (Guo *et al.*, 2007) or had no change (Jaleel *et al.*, 2007).

LRRK2 has been shown to play different roles in the cell; however, little information is available. Based on the data we found from the protein interactions, there was a relationship between LRRK2 and cytoskeletal reorganisation (Gandhi *et al.*, 2008), maintenance functions and cell morphology (Plowey *et al.*, 2008), protein transport through synaptic vesicles (Shin *et al.*, 2008), and the ubiquitination process (Ko *et al.*, 2009). There have also been studies that relate LRRK2 and apoptosis (Ho *et al.*, 2009). Previous studies have shown a relationship between LRRK2 and other PD-related proteins, such as parkin (Ng *et al.*, 2009; W. W. Smith *et al.*, 2005), PINK-1 and DJ-1 (Venderova *et al.*, 2009) or α-synuclein (X. Lin *et al.*, 2009). The interaction of LRRK2 with PQ is not clear. Studies in *Drosophila melanogaster* in which the deletion of kinase domain of LRRK2 did not induce a higher sensitivity to the PQ stimulus has been shown (D. Wang *et al.*, 2008). In contrast, in *Caenorhabditis elegans* studies, the expression of human LRRK2 protein protected against PQ, which increased nematode survival in response to agents that cause mitochondrial dysfunction. However, protection by G2019S, R1441C, or kinase-dead LRRK2 was less effective than wild-type LRRK2 (Saha *et al.*, 2009). In another study with *Caenorhabditits elegans, PINK1* mutant genes have been observed in a minor mitochondrial length and increased PQ sensitivity of the nematode. Moreover, the mutants also displayed defects in axonal outgrowth of a pair of canal-associated neurons. We demonstrated that in the absence of lrk-1 (the *C. elegans* homologue of human LRRK2), all phenotypic aspects of *PINK1* loss-of-function mutants were suppressed (Samann *et al.*, 2009)

5. Conclusion

PQ has been suggested as a potential aetiological factor for the development of PD. We have demonstrated that PQ was able to induce cell death by activating apoptotic machinery. However, PQ also displayed characteristics of autophagy, a degradative mechanism involved in the recycling and turnover of cytoplasmic constituents from eukaryotic cells. Finally, the cells suffered apoptotic death when the PQ remained. Whereas caspase inhibition retarded cell death, autophagy inhibition increased apoptotic cell death induced by PQ. These findings suggest a relationship between autophagy and apoptotic cell death following paraquat exposition and allows us to further investigate and increase our knowledge regarding the toxicity of paraquat and its relationship with the origin of PD.

6. Acknowledgments

Jose M. Bravo-San Pedro was supported by a Junta de Extremadura predoctoral fellowship. Mireia Niso-Santano was supported as a postdoctoral contract of the University of Extremadura. Ruben Gómez-Sánchez was supported by a Spanish Ministerio de Educación predoctoral fellowship. Rosa-Ana González-Polo was supported by a "Miguel Servet" contract (ISCIII, Ministerio de Ciencia e Innovación, Spain). Dr. González-Polo receives research support from ISCIII (Ministerio de Ciencia e Innovación, Spain (CP08/00010, PI11/00040). Dr. José M. Fuentes receives research support from the Ministerio de Ciencia e Innovación, Spain (SAF2010-14993), FUNDESALUD (PRIS10013) and Consejería, Economía, Comercio e Innovación Junta de Extremadura (GR10054).

7. References

Abdollahi, M., Ranjbar, A., Shadnia, S., Nikfar, S., & Rezaie, A. (2004). Pesticides and oxidative stress: a review. *Med Sci Monit, 10*(6), Jun,pp. RA141-147

Amarante-Mendes, G. P., & Green, D. R. (1999). The regulation of apoptotic cell death. *Braz J Med Biol Res, 32*(9), Sep,pp. 1053-1061

Andersen, J. K. (2001). Does neuronal loss in Parkinson's disease involve programmed cell death? *Bioessays, 23*(7), Jul,pp. 640-646

Anglade, P., Vyas, S., Javoy-Agid, F., Herrero, M. T., Michel, P. P., Marquez, J., Mouatt-Prigent, A., Ruberg, M., Hirsch, E. C., & Agid, Y. (1997). Apoptosis and autophagy in nigral neurons of patients with Parkinson's disease. *Histol Histopathol, 12*(1), Jan,pp. 25-31

Baba, M., Takeshige, K., Baba, N., & Ohsumi, Y. (1994). Ultrastructural analysis of the autophagic process in yeast: detection of autophagosomes and their characterization. *J Cell Biol, 124*(6), Mar,pp. 903-913

Bagchi, D., Bagchi, M., Hassoun, E. A., & Stohs, S. J. (1995). In vitro and in vivo generation of reactive oxygen species, DNA damage and lactate dehydrogenase leakage by selected pesticides. *Toxicology, 104*(1-3), Dec 15,pp. 129-140

Bandyopadhyay, S., & Cookson, M. R. (2004). Evolutionary and functional relationships within the DJ1 superfamily. *BMC Evol Biol, 4*Feb 19,pp. 6

Bandyopadhyay, U., & Cuervo, A. M. (2007). Chaperone-mediated autophagy in aging and neurodegeneration: lessons from alpha-synuclein. *Exp Gerontol, 42*(1-2), Jan-Feb,pp. 120-128

Bonifati, V., Rizzu, P., van Baren, M. J., Schaap, O., Breedveld, G. J., Krieger, E., Dekker, M. C., Squitieri, F., Ibanez, P., Joosse, M., van Dongen, J. W., Vanacore, N., van Swieten, J. C., Brice, A., Meco, G., van Duijn, C. M., Oostra, B. A., & Heutink, P. (2003). Mutations in the DJ-1 gene associated with autosomal recessive early-onset parkinsonism. *Science, 299*(5604), Jan 10,pp. 256-259

Bonneh-Barkay, D., Langston, W. J., & Di Monte, D. A. (2005). Toxicity of redox cycling pesticides in primary mesencephalic cultures. *Antioxid Redox Signal, 7*(5-6), May-Jun,pp. 649-653

Boya, P., Gonzalez-Polo, R. A., Casares, N., Perfettini, J. L., Dessen, P., Larochette, N., Metivier, D., Meley, D., Souquere, S., Yoshimori, T., Pierron, G., Codogno, P., & Kroemer, G. (2005). Inhibition of macroautophagy triggers apoptosis. *Mol Cell Biol, 25*(3), Feb,pp. 1025-1040

Bus, J. S., & Gibson, J. E. (1984). Paraquat: model for oxidant-initiated toxicity. *Environ Health Perspect, 55*Apr,pp. 37-46

Butler, D., & Bahr, B. A. (2006). Oxidative stress and lysosomes: CNS-related consequences and implications for lysosomal enhancement strategies and induction of autophagy. *Antioxid Redox Signal, 8*(1-2), Jan-Feb,pp. 185-196

Canet-Aviles, R. M., Wilson, M. A., Miller, D. W., Ahmad, R., McLendon, C., Bandyopadhyay, S., Baptista, M. J., Ringe, D., Petsko, G. A., & Cookson, M. R. (2004). The Parkinson's disease protein DJ-1 is neuroprotective due to cysteine-sulfinic acid-driven mitochondrial localization. *Proc Natl Acad Sci U S A, 101*(24), Jun 15,pp. 9103-9108

Cappelletti, G., Maggioni, M. G., & Maci, R. (1998). Apoptosis in human lung epithelial cells: triggering by paraquat and modulation by antioxidants. *Cell Biol Int, 22*(9-10), 671-678

Clark, I. E., Dodson, M. W., Jiang, C., Cao, J. H., Huh, J. R., Seol, J. H., Yoo, S. J., Hay, B. A., & Guo, M. (2006). Drosophila pink1 is required for mitochondrial function and interacts genetically with parkin. *Nature, 441*(7097), Jun 29,pp. 1162-1166

Costello, S., Cockburn, M., Bronstein, J., Zhang, X., & Ritz, B. (2009). Parkinson's disease and residential exposure to maneb and paraquat from agricultural applications in the central valley of California. *Am J Epidemiol, 169*(8), Apr 15,pp. 919-926

Chinta, S. J., Rane, A., Poksay, K. S., Bredesen, D. E., Andersen, J. K., & Rao, R. V. (2008). Coupling endoplasmic reticulum stress to the cell death program in dopaminergic cells: effect of paraquat. *Neuromolecular Med, 10*(4), 333-342

Choi, W. S., Yoon, S. Y., Oh, T. H., Choi, E. J., O'Malley, K. L., & Oh, Y. J. (1999). Two distinct mechanisms are involved in 6-hydroxydopamine- and MPP+-induced dopaminergic neuronal cell death: role of caspases, ROS, and JNK. *J Neurosci Res, 57*(1), Jul 1,pp. 86-94

Daniel, J. W., & Gage, J. C. (1966). Absorption and excretion of diquat and paraquat in rats. *Br J Ind Med, 23*(2), Apr,pp. 133-136

Debnath, J., Baehrecke, E. H., & Kroemer, G. (2005). Does autophagy contribute to cell death? *Autophagy, 1*(2), Jul,pp. 66-74

Di Monte, D., Sandy, M. S., Ekstrom, G., & Smith, M. T. (1986). Comparative studies on the mechanisms of paraquat and 1-methyl-4-phenylpyridine (MPP+) cytotoxicity. *Biochem Biophys Res Commun, 137*(1), May 29,pp. 303-309

Ding, Q., & Keller, J. N. (2001). Proteasome inhibition in oxidative stress neurotoxicity: implications for heat shock proteins. *J Neurochem, 77*(4), May,pp. 1010-1017

Dinis-Oliveira, R. J., Duarte, J. A., Sanchez-Navarro, A., Remiao, F., Bastos, M. L., & Carvalho, F. (2008). Paraquat poisonings: mechanisms of lung toxicity, clinical features, and treatment. *Crit Rev Toxicol, 38*(1), 13-71

Dinis-Oliveira, R. J., Remiao, F., Carmo, H., Duarte, J. A., Navarro, A. S., Bastos, M. L., & Carvalho, F. (2006). Paraquat exposure as an etiological factor of Parkinson's disease. *Neurotoxicology, 27*(6), Dec,pp. 1110-1122

Drechsel, D. A., & Patel, M. (2008). Role of reactive oxygen species in the neurotoxicity of environmental agents implicated in Parkinson's disease. *Free Radic Biol Med, 44*(11), Jun 1,pp. 1873-1886

Dyllick-Brenzinger, M., D'Souza, C. A., Dahlmann, B., Kloetzel, P. M., & Tandon, A. (2010). Reciprocal effects of alpha-synuclein overexpression and proteasome inhibition in neuronal cells and tissue. *Neurotox Res, 17*(3), Apr,pp. 215-227

Ethell, D. W., & Buhler, L. A. (2003). Fas ligand-mediated apoptosis in degenerative disorders of the brain. *J Clin Immunol, 23*(6), Nov,pp. 439-446

Fabisiak, J. P., Kagan, V. E., Ritov, V. B., Johnson, D. E., & Lazo, J. S. (1997). Bcl-2 inhibits selective oxidation and externalization of phosphatidylserine during paraquat-induced apoptosis. *Am J Physiol, 272*(2 Pt 1), Feb,pp. C675-684

Fall, C. P., & Bennett, J. P., Jr. (1999). Characterization and time course of MPP+ -induced apoptosis in human SH-SY5Y neuroblastoma cells. *J Neurosci Res, 55*(5), Mar 1,pp. 620-628

Fei, Q., McCormack, A. L., Di Monte, D. A., & Ethell, D. W. (2008). Paraquat neurotoxicity is mediated by a Bak-dependent mechanism. *J Biol Chem, 283*(6), Feb 8,pp. 3357-3364

Fengsrud, M., Roos, N., Berg, T., Liou, W., Slot, J. W., & Seglen, P. O. (1995). Ultrastructural and immunocytochemical characterization of autophagic vacuoles in isolated hepatocytes: effects of vinblastine and asparagine on vacuole distributions. *Exp Cell Res, 221*(2), Dec,pp. 504-519

Filonova, L. H., Bozhkov, P. V., Brukhin, V. B., Daniel, G., Zhivotovsky, B., & von Arnold, S. (2000). Two waves of programmed cell death occur during formation and development of somatic embryos in the gymnosperm, Norway spruce. *J Cell Sci, 113 Pt 24*Dec,pp. 4399-4411

Fixsen, W., Sternberg, P., Ellis, H., & Horvitz, R. (1985). Genes that affect cell fates during the development of Caenorhabditis elegans. *Cold Spring Harb Symp Quant Biol, 50*99-104

Formigli, L., Papucci, L., Tani, A., Schiavone, N., Tempestini, A., Orlandini, G. E., Capaccioli, S., & Orlandini, S. Z. (2000). Aponecrosis: morphological and biochemical exploration of a syncretic process of cell death sharing apoptosis and necrosis. *J Cell Physiol, 182*(1), Jan,pp. 41-49

Freude, B., Masters, T. N., Robicsek, F., Fokin, A., Kostin, S., Zimmermann, R., Ullmann, C., Lorenz-Meyer, S., & Schaper, J. (2000). Apoptosis is initiated by myocardial ischemia and executed during reperfusion. *J Mol Cell Cardiol, 32*(2), Feb,pp. 197-208

Fukushima, T., Yamada, K., Isobe, A., Shiwaku, K., & Yamane, Y. (1993). Mechanism of cytotoxicity of paraquat. I. NADH oxidation and paraquat radical formation via complex I. *Exp Toxicol Pathol, 45*(5-6), Oct,pp. 345-349

Funayama, M., Hasegawa, K., Kowa, H., Saito, M., Tsuji, S., & Obata, F. (2002). A new locus for Parkinson's disease (PARK8) maps to chromosome 12p11.2-q13.1. *Ann Neurol, 51*(3), Mar,pp. 296-301

Gandhi, P. N., Wang, X., Zhu, X., Chen, S. G., & Wilson-Delfosse, A. L. (2008). The Roc domain of leucine-rich repeat kinase 2 is sufficient for interaction with microtubules. *J Neurosci Res, 86*(8), Jun,pp. 1711-1720

Gegg, M. E., Cooper, J. M., Schapira, A. H., & Taanman, J. W. (2009). Silencing of PINK1 expression affects mitochondrial DNA and oxidative phosphorylation in dopaminergic cells. *PLoS One, 4*(3), e4756

Geske, F. J., Lieberman, R., Strange, R., & Gerschenson, L. E. (2001). Early stages of p53-induced apoptosis are reversible. *Cell Death Differ, 8*(2), Feb,pp. 182-191

Goers, J., Manning-Bog, A. B., McCormack, A. L., Millett, I. S., Doniach, S., Di Monte, D. A., Uversky, V. N., & Fink, A. L. (2003). Nuclear localization of alpha-synuclein and its interaction with histones. *Biochemistry, 42*(28), Jul 22,pp. 8465-8471

Gomez-Sanchez, R., Bravo-San Pedro, J. M., Niso-Santano, M., Soler, G., Fuentes, J. M., & Gonzalez-Polo, R. A. (2010). The neuroprotective effect of talipexole from paraquat-induced cell death in dopaminergic neuronal cells. *Neurotoxicology, 31*(6), Dec,pp. 701-708

Gonzalez-Polo, R., Niso-Santano, M., Moran, J. M., Ortiz-Ortiz, M. A., Bravo-San Pedro, J. M., Soler, G., & Fuentes, J. M. (2009). Silencing DJ-1 reveals its contribution in paraquat-induced autophagy. *J Neurochem, 109*(3), May,pp. 889-898

Gonzalez-Polo, R. A., Niso-Santano, M., Ortiz-Ortiz, M. A., Gomez-Martin, A., Moran, J. M., Garcia-Rubio, L., Francisco-Morcillo, J., Zaragoza, C., Soler, G., & Fuentes, J. M. (2007a). Inhibition of paraquat-induced autophagy accelerates the apoptotic cell death in neuroblastoma SH-SY5Y cells. *Toxicol Sci, 97*(2), Jun,pp. 448-458

Gonzalez-Polo, R. A., Niso-Santano, M., Ortiz-Ortiz, M. A., Gomez-Martin, A., Moran, J. M., Garcia-Rubio, L., Francisco-Morcillo, J., Zaragoza, C., Soler, G., & Fuentes, J. M. (2007b). Relationship between autophagy and apoptotic cell death in human neuroblastoma cells treated with paraquat: could autophagy be a "brake" in paraquat-induced apoptotic death? *Autophagy, 3*(4), Jul-Aug,pp. 366-367

Gonzalez-Polo, R. A., Rodriguez-Martin, A., Moran, J. M., Niso, M., Soler, G., & Fuentes, J. M. (2004). Paraquat-induced apoptotic cell death in cerebellar granule cells. *Brain Res, 1011*(2), Jun 18,pp. 170-176

Grant, H., Lantos, P. L., & Parkinson, C. (1980). Cerebral damage in paraquat poisoning. *Histopathology, 4*(2), Mar,pp. 185-195

Gray, J. P., Heck, D. E., Mishin, V., Smith, P. J., Hong, J. Y., Thiruchelvam, M., Cory-Slechta, D. A., Laskin, D. L., & Laskin, J. D. (2007). Paraquat increases cyanide-insensitive respiration in murine lung epithelial cells by activating an NAD(P)H:paraquat oxidoreductase: identification of the enzyme as thioredoxin reductase. *J Biol Chem, 282*(11), Mar 16,pp. 7939-7949

Greggio, E., Jain, S., Kingsbury, A., Bandopadhyay, R., Lewis, P., Kaganovich, A., van der Brug, M. P., Beilina, A., Blackinton, J., Thomas, K. J., Ahmad, R., Miller, D. W., Kesavapany, S., Singleton, A., Lees, A., Harvey, R. J., Harvey, K., & Cookson, M. R.

(2006). Kinase activity is required for the toxic effects of mutant LRRK2/dardarin. *Neurobiol Dis, 23*(2), Aug,pp. 329-341

Gross, A., McDonnell, J. M., & Korsmeyer, S. J. (1999). BCL-2 family members and the mitochondria in apoptosis. *Genes Dev, 13*(15), Aug 1,pp. 1899-1911

Grunewald, A., Gegg, M. E., Taanman, J. W., King, R. H., Kock, N., Klein, C., & Schapira, A. H. (2009). Differential effects of PINK1 nonsense and missense mutations on mitochondrial function and morphology. *Exp Neurol, 219*(1), Sep,pp. 266-273

Grunewald, A., Voges, L., Rakovic, A., Kasten, M., Vandebona, H., Hemmelmann, C., Lohmann, K., Orolicki, S., Ramirez, A., Schapira, A. H., Pramstaller, P. P., Sue, C. M., & Klein, C. (2010). Mutant Parkin impairs mitochondrial function and morphology in human fibroblasts. *PLoS One, 5*(9), e12962

Guo, L., Gandhi, P. N., Wang, W., Petersen, R. B., Wilson-Delfosse, A. L., & Chen, S. G. (2007). The Parkinson's disease-associated protein, leucine-rich repeat kinase 2 (LRRK2), is an authentic GTPase that stimulates kinase activity. *Exp Cell Res, 313*(16), Oct 1,pp. 3658-3670

Hague, S., Rogaeva, E., Hernandez, D., Gulick, C., Singleton, A., Hanson, M., Johnson, J., Weiser, R., Gallardo, M., Ravina, B., Gwinn-Hardy, K., Crawley, A., St George-Hyslop, P. H., Lang, A. E., Heutink, P., Bonifati, V., & Hardy, J. (2003). Early-onset Parkinson's disease caused by a compound heterozygous DJ-1 mutation. *Ann Neurol, 54*(2), Aug,pp. 271-274

Haley, T. J. (1979). Review of the toxicology of paraquat (1,1'-dimethyl-4,4'-bipyridinium chloride). *Clin Toxicol, 14*(1), 1-46

Hariri, M., Millane, G., Guimond, M. P., Guay, G., Dennis, J. W., & Nabi, I. R. (2000). Biogenesis of multilamellar bodies via autophagy. *Mol Biol Cell, 11*(1), Jan,pp. 255-268

Hartmann, A., Hunot, S., Michel, P. P., Muriel, M. P., Vyas, S., Faucheux, B. A., Mouatt-Prigent, A., Turmel, H., Srinivasan, A., Ruberg, M., Evan, G. I., Agid, Y., & Hirsch, E. C. (2000). Caspase-3: A vulnerability factor and final effector in apoptotic death of dopaminergic neurons in Parkinson's disease. *Proc Natl Acad Sci U S A, 97*(6), Mar 14,pp. 2875-2880

Hattori, N., & Mizuno, Y. (2004). Pathogenetic mechanisms of parkin in Parkinson's disease. *Lancet, 364*(9435), Aug 21-27,pp. 722-724

Hertzman, C., Wiens, M., Bowering, D., Snow, B., & Calne, D. (1990). Parkinson's disease: a case-control study of occupational and environmental risk factors. *Am J Ind Med, 17*(3), 349-355

Ho, C. C., Rideout, H. J., Ribe, E., Troy, C. M., & Dauer, W. T. (2009). The Parkinson disease protein leucine-rich repeat kinase 2 transduces death signals via Fas-associated protein with death domain and caspase-8 in a cellular model of neurodegeneration. *J Neurosci, 29*(4), Jan 28,pp. 1011-1016

Hoeppner, D. J., Hengartner, M. O., & Schnabel, R. (2001). Engulfment genes cooperate with ced-3 to promote cell death in Caenorhabditis elegans. *Nature, 412*(6843), Jul 12,pp. 202-206

Holtz, W. A., & O'Malley, K. L. (2003). Parkinsonian mimetics induce aspects of unfolded protein response in death of dopaminergic neurons. *J Biol Chem, 278*(21), May 23,pp. 19367-19377

Igney, F. H., & Krammer, P. H. (2002). Death and anti-death: tumour resistance to apoptosis. *Nat Rev Cancer, 2*(4), Apr,pp. 277-288

Iwata, A., Christianson, J. C., Bucci, M., Ellerby, L. M., Nukina, N., Forno, L. S., & Kopito, R. R. (2005). Increased susceptibility of cytoplasmic over nuclear polyglutamine aggregates to autophagic degradation. *Proc Natl Acad Sci U S A, 102*(37), Sep 13,pp. 13135-13140

Jaleel, M., Nichols, R. J., Deak, M., Campbell, D. G., Gillardon, F., Knebel, A., & Alessi, D. R. (2007). LRRK2 phosphorylates moesin at threonine-558: characterization of how Parkinson's disease mutants affect kinase activity. *Biochem J, 405*(2), Jul 15,pp. 307-317

Jenner, P. (2003). Oxidative stress in Parkinson's disease. *Ann Neurol, 53 Suppl 3*S26-36; discussion S36-28

Kachergus, J., Mata, I. F., Hulihan, M., Taylor, J. P., Lincoln, S., Aasly, J., Gibson, J. M., Ross, O. A., Lynch, T., Wiley, J., Payami, H., Nutt, J., Maraganore, D. M., Czyzewski, K., Styczynska, M., Wszolek, Z. K., Farrer, M. J., & Toft, M. (2005). Identification of a novel LRRK2 mutation linked to autosomal dominant parkinsonism: evidence of a common founder across European populations. *Am J Hum Genet, 76*(4), Apr,pp. 672-680

Kegel, K. B., Kim, M., Sapp, E., McIntyre, C., Castano, J. G., Aronin, N., & DiFiglia, M. (2000). Huntingtin expression stimulates endosomal-lysosomal activity, endosome tubulation, and autophagy. *J Neurosci, 20*(19), Oct 1,pp. 7268-7278

Kerr, J. F., Winterford, C. M., & Harmon, B. V. (1994). Apoptosis. Its significance in cancer and cancer therapy. *Cancer, 73*(8), Apr 15,pp. 2013-2026

Kerr, J. F., Wyllie, A. H., & Currie, A. R. (1972). Apoptosis: a basic biological phenomenon with wide-ranging implications in tissue kinetics. *Br J Cancer, 26*(4), Aug,pp. 239-257

Kitada, T., Asakawa, S., Hattori, N., Matsumine, H., Yamamura, Y., Minoshima, S., Yokochi, M., Mizuno, Y., & Shimizu, N. (1998). Mutations in the parkin gene cause autosomal recessive juvenile parkinsonism. *Nature, 392*(6676), Apr 9,pp. 605-608

Kitazawa, Y., Matsubara, M., Takeyama, N., & Tanaka, T. (1991). The role of xanthine oxidase in paraquat intoxication. *Arch Biochem Biophys, 288*(1), Jul,pp. 220-224

Klintworth, H., Newhouse, K., Li, T., Choi, W. S., Faigle, R., & Xia, Z. (2007). Activation of c-Jun N-terminal protein kinase is a common mechanism underlying paraquat- and rotenone-induced dopaminergic cell apoptosis. *Toxicol Sci, 97*(1), May,pp. 149-162

Klionsky, D. J., Cuervo, A. M., Dunn, W. A., Jr., Levine, B., van der Klei, I., & Seglen, P. O. (2007). How shall I eat thee? *Autophagy, 3*(5), Sep-Oct,pp. 413-416

Klionsky, D. J., & Emr, S. D. (2000). Autophagy as a regulated pathway of cellular degradation. *Science, 290*(5497), Dec 1,pp. 1717-1721

Ko, H. S., Bailey, R., Smith, W. W., Liu, Z., Shin, J. H., Lee, Y. I., Zhang, Y. J., Jiang, H., Ross, C. A., Moore, D. J., Patterson, C., Petrucelli, L., Dawson, T. M., & Dawson, V. L. (2009). CHIP regulates leucine-rich repeat kinase-2 ubiquitination, degradation, and toxicity. *Proc Natl Acad Sci U S A, 106*(8), Feb 24,pp. 2897-2902

Kondo, Y., & Kondo, S. (2006). Autophagy and cancer therapy. *Autophagy, 2*(2), Apr-Jun,pp. 85-90

Kwon, H. J., Heo, J. Y., Shim, J. H., Park, J. H., Seo, K. S., Ryu, M. J., Han, J. S., Shong, M., Son, J. H., & Kweon, G. R. (2011). DJ-1 mediates paraquat-induced dopaminergic neuronal cell death. *Toxicol Lett, 202*(2), Apr 25,pp. 85-92

Lam, Y. A., Lawson, T. G., Velayutham, M., Zweier, J. L., & Pickart, C. M. (2002). A proteasomal ATPase subunit recognizes the polyubiquitin degradation signal. *Nature, 416*(6882), Apr 18,pp. 763-767

Lavara-Culebras, E., & Paricio, N. (2007). Drosophila DJ-1 mutants are sensitive to oxidative stress and show reduced lifespan and motor deficits. *Gene, 400*(1-2), Oct 1,pp. 158-165

Leist, M., & Jaattela, M. (2001). Four deaths and a funeral: from caspases to alternative mechanisms. *Nat Rev Mol Cell Biol, 2*(8), Aug,pp. 589-598

Li, C. J., Friedman, D. J., Wang, C., Metelev, V., & Pardee, A. B. (1995). Induction of apoptosis in uninfected lymphocytes by HIV-1 Tat protein. *Science, 268*(5209), Apr 21,pp. 429-431

Li, X., & Sun, A. Y. (1999). Paraquat induced activation of transcription factor AP-1 and apoptosis in PC12 cells. *J Neural Transm, 106*(1), 1-21

Lin, W., & Kang, U. J. (2008). Characterization of PINK1 processing, stability, and subcellular localization. *J Neurochem, 106*(1), Jul,pp. 464-474

Lin, X., Parisiadou, L., Gu, X. L., Wang, L., Shim, H., Sun, L., Xie, C., Long, C. X., Yang, W. J., Ding, J., Chen, Z. Z., Gallant, P. E., Tao-Cheng, J. H., Rudow, G., Troncoso, J. C., Liu, Z., Li, Z., & Cai, H. (2009). Leucine-rich repeat kinase 2 regulates the progression of neuropathology induced by Parkinson's-disease-related mutant alpha-synuclein. *Neuron, 64*(6), Dec 24,pp. 807-827

Liochev, S. I., Hausladen, A., Beyer, W. F., Jr., & Fridovich, I. (1994). NADPH: ferredoxin oxidoreductase acts as a paraquat diaphorase and is a member of the soxRS regulon. *Proc Natl Acad Sci U S A, 91*(4), Feb 15,pp. 1328-1331

Liou, H. H., Tsai, M. C., Chen, C. J., Jeng, J. S., Chang, Y. C., Chen, S. Y., & Chen, R. C. (1997). Environmental risk factors and Parkinson's disease: a case-control study in Taiwan. *Neurology, 48*(6), Jun,pp. 1583-1588

Loo, D. T., Copani, A., Pike, C. J., Whittemore, E. R., Walencewicz, A. J., & Cotman, C. W. (1993). Apoptosis is induced by beta-amyloid in cultured central nervous system neurons. *Proc Natl Acad Sci U S A, 90*(17), Sep 1,pp. 7951-7955

Lum, J. J., Bauer, D. E., Kong, M., Harris, M. H., Li, C., Lindsten, T., & Thompson, C. B. (2005). Growth factor regulation of autophagy and cell survival in the absence of apoptosis. *Cell, 120*(2), Jan 28,pp. 237-248

Manning-Bog, A. B., McCormack, A. L., Li, J., Uversky, V. N., Fink, A. L., & Di Monte, D. A. (2002). The herbicide paraquat causes up-regulation and aggregation of alpha-synuclein in mice: paraquat and alpha-synuclein. *J Biol Chem, 277*(3), Jan 18,pp. 1641-1644

Martinez-Vicente, M., & Cuervo, A. M. (2007). Autophagy and neurodegeneration: when the cleaning crew goes on strike. *Lancet Neurol, 6*(4), Apr,pp. 352-361

Martinvalet, D., Zhu, P., & Lieberman, J. (2005). Granzyme A induces caspase-independent mitochondrial damage, a required first step for apoptosis. *Immunity, 22*(3), Mar,pp. 355-370

Masliah, E., Rockenstein, E., Veinbergs, I., Mallory, M., Hashimoto, M., Takeda, A., Sagara, Y., Sisk, A., & Mucke, L. (2000). Dopaminergic loss and inclusion body formation in alpha-synuclein mice: implications for neurodegenerative disorders. *Science, 287*(5456), Feb 18,pp. 1265-1269

Massey, A. C., Kaushik, S., Sovak, G., Kiffin, R., & Cuervo, A. M. (2006). Consequences of the selective blockage of chaperone-mediated autophagy. *Proc Natl Acad Sci U S A, 103*(15), Apr 11,pp. 5805-5810

Matsumine, H., Saito, M., Shimoda-Matsubayashi, S., Tanaka, H., Ishikawa, A., Nakagawa-Hattori, Y., Yokochi, M., Kobayashi, T., Igarashi, S., Takano, H., Sanpei, K., Koike, R., Mori, H., Kondo, T., Mizutani, Y., Schaffer, A. A., Yamamura, Y., Nakamura, S., Kuzuhara, S., Tsuji, S., & Mizuno, Y. (1997). Localization of a gene for an autosomal recessive form of juvenile Parkinsonism to chromosome 6q25.2-27. *Am J Hum Genet, 60*(3), Mar,pp. 588-596

Mattson, M. P. (2006). Neuronal life-and-death signaling, apoptosis, and neurodegenerative disorders. *Antioxid Redox Signal, 8*(11-12), Nov-Dec,pp. 1997-2006

McCarthy, S., Somayajulu, M., Sikorska, M., Borowy-Borowski, H., & Pandey, S. (2004). Paraquat induces oxidative stress and neuronal cell death; neuroprotection by water-soluble Coenzyme Q10. *Toxicol Appl Pharmacol, 201*(1), Nov 15,pp. 21-31

McCormack, A. L., Thiruchelvam, M., Manning-Bog, A. B., Thiffault, C., Langston, J. W., Cory-Slechta, D. A., & Di Monte, D. A. (2002). Environmental risk factors and Parkinson's disease: selective degeneration of nigral dopaminergic neurons caused by the herbicide paraquat. *Neurobiol Dis, 10*(2), Jul,pp. 119-127

McNaught, K. S., Olanow, C. W., Halliwell, B., Isacson, O., & Jenner, P. (2001). Failure of the ubiquitin-proteasome system in Parkinson's disease. *Nat Rev Neurosci, 2*(8), Aug,pp. 589-594

Menzies, F. M., Ravikumar, B., & Rubinsztein, D. C. (2006). Protective roles for induction of autophagy in multiple proteinopathies. *Autophagy, 2*(3), Jul-Sep,pp. 224-225

Menzies, F. M., Yenisetti, S. C., & Min, K. T. (2005). Roles of Drosophila DJ-1 in survival of dopaminergic neurons and oxidative stress. *Curr Biol, 15*(17), Sep 6,pp. 1578-1582

Meredith, G. E., Totterdell, S., Petroske, E., Santa Cruz, K., Callison, R. C., Jr., & Lau, Y. S. (2002). Lysosomal malfunction accompanies alpha-synuclein aggregation in a progressive mouse model of Parkinson's disease. *Brain Res, 956*(1), Nov 22,pp. 156-165

Miller, D. W., Ahmad, R., Hague, S., Baptista, M. J., Canet-Aviles, R., McLendon, C., Carter, D. M., Zhu, P. P., Stadler, J., Chandran, J., Klinefelter, G. R., Blackstone, C., & Cookson, M. R. (2003). L166P mutant DJ-1, causative for recessive Parkinson's disease, is degraded through the ubiquitin-proteasome system. *J Biol Chem, 278*(38), Sep 19,pp. 36588-36595

Mizushima, N., Yamamoto, A., Hatano, M., Kobayashi, Y., Kabeya, Y., Suzuki, K., Tokuhisa, T., Ohsumi, Y., & Yoshimori, T. (2001). Dissection of autophagosome formation using Apg5-deficient mouse embryonic stem cells. *J Cell Biol, 152*(4), Feb 19,pp. 657-668

Mollace, V., Iannone, M., Muscoli, C., Palma, E., Granato, T., Rispoli, V., Nistico, R., Rotiroti, D., & Salvemini, D. (2003). The role of oxidative stress in paraquat-induced neurotoxicity in rats: protection by non peptidyl superoxide dismutase mimetic. *Neurosci Lett, 335*(3), Jan 2,pp. 163-166

Moore, D. J., Zhang, L., Dawson, T. M., & Dawson, V. L. (2003). A missense mutation (L166P) in DJ-1, linked to familial Parkinson's disease, confers reduced protein stability and impairs homo-oligomerization. *J Neurochem, 87*(6), Dec,pp. 1558-1567

Moran, J. M., Gonzalez-Polo, R. A., Ortiz-Ortiz, M. A., Niso-Santano, M., Soler, G., & Fuentes, J. M. (2008). Identification of genes associated with paraquat-induced toxicity in SH-SY5Y cells by PCR array focused on apoptotic pathways. *J Toxicol Environ Health A, 71*(22), 1457-1467

Nagakubo, D., Taira, T., Kitaura, H., Ikeda, M., Tamai, K., Iguchi-Ariga, S. M., & Ariga, H. (1997). DJ-1, a novel oncogene which transforms mouse NIH3T3 cells in cooperation with ras. *Biochem Biophys Res Commun, 231*(2), Feb 13,pp. 509-513

Nakai, A., Yamaguchi, O., Takeda, T., Higuchi, Y., Hikoso, S., Taniike, M., Omiya, S., Mizote, I., Matsumura, Y., Asahi, M., Nishida, K., Hori, M., Mizushima, N., & Otsu, K. (2007). The role of autophagy in cardiomyocytes in the basal state and in response to hemodynamic stress. *Nat Med, 13*(5), May,pp. 619-624

Newhouse, K., Hsuan, S. L., Chang, S. H., Cai, B., Wang, Y., & Xia, Z. (2004). Rotenone-induced apoptosis is mediated by p38 and JNK MAP kinases in human dopaminergic SH-SY5Y cells. *Toxicol Sci, 79*(1), May,pp. 137-146

Ng, C. H., Mok, S. Z., Koh, C., Ouyang, X., Fivaz, M. L., Tan, E. K., Dawson, V. L., Dawson, T. M., Yu, F., & Lim, K. L. (2009). Parkin protects against LRRK2 G2019S mutant-induced dopaminergic neurodegeneration in Drosophila. *J Neurosci, 29*(36), Sep 9,pp. 11257-11262

Niso-Santano, M., Bravo-San Pedro, J. M., Gomez-Sanchez, R., Climent, V., Soler, G., Fuentes, J. M., & Gonzalez-Polo, R. A. (2011). ASK1 overexpression accelerates paraquat-induced autophagy via endoplasmic reticulum stress. *Toxicol Sci, 119*(1), Jan,pp. 156-168

Niso-Santano, M., Gonzalez-Polo, R. A., Bravo-San Pedro, J. M., Gomez-Sanchez, R., Lastres-Becker, I., Ortiz-Ortiz, M. A., Soler, G., Moran, J. M., Cuadrado, A., & Fuentes, J. M. (2010). Activation of apoptosis signal-regulating kinase 1 is a key factor in paraquat-induced cell death: modulation by the Nrf2/Trx axis. *Free Radic Biol Med, 48*(10), May 15,pp. 1370-1381

Niso-Santano, M., Moran, J. M., Garcia-Rubio, L., Gomez-Martin, A., Gonzalez-Polo, R. A., Soler, G., & Fuentes, J. M. (2006). Low concentrations of paraquat induces early activation of extracellular signal-regulated kinase 1/2, protein kinase B, and c-Jun N-terminal kinase 1/2 pathways: role of c-Jun N-terminal kinase in paraquat-induced cell death. *Toxicol Sci, 92*(2), Aug,pp. 507-515

Nixon, R. A., Wegiel, J., Kumar, A., Yu, W. H., Peterhoff, C., Cataldo, A., & Cuervo, A. M. (2005). Extensive involvement of autophagy in Alzheimer disease: an immuno-electron microscopy study. *J Neuropathol Exp Neurol, 64*(2), Feb,pp. 113-122

Norbury, C. J., & Hickson, I. D. (2001). Cellular responses to DNA damage. *Annu Rev Pharmacol Toxicol, 41*367-401

Norris, E. H., Uryu, K., Leight, S., Giasson, B. I., Trojanowski, J. Q., & Lee, V. M. (2007). Pesticide exposure exacerbates alpha-synucleinopathy in an A53T transgenic mouse model. *Am J Pathol, 170*(2), Feb,pp. 658-666

Olanow, C. W. (2007). The pathogenesis of cell death in Parkinson's disease--2007. *Mov Disord, 22 Suppl 17*Sep,pp. S335-342

Paisan-Ruiz, C., Jain, S., Evans, E. W., Gilks, W. P., Simon, J., van der Brug, M., Lopez de Munain, A., Aparicio, S., Gil, A. M., Khan, N., Johnson, J., Martinez, J. R., Nicholl, D., Carrera, I. M., Pena, A. S., de Silva, R., Lees, A., Marti-Masso, J. F., Perez-Tur, J., Wood, N. W., & Singleton, A. B. (2004). Cloning of the gene containing mutations that cause PARK8-linked Parkinson's disease. *Neuron, 44*(4), Nov 18,pp. 595-600

Pan, T., Kondo, S., Le, W., & Jankovic, J. (2008). The role of autophagy-lysosome pathway in neurodegeneration associated with Parkinson's disease. *Brain, 131*(Pt 8), Aug,pp. 1969-1978

Patel, M., Day, B. J., Crapo, J. D., Fridovich, I., & McNamara, J. O. (1996). Requirement for superoxide in excitotoxic cell death. *Neuron, 16*(2), Feb,pp. 345-355

Peng, J., Mao, X. O., Stevenson, F. F., Hsu, M., & Andersen, J. K. (2004). The herbicide paraquat induces dopaminergic nigral apoptosis through sustained activation of the JNK pathway. *J Biol Chem, 279*(31), Jul 30,pp. 32626-32632

Plowey, E. D., Cherra, S. J., 3rd, Liu, Y. J., & Chu, C. T. (2008). Role of autophagy in G2019S-LRRK2-associated neurite shortening in differentiated SH-SY5Y cells. *J Neurochem, 105*(3), May,pp. 1048-1056

Polymeropoulos, M. H., Lavedan, C., Leroy, E., Ide, S. E., Dehejia, A., Dutra, A., Pike, B., Root, H., Rubenstein, J., Boyer, R., Stenroos, E. S., Chandrasekharappa, S., Athanassiadou, A., Papapetropoulos, T., Johnson, W. G., Lazzarini, A. M., Duvoisin, R. C., Di Iorio, G., Golbe, L. I., & Nussbaum, R. L. (1997). Mutation in the alpha-synuclein gene identified in families with Parkinson's disease. *Science, 276*(5321), Jun 27,pp. 2045-2047

Prigione, A., Piazza, F., Brighina, L., Begni, B., Galbussera, A., Difrancesco, J. C., Andreoni, S., Piolti, R., & Ferrarese, C. (2010). Alpha-synuclein nitration and autophagy response are induced in peripheral blood cells from patients with Parkinson disease. *Neurosci Lett, 477*(1), Jun 14,pp. 6-10

Ravikumar, B., Berger, Z., Vacher, C., O'Kane, C. J., & Rubinsztein, D. C. (2006). Rapamycin pre-treatment protects against apoptosis. *Hum Mol Genet, 15*(7), Apr 1,pp. 1209-1216

Ravikumar, B., & Rubinsztein, D. C. (2004). Can autophagy protect against neurodegeneration caused by aggregate-prone proteins? *Neuroreport, 15*(16), Nov 15,pp. 2443-2445

Reddien, P. W., Cameron, S., & Horvitz, H. R. (2001). Phagocytosis promotes programmed cell death in C. elegans. *Nature, 412*(6843), Jul 12,pp. 198-202

Richardson, J. R., Quan, Y., Sherer, T. B., Greenamyre, J. T., & Miller, G. W. (2005). Paraquat neurotoxicity is distinct from that of MPTP and rotenone. *Toxicol Sci, 88*(1), Nov,pp. 193-201

Rideout, H. J., Lang-Rollin, I., & Stefanis, L. (2004). Involvement of macroautophagy in the dissolution of neuronal inclusions. *Int J Biochem Cell Biol, 36*(12), Dec,pp. 2551-2562

Ryu, E. J., Harding, H. P., Angelastro, J. M., Vitolo, O. V., Ron, D., & Greene, L. A. (2002). Endoplasmic reticulum stress and the unfolded protein response in cellular models of Parkinson's disease. *J Neurosci, 22*(24), Dec 15,pp. 10690-10698

Saha, S., Guillily, M. D., Ferree, A., Lanceta, J., Chan, D., Ghosh, J., Hsu, C. H., Segal, L., Raghavan, K., Matsumoto, K., Hisamoto, N., Kuwahara, T., Iwatsubo, T., Moore, L., Goldstein, L., Cookson, M., & Wolozin, B. (2009). LRRK2 modulates vulnerability to mitochondrial dysfunction in Caenorhabditis elegans. *J Neurosci, 29*(29), Jul 22,pp. 9210-9218

Sakai, M., Yamagami, K., Kitazawa, Y., Takeyama, N., & Tanaka, T. (1995). Xanthine oxidase mediates paraquat-induced toxicity on cultured endothelial cell. *Pharmacol Toxicol, 77*(1), Jul,pp. 36-40

Samann, J., Hegermann, J., von Gromoff, E., Eimer, S., Baumeister, R., & Schmidt, E. (2009). Caenorhabditits elegans LRK-1 and PINK-1 act antagonistically in stress response and neurite outgrowth. *J Biol Chem, 284*(24), Jun 12,pp. 16482-16491

Sapp, E., Schwarz, C., Chase, K., Bhide, P. G., Young, A. B., Penney, J., Vonsattel, J. P., Aronin, N., & DiFiglia, M. (1997). Huntingtin localization in brains of normal and Huntington's disease patients. *Ann Neurol, 42*(4), Oct,pp. 604-612

Sattler, T., & Mayer, A. (2000). Cell-free reconstitution of microautophagic vacuole invagination and vesicle formation. *J Cell Biol, 151*(3), Oct 30,pp. 529-538

Schapira, A. H., Cooper, J. M., Dexter, D., Jenner, P., Clark, J. B., & Marsden, C. D. (1989). Mitochondrial complex I deficiency in Parkinson's disease. *Lancet, 1*(8649), Jun 3,pp. 1269

Shimura, H., Hattori, N., Kubo, S., Mizuno, Y., Asakawa, S., Minoshima, S., Shimizu, N., Iwai, K., Chiba, T., Tanaka, K., & Suzuki, T. (2000). Familial Parkinson disease gene product, parkin, is a ubiquitin-protein ligase. *Nat Genet, 25*(3), Jul,pp. 302-305

Shin, N., Jeong, H., Kwon, J., Heo, H. Y., Kwon, J. J., Yun, H. J., Kim, C. H., Han, B. S., Tong, Y., Shen, J., Hatano, T., Hattori, N., Kim, K. S., Chang, S., & Seol, W. (2008). LRRK2 regulates synaptic vesicle endocytosis. *Exp Cell Res, 314*(10), Jun 10,pp. 2055-2065

Smith, J. G. (1988). Paraquat poisoning by skin absorption: a review. *Hum Toxicol, 7*(1), Jan,pp. 15-19

Smith, W. W., Pei, Z., Jiang, H., Moore, D. J., Liang, Y., West, A. B., Dawson, V. L., Dawson, T. M., & Ross, C. A. (2005). Leucine-rich repeat kinase 2 (LRRK2) interacts with parkin, and mutant LRRK2 induces neuronal degeneration. *Proc Natl Acad Sci U S A, 102*(51), Dec 20,pp. 18676-18681

Song, C., Kanthasamy, A., Jin, H., Anantharam, V., & Kanthasamy, A. G. Paraquat induces epigenetic changes by promoting histone acetylation in cell culture models of dopaminergic degeneration. *Neurotoxicology*Jul 12,pp.

Sperandio, S., de Belle, I., & Bredesen, D. E. (2000). An alternative, nonapoptotic form of programmed cell death. *Proc Natl Acad Sci U S A, 97*(26), Dec 19,pp. 14376-14381

Spillantini, M. G., Schmidt, M. L., Lee, V. M., Trojanowski, J. Q., Jakes, R., & Goedert, M. (1997). Alpha-synuclein in Lewy bodies. *Nature, 388*(6645), Aug 28,pp. 839-840

Suzuki, K., Kirisako, T., Kamada, Y., Mizushima, N., Noda, T., & Ohsumi, Y. (2001). The pre-autophagosomal structure organized by concerted functions of APG genes is essential for autophagosome formation. *EMBO J, 20*(21), Nov 1,pp. 5971-5981

Tanner, C. M., Kamel, F., Ross, G. W., Hoppin, J. A., Goldman, S. M., Korell, M., Marras, C., Bhudhikanok, G. S., Kasten, M., Chade, A. R., Comyns, K., Richards, M. B., Meng, C., Priestley, B., Fernandez, H. H., Cambi, F., Umbach, D. M., Blair, A., Sandler, D. P., & Langston, J. W. (2011). Rotenone, paraquat, and Parkinson's disease. *Environ Health Perspect, 119*(6), Jun,pp. 866-872

Trojanowski, J. Q., & Lee, V. M. (2000). "Fatal attractions" of proteins. A comprehensive hypothetical mechanism underlying Alzheimer's disease and other neurodegenerative disorders. *Ann N Y Acad Sci, 92*462-67

Uversky, V. N., Li, J., & Fink, A. L. (2001). Pesticides directly accelerate the rate of alpha-synuclein fibril formation: a possible factor in Parkinson's disease. *FEBS Lett, 500*(3), Jul 6,pp. 105-108

Valente, E. M., Salvi, S., Ialongo, T., Marongiu, R., Elia, A. E., Caputo, V., Romito, L., Albanese, A., Dallapiccola, B., & Bentivoglio, A. R. (2004). PINK1 mutations are associated with sporadic early-onset parkinsonism. *Ann Neurol, 56*(3), Sep,pp. 336-341

Venderova, K., Kabbach, G., Abdel-Messih, E., Zhang, Y., Parks, R. J., Imai, Y., Gehrke, S., Ngsee, J., Lavoie, M. J., Slack, R. S., Rao, Y., Zhang, Z., Lu, B., Haque, M. E., & Park,

D. S. (2009). Leucine-Rich Repeat Kinase 2 interacts with Parkin, DJ-1 and PINK-1 in a Drosophila melanogaster model of Parkinson's disease. *Hum Mol Genet, 18*(22), Nov 15,pp. 4390-4404

Walls, K. C., Ghosh, A. P., Franklin, A. V., Klocke, B. J., Ballestas, M., Shacka, J. J., Zhang, J., & Roth, K. A. (2010). Lysosome dysfunction triggers Atg7-dependent neural apoptosis. *J Biol Chem, 285*(14), Apr 2,pp. 10497-10507

Wang, C., Ko, H. S., Thomas, B., Tsang, F., Chew, K. C., Tay, S. P., Ho, M. W., Lim, T. M., Soong, T. W., Pletnikova, O., Troncoso, J., Dawson, V. L., Dawson, T. M., & Lim, K. L. (2005). Stress-induced alterations in parkin solubility promote parkin aggregation and compromise parkin's protective function. *Hum Mol Genet, 14*(24), Dec 15,pp. 3885-3897

Wang, D., Tang, B., Zhao, G., Pan, Q., Xia, K., Bodmer, R., & Zhang, Z. (2008). Dispensable role of Drosophila ortholog of LRRK2 kinase activity in survival of dopaminergic neurons. *Mol Neurodegener, 33*

West, A. B., Moore, D. J., Biskup, S., Bugayenko, A., Smith, W. W., Ross, C. A., Dawson, V. L., & Dawson, T. M. (2005). Parkinson's disease-associated mutations in leucine-rich repeat kinase 2 augment kinase activity. *Proc Natl Acad Sci U S A, 102*(46), Nov 15,pp. 16842-16847

Worth, A., Thrasher, A. J., & Gaspar, H. B. (2006). Autoimmune lymphoproliferative syndrome: molecular basis of disease and clinical phenotype. *Br J Haematol, 133*(2), Apr,pp. 124-140

Yang, W., Chen, L., Ding, Y., Zhuang, X., & Kang, U. J. (2007). Paraquat induces dopaminergic dysfunction and proteasome impairment in DJ-1-deficient mice. *Hum Mol Genet, 16*(23), Dec 1,pp. 2900-2910

Yang, W., & Tiffany-Castiglioni, E. (2007). The bipyridyl herbicide paraquat induces proteasome dysfunction in human neuroblastoma SH-SY5Y cells. *J Toxicol Environ Health A, 70*(21), Nov,pp. 1849-1857

Yang, W., & Tiffany-Castiglioni, E. (2008). Paraquat-induced apoptosis in human neuroblastoma SH-SY5Y cells: involvement of p53 and mitochondria. *J Toxicol Environ Health A, 71*(4), 289-299

Yang, W., Tiffany-Castiglioni, E., Koh, H. C., & Son, I. H. (2009). Paraquat activates the IRE1/ASK1/JNK cascade associated with apoptosis in human neuroblastoma SH-SY5Y cells. *Toxicol Lett, 191*(2-3), Dec 15,pp. 203-210

Zeiss, C. J. (2003). The apoptosis-necrosis continuum: insights from genetically altered mice. *Vet Pathol, 40*(5), Sep,pp. 481-495

Zheng, L., Marcusson, J., & Terman, A. (2006). Oxidative stress and Alzheimer disease: the autophagy connection? *Autophagy, 2*(2), Apr-Jun,pp. 143-145

Zimprich, A., Biskup, S., Leitner, P., Lichtner, P., Farrer, M., Lincoln, S., Kachergus, J., Hulihan, M., Uitti, R. J., Calne, D. B., Stoessl, A. J., Pfeiffer, R. F., Patenge, N., Carbajal, I. C., Vieregge, P., Asmus, F., Muller-Myhsok, B., Dickson, D. W., Meitinger, T., Strom, T. M., Wszolek, Z. K., & Gasser, T. (2004). Mutations in LRRK2 cause autosomal-dominant parkinsonism with pleomorphic pathology. *Neuron, 44*(4), Nov 18,pp. 601-607

12

Prediction of Toxicity, Sensory Responses and Biological Responses with the Abraham Model

William E. Acree, Jr.[1], Laura M. Grubbs[1] and Michael H. Abraham[2]
[1]*University of North Texas,*
[2]*University College London,*
[1]*United States*
[2]*United Kingdom*

1. Introduction

Modern drug testing and design includes experimental *in vivo* and *in vitro* measurements, combined with *in silico* computations that enable prediction of the drug candidate's ADMET (adsorption, distribution, metabolism, elimination and toxicity) properties in the initial stages of drug discovery. Recent estimates place the discovery and development cost of a small drug molecule close to US $1.3 billion, from the time of conception to the time when the drug finally reaches the market place. Less than one-fourth of conceived drug candidates proceed to clinical trial stage testing, and of the compounds that enter clinical development less than one-tenth actually receive government approval. Reasons for the low success percentage include poor efficacy, low solubility, unsatisfactory bioavailability, unfavorable pharmacokinetic properties, toxicity concerns and drug-drug interactions, degradation and poor shelf-life stability. Unfavorable pharmacokinetic and ADME properties, toxicity and adverse side effects account for up to two-thirds of drug failures.

Safety evaluation of drug candidates is crucial in the early stages of drug discovery and development. For drug development, safety requires that the potential drug molecule have sufficient selectivity for the desired target receptor so that an adequate dose range can be found where the intended pharmacological action is essentially the only physiological effect exhibited by the drug candidate. Pharmaceutical compounds often exhibit the desired therapeutic action at one concentration range, but may be quite toxic or even lethal at higher dosages and concentrations. Drug induced liver injury (DILI) is the most frequent reason for discontinuation of new drug candidates. Drug-induced liver injuries are classified as predicted/intrinsic or idiosyncratic depending upon whether the injury is dose dependent. Predictable DILIs are dose-dependent, and the injury is largely reversible once the medication is discontinued. Idiosyncratic DILIs, on the other hand, are independent of drug dosage level and believed to be related in part to individual's hypersensitivity or immune system reactions to the medication. Idiosyncratic DILIs depend upon the individual's potential genetic and epigenetic constitution, and immunological responses (Ozer *et al.*, 2010). Examples of drug and/or drug candidates that either failed in late stage clinical testing or were removed from the market because of drug-induced liver injury concerns include: ximelagatran (an anticoagulant that was promoted extensively as a replacement for warfarin, withdrawn in from US market in 2006); troglitazone (an anti-diabetic and anti-inflammatory drug, withdrawn from the UK market in 1997 and US market in 2000); ebrotidine (an H2-reciptor antagonist, marketed in Spain in 1997, withdrawn from the market in 1998); ticrynafen (a diuretic drug used in treatment of hypertension, withdrawn from US market in 1979); benoxaprofen (a nonsteroidal anti-inflammatory drug, withdrawn from US market in 1982); ibufenac (nonsteroidal anti-inflammatory drug used for the treatment of Rheumatoid arithritis, withdrawn from UK market in 1970) and bromfenac (a nonsteroidal anti-inflammatory drug introduced in 1997 as a short-term analgesic for orthopedic pain, withdrawn from the market in 1998) (Lamment *et al.*, 2008; Andrade *et al.*, 1999; Goldkind and Laine, 2006). Other drugs, such as valproic acid, ketoconazole, nicotinic acid, rifampin, chlorzoxazone, isoniazid, dantrolene, nefazodone, telethromycin, nevirapine, atomoxetine and inflixmab have received strong heptatoxicity warnings from the U.S. Food and Drug Administration (Lamment *et al.*, 2008). Sibutramine and phenylpropanolamine, used in the treatment of obesity, were removed from the U.S. market due to adverse effects associated with cardiovascular disease and hemorrhagic stroke, respectively. (Chaput and Tremblay, 2010). Additional drugs withdrawn from the market for cardiovascular toxicities and concerns include: rotecoxib (used to relieve acute pain and symptoms of chronic inflammation, removed from market in 2005) and valdecoxib (used to relieve acute pain and symptoms of chronic inflammation, removed from market in 2005) (Shi and Klotz, 2008).

Toxicity screening identifies drug candidates that exhibit predictable/intrinsic drug-induced liver injury. Idiosyncratic DILI occurs infrequently and only in treated patients which are highly susceptible to the given pharmaceutical compound. Conventional preclinical safety testing is not the best method to detect idiosyncratic DILI. Fourches and coworkers (2010) examined the possibility of using laboratory test animals as viable means to screen drug candidates for possible drug-induced liver injuries. The authors compiled a data set of 951 compounds reported to induce a wide range of liver effects in humans and in different animal species. Of the 951 compounds considered, 650 had been identified as causing liver effects in humans, 685 had been reported in the literature as causing liver effects in rodents, and only 166 had shown liver effects in nonrodents. The concordance between two species, CONC(species A, species) was defined as

$$CONC(species\,A + species B) = \frac{(Toxic\ for\, both\, A\, and\, B) + (Nontoxic\ for\, both\, A\, and\, B)}{Total\, number\ of\ compounds\, studied} \quad (1)$$

as the number of compounds that exhibited toxicity for both animal species plus the number of compounds that showed notoxicity for both animal species divided by the total number of compounds considered. Equation 1 was applied to the liver effect data gathered from the published literature. The authors found a relatively low concordance of between 39 % to 44 % between different species - for human + rodents the concordance was equal to 44.2 % ((402 + 18)/951); and for human + nonrodents that concordance was equal to 39.9 % ((122+257)/951). Animal testing, while informative, does not necessarily provide an accurate indication of the pharmaceutical compound's likelihood to produce a liver effect in humans. For the concordance calculations it was assumed that the pharmaceutical compound had been tested on all three species groups. The above calculations further underscore the importance of finding suitable testing methods and models for use in drug discovery.

Drug safety considerations also include unwanted side effects, and the impact that the pharmaceutical product will have on environment. A significant fraction of the pharmaceutically-active compounds sold each year find their way into the environment as the result of human/animal urine and feces excretion (excreted unchanged drugs or as drug metabolites), direct disposal of unused household drugs by flushing into sewage systems, accidental spills and releases from manufacturing production sites, and underground leakage from municipal sewage systems and infrastructures. Dietrich and coworkers (2010) recently examined the environmental impact that four pharmaceutical compounds (carbamazepine, diclofenac, 17α-ethinylestradiol and metoprolol) had on the growth and reproduction of *Daphnia Magna* after exposure to the individual drugs and drug mixtures at environmentally relevant concentrations. The authors found that effects were still detectable even several generations after first exposure to the pharmaceutical compound. The *Daphnia Magna* had not developed complete resistance to the compound. In the case of metoprolol, both the body length of the females at first reproduction and the number of offspring per female were significantly less than the control group. The same body length pattern was observed for females in the third and fourth generations. No difference in female body length was observed in the first, second and fifth generations. The number of offspring per female was also reduced for the fourth generation. Experimental data further revealed that drugs acting in combination can lead to impairments that are not predicted by the response to single substances alone. The authors noted that aquatic organisms may not evolve a total resistance to pharmaceuticals in natural aquatic systems, presumably due to high fitness costs. One cannot exclude the potential long-term harmful effects that pharmaceuticals might have on the environment. The Chapter will focus on the predicting the toxicity, sensory response and biological response of organic and drug molecules using the Abraham solvation parameter model.

2. Abraham solvation parameter model

The Abraham general solvation model is one of the more useful approaches for the analysis and prediction of the adsorption, distribution and toxicological properties of potential drug candidates. The method relies on two linear free energy relationships (lfers), one for transfer processes occurring within condensed phases (Abraham, 1993a,b; Abraham *et al.*, 2004):

$$SP = c + e \cdot \mathbf{E} + s \cdot \mathbf{S} + a \cdot \mathbf{A} + b \cdot \mathbf{B} + v \cdot \mathbf{V} \tag{2}$$

and one for processes involving gas-to-condensed phase transfer

$$SP = c + e \cdot \mathbf{E} + s \cdot \mathbf{S} + a \cdot \mathbf{A} + b \cdot \mathbf{B} + l \cdot \mathbf{L} \tag{3}$$

The dependent variable, SP, is some property of a series of solutes in a fixed phase, which in the present study will include the logarithm of drug's water-to-organic solvent (log P) and blood-to-tissue partition coefficients, the logarithm of the drug's molar solubility in an organic solvent divided by its aqueous molar solubility (log $C_{solute,org}/C_{solute,water}$), the logarithm of the drug's plasma-to-milk partition coefficient, percent human intestinal absorption and the logarithm of the kinetic constant for human intestinal absorption, and the logarithm of the human skin permeability coefficient (log k_p). The independent variables, or descriptors, are solute properties as follows: **E** and **S** refer to the excess molar refraction and dipolarity/polarizability descriptors of the solute, respectively, **A** and **B** are measures of the solute hydrogen-bond acidity and basicity, **V** is the McGowan volume of the solute and **L** is the logarithm of the solute gas phase dimensionless Ostwald partition coefficient into hexadecane at 298 K. For a number of partitions into solvents that contain large amounts of water at saturation, an alternative hydrogen bond basicity parameter, $\mathbf{B}^o$, is used for specific classes of solute: alkylpyridines, alkylanilines, and sulfoxides. Several of the published Abraham model equations for predicting the toxicity of organic compounds to different aquatic organisms use the $\mathbf{B}^o$ solute descriptor, rather than the **B** descriptor.

Equations 1 and 2 contain the following three quantities: (a) measured solute properties; (b) calculated solute descriptors; and (c) calculated equation coefficients. Knowledge of any two quantities permits calculation of the third quantity through the solving of simultaneous equations and regression analysis. Solute descriptors are calculated from measured partition coefficient ($P_{solute,system}$), chromatographic retention factor (k′) and molar solubility ($C_{solute,solvent}$) data for the solutes dissolved in partitioning systems and in organic solvents having known equation coefficients. Generally partition coefficient, chromatographic retention factor and molar solubility measurements are fairly accurate, and it is good practice to base the solute descriptor computations on observed values having minimal experimental uncertainty. The computation is depicted graphically in Figure 1 by the unidirectional arrows that indicate the direction of the calculation using the known equation coefficients that connect the measured and solute descriptors. Measured $P_{solute,system}$ and $C_{solute,solvent}$ values yield solute descriptors. The unidirectional red arrows originating from the center solute descriptor circle represent the equation coefficients that have been reported for nasal pungency, aquatic toxicity, upper respiratory irritation and inhalation anesthesia Abraham model correlations. Plasma-to-milk partition ratio predictions are achieved (Abraham *et al.*, 2009a) through an artificial neural network with five inputs, 14 nodes in the hidden layer and one node in the output layer. Linear analysis of the plasma-to-milk partition ratios for 179 drugs and hydrophobic environmental pollutants revealed that drug molecules preferentially partition into the aqueous and protein phases of milk. Hydrophobic environmental pollutants, on the other hand, partition into the fat phase.

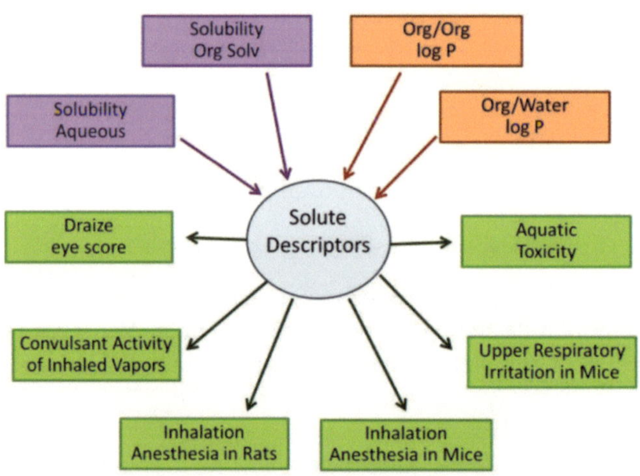

Fig. 1. Outline illustrating the calculation of Abraham solute descriptors from experimental partition coefficient and solubility data, and then using the calculated values to estimate sensory and biological responses, such as toxicity of organic chemicals to aquatic organisms, Draize eye scores, convulsant activity of inhaled vapors, upper respiratory irritation in mice, and inhalation anesthesia in rats and mice.

Prediction of the fore-mentioned toxicities, and sensory and biological responses does require a prior knowledge of the Abraham solute descriptors for the drug candidate of interest. The descriptors **E** and **V** are quite easily obtained. **V** can be calculated from atom and bond contributions as outlined previously (Abraham and McGowan, 1987). The atom contributions are given in Table 1; note that the numerical values are in $cm^3\ mol^{-1}$. A value of 6.56 $cm^3\ mol^{-1}$ is subtracted for each bond in the molecule; irrespective of whether the bond is a single, double or triple bond. For complicated molecules it is time consuming to count the number of bonds, Bn, but this can be calculated from the algorithm given by Abraham (1993a)

$$Bn = Nt - 1 + R \quad (4)$$

where Nt is the total number of atoms in the molecule and R is the number of rings.

C	16.35		N	14.39		O	12.43
Si	26.83		P	24.87		S	22.91
Ge	31.02		As	29.42		Se	27.81
Sn	39.35		Sb	37.74		Te	36.14
Pb	43.44		Bi	42.19			
H	8.71		He	6.76		B	18.32
F	10.48		Ne	8.51		Hg	34.00
Cl	20.95		Ar	19.00			
Br	26.21		Kr	24.60			
I	34.53		Xe	32.90			
			Rn	38.40			

Table 1. Atom contributions to the McGowan volume, in $cm^3\ mol^{-1}$

Once **V** is available, **E** can be obtained from the compound refractive index at 20°C. If the compound is not liquid at room temperature or if the refractive index is not known the latter can be calculated using the freeware software of Advanced Chemistry Development (ACD). An Excel spreadsheet for the calculation of V and E from refractive index is available from the authors. Since E is almost an additive property, it can also be obtained by the summation of fragments, either by hand, or through a commercial software program (ADME Boxes, 2010). The remaining four descriptors **S**, **A**, **B**, and **L** can be determined by regression analysis of experimental water-to-organic solvent partition coefficient data, chromatographic retention factor data, and molar solubility data in accordance to Eqns 1 and 2. Solute descriptors are available for more than 4,000 organic, organometallic and inorganic solutes. Large compilations are available in one published review article (Abraham *et al.*, 1993a), and in the supporting material that has accompanied several of our published papers (Abraham *et al.*, 2006; Abraham *et al.*, 2009b; Mintz *et al.*, 2007).

Experimental data-based solute descriptors have been obtained for a number of pharmaceutical compounds, for example 230 compounds in an analysis of blood-brain distribution (Abraham et al., 2006). Zissimos *et al.* (2002a) calculated the **S**, **A** and **B** solute descriptors of thirteen pharmaceutical compounds (propranolol, tetracaine, papaverine, trytamine, diclorfenac, chloropromazine, ibuprofen, lidocaine, deprenyl, desipramine, fluoxetine, procaine, and miconazole) from measured water-to-octanol, water-to-chloroform, water-to-cyclohexane and water-to-toluene partition coefficient data. Equation coefficients for the four water-to-organic solvent partition coefficients were known. Four mathematical methods based on the Microsoft Solver Progam, the Triplex Program, Descfit/SIMPLEX minimization and Reverse Regression were investigated. The authors (Zissimos *et al.*, 2002b) later illustrated the calculation methods using experimental data from seven high performance liquid chromatographic systems. Solute descriptors of acetylsalicylic acid (Charlton *et al.*, 2003), naproxen (Daniels *et al.*, 2004a), ketoprofen (Daniels *et al.*, 2004b) and ibuprofen (Stovall *et al.*, 2005) have been calculated based on the measured solubilities of the respective drugs in water and in organic solvents.

Abraham model correlations for predicting blood-to-body organ/tissue partition coefficients and the chemical toxicity of organic compounds towards aquatic organisms involve chemical transfer between two condensed phases. Predictive expressions for such solute properties do not contain the Abraham model L solute descriptor. There are however published Abraham model correlations for estimating important sensory and biology responses (such as convulsant activity of inhaled vapors, upper respiratory irritation in mice, inhalation anesthesia in rats and in mice) that do involve solute transfer from the gas phase. To calculate the L solute descriptor one must convert water-to-organic solvent partition coefficient data, P, into gas-to-organic solvent partition coefficients, K,

$$\text{Log K} = \log \text{P} + \log \text{K}_w \tag{5}$$

and water-to-organic solvent solubility ratios, $C_{solute,organic}/C_{solute,water}$, into gas-to-organic solvent solubility ratios, $C_{solute,organic}/C_{solute,gas}$,

$$C_{solute,organic}/C_{solute,gas} = C_{solute,organic}/C_{solute,water} * C_{solute,water}/C_{solute,gas} \tag{6}$$

where $C_{solute,water}/C_{solute,gas}$ is the gas-to-water partition coefficient, usually denoted as K_w. The water-to-organic solvent and gas-to-organic solvent partition coefficient equations are combined in the solute descriptor computations. If log K_w is not known, it can be used as another parameter to be determined. This increases the number of unknowns from four (**S**, **A**, **B** and **L**) to five (**S**, **A**, **B**, **L**, and K_w), but the number of equations is increased significantly as well. Numerical values of the four solute descriptors and K_w can be easily calculated Microsoft Solver. The computations are described in greater detail elsewhere (Abraham *et al.*, 2004; Abraham *et al.*, 2010). The calculated value of the L descriptor can be checked against an Abraham model correlation for estimating the L solute descriptor

$$\mathbf{L} = -\,0.882 + 1.183\,\mathbf{E} + 0.839\,\mathbf{S} + 0.454\,\mathbf{A} + 0.157\,\mathbf{B} + 3.505\,\mathbf{V} \tag{7}$$

$$(N = 4785, SD = 0.31, R^2 = 0.992, F = 115279)$$

from known values of **E, S, A, B** and **V**. Van Noort *et al.* (2010) cited a personnel communication from Dr. Abraham as the source of Eqn. 7. If one is unable to locate sufficient experimental data for performing the fore-mentioned regression analysis, commercial software (ADME Boxes, version*, 2010) is available for estimating the molecular solute descriptors from the structure of the compound. Several correlations (Jover *et al.*, 2004; Zissimos *et al.*, 2002; Lamarche *et al.*, 2001; Platts *et al.*, 1999; Platts *et al.*, 2000) have been reported for calculating the Abraham solute descriptors from the more structure-based, topological-based and/or quantum-based descriptors used in other QSAR and LFER treatments.

3. Presence and toxicity of pharmaceutical compounds in the environment

A significant fraction of the pharmaceutically-active compounds sold each year find their way into the environment as the result of human/animal urine and feces excretion (excreted unchanged drugs or as drug metabolites), direct disposal of unused household drugs by flushing into sewage systems, accidental spills and releases from manufacturing production sites, and underground leakage from municipal sewage systems and infrastructures. While most pharmaceutical compounds are designed to target specific metabolic pathways in humans and domestic animals, their action on non-target organisms may become detrimental even at very low concentrations. The occurrence of pharmaceutical residues and metabolites in the environment is a significant public and scientific concern. If not addressed, pharmaceutical pollution will become even a bigger problem as the world's increasing and aging population purchases more prescription and more self-prescribed over-the-counter medicines to improve the quality of life.

There have been very few published studies that have attempted to estimate the quantity of each pharmaceutical compound that will be released each year into the environment. Escher and coworkers (2011) evaluated the ecotoxicological potential of the 100 pharmaceutical compounds expected to occur in highest concentration in the wastewater effluent from both a general hospital and a psychiatric center in Switzerland. The authors based the calculated drug concentrations on the hospital's records of the drugs administered in 2007, the number of patients admitted, the days of hospital care, and the water usage records for the main hospital wing that houses patients and here pharmaceuticals are excreted. Amounts of the active drugs excreted unchanged in urine and feces were based on published excretion rates taken from the pharmaceutical literature. Table 2 gives the usage pattern of 25 pharmaceutical compounds, expressed as predicted effluent concentration in the hospital wastewater. The predicted concentration is compared to compound's estimated baseline toxicity towards green algae (*Pseudokirchneriella subcapitata*), which was calculated from Eqn. 8

$$-\text{Log } EC_{50} \text{ (Molar)} = 0.95 \log D_{\text{lipw(at pH = 7)}} + 1.53 \tag{8}$$

using the drug molecule's water-to-lipid partition coefficient measured at an aqueous phase pH of 7. The "baseline" concentration would be the concentration of the pharmaceutical compound needed for the toxicity endpoint to be observed assuming a nonspecific narcosis mechanism. In the case of the green algae, the toxicity endpoint corresponds to the molar concentration of the tested drug substance at which the cell density, biomass, or O_2 production is 50 % of that of the untreated algae after a 72 to 96 hour exposure to the drug.

The authors also reported predictive equations for estimating the baseline median lethal concentration for fish (*Pimephales promelas*, 96-hr endpoint)

$$-\text{Log } LC_{50} \text{ (Molar)} = 0.81 \log D_{\text{lipw(at pH = 7)}} + 1.65 \tag{9}$$

and the baseline effective concentration for mobility inhibition for water fleas (*Daphnia magna*, 48-hr. endpoint)

$$-\text{Log } EC_{50} \text{ (Molar)} = 0.90 \log D_{\text{lipw(at pH = 7)}} + 1.61 \tag{10}$$

Pharmaceutical Compound	PEC_{HWW} (µg/L)	$PNEC_{HWW}$ (µg/L)	PEC versus PNEC
Amiodarone	0.80	0.009	PEC Greater
Clotrimazole	0.90	0.014	PEC Greater
Trionavir	1.00	0.028	PEC Greater
Progesterone	15.85	1.40	PEC Greater
Meclozine	0.77	0.12	PEC Greater
Atorvastatin	0.99	0.16	PEC Greater
Isoflurane	94	29.8	PEC Greater
Tribenoside	0.79	0.26	PEC Greater
Ibuprofen	11.40	6.60	PEC Greater
Clopidogrel	1.74	1.60	PEC Greater
Amoxicillin	499	625	PEC Smaller
Diclofenac	2.35	3.30	PEC Smaller
Floxacillin	38.9	233	PEC Smaller
Salicylic acid	17.2	134	PEC Smaller
Paracetamol	64	583	PEC Smaller
Thiopental	21	201	PEC Smaller
Oxazepam	1.84	32	PEC Smaller
Clarithromycin	5.41	122	PEC Smaller
Rifampicin	0.59	16	PEC Smaller
Tramadol	1.92	57	PEC Smaller
Carbazmazepine	0.50	18	PEC Smaller
Tetracaine	0.48	18	PEC Smaller
Metoclopramide	3.27	136	PEC Smaller
Prednisolone	2.10	139	PEC Smaller
Erythomycin	1.40	132	PEC Smaller

Table 2. Predicted Effluent Concentration of Pharmaceutical Compounds in the Wastewater of a General Hospital, PEC_{HWW} (in µg/L) and the Predicted No Effect Concentration of the Pharmaceutical Compound to Green Algae, $PNEC_{HWW}$ (in µg/L)

Pharmaceutical Compound	PEC_{HWW} (μg/L)	$PNEC_{HWW}$ (μg/L)	PEC versus PNEC
Ritonavir	0.86	0.03	PEC Greater
Clotrimazole	0.39	0.01	PEC Greater
Diclofenac	73.0	3.31	PEC Greater
Mefanamic acid	5.38	0.78	PEC Greater
Lopinavir	0.26	0.05	PEC Greater
Nefinavir	0.71	0.16	PEC Greater
Ibuprofen	26.3	6.62	PEC Greater
Clorprothixen	2.53	0.91	PEC Greater
Trimipramine	0.63	0.49	PEC Greater
Meclozin	0.11	0.12	PEC Smaller
Nevirapine	0.98	1.30	PEC Smaller
Venlafaxine	24.6	35.5	PEC Smaller
Promazine	1.67	2.70	PEC Smaller
Olanazpine	8.41	14.9	PEC Smaller
Levomepromazine	1.15	2.40	PEC Smaller
Clopidogrel	0.72	1.60	PEC Smaller
Methadone	3.75	10.5	PEC Smaller
Carbamazepine	5.00	17.7	PEC Smaller
Oxazepam	7.24	32.5	PEC Smaller
Hexitidine	0.21	1.00	PEC Smaller
Duloxetine	0.38	2.30	PEC Smaller
Valproate	4.05	51	PEC Smaller
Fluoxetine	0.54	6.90	PEC Smaller
Lamotrigine	0.65	8.70	PEC Smaller
Clozapine	0.97	16	PEC Smaller
Diazepam	0.48	10	PEC Smaller
Tramadol	2.60	57	PEC Smaller
Pravastatin	3.39	77	PEC Smaller
Amoxacillin	22.8	625	PEC Smaller
Doxepin	0.17	4.90	PEC Smaller
Citolopram	0.51	17	PEC Smaller
Paracetamol	9.61	583	PEC Smaller
Clomethiazole	0.28	23	PEC Smaller

Table 3. Predicted Effluent Concentration of Pharmaceutical Compounds in the Wastewater of a Psychiatric Hospital, PEC_{HWW} (in μg/L) and the Predicted No Effect Concentration of the Pharmaceutical Compound to Green Algae, $PNEC_{HWW}$ (in μg/L)

Most published baseline toxicity QSAR models were derived for neutral organic molecules and require the water-to-octanol partition coefficient, $K_{o/w}$ as the input parameter. For compounds that can ionize, the water-to-octanol partition coefficient is an unsuitable measure of bioaccumulation and chemical uptake into biomembranes, the target site for baseline toxicants. Of the 10 of 25 pharmaceutical compounds listed in Table 2 have a predicted effluent concentration greater predicted no effect value, PNEC value. These 10 compounds would be expected to exhibit toxicity towards the green algae if the algae where exposed to the hospital wastewater for 72 to 96 hours. The drug concentrations in the hospital wastewater would be significantly reduced once the effluent entered the general sewer system. Table 3 provides the predicted effluent concentration and calculated PNEC values of 33 pharmaceutical expected to be present in the wastewater from a psychiatric hospital. The pharmaceutical concentrations were based on hospital records of the 2,008 patients who received 70,855 days of stationary care treatment. Many of the individuals who received treatment had acute psychiatric disorders that required strong medication. Nine of the 33 drugs listed have predicted effluent concentrations in excess of the PNEC value for green algae. Readers are reminded that the "baseline" concentration assumes a nonspecific narcosis mechanism, and that if the compound exhibits a reactive or other specific mode of toxic mechanism, the concentration would be much less.

Since 1980, the U.S. Food and Drug Administration has required that environmental risk assessments be conducted on pharmaceutical compounds intended for human and veterinary use before the product can be marketed. Similar regulations were introduced by the European Union in 1997. The environmental impact tests are generally short-term studies that focus predominately on mortality as the toxicity endpoint for fish, daphnids, algae, plants, bacteria, earthworms, and select invertebrates (Khetan and Colins, 2007). There have been very few experimental studies directed towards determining the no effect concentration (NEC) of pharmaceutical compounds, and even fewer studies involving mixtures of pharmaceutical compounds. The limited experimental data available shows that the NEC is highly dependent upon animal and/or organism type, and on the specific endpoint being considered. For example, the NEC for ibuprofen for 21 day growth for freshwater gastropod (*Planorbis carinatus*) is 1.02 mg/L; the NEC for 21 day reproduction for *Daphnia magna* is less than 1.23 mg/L; the NEC for 30 day survival of Japanese medaka (*Oryzias latipes*) is 0.1 mg/L; the NEC for 90 day survival of Japanese medaka is 0.1 μg/L. Mortality due to ibuprofen exposure was found to increase as the medaka fish matured (Han *et al.*, 2010). More experimental NEC data is needed in order to properly perform environmental risk analyses. Until such data becomes available, one must rely on whatever acute toxicity data that one find and on *in silico* methods that allow one to predict missing experimental values from molecular structure considerations and from easy to measure physical properties.

4. Abraham model: Prediction of environmental toxicity of pharmaceutical compounds

Significant quantities of pharmaceutical drugs and personal healthcare products are discarded each year. The discarded chemicals find their way into the environment, and many end up in the natural waterways where they can have an adverse effect on marine life and other aquatic organisms. Standard test methods and experimental protocols have been established for determining the median mortality lethal concentration, LC_{50}, for evaluating the chronic toxicity, for determining decreased population growth, and for quantifying developmental toxicity at various life stages for several different aquatic organisms. Experimental determinations are often very expensive and time-consuming as several factors may need to be carefully controlled in order to adhere to the established, recommended experimental protocol.

Aquatic toxicity data are available for relatively few organic, organometallic, and inorganic compounds. To address this concern, researchers have developed predictive methods as a means to estimate toxicities in the absence of experimental data. Derived correlations have shown varying degrees of success in their ability to predict the aquatic toxicity of different chemical compounds. In general, predictive methods are much better at estimating the aquatic toxicities of compounds that act through noncovalent or nonspecific modes of action. Nonpolar narcosis and polar narcosis are two such modes of nonspecific action. Nonpolar narcotic toxicity is often referred to as "baseline" or minimum toxicity. Polar narcotics exhibit effects similar to nonpolar narcotics; however, their observed toxicities are slightly more than "baseline" toxicity. Most industrial organic compounds have either a nonpolar or polar narcotic mode of action, which lacks covalent interactions between toxicant and organism. Predictive methods are generally less successful in predicting the toxicity of compounds whose action mechanism involves electro(nucleo)philic covalent reactivity or receptor-mediated functional toxicity. An example of a reactive toxicity mechanism would be alkane isothiocyanates that act as Michael-type acceptors, and undergo N-hydro-C-mercapto addition to cellular thiol functional groups (Schultz *et al.*, 2008).

The Abraham general solvation parameter model has proofed quite successful in predicting the toxicity of organic compounds to various aquatic organisms. Hoover and coworkers (Hoover *et al.*, 2005) published Abraham model correlations for describing the nonspecific aquatic toxicity of organic compounds to:

Fathead minnow:

$$-\log LC_{50}\,(\text{Molar, 96 hr}) = 0.996 + 0.418\,\mathbf{E} - 0.182\,\mathbf{S} + 0.417\,\mathbf{A} - 3.574\,\mathbf{B} + 3.377\,\mathbf{V} \quad (11)$$
$$(N = 196, SD = 0.276, R^2 = 0.953, F = 779.4)$$

Guppy:

$$-\log LC_{50}\,(\text{Molar, 96 hr}) = 0.811 + 0.782\,\mathbf{E} - 0.230\,\mathbf{S} + 0.341\,\mathbf{A} - 3.050\,\mathbf{B} + 3.250\,\mathbf{V} \quad (12)$$
$$(N = 148, SD = 0.280, R^2 = 0.946, F = 493.1)$$

Bluegill:

$$-\log LC_{50}\,(\text{Molar, 96 hr}) = 0.903 + 0.583\,\mathbf{E} - 0.127\,\mathbf{S} + 1.238\,\mathbf{A} - 3.918\,\mathbf{B} + 3.306\,\mathbf{V} \quad (13)$$
$$(N = 66, SD = 0.272, R^2 = 0.968, F = 359.8)$$

Goldfish:

$$-\log LC_{50}\,(\text{Molar, 96 hr}) = 0.922 - 0.653\,\mathbf{E} + 1.872\,\mathbf{S} + -0.329\,\mathbf{A} - 4.516\,\mathbf{B} + 3.078\,\mathbf{V} \quad (14)$$
$$(N = 51, SD = 0.277, R^2 = 0.966, F = 253.7)$$

Golden orfe:

$$-\log LC_{50}\,(\text{Molar, 96 hr}) = -0.137 + 0.931\,\mathbf{E} + 0.379\,\mathbf{S} + 0.951\,\mathbf{A} - 2.392\,\mathbf{B} + 3.244\,\mathbf{V} \quad (15)$$
$$(N = 49, SD = 0.269, R^2 = 0.935, F = 127.0)$$

and *Medaka high-eyes:*

$$-\log LC_{50}\ (\text{Molar, 96 hr}) = -0.176 + 1.046\ \mathbf{E} + 0.272\ \mathbf{S} + 0.931\ \mathbf{A} - 2.178\ \mathbf{B} + 3.155\ \mathbf{V} \quad (16)$$
$$(N= 44, SD = 0.277, R^2 = 0.960, F = 181.8)$$

$$-\log LC_{50}\ (\text{Molar, 48 hr}) = 0.834 + 1.047\ \mathbf{E} - 0.380\ \mathbf{S} + 0.806\ \mathbf{A} - 2.182\ \mathbf{B} + 2.667\ \mathbf{V} \quad (17)$$
$$(N= 50, SD = 0.292, R^2 = 0.938, F = 132.8)$$

The Abraham model described the median lethal toxicity (LC_{50}) to within an average standard deviation of SD = 0.279 log units. The derived correlations pertain to chemicals that exhibit a narcosis mode-of-toxic action, and can be used to estimate the baseline toxicity of reactive compounds and to identify compounds whose mode-of-toxic action is something other than nonpolar and/or polar narcosis. For example, in the case of the fathead minnow database, Hoover *et al.* (2005) noted that 1,3-dinitrobenzene, 1,4-dinitrobenzene, 2-chlorophenol, resorcinol, catechol, 2-methylimidazole, pyridine, 2-chloroaniline, acrolein and caffeine were outliers, suggesting that their mode of action involved some type of chemical specific toxicity. These observations are in accord with the earlier observations of Ramos *et al.* (1998) and Gunatilleka and Poole (1999).

In a follow-up study (Hoover *et al.*, 2007) the authors reported Abraham model expressions for correlating the median effective concentration for immobility of organic compounds to three species of water fleas:

Daphnia magna:

$$-\log LC_{50}\ (\text{Molar, 24 hr}) = 0.915 + 0.354\ \mathbf{E} + 0.171\ \mathbf{S} + 0.420\ \mathbf{A} - 3.935\ \mathbf{B} + 3.521\ \mathbf{V} \quad (18)$$
$$(N= 107, SD = 0.274, R^2 = 0.953, F = 410.0)$$

$$-\log LC_{50}\ (\text{Molar, 48 hr}) = 0.841 + 0.528\ \mathbf{E} - 0.025\ \mathbf{S} + 0.219\ \mathbf{A} - 3.703\ \mathbf{B} + 3.591\ \mathbf{V} \quad (19)$$
$$(N= 97, SD = 0.289, R^2 = 0.964, F = 475.4)$$

Ceriodaphnia dubia:

$$-\log LC_{50}\ (\text{Molar, 24 hr \& 48 hr combined}) = 2.234 + 0.373\ \mathbf{E} - 0.040\ \mathbf{S} - 0.437\ \mathbf{A} - 3.276\ \mathbf{B} + 2.763\ \mathbf{V} \quad (20)$$
$$(N= 44, SD = 0.253, R^2 = 0.936, F = 111.0)$$

Daphnia pulex:

$$-\log LC_{50}\ (\text{Molar, 24 hr \& 48 hr combined}) = 0.502 + 0.396\ \mathbf{E} + 0.309\ \mathbf{S} + 0.542\ \mathbf{A} - 3.457\ \mathbf{B} + 3.527\ \mathbf{V} \quad (21)$$
$$(N= 45, SD = 0.311, R^2 = 0.962, F = 233.2)$$

The data sets used in deriving Eqns. 18 – 21 included experimental log EC_{50} values for water flea immobility and for water flea death. The two toxicity endpoints were taken to be equivalent. Insufficient experimental details were given in many of the referenced papers for Hoover *et al.* to decide whether the water fleas were truly dead, or whether they were severely immobilized but still barely alive. Often, individual authors have reported the numerical value as a median immobilization effective concentration at the time of measurement, and in a later paper, the same authors referred to the same measured value as the median lethal molar concentration, and vice versa. Von der Ohe *et al.* (2005) made similar observations regarding the published toxicity data for water fleas in their statement ".... some studies use mortality (LC_{50}) and immobilization (EC_{50}, effective concentration 50%) as identical endpoints in the context of daphnid toxicity". Von der Ohe *et al.* made no attempt to distinguish between the two. For notational purposes, we have denoted the experimental toxicity data for water fleas as -log LC_{50} in the chapter. We think that this notation is consistent with how research groups in most countries are interpreting the endpoint.

Organic compounds used in deriving the fore-mentioned water flea correlations were for the most common industrial organic solvents. Hoover *et al.* (2007) did find published toxicity data for six antibiotics to both *Daphnia magna* and *Ceriodaphnia dubia* (Isidori *et al.* 2005). Solute descriptors are available for three of the six compounds. One of the compounds, ofloxacin, has a carboxylic acid functional group, and would not be expected to fall on the toxicity correlation for nonpolar-polar narcotic compounds to daphnids. Solute descriptors for the remaining two compounds, erythromycin (**E** = 1.97, **S** = 3.55, **A** = 1.02, **B** = 4.71, and **V** = 5.77) and clarithromycin (**E** = 2.72, **S** = 3.65, **A** = 1.00, **B** = 4.98, and **V** = 5.914), differ considerably from the the compounds used in deriving Eqns. 18-21. There was no obvious structural reason for the authors to exclude erythromycin and clarithromycin from the database; however, except that they did not want the calculated equation coefficients to be influenced by two compounds so much larger than the other compounds in the database and the calculated solute descriptors for both antibiotics were based on very limited number of experimental observations. Inclusion of erythromycin (-log LC_{50} = 4.51 for *Daphnia magna* and -log LC_{50} = 4.86 for *Ceriodaphnia dubia*) and clarithromycin (-logLC_{50} = 4.60 for *Ceriodaphnia dubia* and -log LC_{50} = 4.46 for *Daphnia magna*) in the regression analyses yielded:

Daphnia magna:

$$-\log LC_{50}\ (\text{Molar, 24 hr}) = 0.896 + 0.597\,\mathbf{E} - 0.089\,\mathbf{S} + 0.462\,\mathbf{A} - 3.757\,\mathbf{B} + 3.460\,\mathbf{V} \qquad (22)$$

Ceriodaphnia dubia:

$$-\log LC_{50}\ (\text{Molar, 24 hr}) = 1.983 + 0.373\,\mathbf{E} + 0.077\,\mathbf{S} - 0.576\,\mathbf{A} - 3.076\,\mathbf{B} + 2.918\,\mathbf{V} \qquad (23)$$

Both correlations are quite good. The one additional compound had little effect on the statistics, SD = 0.253 (data set B correlation in Hoover *et al.*, 2007) versus SD = 0.253 for *Daphnia magna* and SD = 0.256 versus SD = 0.253 for *Ceriodaphnia dubia*. Abraham model correlations have also been developed for estimating the baseline toxicity of organic compounds to *Tetrahymena pyriformis* (Hoover et al., 2007), *Spirostomum ambiguum* (Hoover *et al.*, 2007), *Psuedomonas putida* (Hoover *et al.*, 2007), *Vibrio fischeri* (Gunatilleka and Poole, 1999) and several tadpole species (Bowen *et al.*, 2006).

5. Methods to remove pharmaceutical products from the environment

The fate and effect of pharmaceutical drugs and healthcare products is not easy to predict. Medical compounds may be for human consumption to combat diseases or treat illnesses, or to relive pain and reduce inflammation. Many anti-inflammatory and analgesic drugs are available commercially without prescription as over-the-counter medications, with an estimated annual consumption of several hundred tons in developed countries. Pharmaceutical products are also used as veterinary medicines to treat illnesses, to promote livestock growth, to increase milk production, to manage reproduction, and to prevent the outbreak of diseases or parasites in densely populated fish farms. Antibiotics and antimicrobials are used to control and prevent diseases caused by microorganisms. Antiparasitic and anthelmintic drugs are approved for the treatment and control of internal and external parasites. The pharmaceutical compounds find their way into the environment by many exposure pathways, human/animal urine and feces excretion, discharge and runoff from fish farms, as shown in Figure 2. Once in the environment, the drugs and their degradation metabolites are adsorbed onto the soil and dissolved into the natural waterways.

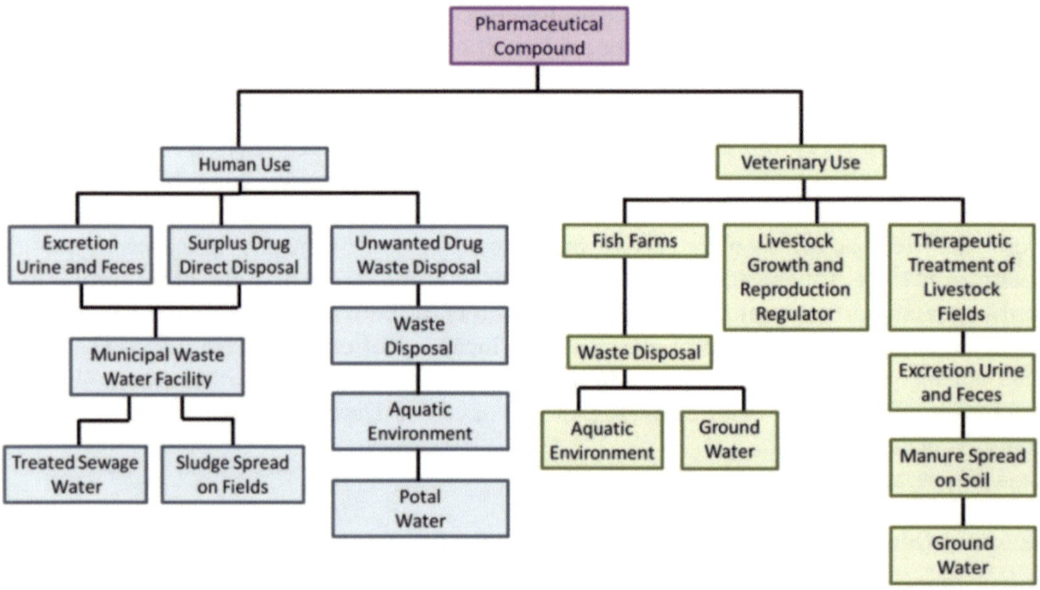

Fig. 2. Environmental occurrence and fate of pharmaceutical compounds used in human treatments and veterinary applications.

Published studies have reported the environmental damage that human and veterinary compounds have on aquatic organisms and microorganisms, on birds and on other forms of wildlife. For example, diclofenac (drug commonly used in ambulatory care) inhibits the microorganisms that comprise lotic river biofilms at a drug concentration level around 100 µg/L (Paje *et al.*, 2002), and damages the kidney and liver cell functions of rainbow trout at concentration levels of 1 µg/L (Triebskorn, *et al.*, 2004). Diclofenac affects nonaquatic organisms as well. India, Pakisan and Nepal banned the manufacture of veterinary formulations of diclofenac to halt the decline of three vulture species that were being poisoned by the diclofenac residues present in domestic livestock carcasses (Taggart *et al.*, 2009). The birds died from kidney failure after eating the diclofenac-tained carcasses. Concerns have also been expressed about the safety of ketoprofen. Naidoo and coworkers (2010a,b) reported vulture mortalities at ketoprofen dosages of 1.5 and 5 mg/kg vulture body weight, which is within the level for cattle treatment. Residues of two fluorquinolone veterinary compounds (enrofloxacin and ciprofloxacin), found in unhatched eggs of giffon vultures (*Gyps fulvus*) and red kites (*Milvus milvus*), are thought to be responsible for the observed severe alterations of embryo cartilage and bones, that prevented normal embryo development and successful egg hatching (Lemus *et al.*, 2009).

Removal of pharmaceutical residues and metabolites in municipal wastewater treatment facilities is a major challenge in reducing the discharge of these chemicals into the environment. Many wastewater facilities use an "activated sludge process" that involves treating the wastewater with air and a biological floc composed of bacteria and protozoans to reduce the organic content. Treatment efficiency for removal of analgesic and anti-inflammatory drugs varies from "very poor" to "complete breakdown" (Kulik *et al.*, 2008), and depends on seasonal conditions, pH, hydraulic retention time and sludge age (Tauxe-Wuersch *et al.*, 2005; Nikolaou *et al.*, 2005).

Advanced treatment processes, in combination with the activated sludge process, results in greater pharmaceutical compound removal from wastewater. Advanced processes that have been applied to the effluent from the activated sludge treatment include sand filtration, ozonation, UV irridation and activated carbon adsorption. Of the fore-mentioned processes, ozonation was found to be the most effective for complete removal for most analgesic and anti-inflammatory drugs. Ozone reactivity depends of the functional groups present in the drug molecule, as well as the reaction conditions. For example, the presence of a carboxylic functional group on an aromatic ring reduces ozone reaction with the aromatic ring carbons. Carboxylic groups are electron withdrawing. Electron-donating substituents, such as -OH groups, facilitate the attack of ozone to aromatic rings. Not all pharmaceutical compounds are reactive with ozone. For such compounds, it may be advantageous to perform the ozonation under alkaline conditions, where hydroxyl radicals are readily abundant. Hydroxyl radicals are highly reactive with a wide range of organic compounds, converting the compound to simplier and less harmful intermediates. With sufficient reaction time and appropriate reaction conditions, hydroxyl radicals can convert organic carbon to CO_2.

Several methods have been successfully employed to generate hydroxyl radicals. Fenton oxidation is an effective treatment for removal of pharmaceutical compounds and other organic contaminants from wastewater samples. The process is based on

$$Fe^{2+} + H_2O_2 \text{------>} Fe^{3+} + OH^- + OH^\cdot \quad (24)$$

the production of hydroxyl radicals from Fenton's reagent (Fe^{2+}/H_2O_2) under acidic conditions, with Fe^{2+} acting as a homogeneous catalyst. Once formed, hydroxyl radicals can oxidize organic matter (i.e. organic pollutants) with kinetic constants in the 10^7 to 10^{10} M^{-1} s^{-1} at 20 ^oC (Edwards *et al.*, 1992; Huang *et al.*, 1993). Fenton's technique has been used both as a wastewater pretreatment prior to the activated sludge process and as a post-treatment method after the activated sludge process. A full-scale pharmaceutical wastewater treatment facility using the Fenton process as the primary treatment method, followed by a sequence of activated sludge processes as the secondary treatment method, has been reported to provide an overall chemical oxygen demand removal efficiency of up to 98 % (Tekin *et al.*, 2006).

UV/H_2O_2 is an effective treatment for removal of pharmaceutical compounds and other organic contaminants from wastewater samples. The effluent is subjected to UV radiation. Some of the dissolved organic will absorb UV light directly, resulting in the destruction of chemical bonds and subsequent breakdown of the organic compound. Hydrogen peroxide is added to treat those compounds that do not degrade quickly or efficiently by direct UV photolysis. Hydrogen peroxide undergoes photolytic cleavage to $OH^\bullet$ radicals

$$H_2O_2 + hv \text{------>} 2\,OH^{\bullet} \tag{25}$$

at a stoichiometric ratio of 1:2, provided that the radiation source has sufficient emission at 190 - 200 nm. Disadvantages of the advanced oxidation processes are the high operating costs that are associated with: (a) high electricity demand (ozone and UV/H_2O_2); (b) the relatively large quantities of oxidants and/or catalysts consumed (ozone, hydrogen peroxide, and iron salts); and (c) maintaining the required pH range (Fenton process).

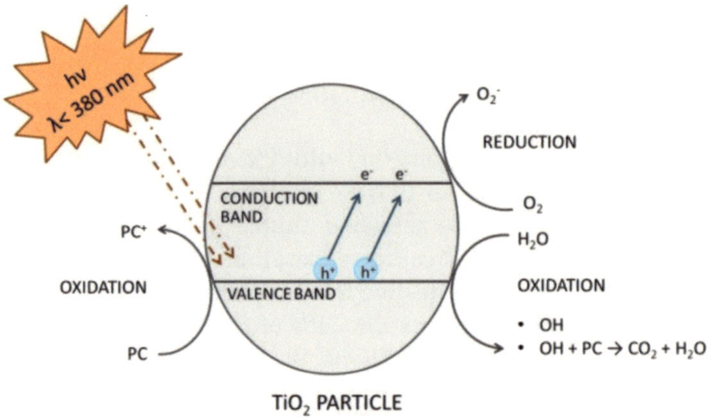

Fig. 3. Basic photocatalyic process involving TiO_2 particle

Photo-catalytic processes involving TiO_2 and/or TiO_2 nanoparticles have also been successful in removing pharmaceutical compounds pharmaceutical compounds (PC) from aqueous solutions. The basic process of photocatalysis consists of ejecting an electron from the valence band (VB) to the conduction band (CB) of the TiO_2 semiconductor

$$TiO_2 + hv \rightarrow e_{cb}^{-} + h_{vb}^{+} \tag{26}$$

creating an h^+ hole in the valence band. This is due to UV irradiation of TiO_2 particles with an energy equal to or greater than the band gap (hv > 3.2 eV). The electron and hole may recombine, or may result in the formation of extremely reactive species (like $^{\bullet}OH$ and O_2^{-*}) at the semi-conductor surface

$$h_{vb}^{+} + H_2O \rightarrow {\cdot}OH + H^+ \tag{27}$$

$$h_{vb}^{+} + OH^{-} \rightarrow {\cdot}OH_{ads} \tag{28}$$

$$e_{cb}^{-} + O_2 \rightarrow O_2^{*-} \tag{29}$$

as depicted in Figure 3, and/or a direct oxidation of the dissolved pharmaceutical compound (PC)

$$h_{vb}^{+} + PC_{ads} \rightarrow PC^{+}{}_{ads} \tag{30}$$

The O_2^{-*} that is produced in reaction scheme 35 undergoes further reactions to form

$$O_2^{-*} + H^+ \rightarrow HO_2^{\cdot} \tag{31}$$

$$H^+ + O_2^{-*} + HO_2^{\cdot} \rightarrow H_2O_2 + O_2 \tag{32}$$

$$H_2O_2 + hv \rightarrow 2 \cdot OH \tag{33}$$

additional hydroxyl radicals that subsequently react with the dissolved pharmaceutical compounds (Gad-Allah *et al.*, 2011). Titanium dioxide is used in the photo-catalytic processes because of its commercial availability and low cost, relatively high photo-catalytic activity, chemical stability resistance to photocorrosion, low toxicity and favorable wide band-gap energy.

Published studies have shown that sonochemical degradation of pharmaceutical and pesticide compounds can be effective for environmental remediation. Sonolytic degradation of pollutants occurs as a result of the continuous formation and collapse of cavitation bubbles on a microsecond time scale. Bubble collapse leads to the formation of a hot nucleus, characterized with extremely high temperatures (thousands of degrees) and pressure (hundreds of atmospheres).

6. Abraham model: Prediction of sensory and biological responses

Drug delivery to the target is an important consideration in drug discovery. The drug must reach the target site in order for the desired therapeutic effect to be achieved. Inhaled aerosols offer significant potential for non-invasive systemic administration of therapeutics but also for direct drug delivery into the diseased lung. Drugs for pulmonary inhalation are typically formulated as solutions, suspensions or dry powders. Aqueous solutions of drugs are common for inhalational therapy (Patton and Byron, 2007). Yet, about 40% of new active substances exhibit low solubility in water, and many fail to become marketed products due to formulation problems related to their high lipophilicity (Tang *et al.*, 2008; Gursoy and Benita, 2004). Formulations for drug delivery to the respiratory system include a wide variety of excipients to assist aerosolisation, solubilise the drug, support drug stability, prevent bacterial contamination or act as a solvent (Shaw, 1999; Forbes *et al.*, 2000). Organic solvents that are used or have been suggested as propellents for inhalation drug delivery systems include semifluorinated alkanes (Tsagogiorgas *et al.*, 2010), binary ethanol-hydrofluoroalkane mixtures (Hoye and Myrdal, 2008), fluorotrichloromethane, dichlorodifluoromethane and 1,2-dichloro-1,1,2,2-tetrafluoroethane (Smyth 2003).

Eye irritation thresholds (EIT), nasal irritation (pungency) thresholds (NPT), and odor detection thresholds (ODT) are related in that together they provide a warning system for unpleasant, noxious and dangerous chemicals or mixtures of chemicals. ODT values should not be confused with odor recognition. The latter area of research was revolutionized by the discovery of the role of odor receptors by Buck and Axel (Nobel Prize in physiology and medicine, 2004). It is now known that there are some 400 different active odor receptors in humans, that a given odor receptor can interact with a number of different chemicals, and that a given chemical can interact with several different odor receptors (Veithen *et al.*, 2009; Veithen *et al.*, 2010). This leads to an almost infinite matrix of interactions, and is a major reason why any connection between molecular structure and odor recognition is limited to rather small groups of chemicals (Sell, 2006). However, the first indication of an odor is given by the detection threshold; only at appreciably higher concentrations of the odorant can it be recognized. Another vital difference between odor detection and odor recognition is that ODT values can be put on a rigorous quantitative scale (Cometto-Muňiz, 2001), whereas odor recognition is qualitative and subject to leaning and memory (Wilson and Stevenson, 2006). As we shall see, it is possible, with some limitations, to obtain equations that connect ODT values with chemical structure in a way that is impossible for odor recognition.

A 'back-up' warning system is provided through nasal irritation (pungency) thresholds, where NPT values are about 10^3 larger than ODT. Nasal pungency occurs through activation of the trigeminal nerve, and so has a different origin to odor itself. Because chemicals that illicit nasal irritation will generally also provoke a response with regard to odor detection, it is not easy to determine NPT values without interference from odor. Cometto-Muňiz and Cain used subjects with no sense of smell, anosmics, in order to obtain NPT values through a rigorous systematic method; a detailed review is available (Cometto-Muňiz *et al.*, 2010). Cometto-Muňiz and Cain also devised a similar rigorous systematic method to obtain eye irritation thresholds (Cometto-Muňiz, 2001). Values of EIT are very close to NPT values. Eye irritation and nasal irritation (or pungency) are together known as sensory irritation. In addition to these human studies, a great deal of work has been carried out on upper respiratory tract irritation in mice. A quantitative scale was devised by Alarie (Alarie, 1966, 1973, 1981, 1988) and developed into a procedure for establishing acceptable exposure limits to airborne chemicals.

Before applying any particular equation to biological activity of VOCs, it is useful to consider various possible models (Abraham, *et al.*, 1994). A number of models were examined; the 'two-stage' model shown in Figure 4 gave a good fit to experimental data, whilst still allowing for unusual or 'outlying' effects. In stage 1, the VOC is transferred from the gas phase to a receptor phase. This transfer will resemble the transfer of chemicals from the gas phase to solvents that have similar chemical properties to the receptor phase. In particular there will be 'selectivity' between VOCs in accordance with their chemical properties and the chemical properties of the receptor phase. In stage 2, the VOC activates the receptor. If this is simply an on-off process, so that all VOCs activate the receptor similarly, then the resultant biological activity will correspond to the selectivity of the VOCs in the first stage, and can then be represented by some structure-activity correlation. However, if some of the VOCs activate the receptor through 'specific' effects, they will appear as outliers to any structure-property correlation. Indeed, if the majority of VOCs act through specific effects, then no reasonable structure-activity correlation will be obtained.

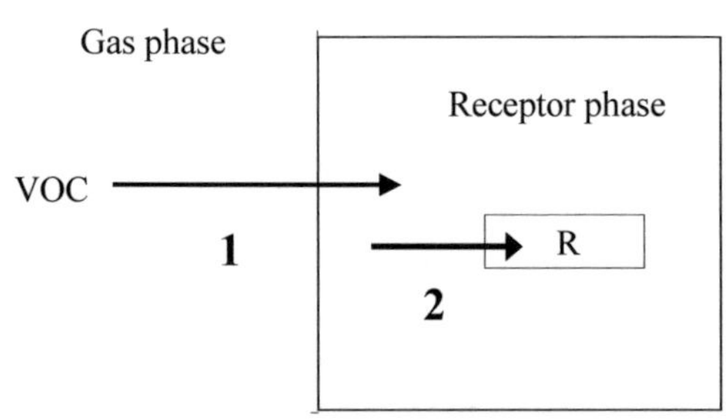

Fig. 4. A two-stage mechanism for the biological activity of gases and vapors; R denotes the receptor.

A stratagem for the analysis of biological activity of VOCs in a given process is therefore to construct some quantitative structure-activity equation that resembles similar equations for the transfer of VOCs from the gas phase to solvents. If the obtained equation is statistically and chemically reasonable, then it may be deduced that stage 1 is the main step. If a reasonable equation is obtained, but with a number of outliers, then stage 1 is probably the main step for most VOCs, but stage 2 is important for the VOCs that are outliers. If no QSAR can be set up, then stage 2 will be the main step for most VOCs. The linear free energy relationship or LFER, Eqn. 3, has been applied to transfers of compounds from the gas phase to a very large number of solvents (Abraham *et al.*, 2010a), and so is well suited as a general equation for the analysis of biological activity of VOCs.

Early work on attempts to correlate ODT values with various VOC properties has been summarized (Abraham, 1996). The first general application of Eqn. 3 to ODT values yielded Eqn. 34 (Abraham *et al.*, 2001; 2002). Note that (1/ODT) is used so that as log (1/ODT) becomes larger, the VOC becomes more potent, and that the units of ODT are ppm. There were a considerable number of outliers, including carboxylic acids, aldehydes, propanone, octan-1-ol, methyl acetate and t-butyl alcohol, suggesting that for many of the VOCs studied stage 2 in Figure 4 is important.

$$\text{Log}\,(1/\text{ODT}) = -5.154 + 0.533\cdot\mathbf{E} + 1.912\cdot\mathbf{S} + 1.276\cdot\mathbf{A} + 1.559\cdot\mathbf{B} + 0.699\cdot\mathbf{L} \quad (34)$$

$$(N= 50, SD = 0.579, R^2 = 0.773, F = 28.7)$$

Aldehydes and carboxylic acids could be included in the correlation through an indicator variable, **H**, that takes the value **H** = 2.0 for aldehydes and carboxylic acids and **H** = 0 for all other VOCs. The correlation could also be improved slightly by use of a parabolic expression in **L**, leading to Eqn. 35 (Abraham *et al.*, 2001; 2002).

$$\text{Log}\,(1/\text{ODT}) = -7.720 - 0.060\cdot\mathbf{E} + 2.080\cdot\mathbf{S} + 2.829\cdot\mathbf{A} + 1.139\cdot\mathbf{B} + \quad (35)$$
$$+2.028\cdot\mathbf{L} - 0.148\cdot\mathbf{L}^2 + 1.000\cdot\mathbf{H}$$

$$(N= 60, SD = 0.598, R^2 = 0.850, F = 44.0)$$

Although Eqn 35 is more general than Eqn 34, it suffers in that it cannot be compared to equations for other processes obtained through the standard Eqn 3. Coefficients for equations that correlate the transfer of compounds from the gas phase to solvents as log *K*, the gas-solvent partition coefficient, are given in Table 4 (Abraham *et al.*, 2010a). The most important coefficients are the s-coefficient that refers to the solvent dipolarity, the a-coefficient that refers to the solvent hydrogen bond basicity, the b-coefficient that refers to the solvent hydrogen bond basicity, and the l-coefficient that is a measure of the solvent hydrophobicity. For a solvent to be a model for stage 1 in the two-stage mechanism, we expect it to exhibit both hydrogen bond acidity and hydrogen bond basicity, since the peptide components of a receptor will include the –CO-NH- entity. In Table 4 we give details of solvents mainly with significant b- and a-coefficients. There is only a rather poor connection between the coefficients in Eqn. 42 and those for the secondary amide solvents in Table 4, suggesting, once again, that for odor thresholds stage 2 must be quite important.

The importance of stage 2 is illustrated by the observations of a 'cut-off' effect in odor detection thresholds (Cometto-Muňiz and Abraham, 2009a, 2009b, 2010a, 2010b). On ascending a homologous series of chemicals, ODT values decrease regularly with increase in the number of carbon atoms in the compounds. That is, the chemicals become more potent. However, a point is reached at which there is no further decrease in ODT or, even, ODTs begin to rebound and increase with increase in carbon chain length (Cometto-Muňiz and Abraham, 2009a, 2010a). This outcome could possibly be due to a size effect. A point is reached at which the VOC becomes too large and the increase in potency, reflected in decreasing ODTs is halted as just described.

Solvent	c	E	s	a	b	l
Methanol	-0.039	-0.338	1.317	3.826	1.396	0.773
Ethanol	0.017	-0.232	0.867	3.894	1.192	0.846
Propan-1-ol	-0.042	-0.246	0.749	3.888	1.076	0.874
Butan-1-ol	-0.004	-0.285	0.768	3.705	0.879	0.890
Pentan-1-ol	-0.002	-0.161	0.535	3.778	0.960	0.900
Hexan-1-ol	-0.014	-0.205	0.583	3.621	0.891	0.913
Heptan-1-ol	-0.056	-0.216	0.554	3.596	0.803	0.933
Octan-1-ol	-0.147	-0.214	0.561	3.507	0.749	0.943
Octan-1-ol (wet)	-0.198	0.002	0.709	3.519	1.429	0.858
Ethylene glycol	-0.887	0.132	1.657	4.457	2.355	0.565
Water	-1.271	0.822	2.743	3.904	4.814	-0.213
N-Methylformamide	-0.249	-0.142	1.661	4.147	0.817	0.739
N-Ethylformamide	-0.220	-0.302	1.743	4.498	0.480	0.824
N-Methylacetamide	-0.197	-0.175	1.608	4.867	0.375	0.837
N-Ethylacetamide	-0.018	-0.157	1.352	4.588	0.357	0.824
Formamide	-0.800	0.310	2.292	4.130	1.933	0.442
Diethylether	0.288	-0.347	0.775	2.985	0.000	0.973
Ethyl acetate	0.182	-0.352	1.316	2.891	0.000	0.916
Propanone	0.127	-0.387	1.733	3.060	0.000	0.866
Dimethylformamide	-0.391	-0.869	2.107	3.774	0.000	1.011
N-Formylmorpholine	-0.437	0.024	2.631	4.318	0.000	0.712
DMSO	-0.556	-0.223	2.903	5.037	0.000	0.719

Table 4. Coefficients in Eqn. 3 for Partition of Compounds from the Gas Phase to dry Solvents, at 298 K

As regards nasal pungency thresholds, a very detailed review is available on the anatomy and physiology of the human upper respiratory tract, the methods that have been used to assess irritation, and the early work on attempts to devise equations that could correlate nasal pungency thresholds (Doty *et al.*, 2004). The first application of Eqn 3 to nasal pungency thresholds used a variety of chemicals including aldehydes and carboxylic acids (Abraham *et al.*, 1998c). Later on, NPT values for several terpenes were included (Abraham *et al.*, 2001) to yield Eqn. 36 (Abraham *et al.*, 2010b) with NPT in ppm; of all the chemicals tested, only acetic acid was an outlier. Note that the term $s \cdot \mathbf{S}$ was statistically not significant and was excluded. Unlike ODT, it seems as though for the compounds studied, stage 1 in the two-stage mechanism is the only important step. This is reflected in that there are several solvents in Table 4 with coefficients quite close to those in Eqn. 36; N-methylformamide is one such solvent, and would be a reasonable model for solubility in a matrix containing a secondary peptide entity.

$$\text{Log}\,(1/\text{NPT}) = -7.700 + 1.543 \cdot \mathbf{S} + 3.296 \cdot \mathbf{A} + 0.876 \cdot \mathbf{B} + 0.816 \cdot \mathbf{L} \quad (36)$$
$$(N = 47, SD = 0.312, R^2 = 0.901, F = 45.0)$$

Along a homologous series of VOCs, the only descriptor in Eqn. 36 that changes significantly is **L.** Since **L** increases regularly along a homologous series, then log 1/(1/NPT) will increase regularly – that is the VOC will become more potent. A very important finding (Cometto-Muňiz *et al.*, 2005a) is that this regular increase does not continue indefinitely. For example, along the series of alkyl acetates log (1/NPT) increases up to octyl acetate, but decyl acetate cannot be detected. This is not due to decyl acetate having too low a vapor pressure to be detected, but is a biological 'cut-off' effect. One possibility (Cometto-Muňiz *et al.*, 2005a) is that for homologous series, the cut-off point is reached when the VOC is too large to activate the receptor. The effect of the cut-off point is shown in Figure 5 where log (1/NPT) is plotted against the number of carbon atoms in the n-alkyl group for n-alkyl acetates. A similar situation is obtained for the series of carboxylic acids, where the irritation potency increases as far as octanoic acid which now exhibits the cut-off effect. However, the compounds phenethyl alcohol, vanillin and coumarin also failed to provoke nasal irritation which suggests that stage 1 in the two-stage process is not always the limiting step. Two other equations for NPT have been reported (Famini *et al.*, 2002; Luan *et al.*, 2010) but the equations contain fewer compounds than Eqn. 36 and neither of them have improved statistics.

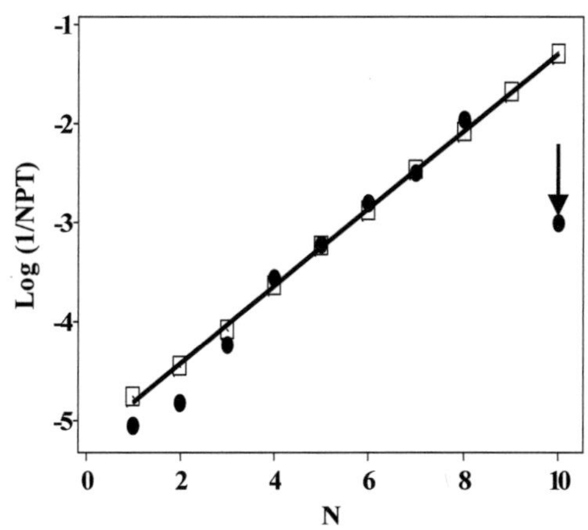

Fig. 5. A plot of log (1/NPT) for n-alkyl acetates against N, the number of carbon atoms in the n-alkyl group; • observed values, □ calculated values from Eqn 36.

A related property to eye irritation in humans is the Draize rabbit eye irritation test (Draize *et al.*, 1944). A given substance is applied to the eye of a living rabbit, and the effects of the substance on various parts of the eye are graded and used to derive an eye irritation score.

All kinds of substances have been applied, including soaps, detergents, aqueous solutions of acids and bases, and various solids. The test is so distressing to the animal that it has largely been phased out, but Draize scores of chemicals as the pure liquid are of value and were used to develop a quantitative structure-activity relationship (Abraham *et al.*, 1998a). It was reasoned that if Draize scores of the pure liquids, DES, were mainly due to a transport mechanism, for example step 1 in Figure 4, then they could be converted into an effect for the corresponding vapors through DES / P^o = *K*. Here *K* is a gas to solvent phase equilibrium or partition coefficient, P^o is the saturated vapor pressure of the pure liquid in ppm at 298 K, and DES/ P^o is equivalent to the solubility of a gaseous VOC in the appropriate receptor phase.

Values of DES for 38 liquids were converted into DES/ P^o and the latter regressed against the Abraham descriptors. The point for propylene carbonate was excluded and for the remaining 37 compounds Eqn. 37 was obtained; the term in $e \cdot \mathbf{E}$ was not significant and was excluded. The coefficients in Eqn. 37 quite resemble those for solubility in N-methylformamide, Table 4, and this suggests that the assumption of a mainly transport mechanism is reasonable.

$$\text{Log (DES / P}^o) = -6.955 + 1.046 \cdot \mathbf{S} + 4.437 \cdot \mathbf{A} + 1.350 \cdot \mathbf{B} + 0.754 \cdot \mathbf{L} \quad (37)$$
$$(N = 37, SD = 0.320, R^2 = 0.951, F = 155.9)$$

At that time, values of EIT for only 17 compounds were available, and so an attempt was made to combine the modified Draize scores with EIT values in order to obtain an equation that could be used to predict EIT values in humans (Abraham *et al.*,1998b). It was found that a small adjustment to DES / P^o values by 0.66 was needed in order to combine the two sets of data as in Eqn. 38; SP is either (DES / P^o - 0.66 or EIT). EIT is in units of ppm.

$$\text{Log (SP)} = -7.943 + 1.017 \cdot \mathbf{S} + 3.685 \cdot \mathbf{A} + 1.713 \cdot \mathbf{B} + 0.838 \cdot \mathbf{L} \quad (38)$$
$$(N = 54, SD = 0.338, R^2 = 0.924, F = 149.69)$$

A slightly different procedure was later used to combine DES / P^o values for 68 compounds and 23 EIT values (the nomenclature MMAS was used instead of DES). For all 91 compounds, Eqn. 39 was obtained. Instead of the adjustment of -0.66 to DES / P^o, an indicator variable, **I**, was used; this takes the value **I** = 0 for the EIT compounds, and **I** = 1 for the Draize compounds (Abraham *et al.*, 2003).

$$\text{Log (SP)} = -7.892 - 0.397 \cdot \mathbf{E} + 1.827 \cdot \mathbf{S} + 3.776 \cdot \mathbf{A} + 1.169 \cdot \mathbf{B} + 0.785 \cdot \mathbf{L} + 0.568 \cdot \mathbf{I} \quad (39)$$
$$(N = 91, SD = 0.433, R^2 = 0.936, F = 204.5)$$

The eye irritation thresholds in humans, based on a standardized systematic protocol, were those determined over a number of years (Cometto-Muñiz & Cain, 1991, 1995, 1998; Cometto-Muñiz *et al.*, 1997, 1998a, 1998b).

Later work (Cometto-Muñiz *et al.*, 2005b, 2006, 2007a, 2007b; Cometto-Muñiz and Abraham, 2008) revealed the existence of a cut-off point in EIT on ascending a number of homologous series. Just as with NPT, these cut-off points are not due to the low vapor pressure of higher members of the homologous series, but appear to relate to a lack of activation of the receptor. If this is due to the size of the VOC, then the overall length may be the determining factor, because on ascending a homologous series, both the width and depth of the homologs remain constant. It is interesting that odorant molecular length has been suggested as one factor in the olfactory code (Johnson and Leon, 2000). Whatever the cause of the cut-off point, it renders all equations for the correlation and prediction of EIT subject to a size restriction.

The only animal assay concerning VOCs is the very important 'mouse assay' first introduced by Alarie (Alarie, 1966, 1973, 1981, 1998; Alarie *et al.*, 1980), and developed into a standard test procedure for the estimation of sensory irritation (ASTM, 1984). In the assay, male Swiss-Webster mice are exposed to various vapor concentrations of a VOC and the concentration at which the respiratory rate is reduced by 50% is taken as the end-point and denoted as RD_{50}. An evaluation of the use RD_{50} to establish acceptable exposure levels of VOCs in humans has recently been published (Kuwabara *et al.*, 2007)

There were a number of attempts to relate RD_{50} values for a series of VOCs to physical properties of the VOCs such as the water-octanol partition coefficient, P_{oct}) or the gas-hexadecane partition coefficient, but these relationships were restricted to particular homologous series (Nielsen and Alarie, 1982; Nielsen and Bakbo, 1985; Nielsen and Yamagiwa, 1989; Nielsen *et al.*, 1990). A useful connection was between RD_{50} and the VOC saturated vapor pressure at 310 K, viz: RD_{50} / VP^o = constant (Nielsen and Alarie, 1982). This is known as Ferguson's rule (Ferguson, 1939) and although it was claimed to have a rigorous thermodynamic basis (Brink and Posternak, 1948) it is now known to be only an empirical relationship (Abraham *et al.*, 1994).

RD_{50} values were also obtained using a different strain of mice, male Swiss OF_1 mice (De Ceaurriz *et al.*, 1981) and were used to obtain relationships between log (1/ RD_{50}) and VOC properties such as log P_{oct}, or boiling point for compounds that were classed as nonreactive (Muller and Gref, 1984; Roberts, 1986). The data used previously (Roberts, 1986) were later fitted to Eqn. 3 to yield Eqn 40 for unreactive compounds (Abraham *et al.*, 1990)

$$\text{Log}\,(1/FRD_{50}) = -0.596 + 1.354\cdot\mathbf{S} + 3.188\cdot\mathbf{A} + 0.775\cdot\mathbf{L} \quad (40)$$
$$(N = 39, SD = 0.103, R^2 = 0.980)$$

FRD_{50} is in units of mmol m^{-3}, rather than ppm, but this affects only the constant in Eqn 40. The fine review of Schaper lists RD_{50} values for not only Swiss-Webster mice but also for Swiss OF_1 mice (Schaper, 1993), and an updated equation for Swiss OF_1 mice in terms of RD_{50} was set out (Abraham, 1996).

$$\text{Log}\,(1/RD_{50}) = -6.71 + 1.30\cdot\mathbf{S} + 2.88\cdot\mathbf{A} + 0.76\cdot\mathbf{L} \quad (41)$$
$$(N = 45, SD = 0.140, R^2 = 0.962, F = 350)$$

The Schaper data base was used to test if log (1/RD_{50}) values for nonreactive VOCs could be correlated with gas to solvent partition coefficients, as log *K*, and reasonable correlations were found for a number of solvents (Abraham *et al.*, 1994; Alarie *et al.*, 1995, 1996). In order to analyze values for a wide range of VOCs it was thought important to distinguish compounds that illicit an effect through a 'chemical' mechanism or through a 'physical' mechanism, these terms being equivalent to 'reactive' or 'nonreactive' (Alarie *et al.*, 1998a). The Ferguson rule was used to discriminate between the two classes; if RD_{50} / VP^o > 0.1 the VOC was deemed to act by a physical mechanism (p), and if RD_{50} / VP^o < 0.1 the VOC was considered to act by a chemical mechanism (c). For 58 VOCs acting by a physical mechanism, Eqn 42 was obtained (Alarie *et al.*, 1998b) for Swiss OF_1 mice and Swiss-Webster mice.

$$\text{Log}\,(1/RD_{50}) = -7.049 + 1.437\cdot\mathbf{S} + 2.316\cdot\mathbf{A} + 0.774\cdot\mathbf{L} \quad (42)$$
$$(N = 58, SD = 0.354, R^2 = 0.840, F = 94.5)$$

A more recent analysis has been carried out (Luan *et al.*, 2006), using the previous data and division into physical and chemical mechanisms. For 47 VOCs acting by a physical mechanism, Eqn 43 was obtained.

$$\text{Log}(1/RD_{50}) = -5.550 + 0.043 \cdot Re + 6.329 \cdot RPCG + 0.377 \cdot ICave + 0.049 \cdot CHdonor - 3.826 \cdot RNSB + 0.047 \cdot ZX \quad (43)$$
$$(N = 47, SD = 0.362, R^2 = 0.844, F = 36.1)$$

The statistics of Eqn 43 are not as good as those of Eqn 42, and since some of the descriptors in Eqn 43 are chemically almost impossible to interpret (ICave is the average information content and ZX is the ZX shadow) it has no advantage over Eqn 42. What is of more interest is that it was possible to derive an equation for VOCs acting by a chemical mechanism (Luan *et al.*, 2006),

$$\text{Log}(1/RD_{50}) = 8.438 + 0.214 \cdot PPSA3 + 0.017 \cdot Hf - 22.510 \cdot V^{c}max + 0.229 \cdot BIC + 44.508 \cdot (HDCA + 1/TMSA) + 0.049 \cdot BO^{min}{}_{C} \quad (44)$$
$$(N = 67, SD = 0.626, R^2 = 0.737, F = 28.0)$$

Although, again, Eqn 44 is chemically difficult to interpret, it does show that it is possible to estimate RD_{50} values for VOCs that are reactive and act through a chemical mechanism.

About 20 million patients receive a general anesthetic each year in the USA. In spite of considerable effort the specific site of action of anesthetics is still not well known. However, even if the actual site of action is not known, it is possible that a general mechanism on the lines shown in Figure 4 obtains. In the first stage the anesthetic is transported from the gas phase to a site of action, and in the second stage interaction takes place with a target receptor, a variety of which have been suggested ((Franks, 2006; Zhang *et al.*, 2007; Steele *et al.*, 2007). Then if stage 1 is a major component, we might expect that a QSAR could be constructed for inhalation anesthesia. It is noteworthy that a QSAR on the lines of Eqn. 2 was constructed for aqueous anesthesia as long ago as 1991 (Abraham *et al.*, 1991). Since then, rather little has been achieved in terms of inhalation anesthesia. The usual end point in inhalation anesthesia is the minimum alveolar concentration, MAC, of an inhaled anesthetic agent that prevents movement in 50 % of subjects in response to noxious stimulation. In rats, this is electrical or mechanical stimulation of the tail. MAC values are expressed in atmospheres, and correlations are carried out using log (1/MAC) so that the smaller is MAC the more potent is the anesthetic. It was shown (Sewell and Halsey, 1997) that shape similarity indices gave better fits for log (1/MAC) than did gas to olive oil partition coefficients, but the analysis was restricted to a model for 10 fluoroethanes for which $R^2 = 0.939$ and a different model for 8 halogenated ethers for which $R^2 = 0.984$ was found. A completely different model of inhalation anesthesia.has been put forward (Sewell and Sear, 2004, 2006) in which no consideration is taken as to how a gaseous solute is transported to a receptor, but solute-receptor interactions are calculated. However, two different receptor models were needed, one for a particular set of nonhalogenated compounds and one for a particular set of halogenated compounds, so the generality of the model seems quite restricted.

A QSAR for inhalation anesthesia was eventually obtained using the LFER, Eqn. 3, as follows (Abraham *et al.*, 2008)

$$\text{Log}(1/MAC) = -0.752 - 0.034 \cdot \mathbf{E} + 1.559 \cdot \mathbf{S} + 3.594 \cdot \mathbf{A} + 1.411 \cdot \mathbf{B} + 0.687 \cdot \mathbf{L} \quad (45)$$
$$(N = 148, SD = 0.192, R^2 = 0.985, F = 1856.1)$$

The only compounds not included in Eqn. 45 were 1,1,2,2,3,3,4,4,5,5,6,6-dodecafluorohexane and 2,2,3,3,4,4,5,5,6,6,7,7-dodecafluoroheptan-1-ol which were known to be subject to cut-off effects, and 1-octanol where the observed MAC value was subject to a greater error than usual. Hence Eqn. 45 is a very general equation, and it can be suggested that stage 1 in Figure 4 does indeed represent the main process.

A related biological end point to inhalation anesthesia is that of convulsant activity. It has been observed that a number of compounds expected to exhibit anesthesia actually provoke convulsions in rats (Eger *et al.*, 1999). The end point, as for inhalation anesthesia, is taken as the compound vapor pressure in atm that just induces convulsion, CON. Eqn 3 was applied to the observed data yielding Eqn 46 (Abraham and Acree, 2009)

$$\text{Log}\,(1/\text{CON}) = -0.573 - 0.228 \cdot \mathbf{E} + 1.198 \cdot \mathbf{S} + 3.232 \cdot \mathbf{A} + 3.355 \cdot \mathbf{B} + 0.776 \cdot \mathbf{L} \quad (46)$$
$$(N = 44,\ SD = 0.167,\ R^2 = 0.978,\ F = 344.2)$$

In terms of structural features it was shown that the anesthetics tended to have large hydrogen bond acidities whereas convulsants tended to have zero or small hydrogen bond acidities. The only other notable structural feature was that convulsants had larger values of **L** and anesthetics tended to have smaller values of **L**. Since **L** is somewhat related to size, the convulsants are generally larger than the inhalation anesthetics.

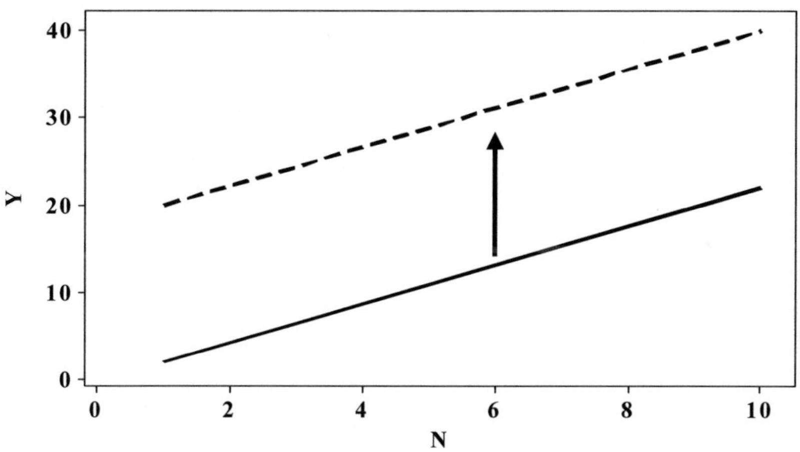

Fig. 6. Plots of VOC activity, **Y**, against VOC carbon number, **N**, illustrating the use of an indicator variable, **I**.

It was pointed out (Abraham *et al.*, 2010c) that a large number of equations on the lines of Eqn. 3 for various biological and toxicological effects of VOCs had been constructed, these equations mainly representing stage 1 in Figure 4. Since this stage refers to the transfer of a VOC from the gas phase to some biological phase, it was argued that it might be possible to amalgamate all these equations into one general equation for the biological and toxicological activity of VOCs. Consider plots of toxicological activity, **Y**, against the number of carbon atoms, **N**, in a homologous series of VOCs. If the two lines are parallel, then a simple indicator variable, **I**, could be used to bring then both on the same line, as shown in Figure 6. If the two lines are not parallel, then after use an indicator variable, they will appear as shown in Figure 7. But even in this situation a general equation (or general line) might be used to correlate both sets of data, albeit with an increase in the regression standard deviation. It remained to be seen exactly how much error was introduced by use of a general equation.

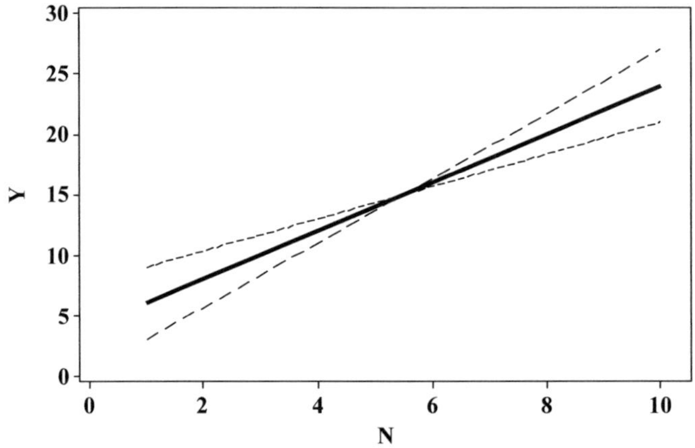

Fig. 7. Plots of VOC activity, **Y**, against VOC carbon number, **N**, showing how a general equation may be used to correlate two sets of data that give rise to lines of different slope.

Various sets of data on toxicological and biological activity, **Y**, for a number of processes were used to construct an equation in which a number of indicator variables, **I**, were used in order to fit all the sets of data into one equation. The result was Eqn. 51 (Abraham *et al.*, 2010c).

$$\mathbf{Y} = -7.805 + 0.056 \cdot \mathbf{E} + 1.587 \cdot \mathbf{S} + 3.431 \cdot \mathbf{A} + 1.440 \cdot \mathbf{B} + 0.754 \cdot \mathbf{L} + 0.553 \cdot \mathbf{Idr} + 2.777 \cdot \mathbf{Iodt} - 0.036 \cdot \mathbf{Inpt} + 6.923 \cdot \mathbf{Imac} + 0.440 \cdot \mathbf{Ird50} + 8.161 \cdot \mathbf{Itad} + 7.437 \cdot \mathbf{Icon} + 4.959 \cdot \mathbf{Idav} \quad (47)$$

$$(N = 643, SD = 0.357, R^2 = 0.992, F = 6083.0)$$

The 'standard' process was taken as eye irritation thresholds, as log (1/EIT) for which no indicator variable was used. The given processes and the corresponding indicator variables are shown in Table 5.

There are two processes listed in Table 5 that have not been considered here. The data on gaseous anesthesia on tadpoles were derived from aqueous anesthesia together with water to gas partition coefficients, and so are indirect data, and the compounds in the data set for inhalation anesthesia on mice cover a very restricted range of descriptors. Of the 720 data points, 77 were outliers. Nearly all of these were VOCs classed as 'reactive' or 'chemical' in respiratory tract irritation in mice, or VOCs that acted by specific effects in odor detection thresholds. The remaining 643 data points all refer to nonreactive VOCs or to VOCs that act through selective and not specific effects. The SD value of 0.357 in Eqn. 47 is quite good by comparison to the various SD values for individual processes, suggesting that the general equation has incorporated these with little loss in accuracy; the predicted standard deviation in Eqn. 47 is only 0.357 log units. The equation is scaled to eye irritation thresholds, but it is noteworthy that the coefficient for the NPT indicator variable is nearly zero. Thus EIT and NPT can be estimated through Eqn. 48 for any nonreactive VOC for which the relevant descriptors are available.

$$\mathbf{Y} = \log(1/EIT) = \log(1/NPT) = -7.805 + 0.056 \cdot \mathbf{E} + 1.587 \cdot \mathbf{S} + 3.431 \cdot \mathbf{A} + 1.440 \cdot \mathbf{B} + 0.754 \cdot \mathbf{L} \quad (48)$$

The Abraham general solvation model provides reasonably accurate mathematical correlations and predicitions for a number of important biological responses, including Eye irritation thresholds (EIT), nasal irritation (pungency) thresholds (NPT), odor detection thresholds (ODT) inhalation anesthesia (rats) and convulsant actictivity (mice).

Activity	Units	**Y**	**I**	VOCs	
				Total	Outliers
Eye irritation thresholds	ppm	log(1/EIT)	None	23	0
EIT from Draize scores	ppm	$\log(D/P^o)$	Idr	72	0
Odor detection thresholds	ppm	log(1/ODT)	Iodt	64	20
Nasal pungency thresholds	ppm	log(1/NPT)	Inpt	48	0
Inhalation anesthesia (rats)	atm	log(1/MAC)	Imac	147	0
Respiratory irritation (mice)	ppm	$\log(1/RD_{50})$	Ird50	147	53
Gaseous anesthesia (tadpoles)	mol/L	log(1/C)	Itad	130	4
Convulsant activity (rats)	atm	log(1/CON)	Icon	44	0
Inhalation anesthesia (mice)	vol %	log(1/vol)	Idav	45	0
Total				720	77

Table 5. Toxicological and Biological Data on VOCs used to construct Eqn. 47

7. References

Abraham, M. H. & McGowan, J. C. (1987) The use of characteristic volumes to measure cavity terms in reversed phase liquid chromatography. *Chromatographia* 23 (4) 243–246.

Abraham, M. H.; Lieb, W. R. & Franks, N. P. (1991) The role of hydrogen bonding in general anesthesia. *Journal of Pharmaceutical Sciences* 80 (8) 719-724.

Abraham, M. H. (1993a) Scales of solute hydrogen-bonding: their construction and application to physicochemical and biochemical processes. *Chemical Society Reviews* 22 (2) 73-83.

Abraham, M. H. (1993b) Application of solvation equations to chemical and biochemical processes. *Pure and Applied Chemistry* 65 (12) 2503-2512.

Abraham, M. H. & Acree, W. E., Jr.(2009) Prediction of convulsant activity of gases and vapors. *European Journal of Medicinal Chemistry* 44 (2) 885-890.

Abraham, M. H.; Nielsen, G. D. & Alarie, Y. (1994) The Ferguson principle and an analysis of biological activity of gases and vapors. *Journal of Pharmaceutical Sciences* 83 (5) 680-688.

Abraham, M. H. (1996) The potency of gases and vapors: QSARs - anesthesia, sensory irritation and odor, in Indoor Air and Human Health, Ed R. B. Gammage and B. A. Berven, 2nd Ed., CRC Lewis Publishers, Boca Raton, USA.

Abraham, M. H.; Kumarsingh, R.; Cometto-Muñiz, J. E. & Cain, W. S. (1998a) A quantitative structure-activity relationship for a Draize eye irritation database. *Toxicology in Vitro* 12 (3) 201-207.

Abraham, M. H.; Kumarsingh, R.; Cometto-Muñiz, J. E. & Cain, W. S. (1998b) Draize eye scores and eye irritation thresholds in man combined into one quantitative structure-activity relationship. *Toxicology in Vitro* 12 (4) 403-408.

Abraham, M. H.; Kumarsingh, R.; Cometto-Muñiz, J. E. & Cain, W. S. (1998c) An algorithm for nasal pungency thresholds in man. *Archives of Toxicology* 72 (4) 227-232.

Abraham, M. H.; Gola, J. M. R.; Cometto-Muñiz, J. E.& Cain, W. S. (2001) The correlation and prediction of VOC thresholds for nasal pungency, eye irritation and odour in humans. *Indoor Built Environment* 10 (3-4) 252-257.

Abraham, M. H.; Gola, J. M. R.; Cometto-Muñiz, J. E.& Cain, W. S. (2002) A model for odour thresholds. *Chemical Senses* 27 (2) 95-104.

Abraham, M. H.; Hassanisadi, M.; Jalali-Heravi, M.; Ghafourian, T.; Cain, W. S. & Cometto-Muñiz, J. E. (2003) Draize rabbit eye test compatibility with eye irritation thresholds in humans: a quantitative structure-activity relationship analysis. *Toxicological Sciences* 76 (2) 384-391.

Abraham, M. H.; Ibrahim, A. & Zissimos, A. M. (2004) Determination of sets of solute descriptors from chromatographic measurements. *Journal of Chromatography, A* 1037 (1-2) 29-47.

Abraham, M. H.; Ibrahim, A.; Zhao, Y.; Acree, W. E., Jr. (2006) A data base for partition of volatile organic compounds and drugs from blood/plasma/serum to brain, and an LFER analysis of the data. *Journal of Pharmaceutical Sciences* 95 (10) 2091-2100.

Abraham, M. H.; Acree, W. E., Jr.; Mintz, C. & Payne, S. (2008) Effect of anesthetic structure on inhalation anesthesia: implications for the mechanism. *Journal of Pharmaceutical Sciences* 97 (6) 2373-2384.

Abraham, M. H.; Gil-Lostes, J. & Fatemi, M. (2009a) Prediction of milk/plasma concentration ratios of drugs and environmental pollutants. *European Journal of Medicinal Chemistry* 44 (6) 2452-2458.

Abraham, M. H.; Acree, W. E., Jr. & Cometto-Muñiz, J. E. (2009b) Partition of compounds from water and from air into amides. *New Journal of Chemistry* 33 (10) 2034-2043.

Abraham, M.H.; Smith, R.E.; Luchtefeld, R.; Boorem, A.J.; Luo, R. & Acree, W.E., Jr., (2010a) Prediction of solubility of drugs and other compounds in organic solvents. *Journal of Pharmaceutical Sciences* 99 (3) 1500-1515.

Abraham, M. H.; Sánchez-Moreno, R.; Gil-Lostes, J.; Cometto-Muñiz, J. E. & Cain, W. S. (2010b) Physicochemical modeling of sensory irritation in humans and experimental animals, Chapter 25, pp 378-389, in Toxicology of the Nose and Upper Airways, Ed. J. B. Morris and D. J. Shusterman, Informa Healthcare, New York, USA.

Abraham, M. H.; Sánchez-Moreno, R.; Gil-Lostes, J.; Acree, W. E. Jr, Cometto-Muñiz, J. E. & Cain, W. S. (2010c)The biological and toxicological activity of gases and vapors, Toxicology in Vitro, 24 (2) 357-362.

ADME Boxes, version* (2010) Advanced Chemistry Development, 110 Yonge Street, 14th Floor, Toronto, Ontario, M5C 1T4, Canada.

Alarie, Y. (1966) Irritating properties of airborne materials to the upper respiratory tract. *Archives Environmental Health* 13 (4) 433-449.

Alarie, Y.(1973) Sensory irritation by airborne chemicals. *C.R.C. Critical Reviews in Toxicology* 2 (3) 299-363.

Alarie, Y. (1981) Dose-response analysis in animal studies: prediction of human response. *Environmental Health Perspective* 42 (Dec) 9-13.

Alarie, Y. (1998) Computer-based bioassay for evaluation of sensory irritation of airborne chemicals and its limit of detection. *Archives of Toxicology* 72 (5) 277-282.

Alarie, Y.; Kane, L. & Barrow, C. (1980) Sensory irritation: the use of an animal model to establish acceptable exposure to airborne chemical irritants. in Toxicology: Principles and Practice, Vol 1, Ed Reeves, A. L., John Wiley & Sons, Inc, New York.

Alarie, Y.; Nielsen, G. D.; Andonian-Haftvan, J. & Abraham, M. H. (1995) Physicochemical properties of nonreactive volatile organic chemicals to estimate RD50: alternatives to animal studies. *Toxicology and Applied Pharmacology* 134 (1) 92-99.

Alarie, Y.; Schaper, M.; Nielsen, G. D. & Abraham, M. H. (1996) Estimating the sensory irritating potency of airborne nonreactive volatile organic chemicals and their mixtures. *SAR and QSAR in Environmental Research* 5 (3) 151-165.

Alarie, Y.; Nielsen, G. D. & Abraham, M. H. (1998a) A theoretical approach to the Ferguson principle and its use with non-reactive and reactive airborne chemicals. *Pharmacology and Toxicology* 83 (6) 270-279.

Alarie, Y.; Schaper, M.; Nielsen, G. D. & Abraham, M. H. (1998b) Structure-activity relationships of volatile organic compounds as sensory irritants *Archives of Toxicology* 72 (3) 125-140.

American Society for Testing and Materials (1984) Standard test method for estimating sensory irritancy of airborne chemicals. Designation: E981-84. American Society for Testing and Materials. Philadelphia, Pa, USA.

Andrade, R.J.; Lucena, M.I.; Martin-Vivaldi, R.; Fernandez, M.C.; Nogueras, F.; Pelaez, G.; Gomez-Outes, A.; Garcia-Escano, M.D.; Bellot, V. & Hervas, A. (1999) Acute liver injury associated with the use of ebrotidine, a new H2-receptor antagonist, *Journal of Hepatology* 31 (4) 641-646.

Bowen, K.R.; Flanagan, K.B.; Acree, W.E. Jr.; Abraham, M.H. & Rafols, C. (2006) Correlation of the toxicity of organic compounds to tadpoles using the Abraham model. *Science of the Total Environmen* 371 (1-3) 99-109.

Brink, F. & Posternak, J. M. (1948) Thermodynamic analysis of the relative effectiveness of narcotics. *Journal of Cell Comparative Physiology* 32, 211-233.

Chaput, J.-P. & Tremblay, A. (2010) Well-being of obese individuals: therapeutic perspectives. *Future Medicinal Chemistry* 2 (12) 1729-1733.

Charlton, A.K.; Daniels, C.R.; Acree, W.E., Jr. & Abraham, M.H. (2003) Solubility of Crystalline Nonelectrolyte Solutes in Organic Solvents: Mathematical Correlation of Acetylsalicylic Acid Solubilities with the Abraham General Solvation Model. *Journal of Solution Chemistry* 32 (12) 1087-1102.

Cometto-Muñiz J.E., (2001) Physicochemical basis for odor and irritation potency of VOCs. In: Indoor Air Quality Handbook, (Spengler, J.D. et al., eds.), pp 20.1-20.21. New York: McGraw-Hill.

Cometto-Muñiz J.E. & Abraham, M. H. (2008) A cut-off in ocular chemesthesis from vapors of homologous alkylbenzenes and 2-ketones as revealed by concentration-detection functions. *Toxicology and Applied Pharmacology* 230 (3) 298-303.

Cometto-Muñiz J.E. & Abraham, M. H. (2009a) Olfactory detectability of homologous n-alkylbenzenes as reflected by concentration-detection functions in humans. *Neuroscience* 161 (1) 236-248.

Cometto-Muñiz J.E. & Abraham, M. H. (2009b) Olfactory psychometric functions for homologous 2-ketones. *Behavioural Brain Research* 201 (1) 207-215.

Cometto-Muñiz J.E. & Abraham, M. H. (2010a) Structure-activity relationships on the odor detectability of homologous carboxylic acids by humans. *Experimental Brain Research* 207 (1-2) 75-84.

Cometto-Muñiz J.E. & Abraham, M. H. (2010b) Odor detection by humans of lineal aliphatic aldehydes and helional as gauged by dose-response functions. *Chemical Senses* 35 (4) 289-299.

Cometto-Muñiz, J. E. & Cain, W. S. (1991) Nasal pungency, odor and eye irritation thresholds for homologous acetates. *Pharmacology, Biochemistry and Behavior* 39 (4) 983-989.

Cometto-Muñiz, J. E. & Cain, W. S. (1995) Relative sensitivity of the ocular trigeminal, nasal trigeminal, and olfactory systems to airborne chemicals. *Chemical Senses* 20 (2) 191-198.

Cometto-Muñiz, J. E. & Cain, W. S. (1998) Trigeminal and olfactory sensitivity: comparison of modalities and methods of measurement. *International Archives of Occupational and Environmental Health* 71 (2) 105-110.

Cometto-Muñiz, J. E.; Cain, W. S. & Hudnell, H. K. (1997) Agonistic sensory effects of airborne chemicals in mixtures: odor, nasal pungency, and eye irritation. *Perception & Psychophysics* 59 (5) 665-674.

Cometto-Muñiz, J. E.; Cain, W. S.; Abraham, M. H. & Kumarsingh, R. (1998a) Sensory properties of selected terpenes. Thresholds for odor, nasal pungency, nasal localizations and eye irritation. Annals of the New York Academy of Sciences 855 (Olfaction and Taste XII) 648-651.

Cometto-Muñiz, J. E.; Cain, W. S.; Abraham, M. H. & Kumarsingh, R. (1998b) Trigeminal and olfactory chemosensory impact of selected terpenes. *Pharmacology and Biochemistry and Behaviour* 60 (3) 765-770.

Cometto-Muñiz, J. E.; Cain, W. S. & Abraham, M. H. (2005a) Determinants for nasal trigeminal detection of volatile organic compounds. *Chemical Senses* 30 (8) 627-642.

Cometto-Muñiz, J. E.; Cain, W. S. & Abraham, M. H. (2005b) Molecular restrictions for human eye irritation by chemical vapors. *Toxicology and Applied Pharmacology* 207 (3) 232-243.

Cometto-Muñiz, J. E.; Cain, W. S.; Abraham, M. H. & Sánchez-Moreno, R. (2006) Chemical boundaries for detection of eye irritation in humans from homologous vapors. *Toxicological Sciences* 91 (2) 600-609.

Cometto-Muñiz, J. E.; Cain, W. S.; Abraham, M. H. & Sánchez-Moreno, R. (2007a) Cutoff in detection of eye irritation from vapors of homologous carboxylic acids and aliphatic aldehydes. *Neuroscience* 145 (3) 1130-1137.

Cometto-Muñiz, J. E.; Cain, W. S.; Abraham, M. H. & Sánchez-Moreno, R. (2007b) Concentration-detection functions for eye irritation evoked by homologous n-alcohols and acetates approaching a cut-off point. *Experimental Brain Research* 182 (1) 71-79.

Cometto-Muñiz, J. E.; Cain, W. S.; Abraham, M. H.; Sánchez-Moreno, R. & Gil-Lostes, J. (2010)Nasal Chemosensory Irritation in Humans, Chapter 12, pp 187-202, in Toxicology of the Nose and Upper Airways, Ed. J. B. Morris and D. J. Shusterman, Informa Healthcare, New York, USA.

Daniels, C.R.; Charlton, A.K.; Wold, R.M.; Pustejovsky, E.; Furman, A.N.; Bilbrey, A.C.; Love, J.N.; Garza, J.A.; Acree, W.E. Jr. & Abraham, M.H. (2004a) Mathematical correlation of naproxen solubilities in organic solvents with the Abraham solvation parameter model. *Physics and Chemistry of Liquids* 42 (5) 481-491.

Daniels, C.R.; Charlton, A.K.; Acree, W.E. Jr. & Abraham, M.H. (2004b) Thermochemical behavior of dissolved Carboxylic Acid solutes: Part 2 - Mathematical Correlation of Ketoprofen Solubilities with the Abraham General Solvation Model. *Physics and Chemistry of Liquids* 42 (3) 305-312.

De Ceaurriz, J. C.; Micillino, J. C.; Bonnet , P. & Guenier, J. P. (1981) Sensory irritation caused by various industrial airborne chemicals. *Toxicology Letters* 9 (2)137-143.

Diettrich, S.; Ploessi, F.; Bracher, F. & Laforsch, C. (2010) Single and combined toxicity of pharmaceuticals at environmentally relevant concentrations in Daphnia Magna – a multigeneration study. *Chemosphere* 79 (1) 60-66.

Doty, R. L.; Cometto-Muñiz, J. E.; Jalowayski, A. A.; Dalton, P.; Kendal-Reed, M. & Hodgson, M. (2004) Assessment of Upper Respiratory Tract and Ocular Irritative Effects of Volatile Chemicals in Humans. *Critical Reviews in Toxicology* 43 (2) 85-142.

Draize, J. H.; Woodward, G. & Calvery, H. O. (1944) Methods for the study of irritation and toxicity of substances applied topically to the skin and mucous membranes. *Journal of Pharmacology* 82 (3), 377-390.

Edwards, J.O. & Curci, R. (1992) Fenton type activation and chemistry of hydroxyl radical. In: *Catalytic oxidation with hydrogen peroxide as oxidant.* Struckul (ed.), Kluwer Academic Publishers, Netherlands, pp. 97–151.

Escher, B.I.; Baumgartner, B.; Koller, M.; Treyer, K.; Lienent, J. & McAndell, C. S. (2011) Environmental Toxicology and Risk Assessment of Pharmaceuticals from Hospital Wastewaters. *Water Research* 45 (1) 75-92.

Eger II, E. I.; Koblin, D. D.; Sonner, J.; Gong, D.; Laster, M. J.; Ionescu, P.; Halsey, M. J. & Hudlicky, T. (1999) Nonimmobilizers and transitional compounds may produce convulsions by two mechanisms. *Anesthesia & Analgesia* 88 (4) 884-892.

Famini, G. R.; Agular, D.; Payne, M. A.; Rodriquez, R. & Wilson, L. Y. (2002) Using the theoretical linear solvation energy relationships to correlate and to predict nasal pungency thresholds. *Journal of Molecular Graphics & Modelling* 20 (4) 277-280.

Ferguson, J. (1939) The use of chemical potentials as indices of toxicity. *Proceedings of the Royal Society of London, Series B* 127, 387-404.

Forbes, B.; Hashmi, N.; Martin G.P. & Lansley, A.B. (2000) Formulation of inhaled medicines: effect of delivery vehicle on immortalized epithelial cells. *Journal of Aerosol Medicine* 13 (3) 281–288.

Fourches, D.; Barnes, J.C.; Day, N.C.; Bradley, P.; Reed, J.Z. & Tropsha, A. (2010) Cheminformatics analysis of assertations mined from literature that describe drug-induced liver injury in different species. *Chemical Research in Toxicology* 23 (1) 171-183.

Franks, N. P. (2006) Molecular targets underlying general anesthesia. *British Journal of Pharmacology* 147 (Suppl. 1) S72-S81.

Gad-Allah, T.A.; Ali, M.E.M. & Badawy, M.I. (2011). Photocatytic oxidation of ciprofloxacin under simulated sunlight. *Journal of Hazardous Materials* 186 (1) 751-755.

Goldkind, L. & Laine, L. (2006) A systematic review of NSAIDs withdrawn from the market due to hepatotoxicity: lessons learned from the bromfenac experience. *Pharmacoepidemiology and Drug Safety* 15 (4), 213-220.

Gunatilleka, A.D. & Poole, C.F. (1999) Models for estimating the non-specific aquatic toxicity of organic compounds. *Analytical Communications* 36 (6) 235-242.

Gursoy, R.N. & Benita, S. (2004) Self-emulsifying drug delivery systems (SEDDS) for improved oral delivery of lipophilic drugs. *Biomedicine and Pharmacotherapy* 58 (3) 173–182.

Han, S.; Choi, K.; Kim, J.; Ji, K.; Kim, S.; Ahn, B.; Yun, J.; Choi, K.; Khim, J.S.; Zhang, X. & Glesy, J.P. (2010) Endocrine disruption and consequences of chronic exposure to ibuprofen in Japanese medaka (Oryzias latipes) and freshwater cladocerans Daphnia magna and Moina macrocopa. *Aquatic Toxicology* 98 (3) 256-264.

Hoover, K.R.; Acree, W.E. Jr. & Abraham, M.H. (2005) Chemical toxicity correlations for several fish species based on the Abraham solvation parameter model. *Chemical Research in Toxicology* 18 (9) 1497-1505.

Hoover, K.R.; Flanagan, K.B.; Acree, W.E. Jr. & Abraham, Michael H. (2007) Chemical toxicity correlations for several protozoas, bacteria, and water fleas based on the Abraham solvation parameter model. *Journal of Environmental Engineering and Science* 6 (2) 165-174.

Hoye, J.A. & Myrdal, P.B. (2008) Measurement and correlation of solute solubility in HFA-134a/ethanol systems. *International Journal of Pharmaceutics* 362 (1-2), 184-188.

Huang, C.P., Dong, C. & Tang, Z. (1993) Advanced chemical oxidation: its present role and potential in hazardous waste treatment. *Waste Mangement* 13 (5-7), 361–377.

Isidori, M.; Lavorgna, M.; Nardelli, A.; Pascarella, L. & Parrella, A. (2005) Toxic and genotoxic evaluation of six antibiotics on nontarget organisms. *Science of the Total Environment* 346 (1-3) 87–98.

Johnson, B. A. & Leon, M. (2000) Odorant Molecular Length: One Aspect of the Olfactory Code. *Journal of Comparative Neurology* 426 (2) 330-338.

Jover, J.; Bosque, R. & Sales, J. (2004) Determination of the Abraham solute descriptors from molecular structure. *Journal of Chemical Information and Computer Science* 44 (3) 1098-1106.

Khetan, S.K. & Colins, T.J. (2007) Human pharmaceuticals in the aquatic environment: a challenge to green chemistry. *Chemical Reviews* 107 (6) 2319-2364.

Kulik, N.; Trapido, M.; Goi, A.; Veressinina, Y. & Munter, Y. (2008) Combined chemical treatment of pharmaceutical effluents from medical ointment production. *Chemosphere*, 70 (8) 1525-1531.

Kuwabara, Y.; Alexeeff, G. V.; Broadwin, R. & Salmon, A.G. (2007) Evaluation and Application of the RD_{50} for determining acceptable exposure levels of airborne sensory irritants for the general public. *Environmental Health Perspective* 115 (11) 1609-1616.

Lamarche, O.; Platts, J.A. & Hersey, A. (2001) Theoretical prediction of the polarity/polarizability parameter π_2^H. *Physical Chemistry Chemical Physics* 3 (14), 2747-2753.

Lammert, C.; Einarsson, S.; Saha, C.; Niklasson, A.; Bjornsson, E. & Chalasani, N. (2008) Relationship between daily dose of oral medications and idiosyncratic drug-induced liver injury: search for signals. *Hepatology* 47 (6) 2003-2009.

Lemus, J. A.; Blanco, G.; Arroyo, B.; Martinez, F.; Grande, J. (2009) Fatal embryo chondral damage associated with fluoroquinolones in eggs of threatened avian scavengers. *Environmental Pollution* 157 (8-9) 2421-2427.

Luan, F. G.; Guo, L.; Cheng, Y.; Li, X. & Xu, X (2010) QSAR relationship between nasal pungency thresholds of volatile organic compounds and their molecular structure. *Yantai Daxue Xuebao, Ziran Kexue Yu Gongchengban* 23 (4) 272-276.

Luan, F.; Ma, W.; Zhang, X.; Zhang, H.; Liu, M.; Hu, Z. & Fan, B. T. (2006) Quantitative structure-activity relationship models for prediction of sensory irritants (log RD50) of volatile organic chemicals. *Chemosphere* 63 (7) 1142-1153.

Mintz, C.; Clark, M.; Acree, W. E., Jr. & Abraham, M. H. (2007) Enthalpy of solvation correlations for gaseous solutes dissolved in water and in 1-octanol based on the Abraham model, *Journal of Chemical Information and Modeling* 47 (1) 115-121.

Morris, J. B. & Shusterman (2010) Toxicology of the Nose and Upper Airways, Informa Healthcare, New York, USA.

Muller, J. & Gref, G. (1984) Recherche de relations entre toxicite de molecules d'interet industriel et proprietes physico-chimiques: test d'irritation des voies aeriennes superieures applique a quatre familles chimique. *Food and Chemical Toxicology* 22 (8) 661-664.

Naidoo, V.; Venter, L.; Wolter, K.; Taggart, M. & Cuthbert, R, (2010a) The toxicokinetics of ketoprofen in Gyps coprotheres: toxicity due to zero-order metabolism. *Archives of Toxicology*, 84 (10) 761-766.

Naidoo, V.; Wolter, K.; Cromarty, D.; Diekmann, M.; Duncan, N.; Meharg, A. A.; Taggart, M. A.; Venter, L. & Cuthbert, R. (2010b) Toxicity of non-steroidal anti-inflammatory drugs to Gyps vultures: a new threat from ketoprofen. *Biology Letters* 6 (3) 339-341.

Nielsen, G. D. & Alarie, Y. (1982) Sensory irritation, pulmonary irritation, and respiratory simulation by airborne benzene and alkylbenzenes: prediction of safe industrial exposure levels and correlation with their thermodynamic properties. *Toxicology and Applied Pharmacology* 65 (3) 459-477.

Nielsen, G. D. & Bakbo, J. V. (1985) Sensory irritating effects of allyl halides and a role for hydrogen bonding as a likely feature of the receptor site. *Acta Pharmacologica et Toxicologica* 57 (2) 106-116.

Nielsen, G. D. & Yamagiwa, M. (1989) Structure-activity relationships of airway irritating aliphatic amines. Receptor activation mechanisms and predicted industrial exposure limits. *Chemico-Biological Interactions* 71 (2-3) 223-244.

Nielsen, G. D.; Thomsen, E. S. & Alarie, Y. (1990) Sensory irritant receptor compartment properties. *Acta Pharmaceutica Nordica* 1 (2) 31-44.

Nikolaou, A.; Meric, S. & Fatta, D. (2005) Occurrence patterns of pharmaceuticals in water and wastewater environments. *Analytical and Bioanalytical Chemistry* 387 (4) 1225-1234.

Ozer, J.S.; Chetty, R.; Kenna, G.; Palandra, J.; Zhang, Y.; Lanevschi, A.; Koppiker, N.; Souberbielle, B.E. & Ramaiah, S.K. (2010) Enhancing the utility of alanine aminotransferase as a reference standard biomarker for drug-induced liver injury. *Regulatory Toxicology and Pharmacology* 56 (3) 237-246.

Paje, M.L.; Kuhlicke, U.; Winkler, M. & Neu, T.R. (2002) Inhibition of lotic biofilms by diclofenac. *Applied Microbiology and Biotechnology* 59 (4-5) 488-492.

Patton, J.S. & Byron, P. R. (2007) Inhaling medicines: delivering drugs to the body through the lungs. *National Reviews Drug Discovery* 6 (1) 67–74

Platts, J.A.; Butina, D.; Abraham, M.H. & Hersey, A. (1999) Estimation of molecular linear free energy relation descriptors using a group contribution approach. *Journal of Chemical Information and Computer Sciences* 39 (5) 835-845;

Platts, J.A.; Abraham, M.H.; Butina, D. & Hersey, A. (2000) Estimation of molecular linear free energy relationship descriptors by a group contribution approach. 2. Prediction of partition coefficients. *Journal of Chemical Information and Computer Sciences* 40 (1) 71-80.

Ramos, E.U.; Vaes, W.H.J.; Verhaar, H.J.M. & Hermens, J.L.M. (1998) Quantitative structure-activity relationships for the aquatic toxicity of polar and nonpolar narcotic pollutants. *Journal of Chemical Information and Computer Science* 38 (5) 845-852.

Roberts, D. W. (1986) QSAR for upper respiratary tract irritation. *Chemical-Biological Interactions* 57 (3) 325-345.

Sanderson, H. & Thomsen, M. (2009) Comparative Analysis of pharmaceuticals versus industrial chemicals acute aquatic toxicity classification according to the United Nations classification system for chemicals. Assessment of (Q)SAR predictability of pharmaceuticals acute aquatic toxicity and their predominant acute toxicity mode-of action. *Toxicology Letters* 187 (2) 84-93.

Schaper, M. (1993) Development of a data base for sensory irritants and its use in establishing occupational exposure limits. *American Industrial Hygiene Association Journal* 54 (9) 488-544.

Schultz, T.W.; Yarbrough, J.W. & Pilkington, T.B. (2007) Aquatic toxicity and abiotic thiol reactivity of aliphatic isothiocyanates: Effects of alkyl-size and –shape. *Environmental Toxicology and Pharmacology* 23 (1) 10-17.

Sell, C. S. (2006) On the unpredictability of odor. *Angewandte Chemie International Edition* 45 (38) 6254-6261.

Sewell, J.C. & Halsey, M.J. (1997) Shape similarity indices are the best predictors of substituted fluorethane and ether anaesthesia. *European Journal of Medicinal Chemistry* 32 (9) 731-737.

Sewell, J.C. & Sear, J.W. (2004) Derivation of preliminary three-dimensional pharmacophores for nonhalogenated volatile anesthetics. *Anesthesia & Analgesia* 99 (3) 744-751.

Sewell, J.C. & Sear, J.W. (2006) Determinants of volatile general anesthetic potency. A preliminary three-dimensional pharmacophore for halogenated anesthetics. *Anesthesia & Analgesia* 102 (3) 764-771.

Shaw, R.J. (1999) Inhaled corticosteroids for adult asthma: impact of formulation and delivery device on relative pharmacokinetics, efficacy and safety. *Respiratory Medicine* 93 (3) 149–160.

Shi, S. & Klotz, U. (2008) Clinical use and pharmacological properties of Selective COX-2 inhibitors. *European Journal of Clinical Pharmacology* 64 (3) 233-252.

Stovall, D.M.; Givens, C.; Keown, S.; Hoover, K.R.; Rodriguez, E.; Acree, W.E. Jr. & Abraham, M.H. (2005) Solubility of Crystalline Nonelectrolyte Solutes in Organic Solvents: Mathematical Correlation of Ibuprofen Solubilities with the Abraham Solvation Parameter Model. *Physics and Chemisry of Liquids*, 43 (3) 261-268.

Smyth. H.D.C. (2003) The influence of formulation variables on the performance of alternative propellant-driven metered dose inhalers. *Advanced Drug Delivery Reviews* 55(7), 807-828.

Steele, L. M.; Morgan, P. G. & Sendensky, M. M. (2007) Genetics and the mechanisms of action of inhaled anesthetics. *Current Pharmacogenomics* 5 (2) 125-141.

Taggart, M.A.; Senacha, K.R.; Green, R.E.; Cuthbert, R.; Jhala, Y.V.; Meharg, A.A.; Mateo, R. & Pain, D.J. (2009) Analysis of nine NSAIDs in ungulate tissues available to critically endangered vultures in India. *Environmental Science and Technology* 43(12) 4561-4566.

Tang, B.; Cheng, G.; Gu, J.-C. & Xu, J.-C. (2008) Development of solid self-emulsifying drug delivery systems: preparation techniques and dosage forms. *Drug Discovery Today* 13 (13-14) 606–612.

Tauxe-Wuersch, A.; De Alencastro, L.F.; Grandjean, D. & Tarradellas, J. (2005) Occurrence of several acidic drugs in sewage treatment plants in Switzerland and risk assessment. *Water Research* 39 (9) 1761-1772.

Tekin, H.; Bilkay, O.; Ataberk, S.S.; Balta, T.H.; Ceribasi, I.H.; Sanin, F.D.; Dilek, F.B. & Yetis, U. (2006) Use of Fenton oxidation to improve the biodegradability of a pharmaceutical wastewater. *Journal of Hazardous Materials* B136 (2) 258-265.

Triebskorn, R.; Casper, H.; Heyd, A.; Eibemper, R.; Köhler, H.-R. & Schwaiger, J. (2004) Toxic effects of the non-steroidal anti-inflammatory drug diclofenac Part II. Cytological effects in liver, kidney, gills and intestine of rainbow trout (*Oncorhynchus mykiss*). *Aquatic Toxicology* 68 (2) 151-166.

Tsagogiorgas, C.; Krebs, J.; Pukelsheim, M.; Beck, G.; Yard, B.; Theisinger, B.; Quintel, M. & Luecke, T. (2010) Semifluorinated alkanes - A new class of excipients suitable for pulmonary drug delivery. *European Journal of Pharmaceutics and Biopharmaceutics* 76 (1) 75-82.

van Noort, P.C.M.; Haftka, J.J.H. & Parsons, J.R. (2010) Updated Abraham solvation parameters for polychlorinated biphenyls. *Environmental Science and Technology* 44 (18) 7037-7042.

Veithen, A.; Wilkin, F.; Philipeau, M.& Chatelain, P. (2009) Human olfaction: from the nose to receptors. *Perfumer & Flavorist* 34 (11) 36-44.

Veithen, A.; Wilkin, F.; Philipeau, M.: Van Osselaare, C. & Chatelain, P. (2010) From basic science to applications in flavors and fragrances. *Perfumer & Flavorist* 35 (1) 38-43.

Von der Ohe, P.C.; Kühne, R.; Ebert, R.-U.; Altenburger, R.; Liess, M. & Schüürmann, G. (2005) Structure alerts – a new classification model to discriminate excess toxicity from narcotic effect levels of organic compounds in the acute daphnid assay. *Chemical Research in Toxicology* 18 (3) 536–555.

Wilson, D. A. & Stevenson, R. J. (2006) Learning to Smell. Johns Hopkins University | Press, Baltimore, USA.

Zhang, T.; Reddy, K. S. & Johansson, J. S. (2007) Recent advances in understanding fundamental mechanisms of volatile general anesthetic action. *Current Chemical Biology* 1 (3) 296-302.

Zissimos, A.M.; Abraham, M.H.; Barker, M.C.; Box, K.J. & Tam, K.Y. (2002a) Calculation of Abraham descriptors from solvent-water partition coefficients in four different systems; evaluation of different methods of calculation. *Journal of the Chemical Society, Perkin Transactions* 2 (3) 470-477.

Zissimos, A.M.; Abraham, M.H.; Du, C.M.; Valko, K.; Bevan, C.; Reynolds, D.; Wood, J. & Tam, K.Y. (2002b) Calculation of Abraham descriptors from experimental data from seven HPLC systems; evaluation of five different methods of calculation. *Journal of the Chemical Society, Perkin Transactions* 2 (12) 2001-2010.

Zissimos, A.M.; Abraham, M.H.; Klamt, A.; Eckert, F. & Wood, (2002a) A comparison between two general sets of linear free energy descriptors of Abraham and Klamt. *Journal of Chemical Information and Computer Sciences* 42 (6) 1320-1331.

13

Mikania glomerata and *M. laevigata*: Clinical and Toxicological Advances

João Cleverson Gasparetto, Roberto Pontarolo,
Thais M. Guimarães de Francisco and Francinete Ramos Campos
Department of Pharmacy, Universidade Federal do Paraná, Brazil

1. Introduction

Mikania laevigata and *M. glomerata*, commonly known as guaco, are important medicinal plant species used in South America for the treatment of respiratory diseases. In folk medicine, their leaves have ample use due to their balsamic, antiophidic, appetite stimulant, antispasmodic, expectorant, and antimalarial properties, among others (Coimbra, 1942; Lucas, 1942; Neves & Sá, 1991; Alice et al., 1995; Gasparetto et al., 2010; Napimoga & Yatsuda, 2010).

There is also pre-clinical evidence of the anti-inflammatory, anti-allergy, and bronchodilation activities of these species (Fierro et al., 1999; Moura et al., 2002; Suyenaga et al., 2002; Graca et al., 2007a). Due to their important effects, pharmaceutical preparations, including syrup and oral solutions, are freely distributed through various government phytotherapy programs and, thus, are widely used by the population (Gasparetto et al., 2010).

The pharmacological effects of guaco are attributed mainly to the presence of coumarin (1,2-benzopyrone); however, other metabolites have been shown to produce significant pharmacological effects. Studies that have evaluated isolated markers in the mouse model of allergic pneumonitis have demonstrated that coumarin and *o*-coumaric acid are part of the phytocomplex that is responsible for the therapeutic activities of guaco species (Santos et al., 2006). In addition, dihydrocoumarin and syringaldehyde have antioxidant, immunologic and anti-inflammatory properties (Farah & Samuelsson, 1992; Hoult & Paya, 1996; Bortolomeazzi et al., 2007; Stanikunaite et al., 2009; Gu & Xue, 2010). Finally, kaurenoic acid, isolated in high quantities from both species (Fierro et al., 1999; Veneziani et al., 1999; Yatsuda et al., 2005), has been shown to contribute to the effects of guaco through its antimicrobial, antinociceptive, anti-inflammatory and smooth muscle relaxant activities (Block et al., 1998; Costa-Lotufo et al., 2002; Wilkens et al., 2002; Cunha et al., 2003; Cotoras et al., 2004; Tirapelli et al., 2004; Cavalcanti et al., 2006).

The presence of these metabolites is directly related to the benefits of guaco, but studies have shown them to be toxic. Dihydrocoumarin administered to groups of rodents led to carcinogenic activity, ulcers, forestomach inflammation, parathyroid gland hyperplasia and increased nephropathy (National Toxicology Program, 1993a). Kaurenoic acid has been shown to kill sea urchin embryos and to cause hemolysis in mouse and human erythrocytes

(Costa-Lotufo et al., 2002); it also induces DNA breaks, cytogenetic abnormalities in human peripheral blood leukocytes, and positive genotoxic effects in the liver, kidney and spleen of mice (Cavalcanti et al., 2010). In addition, kaurenoic acid has been shown dose-dependent genotoxicity in Chinese hamster lung fibroblast cells (Cavalcanti et al., 2006).

Isolated coumarin has been shown to be carcinogenic, especially in the liver and lungs of rats and mice (Lake, 1999). With long exposure, this substance may change biochemical and hematological parameters and cause ulcers and necrosis, fibrosis, and cytologic alterations in the liver (National Toxicology Program, 1993b). In humans, the majority of tests for mutagenicity and genotoxicity suggest that coumarin is not toxic. This low toxicity is attributed to the mechanism of the detoxification of coumarin, which occurs via the 7-hydroxylation pathway in humans. In rats and mice, the main route is by 3,4-epoxidation, resulting in the formation of toxic metabolites (Lake, 1999).

Considering that the toxic and therapeutic effects of these metabolites are dose dependent, understanding their mechanisms and scientific advances is a key point to validate their therapeutic indications without putting human health at risk. This chapter describes the scientific aspects of guaco, especially the pre-clinical and clinical studies, with a particular emphasis on the pharmacological and toxicological effects of the extracts, preparations and isolated metabolites.

Keywords: *Mikania laevigata, Mikania glomerata,* guaco, toxicity, pharmacological effects, review, coumarin, *o*-coumaric acid and kaurenoic acid.

2. General overview

Mikania glomerata Sprengel and *M. laevigata* Schultz Bip. ex Baker, commonly known as guaco, are medicinal species used to treat several inflammatory and allergic conditions, particularly in the respiratory system due to their bronchodilator properties (Gasparetto et al., 2010).

Both species grow in the same regions and have similar morphological characteristics, which make them hard to distinguish. The leaves are similar, and both species have the characteristic odor of coumarin. The main difference between the species is the flowering period, which occurs in January for *Mikania glomerata* and September for *M. laevigata*. Therefore, humans use these plants without distinction (Lima, 2003; Ritter & Miotto, 2005).

An similar chemical profile has also been described for these plants (Oliveira, 1986; Lima & Biasi, 2002). Therefore, detailed studies of their morphological and anatomical features are necessary to allow botanical identification and quality control of these medicinal species in the absence of another way to make the distinction.

In folk medicine, these plants have a long history of use by rainforest inhabitants, especially by native peoples in South American, who have an ancient tradition of using guaco for the treatment of several diseases. Amazonian tribes have used the crushed leaf topically on skin eruptions and on snakebites. They also consume teas made from the leaves and/or stems against snake venom and to cure fevers, stomach disorders and rheumatism. South American tribes also believe that the aroma of the freshly crushed leaves left around sleeping areas keeps snakes away (Napimoga & Yatsuda, 2010).

In recent decades, guaco has been used as a home and commercial remedy. In popular medicine, the leaves have been widely used due to their tonic, antipyretic, balsamic, antiophidic, appetite stimulant, neuralgia, antispasmodic, expectorant, and antimalarial properties and for the treatment of rheumatism, eczema, influenza, asthma and sore throat.

Guaco can be used as infusion and decoction, but it is most commonly used in the commercialization of crude extracts for medicinal purposes (Coimbra, 1942; Lucas, 1942; Neves & Sá, 1991; Ruppelt et al., 1991; Galvani & Barreneche, 1994; Alice et al., 1995; Matos, 2000; Souza & Felfili, 2006; Botsaris, 2007).

Because of the therapeutic effects attributed to guaco species, syrups and oral solutions are widely used by the South American population and have been distributed in free government phytotherapy programs (Gasparetto et al., 2010). These preparations have been used as an effective natural bronchodilator, expectorant and cough suppressant in treatment of respiratory problems such as bronchitis, pleurisy, cold, flu, coughs and asthma, and sore throats, laryngitis and fever (Napimoga & Yatsuda, 2010).

3. Chemical constituents

Numerous studies have been conducted to evaluate the chemical composition of guaco species. Detailed screenings revealed the presence of alcohols, acids, esters, aldehydes, organic esters, terpenes, diterpenes, triterpenes and steroids, among other metabolites; some of them are associated with the therapeutic effects of guaco (Gasparetto et al., 2010).

A wide variation in metabolite content has been observed among different extracts and pharmaceutical preparations (Gasparetto et al., 2011). In fact, the geographic origins, agronomic aspects, extraction solvent and extraction techniques have been described as crucial factors to obtain a desirable substance. Thus, to maximize the yield of any metabolite and to standardize the extracts, these aspects must be considered (Gasparetto et al., 2010).

In the essential oil of guaco, a variety of compounds have been found, including α-acorenol, α-cadinol, α-copaene, α-humulene, α-muurolol, α-pinene, α-terpinol, β-pinene, β-farnesene, β-bourbonene, β-cubebene, β-elemene, β-caryophyllene, γ- elemene, (E)-β-ocimene, (E)-nerolidol, *p*-cymene, α, β, γ and Δ cardinene, α and TAU- caudynol, epi-α-bisabolol, epi-α-muurolol, aromadendrene, bicyclogermacrene, caryophyllene oxid, citronellyl acetate, coumarin, cubebene, elemol, germacrene-B, germacrene-D, globulol, limonene, linalol, myrcene, nerolidol E, nonanal, sabinene, silvestrene, spathulenol, terpin 4-ol, *trans*-ocymene, *trans*-cariophyllene and 1,4-dimethoxybenzene (Radunz, 2004; Duarte et al., 2005; Rehder et al., 2006).

In hexanic and dichloromethane extracts, the presence of coumarin, *o*-coumaric acid, campesterol, kaurenoic acid, grandiforic acid, stigmasterol, lupeol, lupeol acetate, germacrene, sesquiterpenes, 11-methylbutanoic acid, *ent*-15β-benzoyloxykaur-16(17)-en-19-oic acid, 17-hydroxy-*ent*-kaur-15(16)-en-19-oic acid, β-sitosterol and peroxides has been described (Oliveira et al., 1984; Vilegas et al., 1997a; Vilegas et al., 1997b; Santos et al., 1999; Veneziani et al., 1999; Cabral et al., 2001; Schenkel et al., 2002; Contini et al., 2006).

Hydroalcoholic extracts are the most common preparations that have been commercialized for therapeutic purposes, and the majority of phytochemical assays that have been conducted have been to evaluate their chemical compositions. Thus, using different analytical procedures, the presence of a large number of compounds has been described, including stigmasterol, phytol, 1-ethoxy-1-phenylethanol, 4-hydroxy-3,5-dimethoxybenzaldehyde, hexanoic acid, ethyl hexadecanoate, ethyl linoleoate, kaurenol, an isomer of kaurenoic acid, spathulenol, hexadecanoic acid, 9,12,15-octadecatrienoic acid, cupressenic acid, isopropiloxigrandifloric acid, 2-5-ciclohexadiene-1,4-dione,2,6-bis, 1-octadecene, octadecanoic acid, ester diterpenic, caryophyllene oxide, 10,13-octadecadienoic acid, isobutiloxigrandifloric acid, *trans*-cariofileno, 8,11-octadecadienoic acid, lupeol, lupeol

acetate, benzoylgrandifloric and cinnamoylgrandifloric acids (Oliveira et al., 1993; Moura et al., 2002; Biavatti et al., 2004; Santos, 2005; Yatsuda et al., 2005; Bertolucci et al., 2008; Alves et al., 2009; Bolina et al., 2009; Muceneeki et al., 2009).
In quantitative terms, the most prevalent metabolites of hydroalcoholic extracts are coumarin (1,2-benzopyrone) (Biavatti et al., 2004; Bueno & Bastos, 2009), *o*-coumaric acid (Santos, 2005), dihydrocoumarin (Alves et al., 2009), syringaldehyde (Muceneeki *et al.*, 2009) and kaurenoic acid (Vilegas et al., 1997a; Vilegas et al., 1997b; Yatsuda et al., 2005; Bertolucci et al., 2008). These substances have been associated with the therapeutic effects of guaco because they have anti-inflammatory and bronchodilator properties. The chemical structures of each compound are shown in Figure 1:

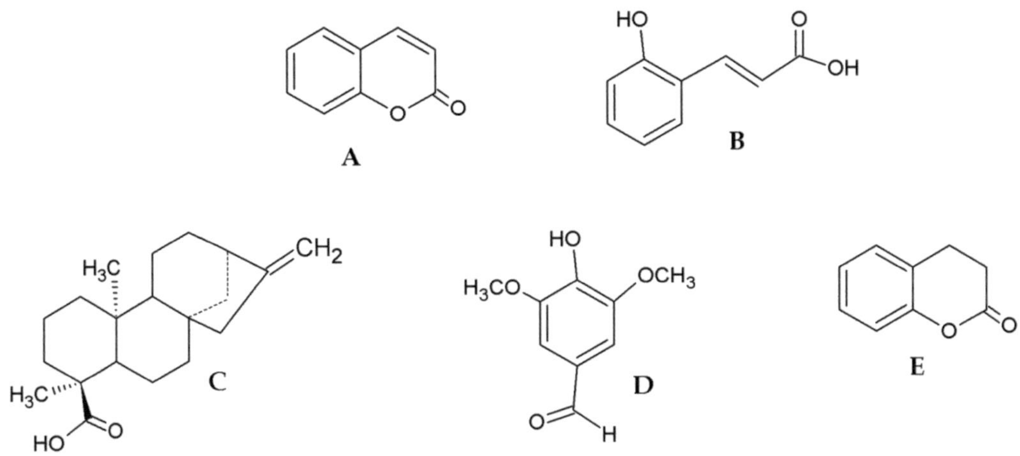

Fig. 1. Chemical structures of the main substances associated with the therapeutic effects of guaco. Data: (A) coumarin, (B) *o*-coumaric acid, (C) kaurenoic acid, (D) syringaldehyde and (E) dihydrocoumarin.

4. Pre-clinical and clinical trials

In addition to the use of guaco in popular medicine, pre-clinical studies have justified the main therapeutic uses of guaco species. Aqueous extracts prepared from several plant parts efficiently inhibit the different toxic, pharmacological, and enzymatic effects induced by the venom of *Bothrops* and *Crotalus* snakes. For example, guaco root extracts reduced the hemorrhage zone stimulated by the intradermal injection of *Bothrops* venom by 80% in rats. This result suggests that there is an interaction between the components of guaco and metalloproteases involving the catalytic sites of these enzymes or essential metal ions, thereby inhibiting their hemorrhagic activities (Maiorano et al., 2005).
Guaco extracts have also been considered to be powerful inhibitors of clotting activity, probably due to the interaction with thrombin-like enzymes. Guaco leaves and stems significantly diminished the coagulant activity induced by *Crotalus* and *Bothrops* venoms, especially the root extract, which led to clotting times of more than 45 min. Root extracts (1:50 *w/w*) also neutralized the edema caused by *Crotalus durissus terrificus* venom by 40%, with additional phospholipase A2 activity inhibition (95%). Nevertheless, no significant inhibition was observed against *Bothrops jararacussu* venom by incubating different ratios of guaco extracts and snake venom (1:50, 1:100 and 1:200 *w/w*) (Maiorano et al., 2005).

The tea of guaco leaves, administered orally in mice, had analgesic and anti-inflammatory activities following the intra-peritoneal administration of 0.1 N acetic acid or the intravenous administration of 0.2 mL Evans blue dye solution. The number of contortions was measured, and after 30 min of acid administration, a reduction of 63% was reached following oral administration of 10 mg/kg of the extract. The inhibition of dye diffusion to the peritoneal cavity was 49%, indicating an anti-inflammatory activity, but this result was not consistent with the analgesic effects (Ruppelt et al., 1991).

The hydroalcoholic extract also affected the inflammatory and oxidative stress caused by a single coal dust intratracheal instillation in rat. Histopathological analyses revealed that animals pretreated subcutaneously with the hydroalcoholic extract (100 mg/kg) had a reduction in lung inflammation, with an additional decrease in protein thiol levels, suggesting that guaco has an important protective effect on the oxidation of thiol groups (Freitas et al., 2008).

With regard to the antiedema activity of guaco, *in vivo* studies conducted in rats treated orally with an extract made from leaves (400 mg/kg) showed a complete reduction in the paw edema induced by carrageenan. A 28.26% decrease in leukocyte migration at the lesion site was also observed (Suyenaga et al., 2002). In mice, the subcutaneous administration of the same extract (3 mg/kg) significantly reduced the vascular permeability and leukocyte adhesion to inflammed tissues with carrageenan-induced peritonitis. The antiedema activity of guaco species has been associated with the inhibition of the pro-inflammatory cytokine production at the inflammatory site (Alves et al., 2009).

The ability of guaco to decrease ulcerative lesions was also tested by treating rats orally with 1000 mg/kg crude hydroalcoholic extract. A 50% decrease in the ulcerative lesions produced by reserpine was achieved, with higher levels of reduction in lesions caused by hypothermic restraint stress (82%), indomethacin (85%) and ethanol (93%). The antisecretory mechanism was confirmed by measuring acid hypersecretion induced by histamine, pentagastrin and bethanechol. Duodenal administration of the hydroalcoholic extract inhibited only the gastric acid secretion induced by bethanechol, a selective agonist of the muscarinic receptors of the parasympathetic nervous system (Bighetti et al., 2005).

The dichloromethane fraction obtained from the ethanolic extract was evaluated in rats for its anti-allergic and anti-inflammatory properties on ovalbumin-induced allergic pleurisy and in models of local inflammation induced by biogenic amines, carrageenan and Platelet-Activating Factor (PAF). The subcutaneous injection of 100 mg/kg of the dichloromethane fraction significantly reduced the plasma exudation, leukocyte infiltration and PAF. Because the pre-treatment of the animals did not alter the pleurisy induced by histamine, serotonin or carrageenan, the fraction was considered effective only for inhibiting immunologic inflammation and not the acute inflammatory response caused by other agents (Fierro et al., 1999).

Guaco also has antidiarrheal effects by decreasing the propulsive movements of the intestinal contents in mice. The percentage distances of the small intestine (from the pylorus to the ceccum) traveled by the charcoal plug were determined. Oral administration of aqueous guaco extract (1000 mg/mL) produced a significant reduction in the distance of the charcoal marker in the animal feces (66.99 ±10.60%). This extract was considered to give an excellent outcome because the reduction was as effective as that produced by loperamide (62.34 ±11.21%), a reference antidiarrheal drug (Salgado et al., 2005).

The antiparasitic effects of lyophilized hydroalcoholic extracts on the growth of *Leishmania amazonensis* and *Trypanosoma cruzi* were also established. By inoculating the parasites in medium containing 100 µg/mL of the extract, approximately 50% growth inhibition was observed for the *Trypanosoma* epimastigote and *Leishmania* promastigote forms. Additionally, under the tested concentration, a nearly complete reduction was achieved for the *Leishmania* amastigote form (97.5 ± 2.6%) (Luize et al., 2005).

Different guaco extracts were also tested for their antimicrobial properties. Using the minimal inhibitory concentration (MIC) assay, the essential oil obtained from guaco leaves had only limited action (MIC values from 300 to >1000 µg/mL) against *Candida albicans* and different serotypes of *Escherichia coli* (Duarte et al., 2005, 2007). Lyophilized hydroalcoholic extracts showed some degree of antibacterial activity, with MIC values of 500 µg/mL for *Staphylococcus aureus,* 250 µg/mL for *Bacillus subtilis,* 500 µg/mL for *Escherichia coli,* >1000 µg/mL for *Pseudomonas aeruginosa,* 500 µg/mL for *Candida krusei* and *C. tropicalis,* and >1000 µg/mL for *C. albicans* and *C. parapsilosis* (Holetz et al., 2002).

The antimicrobial activities of the hexane, ethanolic and ethyl acetate fractions from the ethanolic extract of both guaco species were also evaluated by the MIC and minimum bactericidal concentration (MBC) assays. Negligible activity was observed using ethyl acetate fractions against strains of *Streptococcus mutans, S. cricetus and S. sobrinus.* The ethanolic extract fraction had moderate activity (MIC and MBC values from 25 to > 800 µg/mL) against different strains of *S. cricetus*, *S. sobrinus* and *S. mutans* but no bactericidal activity (MIC and MBC values > 800 µg/mL) against *S. mutans* D1 and P6 strains. Only the hexane fraction showed remarkable antibacterial activity, having the lowest MIC (12.5–100 mg/ml) and MBC (12.5–400 mg/ml) values (Yatsuda et al., 2005).

Regarding the use of guaco for the treatment of respiratory diseases, *in vitro* studies revealed that the hydroalcoholic extract produced dose-dependent relaxation in denuded and intact rat epithelium tracheal precontracted with acetylcholine, with a median effective concentration (EC_{50}) of 1400 µg/mL and a maximum effect (E_{max}) of 95%. The mechanism of relaxation has also been established, leading to the conclusion that the antispasmodic activity of guaco does not depend on epithelium-derived substances but instead involves changes in the cellular mobilization of calcium (Graça et al., 2007a). A dose-dependent relaxation was also observed in human bronchi precontracted with potassium, with a median inhibitory concentration (IC_{50}) of 0.34 mg/mL, supporting the indication that guaco is effective for the treatment of respiratory diseases in which bronchoconstriction is present (Moura et al., 2002).

In addition to guaco extracts, isolated compounds, especially the main metabolites, also have substantial pharmacological effects. Studies conducted in a mouse model of allergy pneumonitis recognized that both coumarin and *o*-coumaric acid are part of the phytocomplex responsible for the therapeutic activities of guaco species because a reduction in the influx of total leukocytes and eosinophils in lung tissue was observed upon treatment with these substances. Anti-inflammatory and antioxidant properties have been described for dihydrocoumarin, reported to be one of the major compounds in hydroalcoholic extracts. Syringaldehyde has been shown to have a moderate antioxidant activity (Bortolomeazzi et al., 2007) and a dose-dependent inhibition of cyclooxygenase-2 (COX-2) activity (IC_{50} = 3.5 µg/mL), thereby contributing to the anti-inflammatory properties of guaco extracts (Farah & Samuelsson, 1992; Stanikunaite et al., 2009).

Kaurenoic acid (*ent*-kaur-16-en-19-oic acid) has lately been of considerable interest relating to the pharmacological activities of guaco species. At a concentration of 0.69 mg/mL, it has *in vitro* activity against trypomastigote forms of *T. cruzi*. It also has a moderate antimicrobial activity against strains of *S. aureus, S. epidermidis, Mycobacterium smegmatis* and *B. cereus.*

However, no antimicrobial action has been reported against Gram negative bacteria such as *E. coli* and *P. aeruginosa* (Silva et al., 2002; Zgoda-Pols et al., 2002).

Using the microculture tetrazolium assay (MTT), it was shown that 78 µM kaurenoic acid led to a 95% growth inhibition of CEM leukemic cells and a 45% growth inhibition of MCF-7 breast and HCT-8 colon cancer cells (Costa-Lotufo et al., 2002). In experiments conducted by the trypan blue dye-exclusion method, 70 µM kaurenoic acid reduced the viability of MCF7 and SKBR3 cells by 40% and 25%, respectively. However, resistance to treatment was observed in the HB4A cell line, demonstrating a selective activity in cancerous cells (Peria et al., 2010).

Kaurenoic acid also contributes to the anti-inflammatory activity of guaco. To determine this effect, lipopolysaccharide (LPS)-induced RAW264.7 macrophages were treated with different concentrations of kaurenoic acid, and a dose-dependent inhibition of nitric oxide production (IC_{50} = 51.73 µM) and prostaglandin E_2 release (IC_{50} = 106.09 µM) was observed. A reduction in the protein levels of COX-2 and the expression of inducible nitric oxide synthase was also seen. Additionally, kaurenoic acid dose-dependently inhibited the LPS-induced activation of the NF-kB mediator as assayed by electrophoretic mobility shift assay (EMSA), and it almost abolished the binding affinity of NF-kB for at 100.0 µM (Choi et al., 2011).

The anti-inflammatory effect of kaurenoic acid on acetic acid-induced colitis in rats has also been proven. Colitis was induced by intracolonic instillation of 2 ml of a 4% (*v/v*) acetic acid solution; 24 h later, the colonic mucosal damage was analyzed microscopically for the severity of mucosal damage, myeloperoxidase (MPO) activity and malondialdehyde (MDA) levels in the colon segments. A significant reduction in the gross damage score (52% and 42%) and wet weight of damaged colon tissue (39% and 32%) were observed in rats that received 100 mg/kg kaurenoic acid by rectal and oral routes, respectively. This effect was confirmed biochemically by a two- to three-fold reduction of the colitis-associated increase in MPO activity, a marker of neutrophilic infiltration, and by a marked decrease in the level of MDA, an indicator of lipoperoxidation in colon tissue. Furthermore, light microscopy revealed a marked decrease of inflammatory cell infiltration and submucosal edema formation in the colon segments of rats treated with kaurenoic acid (Paiva et al., 2002).

The *in vivo* anti-inflammatory effect of 50 mg/kg kaurenoic acid was examined in carrageenan-induced paw edema in mice. Kaurenoic acid dose-dependently reduced paw swelling up to 34.4% 5 h post-induction, demonstrating inhibition in an acute inflammation model. Taken together, the action of kaurenoic acid on COX-2 and inducible nitric oxide synthase expression is one of the mechanisms responsible for its anti-inflammatory properties (Choi et al., 2011).

At 160 µM, kaurenoic acid significantly decreased the contraction of rat uterine muscle precontracted with oxytocin (E_{max} = 83%) and acetylcholine (E_{max} = 91%) (Cunha et al., 2003). At 10 µM and above, kaurenoic acid also had concentration-dependent activity on vascular smooth muscle (endothelium-intact or denuded rat aortic rings) precontracted with phenylephrine and potassium chloride (Tirapelli et al., 2002, 2004). The mechanism of the vasorelaxant action involves the block of extracellular Ca^{2+} influx, but it is partly mediated by the activation of the nitric oxide cyclic GMP pathway and the opening of K^+ channels sensitive to charybdotoxin and 4-aminopyridine. Activation of the endothelial and neuronal nitric oxide synthase isoforms is also required for the relaxant effect induced by kaurenoic acid.

Although several guaco metabolites have been described as having therapeutic relevance, the simple coumarin (1,2 benzopyrone) has been considered to be the main component, and it has been used for the treatment of various clinical conditions. For example, in Brazil, the daily uptake (0.5–5 mg) of this substance has been assured by regulatory agencies (Brasil, 2008), but the recommended doses for the treatment of several diseases can vary largely according to the therapy (Lacy & O´Kennedy, 2004).

Coumarin is an anticoagulant and antithrombotic agent. It has been widely used in combination with troxerrutine to improve peripheral venous and lymphatic circulation and is also used to reduce the swelling caused by lymphatic and venous vessel problems. Pre-clinical studies also revealed that coumarin administered to the rat duodenum (100 mg/kg) produces antiulcerogenic activity by inhibiting the acid secretion mediated by the parasympathetic system (Bighetti et al., 2005).

In clinical trials, coumarin had *in vivo* macrophage-derived actions and has been used as an adjuvant in melanoma therapy and for recurrence prevention (Thornes et al., 1994). In carcinoma, coumarin (100 mg/day) in combination with cimetidine (1200 mg/day) led to metastatic reduction without toxic side effects (Thornes et al., 1982). Patients with metastatic prostate cancer were treated with 3 g of coumarin daily, and stable levels of prostate specific antigen (PSA) were maintained for over 7 years (Lacy & O´Kennedy, 2004).

Coumarin also activates macrophages and cells of the immune system (Hoult & Paya, 1996; Lacy & O´Kennedy, 2004). It has also been reported to reduce acute and chronic protein edema. In rodents, coumarin decreases the swelling caused by thermal damage; in humans, a significant reduction of lymphoedema was confirmed through a double-blind trial involving patients with elephantiasis and postmastectomy (Hoult & Paya, 1996).

Coumarin induces a concentration-dependent relaxation in guinea pig trachea pre-contracted with histamine (EC_{50} = 35.0 µg/mL) or carbachol (EC_{50} = 33.4 µg/mL) (Ramanitrahasimbola et al., 2005). However, this effect was not associated with the antispasmodic activity on rat jejunum and ileum cells isolated from guinea pig (Aboy et al., 2002). Coumarin was also less effective in guinea pig trachea (EC_{50} = 130.8 µg/mL) and endothelium-denuded trachea (EC_{50} = 153.4 µg/mL) pre-contracted with potassium chloride. When coumarin was combined with theophylline, a significant additive relaxing effect on pre-contracted trachea was observed, and this effect was not blocked by propranolol. These results indicate that the bronchodilator effect of coumarin is partly due to endothelium-dependent tracheal relaxation and also mediated through a non-specific tracheal relaxation (Ramanitrahasimbola et al., 2005).

5. Absorption, distribution, metabolism and excretion of coumarin, the main substance of guaco

Coumarin (1,2-benzopyrone) is a naturally occurring compound, which is present in a wide variety of plants, micro-organisms and in some animal species (Lake, 1999). In the 1990s, coumarin was widely used as a trial drug in cancer treatment and is still used to improve peripheral venous and lymphatic circulation, to stimulate the proteolytic effect of macrophages, and to treat edema. As a consequence, the metabolism of coumarin, including the excretion of some of its metabolites, has been widely studied in humans and other animal species.

Following oral administration, coumarin is rapidly absorbed from the gastrointestinal tract and distributed throughout the body (Egan et al., 1990; O´Kennedy & Thornes, 1997). The quick absorption is related to its non-polar characteristics and high partition coefficient (21.5%), which are considered favorable for rapid absorption, suggesting that coumarin should easily cross the lipid bilayer by passive diffusion (Lacy & O'Kennedy, 2004).

In systemic circulation, only 2 to 6% of coumarin molecules remain intact (Ritschel et al., 1979). In the liver, coumarin is converted to 7-hydroxycoumarin by a specific cytochrome P-450-linked mono-oxygenase enzyme (CYP2A6). Then, 7-hydroxycoumarin undergoes a phase II reaction, a glucuronide conjugation, that results in the formation of 7-hydroxycoumarin glucuronide, which is subsequently eliminated in the urine (O´Kennedy & Thornes, 1997; Wang et al., 2005).

In addition to 7-hydroxycoumarin, the formation of other metabolites is possible, and the metabolic pathways are species-specific. Thus, coumarin may be hydroxylated at one of the other five possible positions, carbons 3, 4, 5, 6, and 8, to yield 3-, 4-, 5-, 6- and 8-hydroxycoumarin, respectively. In addition, the lactone ring can also open and lead to the formation of a variety of metabolites, including *o*-hydroxyphenylacetaldehyde, *o*-hydroxyphenylethanol, *o*-hydroxyphenylacetic acid and *o*-hydroxyphenylacetic acid. The formation of 6,7-dihydroxycoumarin, *o*-coumaric acid, *o*-hydroxyphenylpropionic acid and dihydrocoumarin has also been described (Lake, 1999).

In humans, the half-life of intravenously administered coumarin can vary slightly according to the dosage (Ritschel et al., 1976), but its metabolism is usually fast. The low availability along with the short half-life (1.02 hrs peroneal vs. 0.8 hrs intravenous) lead coumarin to be considered as a pro-drug and 7-hydroxycoumarin as the substance with more therapeutic relevance (Lacy & O'Kennedy, 2004). In other species, the half-life of coumarin can vary from 1 to 4 hours and is quickly eliminated from systemic circulation.

The mechanism of the excretion of coumarin and its metabolites also depends of the species. For example, a large amount of biliary excretion has been described followed by a considerable elimination via feces in rats. In the Syrian hamster, rabbit and baboon, elimination is via urine. In humans, the rapid and total excretion via urine suggests that there is little or no biliary excretion (Shilling et al., 1969).

Regarding dermal application, coumarin is amply absorbed, distributed and excreted in the urine and feces of humans and rats. Following the applied dose of 0.02 mg/cm^2, the total absorption was 60% in humans and 72% in rats with a 6-h exposure. The mean plasma half-life of coumarin and its metabolites was approximately 1.7 h for humans and 5 h for rats. As in oral administration, the dermal application of coumarin resulted in the formation of 7-hydroxycoumarin and excretion in the urine as 7-hydroxycoumarin glucuronide. In rats, at least twenty metabolites were found, but only *o*-hydroxyphenylacetic acid was identified (Ford et al., 2001).

In summary, the 7-hydroxylation pathway is characteristic for human and a minor route for rat and mouse, which primarily use the 3,4-epoxidation pathway (Lacy & O'Kennedy, 2004). Another possible route in rat, Syrian hamster, gerbil and human is the 3-hydroxylation pathway leading to the formation of 3-hydroxycoumarin (Lake et al., 1992). The 3-hydroxycoumarin is a minor *in vivo* metabolite in rat and human and a major urinary metabolite in rabbit. The possible metabolic pathways of coumarin are shown in Figure 2.

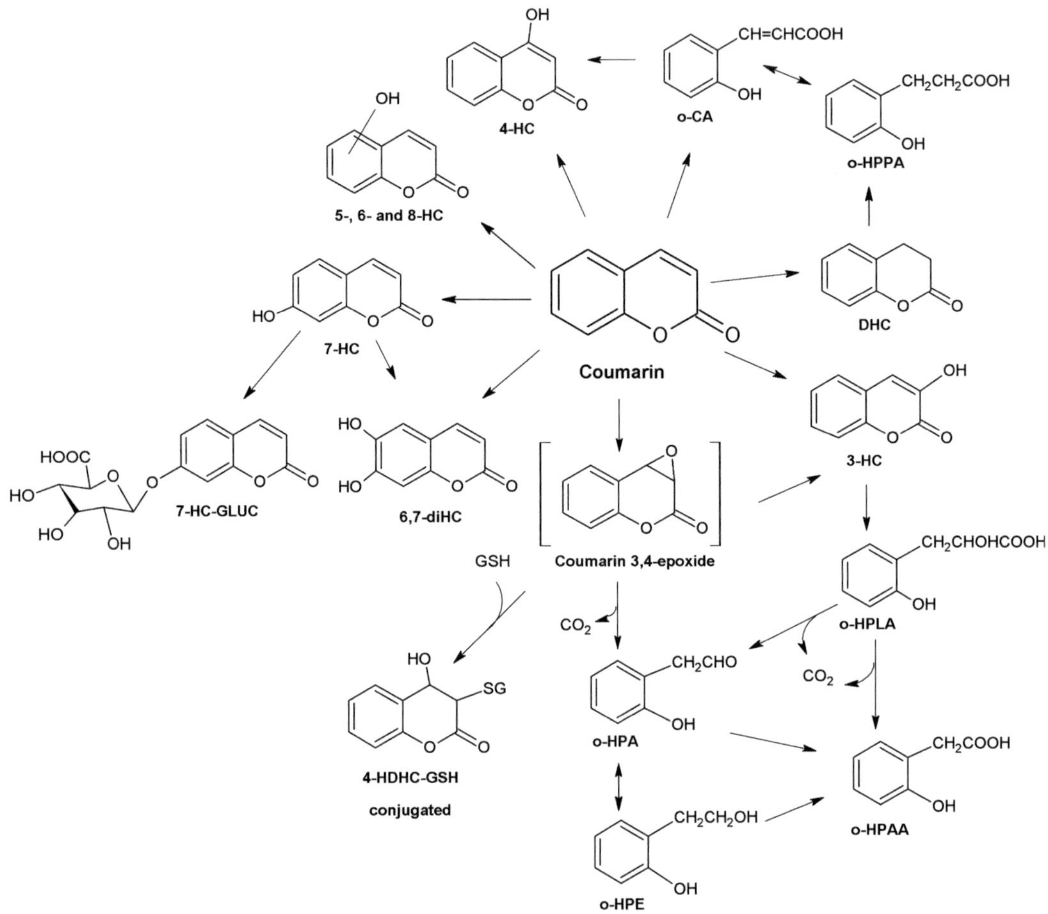

Fig. 2. Pathways of coumarin metabolism. Dihydrocoumarin (DHC); *o*-hydroxyphenylpropionic acid (o-HPPA); *o*-coumaric acid (o-CA); 3, 4, 5, 6, 7 and 8-hydroxycoumarin (HC); 7-hydroxycoumarin glucoronide (7-HC-GLUC); 6,7-dihydroxycoumarin (6,7-diHC); *o*-hydroxyphenylacetic acid (o-HPLA); o-hydroxyphenylacetic acid (o-HPAA); *o*-hydroxyphenylacetaldehyde (o-HPA); *o*-hydroxyphenylethanol (o-HPE); 4-hydroxydihydrocoumarin-glutathione-conjugated (4-HDHC-GSH).

6. Toxicological studies

Guaco species have been widely used by the South America population; thus, several studies, although insufficient, have been done to evaluate the toxicity of the extracts, phytomedicines, and isolated compounds.

The aqueous extract of *M. laevigata* was screened for anti-mutagenic activity using the Salmonella/microsome assay. The infusions was negative for mutagenic activity, showing high percentages of inhibition of mutagenesis induced by mutagens 2-aminofluorene (2AF), in the presence of exogenous metabolism (S9 fraction), for frameshift (TA98) and base pair substitution (TA100) lesions. In addition, these inhibitions were observed against mutagen sodium azide in assays with the TA100 strain, without exogenous metabolism (S9 fraction). A synergistic effect was also observed in frameshift mutagenic events, with direct action in the presence of 4-oxide-1-nitroquinoline and a tendency to a low percentage of action enhancement in the presence of the 2AF mutagen (Fernandes & Vargas, 2003).

In contrast to the outcomes from the Salmonella/microsome trials, studies conducted by the comet assay revealed that guaco extracts have deleterious effects. DNA damage was observed in rat hepatoma cells treated with hydroalcoholic maceration (10 and 20 µL/mL) and infusion (20 and 40 µL/mL) of the leaves. The genotoxic potential of the infusion was also observed by the micronucleous test at a very high concentration (40 µL/mL), suggesting a limitation in the phytotherapeutic use of guaco species (Costa et al., 2008).

Caution is recommended for patients who use lyophilized extracts or medicines containing isolated compounds, such as coumarin and *o*-coumaric acid. Hemorrhaging lung tissue was observed in mice treated with these substances and with the extract. However, this effect was not observed in animals treated with the whole hydroalcoholic extract, leading to the conclusion that some protective effect of the whole extract can be lost during the lyophilization process (Santos et al., 2006).

Because guaco showed an effect against *L. amazonensis* and *T. cruzi*, it was important to assess its toxic effects on mammalian host cells to determine the ratio of selectivity to biological activity. For this purpose, a test of cytotoxicity in sheep erythrocytes was performed using hydroalcoholic extracts of leaves at different concentrations and times of incubation. At 100, 500 and 1000 µg/mL, guaco extracts caused, respectively, 25, 50 and 75% hemolysis in erythrocytes incubated at 120 min. However, the hydroalcoholic extract was not considered cytotoxic to sheep erythrocytes because no significant hemolytic effect was observed at 100 and 500 µg/mL after 60 minutes of incubation (Luize et al., 2005).

The hydroalcoholic extract did not impair the fertility of rats following 52 days of oral treatment with a chronic dose of 3.3 g/kg of animal. In females, no changes in mating, gestation, preimplantation loss, the number of implanted embryos or offspring, weaning and the implantation and resorption indexes were observed using this kind of extract (SÁ et al., 2006). In males, the treatment did not alter body and organ weights and did not interfere in gamete production, serum testosterone levels or food intake (SÁ et al., 2003). Following 90 days of treatment, no significant change was observed in body and organ weights, gamete concentration on the epididymis cauda, serum testosterone level or food consumption, suggesting the absence of toxicity or antifertility activity of the hydroalcoholic extract (SÁ et al., 2010).

The absence of any effect on body weight gain or behavioral patterns in mice subjected to a repeated-dose over 14-, 28- or 60-day treatments (3 mg/kg) indicated that the *M. laevigata* ethanolic extract does not induce significant toxicity. The lack of alterations in hematological parameters, liver cell injury and serum aminotransferases (AST and ALT) was indicative of normal hepatic and biliary function. In addition, there was no change in urea levels, indicating the absence of alterations in the kidney. Additionally, the LD_{50} was found to be almost 75-fold higher than the pharmacological dose tested (Alves et al., 2009).

The potential genotoxicity of the dichloromethane fraction of the hydroalcoholic extract was evaluated on plasmid DNA using an alkaline lysis procedure, in which plasmid DNA was treated with $SnCl_2$ and the *M. glomerata* extract fraction. The role of reactive oxygen species in DNA damage was also evaluated by incubating the extract fraction with sodium benzoate, a hydroxyl radical scavenger. The results showed that the dichloromethane fraction was not genotoxic because this fraction did not damage DNA directly or by producing the hydroxyl radical reactive oxygen species (Moura et al., 2002)

The pharmaceutical preparation of guaco syrup did not produce any disturbances in the hematological or biochemical parameters in rodents following 90 days of treatment with subchronic and chronic doses (75, 150 and 300 mg/kg). Additionally, no evidence of toxicity in the hepatic, renal or pancreatic systems was reported. At reproductive endpoints, no alterations in body and organ weights, sperm, spermatid number, testosterone levels, or sperm morphology were observed after exposure to guaco syrup (Graca et al., 2007a, 2007b).

In humans, only two phase I clinical studies have been conducted to evaluate the clinical safety of guaco syrup. The volunteers (n= 24 - 26) received an oral dose of 15 mL phytomedicine four times a day over 21 to 28 days; after the treatment, any clinically significant changes in coagulation parameters were observed. In some cases, low variations in biochemical, hematological and serological analysis were observed, but none of the volunteers had values out of the established normality limits. Among them, only two volunteers reported mild drowsiness during the treatment, and one reported diarrhea and nausea. However, it is unclear if these effects were caused by guaco ingestion and in addition, clinical, electrocardiographic and laboratory tests did not show any evidence of toxicity. Nevertheless, more conclusive studies should be made because only phytomedicines containing low amounts of guaco extract associated with other plants were evaluated (Soares et al., 2006; Tavares et al., 2006).

The toxicity of the main isolated compounds has also been assessed. For example, kaurenoic acid has been shown to kill sea urchin embryos by inhibiting the first cleavage of the fertilized eggs (IC_{50} = 84.2 μM). Additionally, this compound progressively induced the destruction of embryos in other development stages (IC_{50} = 44.7 μM for blastulae stages and < 10 μM for larvae stages) (Costa-Lotufo et al., 2002).

Kaurenoic acid has been shown to have a weak to negligible capacity for killing human sperm. The estimated ED_{50} for sperm immobilization was 374.1 μg/mL, using 15×10^6 sperm/500 μL (VALENCIA et al., 1986). This compound has also been shown to induce dose-dependent hemolysis of mouse and human erythrocytes with an EC_{50} of 74.0 and 56.4 μM, respectively (Costa-Lotufo et al., 2002).

By the microculture tetrazolium test (MTT) assay, 78 μM kaurenoic acid causes cytotoxicity in CEM leukemic cells, leading to a 95% growth inhibition. This effect was also observed in MCF-7 breast and HCT-8 colon cancer cells, with a growth inhibition of 45% (Costa-lotufo et al., 2002). Moderate antiproliferative effects were also observed in K562, HL60, MDA-MB435 and SF295 human cancer cell lines (IC_{50} = 9.1 - 14.3 μg/mL). Fluorescence microscopy using acridine orange/ethidium bromide staining indicated that kaurenoic acid induced apoptosis and necrosis in HL-60 cell cultures, consistent with the findings described in the MTT assay. However, the antiproliferative effects were not selective to cancer cells because inhibition of lymphocyte proliferation also occurred (IC_{50} = 12.6 μg/mL) (Cavalcanti et al., 2009).

The cytotoxic effects of kaurenoic acid have been partly associated with its partial inhibitory effect on human topo-isomerase (topo) I activity. In contrast, 14-hydroxy-kaurane, xylopic acid, and semi-synthetic derivatives of kaurenoic acid [16*α*-methoxy-(−)-kauran-19-oic acid, 16*α*-methoxy-(−)-kauran-19-oic methyl ester and 16*α*-hydroxy-(−)-kauran-19-oic acid] lack genotoxic and mutagenic effects. This result suggests that the exocyclic double bond (C16) moiety may be the active pharmacophore for the genetic toxicity of kaurenoic acid (Cavalcanti et al., 2009).

At 30 and 60 µg/mL, kaurenoic acid also induces DNA breaks and cytogenetic abnormalities in human peripheral blood leukocytes (PBLs), as evaluated by comet, cytokinesis-block micronucleus and chromosomal aberration assays. Using a yeast cell model, cytotoxic and mutagenic effects of kaurenoic acid were also observed in the XV185-14c strain: there was an increase in the frequencies of point, frameshift, and forward mutations in the stationary phase at high concentrations (0.5–2 µg/mL). However, these effects were more pronounced when cells were treated in the exponential phase than in growth or non-growth conditions (Cavalcanti et al., 2010).

Positive genotoxic effects have also been described testing kaurenoic acid *in vivo* in multiple organs, such as the liver, kidney and spleen of mice (alkaline comet assay). DNA migration in liver cells was considerable at all tested doses (25, 50 and 100 mg/kg, i.p.) and at higher doses (50 and 100 mg/kg) in kidney cells. No DNA breaks were observed after the treatment in spleen cells (Cavalcanti et al., 2010). Finally, genotoxicity in Chinese hamster lung fibroblast cells was also observed using the comet and the micronucleus assays. However, lower concentrations (2.5, 5, and 10 µg/mL) failed to induce significant effects, whereas higher concentrations (30 and 60 µg/mL) lead to an increase in cell damage index and frequency. These data indicated that kaurenoic acid induces dose-dependent genotoxicity (Cavalcanti et al., 2006).

Dihydrocoumarin is one of the most studied guaco metabolites in regards to its toxic effects. In the human TK6 lymphoblastoid cell line, dihydrocoumarin caused an increase in p53 acetylation and cytotoxicity. Flow cytometric analysis to detect annexin V binding to phosphatidylserine demonstrated that dihydrocoumarin also increased apoptosis more than 3-fold over controls. In addition, dihydrocoumarin disrupted epigenetic processes in the yeast *Saccharomyces cerevisiae* and also inhibited several human sirtuin deacetylases (SIRT1 and SIRT2), a class of proteins that control some epigenetic processes and has, interestingly, been implicated in extending the longevity of several organisms (Olaharski et al., 2005).

Toxicity and carcinogenicity studies were also conducted by administering 99% pure dihydrocoumarin to groups of rats and mice in short (16 days), 13-week, and long (2 years) exposures. The short exposure lead to the death all male and female rats treated with 3000 mg/kg of dihydrocoumarin. At 1500 mg/kg, half of the animals died and a gain of body weight was observed; however, there were no clinical findings of organ-specific toxicity or evidence of impaired blood coagulation. A similar finding was also observed in mice groups, however with total mortality observed at a lower body/weight concentration than the rat groups (2250 mg/kg).

Following 13 weeks of administration, groups of 10 male and 10 female rats were studied, and a difference of exposure sensitivity was observed between the groups. In this case, two male and five female rats died after the administration of 1200 mg/kg dihydrocoumarin. The platelet counts were diminished in males receiving 600 mg/kg and in the female groups receiving 300 mg/kg dihydrocoumarin. Hemoglobin and hematocrit values were significantly lower in males that received 300 mg/kg dihydrocoumarin; this dose caused hepatocellular hypertrophy in both sexes. Additionally, the absolute and relative liver and kidney weights were significantly greater than those of the controls following a treatment of 600 mg/kg dihydrocoumarin. In mice groups, mortality was 80% in male and 50% in female receiving 1600 mg/kg dihydrocoumarin. With this exposure, the absolute and relative liver weight in both sexes and the relative kidney weight in males were significantly greater than those of the controls. However, no variation in body weight or changes in hematologic parameters were observed in either sex.

Under long dihydrocoumarin exposure (2 years), carcinogenic activity in male rats was evident based on the increased of incidence of renal tubule adenoma and focal hyperplasia. The transitional cell carcinomas in two males were chemical related. No evidence of carcinogenic activity was observed in female rats receiving 150, 300, or 600 mg/kg dihydrocoumarin. In mice, no evidence of carcinogenic activity was observed in male groups receiving 200, 400 or 800 mg/kg dihydrocoumarin; however, these doses led to an increase in the incidence of hepatocellular adenoma and carcinoma (combined) in females. In addition, ulcers, forestomach inflammation, parathyroid gland hyperplasia, and increased nephropathy were observed in these groups of rodents (National Toxicology Program, 1993a).

Coumarin, a main compound of guaco extracts, is a substance known to cause hepatotoxicity in liver rats. Prior to the existence of any available carcinogenicity and mutagenicity data, it was classified as a toxic substance by the Food and Drug Administration. Thus, it was banned in the USA in 1954 and in the UK in 1965 (Lake, 1999).

Various tests have been conducted to evaluate the toxicity and health effects of coumarin in laboratory animals. For example, doses of 25 mg/kg or higher were reported to produce liver damage in dogs (Felter et al., 2006). In primates (baboons) that received dietary coumarin for 2 years (0 to 67.5 mg/kg/day), no evidence of toxicity from biochemical and histochemical analyses was observed. However, an increase in the relative liver weight occurred at a high dosage, with additional dilatation of the endoplasmic reticulum observed after 10 months of treatment (Felter et al., 2006). The Syrian hamster has also been found to be resistant to coumarin-induced toxicity (Lake, 1999)

In groups of rats and mice, 97% pure coumarin administered orally has toxic effects with a short exposure (16 days), after 13 weeks, and a long (2 years) exposure. All groups of male and female rats died following 16 days of treatment with 400 mg/kg of coumarin. Increases in mean body weight also occurred, but no clinical signs of organ-specific toxicity were observed. Additionally, coagulation parameters were not impaired. In mice, groups of 5 male and 5 female rats were studied, and all 10 mice receiving 600 mg/kg, two male mice receiving 300 mg/kg, and one male mouse receiving 75 mg/kg died. With a short exposure, coagulation parameters were not impaired; however, an increase in the mean body weight and excessive lacrimation, piloerection, bradypnea and ataxia were observed for the 300 mg/kg dose in the first hours of administration (National Toxicology Program, 1993b).

Following 13 weeks of exposure to 300 mg/kg of coumarin, 30% of rats in the male and female groups died. Both groups had increased erythrocyte counts and decreased hemoglobin and erythrocyte mean volumes. Serum levels of total bilirubin and one or more cytoplasmic enzymes were higher than those of control groups. The absolute and relative liver weights also increased significantly following the administration of 150 mg/kg coumarin, and centrilobular hepatocellular degeneration and necrosis, chronic active inflammation, and bile duct hyperplasia were also observed in the liver. In the mice groups, 20% of male and female groups receiving 300 mg/kg coumarin died; similar to rats, coumarin decreased the erythrocyte volume and hemoglobin. Centrilobular hepatocellular hypertrophy was observed in both sexes at 300 mg/kg, and the absolute and relative liver weights increased following treatment with 150 mg/kg coumarin.

During the long (2 years) exposure, groups of 60 male and 60 female rats were treated with coumarin at different dosages, and after 15 months, 10 animals from each group were evaluated. Treatment with 50 mg/kg led to a significant reduction in the activated partial thromboplastin times and the erythrocyte volume and hemoglobin values, and an increase of platelet counts was also observed. With this dose, the values of alanine aminotransferase, sorbitol dehydrogenase, and g-glutamyltransferase significantly increased in males, whereas these effects were observed only from 100 mg/kg in females. Additionally, lesions associated with the administration of coumarin were also observed during the long exposure, which include an increase of the severity of nephropathy, increase of incidences of bile duct and parathyroid gland hyperplasias, increase of the incidences of ulcers, and necrosis, fibrosis, and cytologic alterations in the liver (National Toxicology Program, 1993b). A carcinogenic potential has also been described for coumarin, especially in the liver and lungs of rats and mice. However, the dose–response relationships are nonlinear with tumor formation and hepatic and pulmonary toxicity are associated only with high doses (Lake, 1999).

Regarding the mutagenic and genotoxic potential of coumarin, it showed weak clastogenic activity in Chinese Hamster ovary cells *in vitro*. However, this response was observed only at a very high concentration (10.95 µM). Negative responses were reported in the *Salmonella typhimurium* assay in the TA98, TA1535, TA1537 and TA1538 strains, either with or without metabolic activation. However, gene mutations have been described in the TA100 strain in the presence of a metabolic activating system (S9) (Lake, 1999).

Using the Ames genotoxic assay, coumarin has not been shown to be a mutagenic agent in the TA100 strain assessed without metabolic activation (liver S9 fraction). With metabolic activation, coumarin produces only a weak positive effect at a high concentration. However, this effect has been widely discussed because a greater response was achieved in the presence of liver S9 fraction from untreated Syrian hamsters than from rats treated with Aroclor 1254, a substance used to stimulate coumarin metabolism by the 3,4-epoxidation pathway in rat hepatic microsomes. This result does not correlate with the extent of coumarin metabolism and coumarin-induced liver injury in these species. Because of the differences in their metabolic pathways, a chronic dose of coumarin induces liver lesions and tumor in the rat and not in the Syrian hamster, which appears to be refractory for coumarin-induced hepatotoxicity (Lake, 1999).

In addition, *in vivo* studies have shown that coumarin is unable to induce sex-linked recessive lethal mutations in germ cells of male *Drosophila melanogaster*. Furthermore, no evidence for coumarin-induced genotoxicity has been observed in the *in vivo* micronucleus test in mouse peripheral blood cells. The conclusion is that coumarin is not DNA-reactive and that the induction of tumors at high doses in rodents is attributed to cytotoxicity and regenerative hyperplasia (Felter et al., 2006).

In humans, the majority of tests for mutagenicity and genotoxicity also suggest that coumarin is not a toxic agent (Lake, 1999). The lack of toxicity has been associated with the detoxification mechanism of coumarin, which in humans involves the 7-hydroxylation pathway, a minor route in rats and mice; these rodents use the 3,4-epoxidation pathway instead, which results in toxic metabolite formation (Gasparetto et al., 2011). Thus, the species-specific target organ toxicity has been attributed to the pharmacokinetics of coumarin metabolism, causing rats to be susceptible to liver effects and mice to have toxicity particularly in the lung. Therefore, it is possible to conclude that the use of rats and mice is not an adequate model to compare the metabolism and toxicity of coumarin with humans, due to their particular metabolism. Because *in vitro* genotoxicity studies demonstrated toxicity only at very high doses and no evidence for *in vivo* studies was observed, it is possible to conclude that there is no human health risk from coumarin exposure in natural dietary sources, such guaco species.

7. Conclusion

For centuries, medicinal plants have been used worldwide for the treatment of several diseases. In South American populations, plant products significantly contribute to primary health care and are sometimes the only therapeutic resources of some communities and ethnic groups.

Among the medicinal species used in South America populations, *M. glomerata* and *M. laevigata* are especially important due to their relevant therapeutic properties. In popular medicine, both species have a long history of use, and they are still employed especially for the treatment of respiratory diseases.

Pre-clinical trials have been conducted on guaco extract that have revealed scientific evidence for its anti-inflammatory, anti-allergy, and bronchodilation properties. However, there are currently no clinical studies for assessing the efficacy of guaco extracts and preparations in patients who present respiratory complaints.

Both guaco species have many bioactive compounds that probably contribute to the pharmacological effects. Thus, the properties of guaco should not be attributed only to coumarin because high contents of kaurene diterpenes and cinnamic acid derivatives were found in the extracts. Studies involving the quality control of different brands of guaco phytomedicines and extracts have been conducted and have shown a wide variation in the content of the main metabolites. A number of studies have reported that this discrepancy is due to the geographic origins, agronomic aspects, extractor solvent and extraction techniques of the guaco. Therefore, depending of the region and period of plant collection, the effects and/or toxicity of guaco may change or not be evident.

Regarding the safety of the extracts, phytomedicines and isolated compounds, guaco species did not present significant toxic and genotoxic effects in humans. However, the majority of studies were conducted in rat and mice, which have a unique metabolism, suggesting that new studies must be conducted. Additionally, relevant information on metabolism, bioavailability and toxicity has only been reported for coumarin, without substantial information concerning the other main metabolites.

In general, is possible to conclude that there is a need for clinical studies using standardized phytomedicines or extracts. This may be the most important step to ensure conclusive studies of guaco species. By conducting clinical studies, it will be possible to know the most effective extract for therapeutic purposes and to correlate the metabolite content with its relevance in a pharmacological and toxicological context. Meeting this requirement will guarantee the benefits and safe use of guaco.

8. References

Aboy, A. L.; Ortega, G. G.; Petrovick, P. R.; Langeloh, A. & Bassani, V. L. (2002). Atividade Antiespasmódica de Soluções Extrativas de *Mikania glomerata* Sprengel (guaco). *Acta Farmaceutica Bonaerense*, Vol.21, No.3, (June, 2002), pp. 185-191, ISSN 0326-2383

Alice, C. B.; Siqueira, N. C. S.; Mentz, L. A.; Silva, G. A. A. B. & José, K. F. D. (1995). *Plantas Medicinais de Uso Popular, Atlas Farcacognóstico*, Ulbra, Canoas, Brasil

Alves, C. F.; Alves, V. B. F.; De Assis, I. P.; Clemente-Napimoga, J. T.; Uber-Bucek, E.; Dal-Secco, D.; Cunha, F. Q.; Rehder, V. L. G. & Napimoga, M. H. (2009). Anti-inflammatory Activity and Possible Mechanism of Extract from *Mikania laevigata* in

Carrageenan-induced Peritonitis. *Journal of Pharmacy and Pharmacology*, Vol.61, No.8, (August, 2009), pp.1097-1104, ISSN 0022-3573

Bertolucci, S. K.; Pereira, A. B.; Pinto, J. E.; Aquino Ribeiro, J. A.; Oliveira, A. B. & Braga, F. C. (2008). Development and Validation of an RP-HPLC Method for Quantification of Cinnamic Acid Derivatives and Kaurane-Type Diterpenes in *Mikania laevigata* and *Mikania glomerata*. *Planta Medica*, Vol.75, No.3, (December, 2008), pp. 280-285 ISSN 0032-0943

Biavatti, M. W.; Koerich, C. A.; Henck, C. H.; Zucatelli, E.; Martineli, F. H.; Bresolin, T. B. & Leite, S. N. (2004). Coumarin Content and Physicochemical Profile of *Mikania laevigata* Extracts. *Zeitschrift für Naturforschung*, Vol.59, No.3, (March-April, 2004), pp. 197-200, ISSN 0939-5035

Bighetti, A. E.; Antonio, M. A.; Kohn, L. K.; Rehder, V. L.; Foglio, M. A.; Possenti, A.; Vilela, L. & Carvalho, J. E. (2005). Antiulcerogenic Activity of a Crude Hydroalcoholic Extract and Coumarin Isolated from *Mikania laevigata* Schultz Bip. *Phytomedicine*, Vol.12, No.1, (January, 2005), pp. 72-77, ISSN 0944-7113

Block, L. C.; Scheidt, C.; Quintao, N. L.; Santos, A. R. & Cechinel-Filho, V. (1998). Phytochemical and Pharmacological Analysis of Different Parts of *Wedelia paludosa* DC. (Compositae). *Pharmazie*, Vol.53, No.10, (October, 1998), pp. 716-718, ISSN 0031-7144

Bolina, R. C.; Garcia, E. F. & Duarte, M. G. R. (2009). Estudo Comparativo da Composição Química das Espécies Vegetais *Mikania glomerata* Sprengel e *Mikania laevigata* Schultz Bip. ex Baker. *Revista Brasileira de Farmacognosia*, Vol.19, No.1, (January/March, 2009), pp. 294-298, ISSN 0102-695X

Bortolomeazzi, R.; Sebastianutto, N.; Toniolo, R. & Pizzariello, A. (2007). Comparative Evaluation of the Antioxidant Capacity of Smoke Flavouring Phenols by Crocin Bleaching Inhibition, DPPH Radical Scavenging and Oxidation Potencial. *Food Chemistry*, Vol.100, No.4, (November, 2005), pp. 1481-1489, ISSN 0308-8146

Botsaris, A. S. (2007). Plants Used Traditionally to Treat Malaria in Brazil: The Archives of Flora Medicinal. *Journal of Ethnobiology and Ethnomedicine*, Vol.3, No.1, (May, 2007), pp. 18, ISSN 1746-4269

Brasil (2008). Agência Nacional de Vigilância Sanitária - ANVISA. Instrução Normativa nº 5 de 11 de dezembro de 2008 - Determina a Lista de Registro Simplificado de Fitoterápicos no Brasil. *Diário Oficial da União*, Brasília - DF.

Bueno, P. C. P. & Bastos, J. K. (2009). A Validated Capillary Gas Chromatography Method for Guaco (*Mikania glomerata* S.) Quality Control and Rastreability: From Plant Biomass to Phytomedicines. *Revista Brasileira de Farmacognosia*, Vol.19, No.1, (January-March, 2009), pp. 218-223, ISSN 0102-695X

Cabral, L. M.; Santos, T. C. & Alhaique, F. (2001). Development of a Profitable Procedure for the Extraction of 2-H-1-benzopyran-2-one (coumarin) from *Mikania glomerata*. *Drug Development and Industrial Pharmacy*, Vol.27, No.1, (July, 2009), pp. 103-106, ISSN 1520-5762

Cavalcanti, B. C.; Bezerra, D. P.; Magalhaes, H. I. F.; Moraes, M. O.; Lima, M. A. S.; Silveira, E. R.; Camara, C. A. G.; Rao, V. S.; Pessoa, C. & Costa-Lotufo, L. V. (2009). Kauren-19-oic Acid Induces DNA Damage Followed by Apoptosis in Human Leukemia Cells. *Journal of Applied Toxicology*, Vol.29, No.7, (October, 2009), pp. 560-568, ISSN 0260-437X

Cavalcanti, B. C.; Costa-Lotufo, L. V.; Moraes, M. O.; Burbano, R. R.; Silveira, E. R.; Cunha, K. M.; Rao, V. S.; Moura, D. J.; Rosa, R. M.; Henriques, J. A. & Pessoa, C. (2006). Genotoxicity evaluation of kaurenoic acid, a bioactive diterpenoid present in Copaiba oil. *Food and Chemical Toxicology,* Vol.44, No.3, (March, 2006), pp. 388-392, ISSN 0278-6915

Cavalcanti, B. C.; Ferreira, J. R. O.; Moura, D. J.; Rosa, R. M.; Furtado, G. V.; Burbano, R. R.; Silveira, E. R.; Lima, M. A. S.; Camara, C. A. G.; Saffi, J.; Henriques, J. A. P.; Rao, V. S. N.; Costa-Lotufo, L. V.; Moraes, M. O. & Pessoa, C. (2010). Structure-mutagenicity Relationship of Kaurenoic Acid from *Xylopia sericeae* (Annonaceae). *Mutation Research/Genetic Toxicology and Environmental Mutagenesis*, Vol.701, No.2, (June, 2010), pp. 154-163, ISSN 1383-5718

Choi, R. J.; Shin, E. M.; Jung, H. A.; Choi, J. S. & Kim, Y. S. (2011). Inhibitory Effects of Kaurenoic Acid from *Aralia continentalis* on LPS-induced Inflammatory Response in RAW264.7 macrophages. *Phytomedicine,* Vol. 18, No. 5, (March, 2011), pp. 677-682, ISSN 0944-7113

Coimbra, R. (1942). *Notas de Fitoterapia.* L. C. S. A., Rio de Janeiro, Brasil

Contini, S. H. T.; Santos, P. A.; Veneziani, R. C. S.; Pereira, M. A. S.; Franca, S. C.; Lopes, N. P. & Oliveira, D. C. R. (2006). Differences in Secondary Metabolites from Leaf Extracts of *Mikania glomerata* Sprengel Obtained by Micropropagation and Cuttings. *Revista Brasileira de Farmacognosia,* Vol.16, No.1, (December, 2006), pp. 596-598, ISSN 0102-695X

Costa-Lotufo, L. V.; Cunha, G. M.; Farias, P. A.; Viana, G. S.; Cunha, K. M.; Pessoa, C.; Moraes, M. O.; Silveira, E. R.; Gramosa, N. V. & Rao, V. S. (2002). The Cytotoxic and Embryotoxic Effects of Kaurenoic Acid, a Diterpene Isolated from *Copaifera langsdorffii* Oleo-resin. *Toxicon,* Vol.40, No.8, (April, 2002), pp. 1231-1234, ISSN 0041-0101

Costa, R. J.; Diniz, A.; Mantovani, M. S. & Jordao, B. Q. (2008). *In vitro* Study of Mutagenic Potential of *Bidens pilosa* Linne and *Mikania glomerata* Sprengel Using the Comet and Micronucleus Assays. *Journal of Ethnopharmacology,* Vol. 118, No. 1, (March, 2008), pp. 86-93, ISSN 0378-8741

Cotoras, M.; Folch, C. & Mendoza, L. (2004). Characterization of the Antifungal Activity on *Botrytis cinerea* of the Natural Diterpenoids Kaurenoic Acid and 3β-hydroxy-kaurenoic Acid. *Journal of Agricultural and Food Chemistry,* Vol.52, No.10, (May, 204), pp. 2821-2826, ISSN 0021-8561

Cunha, K. M. A.; Paiva, L. A. F.; Santos, F. A.; Gramosa, N. V.; Silveira, E. R. & Rao, V. S. N. (2003). Smooth Muscle Relaxant Effect of Kaurenoic Acid, a Diterpene from *Copaífera langsdorffii* on Rat Uterus *in vivo. Phytotherapy Research,* Vol.17, No.4, (April, 2003), pp. 320-324, ISSN 0951-418X

Duarte, M. C.; Figueira, G. M.; Sartoratto, A.; Rehder, V. L.; Delarmelina, C. (2005). Anti-Candida activity of Brazilian Medicinal Plants. *Journal of Ethnopharmacology,* Vol.97, No.2, (February, 2005), pp. 305-311, ISSN 0378-8741

Duarte, M. C. T.; Leme, E. E.; Delarmelina, C.; Soares, A. A.; Figueira, G. M. & Sartoratto, A. (2007). Activity of Essencial Oils from Brazilian Medicinal Plants on *Escherichia coli. Journal of Ethnopharmacology,* Vol.111, No.1, (December, 2006), pp. 197-201, ISSN 0378-8741

Egan, D.; O'Kennedy, R.; Moran, E.; Cox, D.; Prosser, E. & Thornes, R. D. (1990). The Pharmacology, Metabolism, Analysis, and Applications of Coumarin and Coumarin-Related Compounds. *Drug Metabolism Reviews*, Vol.22, No.5, (May, 1990), pp. 503-529, ISSN 0360-2532

Farah, M. H. & Samuelsson, G. (1992). Pharmacologically active phenylpropanoids from *Senra incana*. *Planta Medica*, Vol. 58, No.1, (February, 1992), pp.14-18, ISSN 0032-0943

Felter, S. P.; Vassallo, J. D.; Carlton, B. D. & Daston, G. P. A. (2006). Safety Assessment of Coumarin Taking Into Account Species-specificity of Toxicokinetics. *Food and Chemical Toxicology*, Vol.44, No.4, (April, 2006), pp.462-475, ISSN 0278-6915

Fernandes, J. B. & Vargas, V. M. (2003). Mutagenic and Antimutagenic Potential of the Medicinal Plants *M. laevigata* and *C. xanthocarpa*. *Phytotherapy Research*, Vol.17, No.3, (March, 2003), pp. 269-273, ISSN 1099-1573

Fierro, I. M.; Silva, A. C.; S., L. C.; Moura, R. S. & Barja-Fidalgo, C. (1999). Studies on the Anti-allergic Activity of *Mikania glomerata*. *Journal of Ethnopharmacology*, Vol.66, No.1, (July, 1999), pp. 19-24, ISSN 0378-8741

Ford, R. A.; Hawkins, D. R.; Mayo, B. C. & Api, A. M. (2001). The *In vivo* Dermal Absorption and Metabolism of [4-C-14] Coumarin by Rats and by Human Volunteers Under Simulated Conditions of Use in Fragrances. *Food and Chemical Toxicology*, Vol.39, No.2, (February, 2001), pp. 153-162, ISSN 0278-6915

Freitas, T. P.; Silveira, P. C.; Rocha, L. G.; Rezin, G. T.; Rocha, J.; Citadini-Zanette, V.; Romao, P. T.; Dal-Pizzol, F.; Pinho, R. A.; Andrade, V. M. & Streck, E. L. (2008). Effects of *Mikania glomerata* Spreng. and *Mikania laevigata* Schultz Bip. ex Baker (Asteraceae) Extracts on Pulmonary Inflammation and Oxidative Stress Caused by Acute Coal Dust Exposure. *Journal of Medicinal Food*, Vol.11, No.4, (December, 2008), pp. 761-766, ISSN 1096-620X

Galvani, F. R. & Barreneche, M. L. (1994). Levantamento das Espécies Vegetais Utilizadas em Medicina Popular no Município de Uruguaiana (RS). *Revista FZVA*, Vol.1, No.1, pp. 1-14, ISSN 0104-4257

Gasparetto, J. C.; Campos, F. R.; Budel, J. M. & Pontarolo, R. (2010). *Mikania glomerata* e *M. laevigata*: Estudos Agronômicos, Genéticos, Morfoanatômicos, Químicos, Farmacológicos, Toxicológicos e Uso nos Programas de Fitoterapia do Brasil - Uma Revisão. *Revista Brasileira de Farmacognosia*, Vol.20, No.4, (August/September, 2010), pp. 627-640, ISSN 0102-695X

Gasparetto, J. C.; Francisco, T. M. G.; Campos, F. R. & Pontarolo, R. (2011). Development and Validation of Two Methods Based on High Performance Liquid Chromatography-tandem Mass Spectrometry for Determining 1,2 benzopirone, Dihydrocoumarin, *o*-coumaric acid, Syringaldehyde and Kaurenoic Acid in Guaco Extracts and Pharmaceutical Preparations. *Journal of Separation Sciences*, Vol.34, No.1, (January, 2011), pp. 1-9, ISSN 1615-9306

Graca, C.; Baggio, C. H.; Freitas, C. S.; Rattmann, Y. D.; De Souza, L. M.; Cipriani, T. R.; Sassaki, G. L.; Rieck, L.; Pontarolo, R.; Silva-Santos, J. E. & Marques, M. C. (2007a). *In vivo* Assessment of Safety and Mechanisms Underlying *In vitro* Relaxation Induced by *Mikania laevigata* Schultz Bip. ex Baker in the Rat Trachea. *Journal of Ethnopharmacology*, Vol.112, No.3, (March, 2007), pp. 430-439, ISSN 0378-8741

Graca, C.; Freitas, C. S.; Baggio, C. H.; Dalsenter, P. R. & Marques, M. C. (2007b). *Mikania laevigata* Syrup does not Induce Side Effects on Reproductive System of Male Wistar rats. *Journal of Ethnopharmacology*, Vol.111, No.1, (November 2006), pp. 29-32, ISSN 0378-8741

Gu, Y. H. & Xue, K. (2010). Direct Oxidative Cyclization of 3-Arylpropionic Acids Using PIFA or Oxone: Synthesis of 3,4-dihydrocoumarins. *Tetrahedron Letters*, Vol.51, No.1, (January, 2010), pp. 192-196, INSS 0040-4039

Holetz, F. B.; Pessini, G. L.; Sanches, N. R.; Cortez, D. A.; Nakamura, C. V. & Filho, B. P. (2002). Screening of Some Plants Used in the Brazilian Folk Medicine for the Treatment of Infectious Diseases. *Memorial Instituto Oswaldo Cruz*, Vol.97, No.7, (October, 2002), pp. 1027-1031, ISSN 1678-8060

Hoult, J. R. S. & Paya, M. (1996). Pharmacological and Biochemical Actions of Simple Coumarins: Natural Products with Therapeutic Potential. *General Pharmacology*, Vol.27, No.4, (June, 1996), pp.713-722, ISSN 0306-3623

Lacy, A. & O'kennedy, R. (2004). Studies on Coumarins and Coumarin-Related Compounds to Determine their Therapeutic Role in the Treatment of Cancer. *Current Pharmaceutical Design*, Vol.10, No.30, (November, 2004), pp. 3797-3811, ISSN 1381-6128

Lake, B. G. (1999). Coumarin Metabolism, Toxicity, and Carcinogenicity: Relevance for Human Risk Assessment. *Food and Chemical Toxicology*, Vol.37, No.4, (April, 1999), pp. 423-453, ISSN 0278-6915

Lake, B. G.; Gaudin, H.; Price, R. J. & Walters, D. G. (1992). Metabolism of [3-14C] Coumarin to Polar and Covalently Bound Products by Hepatic Microsomes from the Rat, Syrian-Hamster, Gerbil and Humans. *Food and Chemical Toxicology*, Vol.30, No.2, (February, 1992), pp. 105-115, ISSN 0278-6915

Lima, N. P. & Biasi, L. A. (2002). Estaquia semilhenosa e Comparação de Metabólitos Secundários em *Mikania glomerata* Sprengel e *Mikania laevigata* Schultz Bip. Ex Baker. *Scientia Agraria*, Vol.3, No.1-2, pp. 113-132, ISSN 1983-2443

Lima, N. P. E. A. (2003). Estaquia semilhenosa e Análise de Metabólitos Secundários de Guaco (*Mikania glomerata* Sprengel e *Mikania laevigata* Schultz Bip. Ex Baker). *Revista Brasileira de Plantas Medicinais*, Vol.5, No.2, pp. 47-54, ISSN 1516-0572

Lucas, V. (1942). Estudo Farmacognóstico do Guaco *Mikania glomerata* Sprengel. *Revista Flora Medicinal*, Vol.9, No.1, pp. 101-132

Luize, P. S.; Tiuman, T. S.; Morello, L. G.; Ueda-Nakamura, T.; Dias-Filho, B. P.; Cortez, D. A. G.; Mello, J. C. P. & Nakamura, C. V. (2005). Effects of Medicinal Plant Extracts on Growth of *Leishmania* (L.) *amazonensis* and *Trypanosoma cruzi*. *Revista Brasileira de Ciências Farmacêuticas*, Vol.41, No.1, (January/March, 2005), pp. 85-94, ISSN 1516-9332

Maiorano, V. A.; Marcussi, S.; Daher, M. A.; Oliveira, C. Z.; Couto, L. B.; Gomes, O. A.; Franca, S. C.; Soares, A. M. & Pereira, P. S. Antiophidian Properties of the Aqueous Extract of *Mikania glomerata*. *Journal of Ethnopharmacology*, Vol.102, No.3, (August, 2005), pp. 364-370, ISSN 0378-8741

Matos, F. J. A. (2000). *Plantas medicinais: Guia de seleção e emprego de plantas usadas em fitoterapia no nordeste do Brasil*. Imprensa Universitária-UFC, ISBN 978.85.7282.008.X, Fortaleza, Brasil.

Moura, R. S.; Costa, S. S.; Jansen, J. M.; Silva, C. A.; Lopes, C. S.; Bernardo-Filho, M.; Nascimento Da Silva, V.; Criddle, D. N.; Portela, B. N.; Rubenich, L. M.; Araujo, R. G. & Carvalho, L. C. (2002). Bronchodilator Activity of *Mikania glomerata* Sprengel on Human Bronchi and Guinea-Pig Trachea. *Journal of Pharmacy and Pharmacology*, Vol.54, No.2, (February, 2002), pp. 249-256, ISSN 0022-3573

Muceneeki, R. S.; Amorim, C. M.; Cesca, T. G.; Biavatti, M. W. & Bresolin, T. B. (2009). A Simple and Validated LC Method for the Simultaneous Determination of Three Compounds in *Mikania laevigata* Extracts. *Chromatographia*, Vol.69, No.2, (February, 2009), pp. 219-223, ISSN 1612-1112

Napimoga, M. H. & Yatsuda, R. (2010). Scientific Evidence for *Mikania laevigata* and *Mikania glomerata* as a Pharmacological Tool. *Journal of Pharmacy and Pharmacology*, Vol.62, No.7, (March, 2010), pp. 809-820, ISSN 0022-3573

National Toxicology Program. Department of Health and Human Services: USA Government. (1993a). NTP Toxicology and Carcinogenesis Studies of 3,4-Dihydrocoumarin (CAS No. 119-84-6) in F344/N Rats and B6C3F1 Mice (Gavage Studies). *National Toxicology Program Technical Report Series*. Vol.423, (September, 1993), pp. 1-336

National Toxicology Program. Department of Health and Human Services: USA Government. (1993b). NTP Toxicology and Carcinogenesis Studies of Coumarin (CAS No. 91-64-5) in F344/N Rats and B6C3F1 Mice (Gavage Studies). *National Toxicology Program Technical Report Series*. Vol.422, (September, 1993), pp. 1-340

Neves, L. J. & Sá, M. D. F. A. (1991). Contribuição ao Estudo de Plantas Medicinais *Mikania glomerata* Spreng. *Revista Brasileira de Farmácia*, Vol.72, No.2, pp. 42-47, ISSN 0370-372X

O'Kennedy, R. & Thornes, R. D. (1997). *Coumarins: Biology, applications and mode of action.* John Wiley, ISBN 978-0-471-96997-6, Chichester, United Kington.

Olaharski, A. J.; Rine, J.; Marshall, B. L.; Babiarz, J.; Zhang, L. & Verdin, E. (2005). The Flavoring Agent Dihydrocoumarin Reverses Epigenetic Silencing and Inhibits Sirtuin Deacetylases. *PloS Genetic*, Vol.1, No.6, (December, 2005), pp. 689-694, ISSN 1553-7390

Oliveira, F.; Alvarenga, M. A.; Akisue, G. & Akisue, M. K. (1984). Isolamento e Identificação de Componentes Químicos de *Mikania glomerata* Sprengel e de *Mikania laevigata* Schultz Bip. ex Baker. *Revista de Farmácia e Bioquímica da Universidade de São Paulo*, Vol.20, No.2, pp .169-183, ISSN 0370-4726

Oliveira, F. D. E. A. (1986). Morfodiagnose das Folhas e das Partes Reprodutivas de *Mikania Laevigata* Shultz Bip ex Baker. *Revista Brasileira de Farmacognosia*, Vol.1, No.1, pp. 20-34, ISSN 0102-695X

Oliveira, F.; Saito, M. L. & Garcia, L. O. (1993). Caracterização Cromatográfica em Camada Delgada do Extrato Fluido de Guaco - *Mikania glomerata* Sprengel. *Lecta-USF*, Vol.11, No.1, (January/December, 1993), pp. 43-55, ISSN 0104-0987

Paiva, L. A. F.; Gurgel, L. A.; Silva, R. M.; Tome, A. R.; Gramosa, N. V.; Silveira, E. R.; Santos, F. A. & Rao, V. S. N. (2003). Anti-Inflammatory Effect of Kaurenoic Acid, a Diterpene from *Copaifera langsdorffii* on Acetic Acid-induced Colitis in Rats. *Vascular Pharmacology*, Vol.39, No.6, (January, 2003), pp. 303-307, ISSN 1537-1891

Peria, F. M.; Tiezzi, D. G.; Tirapelli, D. P.; Neto, F. S.; Tirapelli, C. R.; Ambrosio, S.; Oliveira, H. F. & Tirapelli, L. (2010). Kaurenoic Acid Antitumor Activity in Breast Cancer

Cells. *Journal of Clinical Oncology*, Vol.28, No.15, (May, 2010), suppl. e13641, ISSN 1527-7755

Radunz, L. L. (2004). *Efeito da temperatura do ar de secagem no teor e na composição dos óleos essenciais de guaco (Mikania glomerata Sprengel) e hortelã-comum (Mentha x villosa Huds).* 90 p. Tese (Doutorado em Engenharia Agrícola) - Programa de Pós-Graduação em Engenharia Agrícola, Universidade Federal de Viçosa, Viçosa, Minas Gerais, Brasil

Ramanitrahasimbola, D.; Rakotondramanana, D. A.; Rasoanaivo, P.; Randriantsoa, A.; Ratsimamanga, S.; Palazzino, G.; Galeffi, C. & Nicoletti, M. (2005) Bronchodilator Activity of *Phymatodes scolopendria* (Burm.) Ching and its Bioactive Constituent. *Journal of Ethnopharmacology*, Vol.102, No.3, (August, 2005), pp. 400-407, ISSN 0378-8741

Rehder, V. L.; Sartoratto, A. & Rodrigues, M. V. N. (2006). Essencial Oils Composition from Leaves, Inflorescences and Seeds of *Mikania laevigata* Schultz Bip. ex Baker and *Mikania glomerata* Sprengel. *Planta Medica,* Vol.8, No.1, (July, 2006), pp. 116-118, ISSN 0032-0943

Ritschel, W. A.; Brady, M. E. & Tan, H. S. (1979). First-pass Effect of Coumarin in Man. *International Journal of Clinical Pharmacology and Biopharmacy*, Vol.17, No.3, pp. 99-103, ISSN 0340-0026

Ritschel, W. A.; Ho Mann, K. A.; Tan, H. S. & Sanders, P. R. (1976). Pharmacokinetics of Coumarin Upon i.v. Administration in Man. *Arzneimittel-Forschung (Drug Research)*, Vol.26, No.7, pp. 1382 - 1387, ISSN 0004-4172

Ritter, M. R. & Miotto, S. T. S. (2005). Taxonomia de *Mikania* Willd. (Asteraceae) no Rio Grande do Sul, Brasil. *Hoehnea*, Vol.32, No.3, (June, 2005), pp. 309-359, ISSN 0073-2877

Ruppelt, B. M.; Pereira, E. F.; Goncalves, L. C. & Pereira, N. A. (1991). Pharmacological Screening of Plants Recommended by Folk Medicine as Anti-Snake Venom: I. Analgesic and Anti-Inflammatory Activities. *Memorial Instituto Oswaldo Cruz*, Vol.86, No.2, pp. 203-205, ISSN 0074-0276

Sá, R. C. S.; Leite, M. N.; Reporedo, M. M. & Almeida, R. N. (2003). Evaluation of Long-term Exposure to *Mikania glomerata*. *Contraception*, Vol.67, No.4, (December, 2002), pp. 327-331, ISSN 0010-7824

Sá, R. C. S.; Leite, M. N.; Peters, V. M.; Guerra, M. O. & Almeida, R. N. (2006). Absence of Mutagenic Effect of *Mikania glomerata* Hydroalcoholic Extract on Adult Wistar rats *in vivo*. *Brazilian Archives of Biology and Technology*, Vol.49, No.4, (July, 2006), pp. 599-604, ISSN 1516-8913

Sá, R. C. S.; Leite, M. N. &Almeida, R. N. (2010). Toxicological Screening of *Mikania glomerata* Spreng., Asteraceae, Extract in Male Wistar Rats Reproductive System, Sperm Production and Testosterone Level After Chronic Treatment. *Brazilian Journal of Pharmacognosy*, Vol.20, No.5, (November, 2010), pp. 718-723, ISSN 0102-695X

Salgado, H. R. N.; Roncari, A. F. F. & Moreira, R. R. D. Antidiarrhoeal Effects of *Mikania glomerata* Spreng. (Asteraceae) Leaf Extract in Mice. *Revista Brasileira de Farmacognosia*, Vol.15, No.3, (July/September, 2005), pp. 205-208, ISSN 0102-695X

Santos, P. A.; Pereira, M. A. S.; França, S. C. & Lopes, N. P. (1999). Esteróides e Cumarina em Calos de *Mikania glomerata* Sprengel. *Revista Brasileira de Ciências Farmacêuticas*, Vol.35, No.2, pp. 231-235, ISSN 1516-9332

Santos, S. C. (2005). *Caracterização cromatográfica de extratos medicinais de guaco: Mikania laevigata SCHULTZ Bip. EX BAKER e Mikania glomerata SPRENGEL e ação de M. laevigata na inflamação alérgica pulmonar*. 81 p. Dissertação (Mestrado em Ciências Farmacêuticas) - Setor de Ciências da Saúde, Universidade do Vale do Itajaí, Itajaí, Santa Catarina, Brasil.

Santos, S. C.; Krueger, C. L.; Steil, A. A.; Krueger, M. R.; Biavatti, M. W. & Wisnewski Junior, A. (2006). LC Characterisation of Guaco Medicinal Extracts, *Mikania laevigata* and *Mikania glomerata*, and their Effects on Allergic Pneumonitis. *Planta Medica*, Vol.72, No.8, (February, 2006), pp. 679-684, ISSN 0032-0943

Schenkel, E. P.; Rücher, G.; Manns, D.; Falkenberg, M. B.; Matzenbacher, N. I.; Sobral, M.; Mentz, L. A.; L., B. S. A. & Heinzmann, B. M. (2002). Screening of Brazilian Plants for the Presence of Peroxides. *Revista Brasileira de Ciências Farmacêuticas*, Vol.38, No.2, (April/June, 2002), pp. 191-196, ISSN 1516-9332

Shilling, W. H.; Crampton, R. F. & Longland, R. C. (1969). Metabolism of Coumarin in Man. *Nature*, Vol.221, No.5181, (February,1969), pp. 664-665, ISSN 0028-0836

Silva, R. Z.; Rios, E. M.; Silva, M. Z.; Leal, L. F.; Yunes, R. A.; Miguel, O. G. & Cechinel-Filho, V. (2002). Investigação Fitoquímica e Avaliação da Atividade Antibacteriana da *Mikania lanuginosa*. *Visão acadêmica*, Vol.3, No.2, (July/December, 2002), pp. 59-64, ISSN 1518-8361

Soares, A. K. A.; Carmo, G. C. C.; Quental, D. P.; Nascimento, D. F.; Bezerra, F. A. F.; Moraes, O. M. & Moraes, M. E. A. (2006). Avaliação da Segurança Clínica de um Fitoterápico Contendo *Mikania glomerata, Grindelia robusta, Copaifera officinalis, Myroxylon toluifera, Nasturtium officinale*, Própolis e Mel em Voluntários Saudáveis. *Revista Brasileira de Farmacognosia*, Vol.16, No.4, pp. 447-454, ISSN 0102-695X

Souza, C. D. & Felfili, J. M. (2006). Uso de Plantas Medicinais na Região de Alto Paraíso de Goiás, GO, Brasil. *Acta Botanica Brasilica*, Vol.20, No.1, (March, 2006), pp. 135-142, ISSN 1677-941X

Stanikunaite, R.; Khan, S. I.; Trappe, J. M. & Ross, S. A. (2009). Cyclooxygenase-2 Inhibitory and Antioxidant Compounds from the Truffle *Elaphomyces granulatus*. *Phytotherapy Research*, Vol.23, No.4, (April, 2009), pp. 575-578, ISSN 1099-1573

Suyenaga, E. S.; Reche, E.; Farias, F. M.; Schapoval, E. E.; Chaves, C. G. & Henriques, A. T. (2002). Antiinflammatory Investigation of Some Species of *Mikania*. *Phytotherapy Research*, Vol.16, No.6, pp. 519-523, ISSN 1099-1573

Tavares, J. P.; Martins, I. L.; Vieira, A. S.; Lima, F. A. V.; Bezerra, F. A. F.; Moraes, M. O. & Moraes, M. E. A. (2006). Estudo de Toxicologia Clínica de um Fitoterápico a Base de Associações de Plantas, Mel e Própolis. *Revista Brasileira de Farmacognosia*, Vol.16, No.3, (July/September, 2006), pp. 350-356, ISSN 0102-695X

Thornes, R. D.; Daly, L.; Lynch, G.; Breslin, B.; Browne, H.; Browne, H. Y.; Corrigan, T.; Daly, P.; Edwards, G.; Gaffney, E.; Henley, J.; Healy, T.; Keane, F.; Lennon, F.; Mcmurray, N.; Oloughlin, S.; Shine, M. & Tanner, A. (1994). Treatment with Coumarin to Prevent or Delay Recurrence of Malignant-Melanoma. *Journal of Cancer Research and Clinical Oncology*, Vol.120, No.1 (March, 1994), pp. S32-S34, ISSN 0171-5216

Thornes, R. D.; Lynch, G. & Sheehan, M. W. (1982). Cimetidine and Coumarin Therapy of Melanoma. *The Lancet*, Vol.320, No.8293, (August, 1982), pp. 328, ISSN 0140-6736

Tirapelli, C. R.; Ambrosio, S. R.; Da Costa, F. B. & De Oliveira, A. M. (2002). Inhibitory Action of Kaurenoic Acid from *Viguiera robusta* (Asteraceae) on Phenylephrine-induced Rat Carotid Contraction. *Fitoterapia,* Vol.73, No.1, (November, 2001), pp. 56-62, ISSN 0367-326X

Tirapelli, C. R.; Ambrosio, S. R.; Da Costa, F. B.; Coutinho, S. T.; De Oliveira, D. C. R. & De Oliveira, A. M. (2004). Analysis of the Mechanisms Underlying the Vasorelaxant Action of Kaurenoic Acid in the Isolated Rat Aorta. *European Journal of Pharmacology,* Vol.492, No.2-3, (May, 2004), pp. 233-241, ISSN 0014-2999

Valencia, A.; Wens, A.; Ponce-Monter, H.; Pedrón, N.; Gallegos, A. J.; Quijano, L.; Calderón, J.; Gómez, F. & Ríos, T. (1986). Zoapatle XII. *In vitro* effect of kaurenoic acid isolated From Montanoa frutescens and two derivatives upon human spermatozoa *Journal of Ethnopharmacology,* Vol.18, No.1, (October, 1986), pp. 89-94, ISSN 0378-8741

Veneziani, R. C. S.; Camilo, D. & Oliveira, R. (1999). Constituents of *Mikania glomerata* Sprengel. *Biochemical Systematics and Ecology,* Vol.27, No.1, (January, 1999), pp. 99-102, ISSN 0305-1978

Vilegas, J. H. Y.; Demarchi, E. & Lancas, F. M. (1997a). Determination of Coumarin and Kaurenoic Acid in *Mikania glomerata* ('guaco') Leaves by Capillary Gas Chromatography. *Phytochemical Analysis,* Vol.8, No.2, (March, 1997), pp. 74-77, ISSN 1099-1565

Vilegas, J. H. Y.; Marchi, E. & Lanças, F. M. (1997b). Extraction of Low-polarity Compounds (with Emphasis on Coumarin and Kaurenoic Acid) from *Mikania glomerata* ("guaco") Leaves. *Phytochemical Analisys,* Vol.8, No.5, (September/October, 1997), pp. 266-270, ISSN 1099-1565

Wang, Q.; Jia, R.; Ye, C.; Garcia, M.; Li, J. B. & Hidalgo, I. J. (2005). Glucuronidation and Sulfation of 7-hydroxycoumarin in Liver Matrices from Human, Dog, Monkey, Rat, and Mouse. *In Vitro Cellular & Developmental Biology-Animal,* Vol.41, No.3-4, (March/April, 2005), pp. 97-103, ISSN 1071-2690

Wilkens, M.; Alarcon, C.; Urzua, A. & Mendoza, L. (2002) Characterization of the Bactericidal Activity of the Natural Diterpene Kaurenoic Acid. *Planta Medica,* Vol.68, No.5, (May, 2002), pp. 452-454, ISSN 0032-0943

Yatsuda, R.; Rosalen, P. L.; Cury, J. A.; Murata, R. M.; Rehder, V. L.; Melo, L. V. & Koo, H. (2005). Effects of *Mikania* genus Plants on Growth and Cell Adherence of *Mutans streptococci. Journal of Ethnopharmacology,* Vol.97, No.2, (January, 2005), pp. 183-189, ISSN 0378-8741

Zgoda-Pols, J. R.; Freyer, A. J.; Killmer, L. B. & Porter, J. R. (2002). Antimicrobial Diterpenes from the Stem Bark of *Mitrephora celebica. Fitoterapia,* Vol.73, No.5, (August, 2002), pp. 434-438, ISSN 0367-326X

14

Evaluation of Drug Toxicity for DNA Vaccine Candidates Against Infectious Diseases: Hepatitis C as Experimental Model

Dania Bacardí, Karelia Cosme, José Suárez,
Yalena Amador-Cañizares and Santiago Dueñas-Carrera
Center for Genetic Engineering and Biotechnology,
Cuba

1. Introduction

Progress in the field of biotechnology has accelerated the development of a broad range of novel vaccines, and the composition of vaccine products has evolved from attenuated or inactivated whole-cell organisms, to protein polysaccharide conjugates, peptides, recombinant proteins, DNA vaccines and viral vectors. More recently, there has been a generation of a wide range of complex vaccine products and vaccine technologies (Buckland, 2005) that are often combined with novel adjuvants (Kovarik & Siegrist, 2001; Litvinov, 2009), administered in new delivery systems, and by new routes of inoculation.

In this context, DNA immunization has arisen as a promising strategy for the development of successful vaccines against infectious agents. In fact, some DNA vaccines have been already registered for application in animals (horses, fishes and dogs) against infection with West Nile virus, Infectious haematopoietic necrosis virus or treating melanoma (Liu, 2011). Moreover, thousands of people have already received DNA vaccine candidates in clinical trials without major adverse events (Alvarez-Lajonchere & Dueñas-Carrera, 2009).

DNA vaccination involves the administration of DNA, generally but not always a plasmid, to a host in order to induce a desired immune response. Once into the host, the DNA is taken up by cells, including antigen presenting cells, and the protein(s) expected to be the target of the immune system is/are expressed, processed and presented to specialized cells for induction of immune response. For this purpose, the DNA vaccine must comprise an eukaryotic expression unit, encompassing an enhancer/promoter region, intron, signal sequence, vaccine gene and a transcriptional terminator (poly A), for driving protein synthesis in the host (Glenting & Wessels, 2005). Frequently, DNA vaccines also include immune stimulatory sequences (ISS) for adding adjuvanticity (Glenting & Wessels, 2005). In addition, a unit for the previous propagation of the DNA in the microbial host, in order to obtain the required amounts for vaccination, is normally present, although some compact variants of DNA vaccines are designed for lacking this unit in the final product (Liu, 2011).

DNA immunization has many possible advantages. No dangerous infectious agents are involved, while the expression of the antigen of interest, in its native form, is possible. DNA vaccines can induce innate and adaptive, both humoral and cell mediated, immune responses. There is a potential for encoding multiple immunogenic epitopes with the purpose of raising protection against several diseases by a single vaccine. Compared with many conventional vaccines, DNA vaccines are relatively stable. Moreover, DNA vaccines are rapid to construct and their manufacture is generic (Liu, 2011).

The above mentioned advantages have resulted attractive for the application of DNA vaccination in the infectious disease field in humans. This immunization strategy has been widely evaluated against a variety of human pathogens; some of them without a current vaccine solution available like hepatitis C virus (HCV) and human immunodeficiency virus (HIV). In fact, DNA immunization has even reached the phase of clinical evaluation in several infectious diseases (Table 1).

The mechanism of action for DNA vaccines and their potential use for therapeutic and preventive purposes imposes relevant challenges for the evaluation of their safety. In addition, knowledge about potential undesirable side effects at long term is still limited. So far, all DNA vaccine candidates entering to clinical evaluation in humans have been previously evaluated for immunogenicity and toxicity in animal models with good results. However, immunogenicity in humans of naked DNA vaccine candidates has not generally fulfilled the expectations. Therefore, several strategies are currently being evaluated for enhancing the immune response, but some of them involve incorporation of components which are potentially able to also increase the toxicity, or might raise the risk for non-controlled or non-desired immune responses. Consequently, evaluation of toxicity related to DNA-based immunization is a continuously challenged field.

Infectious disease
HIV
Influenza
Malaria
HBV
HCV
SARS
Marburg
Ebola
HPV
West Nile virus
Dengue
HSV
Measles

Table 1. Infectious diseases for which DNA vaccines have entered to clinical trials

In this chapter we discuss relevant elements to be considered during the evaluation of toxicity related to DNA vaccines applied to infectious diseases. We will focus on local reactogenicity and systemic toxicity studies, biodistribution, persistence, and integration analysis, as well as immune-related studies for detecting potential adverse events after immunization with DNA-based vaccines candidates against HCV, as a model. We focus on HCV infection since it is a worldwide health problem, causing chronic hepatitis, frequently progressing to cirrhosis and hepatocellular carcinoma. There is no currently available vaccine against this pathogen and current therapies are generally effective in only approximately half of patients treated (Ghany et al., 2009). However, some vaccine candidates against HCV are being currently evaluated on clinical trials; two of them being based on DNA immunization (reviewed by Alvarez-Lajonchere & Dueñas-Carrera, 2009).

2. Safety evaluation

In addition to immunogenicity demonstration, regulatory agencies require sufficient pre-clinical data supporting safety to approve initiation of clinical trials of novel vaccines, including DNA vaccine candidates. The regulatory frame has been abundantly settled (Guidelines for assuring the quality of DNA vaccines, 1998; Guidelines on clinical evaluation of vaccines: regulatory expectations, 2004; Guidelines on nonclinical evaluation of vaccines, 2006). Precisely, the principal aim of non-clinical safety examination is to understand the toxicity of the candidate drug well enough to make judgment that the risk/benefits profile is adequate to initiate clinical trials (Contrera, 1993). Toxicity is complex, and impacted by several factors, such as: the xenobiotic, the dosage, the route, the action mechanism and the products of biotransformation. The distribution of many xenobiotics in the body may only affect certain key organs. Others, however, may damage any cell or tissue it enters in contact with. In addition, the toxicity can result in cellular/biochemical or adverse macromolecular changes. Some examples are: cell substitution, as fibrosis; damage to an enzyme system; interruption of protein synthesis; production of undesired chemical reagents in the cells and damages in the DNA. The distribution of toxic substances and toxic metabolites in the whole body determines the organs and tissues where the toxicity is produced. Many toxic substances are stored in the body, and the most common deposits of storage are fatty structures, the bones and highly vacularized organs involved in blood detoxification, such as the liver and the kidneys.
The safety evaluation involves the experimental studies directed to determine the toxicity, identifying and quantifying effects and establishing parameters (as dose, toxic and lethal concentrations, etc.) of the substances, using *in vivo* or *in vitro* models. With the information provided by these studies and other data, the Evaluation and the Estimate of the Risk are carried out, as determination of the probability and nature of the effects that can be derived from the exposition to the xenobiotics.
As for other vaccination strategies, evaluation of safety in the case of DNA immunization requires several considerations and tests. The lots of vaccine candidates to be used in pre-clinical studies should have been released according to the specifications required for their use in humans. Manufacturers need to establish a reproducible process for producing the DNA vaccine candidate in a sterile and free of endotoxins condition.
The main challenge in establishing a predictive non-clinical safety assessment comes from the fact that vaccines act through complex multi-stage mechanisms. Thus, the detection of the toxicity of vaccines is likely to be more complex than for conventional chemically-derived drug products, because safety concerns regarding the immune response to the vaccine add to the general concerns related to exogenous substances administration. Thus, toxicity testing programs recommended for conventional drug products may not always be applicable to vaccine products.
The non-clinical safety assessment of vaccines represents a new and evolving field. And clearly, consensus is needed among industry, academia, and regulatory authorities regarding the most appropriate approaches to this area. Depending on the target population

and vaccine indication, it may be necessary to conduct special non-clinical safety assessments. In particular, if a target population for the product includes pregnant women or females of reproductive age, reproductive toxicity studies should be considered. A global picture of the pre-clinical studies suggested for DNA vaccines is shown in Table 2.

Type of study	By guideline (EMEA. CPMP/SWP/112/98, 1998)
Single dose toxicity	Should incorporate some safety pharmacology endpoints, and investigate potential efficacy and toxicological consequences where systemic exposure is maximized.
Repeated dose toxicity	It will be required where multiple dosing of human subjects is intended. The route, mode, frequency and duration of administration in the animal studies should mimic the clinical dosing regimen. Where the duration of treatment of patients is long-term, toxicity studies should generally be of 6 months duration. The duration of the recovery phase investigations should be based on the persistence of the gene therapy product and expression of gene product
Immunotoxicity	The potential for stimulating cell mediated or humoral immunity to the nucleic acid, the vector-derived material (e.g. viral protein) or the expressed protein should be investigated. The potential production of anti-DNA antibodies upon nucleic acid administration should be addressed because they could mediate resistance to treatment and/or signal the development of autoimmunity. Formation of neutralizing antibodies to the gene construct, its vector or the expressed gene product should be studied as it may reduce efficacy.
Reproduction and developmental toxicity studies	Embryo-fetal and perinatal toxicity studies may be required depending on the disease and clinical population to be treated, if women of child-bearing potential are to be exposed to gene therapy products.
Genotoxicity and Carcinogenicity/ oncogenicity/tumorigenicity studies	Standard genotoxicity or life-time rodent carcinogenicity studies are not generally required. Depending on the extent of integration of DNA into the host genome and the clinical indication, studies may be required to investigate the potential for tumor formation or disruption of normal gene expression.
Distribution studies	Studies should provide data on all organs, whether target or not. Observation time should cover persistence of signal (i.e. duration of transgene expression and activity) and include time-points for which there is no signal detection, if applicable. The dosing should mimic the clinical use with appropriate safety margins.
Integration studies	Depending on the proposed clinical use (e.g., non-life threatening disease or pediatric use). The likelihood and the possible consequences of vector integration should be evaluated and measures to control potential associated risks should be described and justified.
Local tolerance	A local tolerance study may be required in an appropriate species. However, if the proposed clinical formulation and route of administration have been examined in other animal studies then separate local tolerance studies are not necessary.

Table 2. Pre-clinical studies indicated for DNA vaccines

The toxicological studies in animals constitute one of the main sources of information to study the toxicity of chemical compounds and biotechnology products, including vaccines. DNA vaccines evaluated in toxicological studies should comply with good manufacturing practices (Good manufacturing practices for biological products, 1992; Good manufacturing practices for pharmaceutical products, 2003). In these studies, even the less evident effects of the acute and chronic exposition can be generally evaluated easily. In these assays, the capacity to manipulate the experimental conditions allows the evaluation of many variables in response to toxic substances. These studies are very important to predict the toxicity effects in human susceptible populations. However, important limitations should be remarked regarding to the uncertainty of extrapolation from animals to humans. Particularly, it is difficult to extrapolate data obtained with high dose in animals, to the prospective toxicity of the relatively much smaller administration of therapeutic dose in humans.

The selection of the doses, duration and frequency of the dosage should be based on the proposed clinical regime; the levels and duration of the genetic expression in animal experimental models and in humans should also be considered. Typically, pre-clinical studies are carried out in rodents (mice or rats) and rabbits in a general toxicology "screening" base. Such studies are designed to identify both, intrinsic toxicity of the vaccine candidate, as well as immunotoxicity arising from the host immune response after its administration.

Accumulated data uniformly suggest that DNA vaccines are safe (reviewed by Liu, 2011). Mice and rats have been usually used as "first" species to study the toxicity of DNA vaccines. However, the reliability of a particular animal model in predicting an adverse clinical outcome cannot be established. In addition, the effect of vaccines does not exactly scale up directly on body weight or body surface area, since DNA vaccine candidates are expected to act mostly at the local site of administration to induce an immune response that traffics systemically. For this reason, rabbits are frequently used as "confirmatory" species to evaluate acute and chronic toxicity of DNA vaccine candidates since they are animals large enough to receive a full human dose of the vaccine candidate.

According to current Guidance, local reactogenicity and systemic toxicity studies should test the highest dose of the vaccine candidate planned for human use. In addition, N+1 administrations of the vaccine candidate should be delivered in these studies, with respect to the planned number of immunizations to be applied in humans. Recommended analysis include serum chemistry, haematology and coagulation test, in addition to gross and microscopic histology of different organs, particularly those potentially targeted by DNA immunization. Short-term and persistent toxicity are suggested to be evaluated in separate cohorts of animals 2-3 days and 2-3 weeks after final vaccination.

The U.S. Pharmaceutical Research and Manufacturers Association has recommended that non-clinical toxicologic evaluations should be decided case by case (Stoll, 1987) and regulatory and industry representatives attending the first International Conference on Harmonization of Technical Requirements for Registration of Pharmaceuticals for Human Use also supported this position (ICH, 1997).

2.1 Studies of acute toxicity

From the regulatory point of view, the information provided by the study of acute toxicity is essential for the classification, manipulation and transportation of a product. From the academic point of view, a carefully designed study of acute toxicity provides important information on the mechanism of toxicity, the relationship structure-activity and for the medical warning in the event of poisoning (based on the observed toxic effects (Chan & Hayes, 2001).

In general, these assessments include the evaluation of the oral, dermal and inhalator toxicity, as well as dermal and ophthalmic irritability, all of them guided by international regulations. Other studies should be kept in mind like the pre-natal and post-natal exposition, sensitization and phototoxicity. Depending on different scientific factors, the number and type of necessary acute tests to establish the initial toxicity may vary from a compound to another (Chan & Hayes, 2001; OECD Guidelines for testing of chemicals, 1993). A battery of studies should be designed under different conditions and exposition routes.

The objectives of this type of studies are:

1. to define the intrinsic toxicity of a compound.
2. to evaluate the danger at the target and not target species.
3. to define the most susceptible species.
4. to identify target organs.
5. to provide information for designing and selecting the dose levels for the long term studies.
6. to offer information to the clinical researcher in order to predict, diagnose, and prescribe the treatment for the over exposition to any drugs.

In the case of vaccine regulation, it establishes the employment of at least one animal species, which will be receiving high dose levels for providing an appropriate margin of security in relation to the dose expected to be applied in humans. Therefore, with the toxic signs found in this assessment, the relationship dose-response should be broadly characterized. The histopathology study of the key organs should be also included.

Here, as example, we show some data obtained in an acute toxicity study with CIGB-230, a DNA vaccine candidate, based on a plasmid for DNA immunization expressing HCV structural antigens (Alvarez-Lajonchere et al., 2006), which was planned to be used as a therapeutic vaccine candidate in HCV-infected patients.

In the acute toxicity study, carried out in Sprague-Dawley rats, we explored the effect of intramuscular injection with a high dose of the vaccine candidate CIGB-230, and the application of up to 90 times the planned therapeutic dose to be evaluated in the clinical setting. There were six working groups, 10 animals each (5 females and 5 males); group I: normal saline (control); group II: placebo of GIGB-230 (control); group III: plasmid pIDKE2 in high dose (90 times the planned therapeutic dose); group IV: CIGB-230 in high dose 1 (30 times the planned therapeutic dose); group V: CIGB-230 in high dose 2 (60 times the planned therapeutic dose); group VI: CIGB-230 in high dose 3 (90 times the planned therapeutic dose). The animals consumed food (Figure 1) within the ranks established for the species, which was translated in a progressive increase in body weight in both males and females (Figure 2).

The signs more frequently found were the extramedular hematopoiesis and lymphoid hyperplasia in the spleen, as well as the presence of secondary follicles in the ganglion (Table 3). The first one of these signs has been reported as frequently detected in this species, in which hematopoietic reserve is limited, causing that frequently the spleen and the liver assume this function in a complementary way (Loeb et al., 1978; Greaves, 2000). The presence of lymphoid hyperplasia and of secondary follicles is an indicative of the appropriate function of these organs of the immune system (spleen, liver and inguinal ganglion), demonstrating that, as expected, the treatment with the vaccine candidate in study does not alter the cellular morphology, neither the function of these organs.

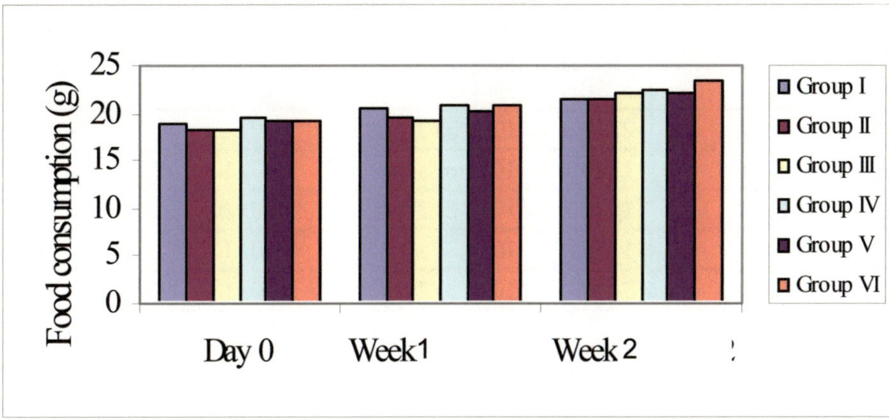

Fig. 1. Behavior of average food consumption in Sprague-Dawley rats. Ten animals per group (5 females and 5 males); group I: normal saline (control); group II: placebo of GIGB-230 (control); group III: plasmid pIDKE2 in high dose (90 times the planned therapeutic dose); group IV: CIGB-230 in high dose 1 (30 times the planned therapeutic dose); group V: CIGB-230 in high dose 2 (60 times the planned therapeutic dose); group VI: CIGB-230 in high dose 3 (90 times the planned therapeutic dose).

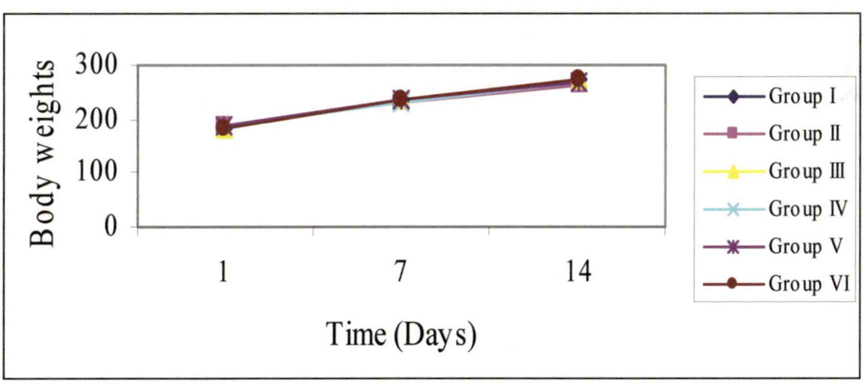

Fig. 2. Behavior of animal body weight (g). Ten animals per group (5 females and 5 males); group I: normal saline (control); group II: placebo of GIGB-230 (control); group III: plasmid pIDKE2 in high dose (90 times the planned therapeutic dose); group IV: CIGB-230 in high dose 1 (30 times the planned therapeutic dose); group V: CIGB-230 in high dose 2 (60 times the planned therapeutic dose); group VI: CIGB-230 in high dose 3 (90 times the planned therapeutic dose).

Another finding observed in spleen was the presence of a germinal center. Given the greater frequency of detection of this sign in the group inoculated with saline solution, it is not probably related with CIGB-230.

Group	Administration Site	Spleen			Mesenteric Ganglion	Liver	
	IF	CG	HE	HL	FS	FN	Mg
I	0/10	5/10	2/10	1/10	10/10	3/10	0/10
II	0/10	2/10	0/10	3/10	10/10	0/10	0/10
III	0/10	1/10	0/10	6/10	10/10	2/10	0/10
IV	0/10	1/10	4/10	8/10	10/10	1/10	1/10
V	1/10	1/10	4/10	8/10	10/10	0/10	0/10
VI	0/10	3/10	0/10	3/10	10/10	0/10	0/10

Legend: HE: Extra-medular hematopoiesis, FN: Centers of necrosis, HL: Lynphoid hyperplasia, Cg: Germinal center, Mg: Microgranulome, FS: Secondary follicle, IF: lymphohistocitary focal Infiltrated

Table 3. Frequency of detection of microscopic findings by organ observed and treatment group.

The thymus showed normal morphology, without evidences of cellular depletion, which corroborates the functionality of this organ, non-altered with the applied treatments. In fact, in the studied lymphoid organs histopathological alterations were not observed, showing reactions common to the antigenic stimulation, characterized by germinal centers at the level of the cortical area in ganglion and in the spleen white pulp.

The site of administration was also object of histopathological study, given the importance of the evaluation of the local response in this type of vaccine. Only one animal in the group V, injected with 60 times the therapeutic dose, presented a lymphohistocitary infiltrate.

Therefore, the study evidenced only some minor findings that were produced by non-specific causes, not related to the administration of the vaccine candidate, or in other cases, findings that are the result of antigenic stimulation, as expected response to the immunization, which is far to be an adverse event, on the contrary, corroborates the pharmacological action of the product and demonstrates that it does not produce undesired alterations on the immune system. The vaccine candidate CIGB-230 did not cause adverse effects or evidenced signs of toxicity for the dosage used, including the maximum dose inoculated (90 times the planned therapeutic dose)

2.2 Studies of local tolerance

The purpose of these studies is to check if the active pharmaceutical ingredient, as well as the excipients, are tolerated in those sites that can be in contact with the medication during the period of application in humans, taking into consideration the administration ways, either accidental or planned as treatment régime. The outlined design in each schedule should distinguish between the traumatic effects as consequence of the administration and those that are derived of the product under evaluation (toxicological or pharmacodynamic effects).

In the studies of local tolerance, the frequency, duration and way of administration should consider the proposed clinical evaluation in humans. Nevertheless, the period of

administration should not exceed the four weeks (ICH M3 (M), 2000; The principles governing medical products to the European Community, 1992).
As vaccines in most cases are administered by intramuscular, subcutaneous or intracutaneous way, the local tolerance in the application site should always be evaluated, using the same formulation that will be administered in the clinical evaluation in humans. In many cases, the potential local effects of the product can be evaluated in the studies to unique dose and of toxicity to repeated dose, but obviously it is necessary to evaluate the local tolerance for separate.
As illustration, here we show some data related to the local tolerance study carried out to the vaccine candidate CIGB-230. In this design, CIGB-230 vaccine candidate and the plasmid pIDKE2, component of this formulation, were used as substance in study. The groups of treatment were: control, inoculated with normal saline; placebo; and groups with CIGB-230 vaccine candidate using 1, 10 and 30 times the therapeutic dose, as well as the satellite group inoculated with 30 times the therapeutic dose. Six inoculations, 72 hours apart, were carried out in all treatment groups. After inoculations, all animals were sacrificed except those corresponding to the satellite group that stayed under clinical observation in order to evaluate the reversion of the possible observed effects. Clinical observation was carried out during 19 days (groups I to VI). In the case of the satellite group, the clinical observation was carried out up to day 40 of the experimental phase. Macroscopic observation and sample extraction was performed during necropsy, in order to evaluate the histopathology at the administration site and other organs, at the moment of the animal sacrifice.

Group	Spleen	Liver	Mesenteric ganglion	Administration site
	HL	FN	FS	IFHL
I	4/5	1/5	5/5	0/5
II	4/5	1/5	5/5	4/5
III	4/5	0/5	5/5	3/5
IV	5/5	0/5	5/5	5/5
V	3/5	0/5	5/5	5/5
VI	5/5	0/5	5/5	5/5
VII	5/5	1/5	5/5	0/5

Group I: normal saline (control); group II: placebo of GIGB-230 (control); group III: CIGB-230 in the planned therapeutic dose; group IV: CIGB-230 10 times the planned therapeutic dose; group V: CIGB-230 30 times the planned therapeutic dose; group VI: plasmid pIDKE2 30 times the planned therapeutic dose; group VII: CIGB-230 30 times the planned therapeutic dose (satellite group). Legend:FN: Centers of necrosis, HL: Lymphoid hyperplasia, FS: Secondary follicle, IFHL: lymphohistocitary focal Infiltrate.

Table 4. Frequency of detection of microscopic findings by organ observed and treatment group at day 20.

Animals consumed food according to the standards established for their species, which led to a gradual increase in body weight. There were neither etiological nor anatomical changes. There was a normal response to stimuli in all animals involved in the study. The macroscopic/microscopic observations confirmed the clinical observations and proved there was no damage related to the substance in trial in any organ of the studied animals. In the histopathologic study, a predominant cellular response consisting in a focal infiltration of histiocytes, lymphocytes and leukocytes, was observed in all groups of treatment (Table 4 and Figure 3), In the spectrum of doses explored in Sprague-Dawley rats, CIGB-230 vaccine candidate was well tolerated by intramuscular injection.

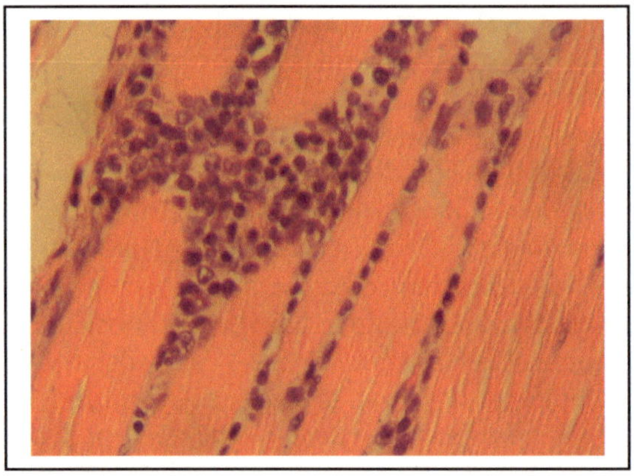

Fig. 3. Lymphohistocitary infiltrate observed in the place of administration of a representative animal.

2.3 Studies of toxicity to repeated dose

The studies of toxicity to repeated dose allow showing the wide scenario of adverse effects of a preparation. The time of duration of these studies may vary, generally from 1 to 4 weeks for short term studies, 3 months in the case of subchronic studies and of 6 to 12 months, classified as chronics. Different variables, associated with the health and the behavior of the used animal species, are followed up, resulting in the ability of detecting the adverse effects caused by the preparation under test.

The results obtained from the studies of toxicity to repeated doses play a fundamental role in the evaluation of the safety of medications, pesticides, nutritious preservatives and other preparations. These offer enough information to predict the long term toxicity of a compound administered in low dose, whenever an appropriate relationship structure-activity exists.

For the evaluation of vaccines in studies of toxicity to repeated doses, the employment of animal species carefully selected, to which apply different dose levels of the product under test is usually required. These studies should always be carried out, even in those cases in which single inoculation of the vaccine is expected in humans. The route and administration frequency will be similar to the proposed clinical schedule, keeping in mind the potential differences of the response in the time between animals and humans. Previous works have evidenced the safety of repeated administration of a plasmid DNA vaccine candidate by different routes in various animal models (Parker et al., 1999; Tuomela et al., 2005). A wide range of doses has been evaluated and in all administration methods, DNA vaccines have been well-tolerated and non-toxic.

In the case of CIGB-230, as previously described (Bacardí et al., 2009), no toxic effects were found after repeated intramuscular injection in Sprague-Dawley rats. The study was conformed by 6 groups: a non-treated group, a placebo one, a satellite group and three groups treated with 5, 15 and 50 times the planned therapeutic dose, respectively. The

satellite group was used to evaluate the reversibility of possible adverse effects, and the non-treated group remained during the whole study with the same lodging and feeding conditions. A daily administration was carried out during 30 days.
Clinical observations led us to confirm the quality of this product; no evidences of ethologic or morphological alterations, which could be attributable to the substance under study, were found. Results from these evaluations proved a normal behavioral pattern in the animals, with feeding consumption rates, weight gain and behavior corresponding to healthy animals of the species, even when they were repeatedly inoculated (30 administrations). This also showed that the repeated administration of the vaccine did not cause metabolic or behavioral alterations which might be translated into adverse effects, thus constituting indirect signals of non-toxicity, given the sensitivity of these parameters to detect alterations produced by the inoculation of exogenous substances. Neither ethologic nor anatomic alterations were observed in the animals used in the study, thus preserving the condition of a normal response versus stimuli in all cases. Macroscopic observations confirmed the clinical observations and evidenced that there was no damage to any of the organs tested. At the time of the clinical pathology assessment (either of hematology or blood biochemistry), no functional and/or structural alterations of tested organs existed. The results suggest full hematopoietic functionality without evidences of alterations produced by the repeated administration of this vaccine candidate. An integral analysis of hemochemical determinations indicates that the repeated inoculation of CIGB-230 in rats does not cause toxic effects on kidneys and liver, which are main target organs given their participation in metabolic and excretion processes (Bacardí et al., 2009).
Histopathological evaluation proved that the single or multiple administration of the product did not induce morphological alterations in the studied organs of rats, also showing full functional morphology in those from the immune system. Therefore, these observations suggest that the inoculation of CIGB-230 does not affect eritropoiesis or the production of white blood cells precursors. Extra-medullar hematopoiesis (mainly observed in the spleen) has been previously described as a result of organ response to moderate stress; additionally, it is a commonly reported finding on this species, which hematopoietic reserve is limited. This finding appeared with equal frequency in the placebo and non-treated group and in those treated with CIGB-230, further supporting its unrelated nature with the administration of the test item. Lymphoid hyperplasia and secondary follicle are signs of adequate functioning of lymphoid organs; this suggests that, as expected, treatment with CIGB-230 does not alter cellular morphology or function of these organs. At the site of administration, most rats showed minimum focal infiltrate of lymphocytes and histiocytes. In the satellite group (VI), the reversion of this finding was observed, because it was present in only four of the animals (Bacardí et al., 2009).
The results demonstrated that CIGB-230 therapeutic vaccine candidate was well tolerated, did not induce either local or systemic adverse alterations at the studied doses, and exhibited no observable toxicity in rats when tested.

2.4 Biodistribution and persistence

One major risk related to DNA immunization is distribution to non-desired tissues and organs, as well as potential integration to the host genome. Long-term persistence might facilitate the integration of plasmid DNA into the host's genome. Moreover, long-term expression could cause long-term skewing of the immune system influencing subsequent immunizations and infections. One study found that DNA delivered into mouse muscle was stably expressed for 19 months, even though no integration could be detected (Wolff et al., 1992).

The biodistribution and persistence of a DNA vaccine is potentially dependent on the formulation (naked DNA or combined with other elements), route of administration and delivery method and should be evaluated. It is suggested that these studies of biodistribution and persistence should be designed to determine whether subjects in DNA vaccine trials are at risk from the long-term expression of the encoded antigen, and/or integration of the plasmid that might increase susceptibility to malignant transformation.

A typical biodistribution/persistence study assesses the presence of plasmid collected from a panel of tissues at multiple time points ranging from a few days to several months post administration. The panel of tissues typically includes the blood, heart, brain, liver, kidney, bone marrow, ovaries/testes, lung, draining lymph nodes, spleen, muscle at the site of administration and subcutis at the injection site (Guidance for Industry Considerations for Plasmid DNA Vaccines for Infectious Disease Indications, 2007).

Up to now, the results obtained in pre-clinical evaluation of DNA vaccine candidates evidence a consistent pattern of rapid clearance of the plasmid regardless of promoter, backbone or inserted genes (Bureau et al., 2004; Tuomela et al., 2005). Similarly, no evidence of integration into the host genomic DNA has been generally observed (Coelho-Castelo 2006; Pal et al., 2006).

Different animal species have been evaluated for this type of studies (Manam et al., 2000; Parker et al., 1999). A short time after administration of the plasmid DNA in mice, the plasmid can be detected in several organs, some of them far from the inoculation site, which indicates a quick dissemination through the body (Hohlweg & Doerfler, 2001; Manam et al., 2000). Sporadically, the plasmid was detected in gonads, but it dissipated rapidly (Manam et al., 2000; Parker et al., 1999). Evidently, when plasmid is transmitted to the gonads, germ line chromosomal integration and germ line transmission may occur, although these phenomena have not been observed so far and due to rapid DNA clearance in the gonads, the risk of these events is expected to be minimal.

In fact, several weeks after injection of the DNA construct, the plasmid could only be detected at the site of injection in mice and rats (Manam et al., 2000). DNA injected in mouse muscle has been reported to persist for up to two years and was expressed at a low, but significant level (Armengol et al., 2004), although persistence and expression seems to be variable.

The level of plasmid DNA at the injection site has been below 100 copies/ µg DNA after initial injection with 100–200 µg DNA (Manam et al., 2000; Parker et al., 1999; Tuomela et al., 2005). Previous work has shown that 30 minutes after intramuscular injection 33% of the initial concentration was present and 60 minutes later less than 1% remained (Kim et al., 2003). The amount of plasmid DNA in organs remote from the injection site was 2–3 orders of magnitude lower than at the injection site (Kim et al., 2003). When de administration was carried out by intravenous route, plasmid DNA was initially distributed at a relatively low amount to all tissues examined, except the gonads and brain, in which no plasmid DNA was detected. However, plasmid DNA was rapidly cleared (Parker et al., 1999; Tuomela et al., 2005). Less than 1% of the initial concentration was detected in blood 30 minutes post-administration in mice, and no plasmid was detected 60 minutes post-administration (Kim et al., 2003). These results indicate that most DNA administered seems to be degraded by extracellular nucleases and only a minor amount is taken up by cells. This situation causes that high-dose levels of plasmid are usually required for DNA immunization when naked DNA is employed.

Despite the relatively prolonged antigenic stimuli generated by DNA immunization due to gene expression for a period of time, for therapeutic DNA vaccine candidates against infectious agents several immunizations might be required in order to reach the sustained clearance of the pathogen. In this scenario, DNA might accumulate in higher amounts in the body which increases the risk for undesired events. In such cases, biodistribution and integration studies should be performed, taking into account the predicted immunization schedule in humans.

In the case of CIGB-230, the biodistribution study conducted demonstrated that after repeated intramuscular administration in mice, plasmid was readily detected in blood, as well as in all evaluated organs, except pancreas, as early as 1 h after inoculation (Bacardí et al., 2009). This wide organ distribution is consistent with the above mentioned results regardless of the animal model or the method and route of administration. So far, the knowledge regarding the actual mechanisms by which administered DNA distributes widely throughout the body is scarce. The DNA is probably efficiently transported to all organs by the blood. In this case, highly vascularized organs, as well as those involved in blood detoxification and recycling, such as the liver and kidneys should receive the highest amount of DNA. We were able to detect plasmid in liver, as well as in kidney samples, 1 h after the eighth inoculation. However, 17 h later, the signal could no longer be detected in kidney, whereas it remained in the liver. In this sense, either of two speculations can be raised: 1) clearance kinetics is faster in the kidneys or 2) there is a preference for the plasmid to distribute in greater quantity to the liver in our experimental conditions. Elevated levels of plasmid DNA have been found in the hepatic tissue during the first hours after intravenous (Kobayashi et al., 2001) and intranasal (Oh et al., 2001) inoculation in mice; consequently, the extensive uptake of naked DNA by the liver appears to be a common feature, in which the scavenger receptors play an important role. On the contrary, accumulated data regarding renal tissue are more heterogeneous. Some investigators were not able to detect plasmid copies in the renal tissue after 24 h of DNA inoculation formulated with poloxamer 188 in mice and rabbits (Quezada et al., 2004), nevertheless other work inoculating DNA-PEI complexes intravenously in mice, detected plasmid in kidneys even several days post-inoculation, evidencing the importance of formulation and route of administration (Jeong et al., 2007).

On the other hand, we observed a rapid diffusion of the plasmid to the ovaries, because it was present at detectable levels 1 h after the eighth inoculation. At the same time, the clearance kinetic in these organs was fast, because it could not be detected 17 h later (Bacardi et al., 2009).

Being the injection site for CIGB-230, the muscle receives the highest amount of DNA. As expected, 1 h after the eighth inoculation we could detect it in the inoculation site. Seventeen hours later, we still detected a positive signal, which persisted 30 days after 7 doses in all the evaluated mice, but it was not detected at a later time (Bacardi et al., 2009). In a previous study (Acosta-Rivero et al., 2006), we could detect HCV E2 protein expression in the muscle cells of the inoculation site as early as 72 h post-inoculation of CIGB-230 in BALB/c mice, under the same conditions described in the biodistribution study. In addition to the non-detection of the plasmid, three months after the last immunization antigen expression was not detected (Bacardi et al., 2009).

Several strategies, based on improvement on formulation or delivery vehicles have been or are currently being evaluated as alternative for reducing DNA dose levels or in order to increase immunogenicity of DNA vaccine candidates (Liu, 2011). However, although some of these strategies have succeeded at increasing the ability of DNA to reach the intracellular space as well as enhance immunogenicity, the risk for greater possibility of an undesired integration event is also bigger.

Integration of plasmid DNA into the recipient's genome appears the major point into the safety issues of DNA vaccination. Integration may occur randomly or by homologous recombination and could lead to activation of oncogenes, inactivation of tumor suppressor genes, or, when integrated into the chromosomal DNA of germ line cells, to vertical transmission.

Techniques for sensitive and precise detection of DNA integration have been developed. High molecular weight DNA is isolated and purified from non-integrated plasmid using pulsed-field gel electrophoresis, followed by detection and quantification of the plasmid with real time PCR. A recommendation is given that the sensitivity of this assay be sufficient to quantify <100 copies of plasmid per microgram of host DNA. A claim of "non-persistence" requires that the amount of plasmid at each site falls below this limit of quantification (Guidance for Industry Considerations for Plasmid DNA Vaccines for Infectious Disease Indications, 2007). In a previous work, the sensitivity of the PCR has been approximately 1 plasmid copy per μg DNA, representing approximately 150,000 nuclei and all detectable plasmid DNA in treated muscle tissue has been generally extrachromosomal (Ledwith et al., 2000). Thus, random integration might have occurred, but at frequencies of <1–8 copies in 150,000 nuclei. (Ledwith et al., 2000), which would be at least three orders of magnitude below the spontaneous mutation rate of gene-inactivating mutations. Therefore, in a case like this, the risk of mutation due to plasmid integration following intramuscular inoculation is negligible.

In contrast to the study mentioned above, Wang et al, using a newly developed PCR assay, identified four independent integration events upon plasmid injection followed by elecroporation *in vivo* (Wang et al., 2004). This PCR uses a vector-specific primer and a genomic primer based on repetitive DNA. The PCR detects covalent junction of plasmid to-genomic DNA sequences after repeated rounds of gel purification to remove free plasmid DNA. Electroporation markedly increased plasmid tissue levels and its association with genomic DNA after gel-purification approximately 980 copies of plasmid DNA were found to be associated with 1 μg of high molecular weight genomic DNA, whereas for the muscle DNA samples from non electroporated mice, only 17 copies/μg DNA were found (Wang et al., 2004). Therefore, the risk of DNA integration into the genome exists. Thus, for each new DNA vaccine candidate to be used, integration should be considered. Depending on the extent of integration of DNA into the host genome and the clinical indication, studies may be required to investigate the potential for tumor formation or disruption of normal gene expression.

2.5 Mutagenicity and carcinogenicity studies

Studies should be carried out in order to evaluate the potential damage to the host genetic material as consequence from the exposition to the DNA vaccine preparation. Particularly, mutagenicity/carcinogenic studies allow identifying possibly dangerous compounds at this level.

Tumors can be induced by numerous agents, including radiations, biological agents and chemical substances of diverse origin. Malignant transformation originates from alterations in the cellular genetic program or from changes in the information contained in the cells and its subsequent fixation and replication. Carcinogenicity studies identify these undesired events and are necessary when medications will be administered for 6 months or more in humans, or for those frequently used in an intermittent way in chronic or recurrent treatments. In addition, these tests should be carried out if drugs under evaluation are planned to be administered by short time but there is previous demonstration or known risk of possible carcinogenicity, and accumulation of the product or their metabolites in tissues may rise with possible undesired physiopathologic responses (ICH, 1995).
The experimental design for this type of studies involves carrying out specific evaluations taking into account characteristic of the product, duration of the clinical treatment, target population, biological activity, and expression of receptors in normal and malignant cells. Several established carcinogenicity criteria are increases in malignant tumors in treated animals, increases in the combination of benign and malignant tumors, tumors appearance in non usual sites, rare tumors for the animal species, tumors detection at early ages.
A standard battery of genotoxicity and conventional carcinogenicity studies are not generally applicable to DNA-vaccines. However, genotoxicity studies may be required to address a concern about a specific impurity or novel chemical component, e.g. a complexing material that has not been tested previously (Guidelines for assuring the quality and nonclinical safety evaluation of DNA vaccines, 2005). The main risk for mutagenic/carcinogenic activity for DNA vaccine preparation comes from the persistence of the DNA in the host, and the potential for integration into the genome. Therefore, mutagenic/carcinogenicity studies in DNA vaccination are related to the integration studies and are particularly required if integration events are detected. In addition, for non-naked DNA vaccine preparations, even in the case of non-integration events detected, the presence of potentially dangerous compounds in the preparation should be evaluated according to the above mentioned criteria. This is particularly relevant when DNA vaccine preparation is planned to be employed in several doses or the duration of treatment is expected to be long, like in chronic infectious diseases such as hepatitis B and C.

2.6 Immunotoxicity

We recommend that vaccine immunogenicity be assessed in a relevant animal model whenever possible. This may include the evaluation of antigen-specific antibody titers, seroconversion rates, activation of cytokine secreting cells, and/or measures of cell-mediated immune responses. In this sense, the immune system represents an important and potential target organ for toxicity, which is similar in organization, cell types and functions in both man and animals, and thus represents a relevant parameter in the risk assessment process.
The mechanism of action in DNA vaccination is the induction of a relevant immune response against a target. Therefore, the way this occurs in the host is very relevant and should be evaluated carefully since undesired effects might arise at the immunological level due to vaccination. Immunotoxicity (e.g. immunosuppression, myelotoxicity, allergy, or autoimmunity) studies are required to assess the immunogenic potential of a product. Some indicative of immune affections should be observed: inflammatory reactions (stimulation), variation in the expression of the surface antigens in target cells (autoinmune potential), and long term immunological effects.

Published preclinical studies indicate that DNA vaccination can activate autoreactive B cells to secrete IgG anti-DNA autoantibodies. However, the magnitude and duration of this response appears to be insufficient to cause disease in normal animals or accelerate disease in autoimmune-prone mice. Preclinical studies suggest that systemic autoimmunity is unlikely to result from DNA vaccination. Similarly, the absence of an immune response against cells expressing the vaccine-encoded antigen (including muscle cells and dendritic cells) suggests that an autoimmune response directed against tissues in which such cells reside is unlikely. Yet the possibility persists that DNA vaccines might idiosyncratically cause or worsen organ-specific autoimmunity by encoding antigens (including cryptic antigens) that cross-react with self (Guidance for Industry Considerations for Plasmid DNA Vaccines for Infectious Disease Indications, 2007).

In non-clinical and clinical investigations to date, tolerance has not been observed in adult animals and humans, and the initial concern may have been overstated. Tolerance can be induced in neonatal mice; this may be because the mouse immune system at birth is immature. If development of tolerance is a concern for a specific product, a more relevant animal model is desirable.

A case by case approach to evaluate immunotoxicity of DNA vaccines, based on the potential similarity of expressed antigens to natural human proteins and immune response in animal models should be explored. General welfare of animals in preclinical immunogenicity and toxicity studies continue to be carefully monitored. At least limited immunotoxicological assessment should be performed in all toxicity studies. This evaluation is based on two sources of information, one coming from routine toxicity parameters and the other from specific immunological tests in multiple species.

Parameters determined in all the toxicity studies and which enable the toxicologist to detect some aspects of potential immunotoxicity, if present, are the following:

- White blood cells and differential count;
- plasma globulin level;
- routine histopathological examinations. These include: weighing the thymus and spleen, histo-pathological examination of the thymus, spleen, hilar and mesenteric lymph nodes and femoral bone marrow.
- Specific immune parameters are also examined to assist decision making and include:
- femoral bone marrow cellularity (rat only), in all the toxicity studies including the 1-month toxicity studies;
- total plasma immunoglobulins (IgG and IgM) in all the species using radial immunodiffusion method, in conjunction with the clinical chemistry examinations; and
- histopathological examination of the popliteal lymph nodes in all the toxicity studies, whatever the species; special attention is paid to all the other lymph nodes which are occasionally present on the slides (retromandibular, parathymic) and to the bronchial- and gut-associated lymphoid tissues.

The results of the lymphoid organs and bone marrow histopathological examinations are analyzed together with information from all other organs/tissues. This assists the pathologist to discriminate between primary lymphoid system lesions (direct immunotoxic effect) and secondary lymphoid system lesions (indirect immunotoxic effect). The latter, in the case of treatment-induced stress, can be frequently observed in toxicity studies. These special immunotoxicity studies require careful monitoring of all changes, which are stress and malnutrition status-related information, often neglected in routine histopathological examination. Special immune function tests might be selected and include measurement of plaque forming cell (PFC) and serum antibody titers to keyhole lympet hemocyanin (KLH), lymphocyte transformation, mixed lymphocyte responses, blood lymphocyte phenotyping and natural killer cell cytotoxicity (Dean et al., 1998).

Frequently, cytokines are used as immune modulators in DNA immunization, co-expressed to the antigen targeted to elicit immune response or in other variants. In such cases, preclinical studies in animal species responsive to the encoded human cytokine(s) or models using homologous animal gene(s) are encouraged. Such studies should assess whether modulation of cellular or humoral components of the immune system might result in unintended adverse consequences, such as generalized immunosuppression, chronic inflammation, autoimmunity or other immunopathology (Guidance for Industry Considerations for Plasmid DNA Vaccines for Infectious Disease Indications, 2007).

In the therapeutic setting, where DNA vaccination is expected to dramatically change the context of the immune response in order to reach for instance the clearance of a chronic pathogen like HCV, uncontrolled or undesired immune response is a theoretical risk. However, DNA vaccination has been safe and well tolerated, with no evidence of this side-effect; even when specific immune response has been elicit de novo against HCV antigens (Alvarez-Lajonchere et al., 2009; Castellanos et al., 2010). In general, immunopathological reactions such as general immunosuppression or uncontrolled inflammation have not been observed in humans inoculated with DNA vaccines so far.

2.7 Study of reproductive function and perinatal toxicity

These studies intend to give general information on the effects of a substance on the female/male reproductive system, such as gonadal function, estral cycle, behavior of mating, conception, childbirth and nursing. They can be carried out in one or two generations. In these studies, assessment of the growth and development of the descendant is carried out. Teratogenic potential (property of causing permanent structural and functional abnormalities during the period of embryonic development) is also evaluated, as well as any potential danger for the neonate due to exposition of the mother to a substance during pregnancy is also investigated.

Worldwide harmonized guidelines for reproductive testing have been established (ICH (1996): Detection of Toxicity to Reproduction from Medicinal Products; ICH (1996): Reproductive Toxicity: Male Fertility Studies). Generally, animal studies have been conducted in three segments: in adults, in pregnant animals, and in pregnant and lactating animals.

In the case of DNA vaccines against infectious agents, they are expected to be administered to different populations, including people at fertile ages and potentially pregnant women. Therefore, these studies are required before general application of a DNA vaccine. However, these studies may not be required prior to clinical studies in populations with life-threatening diseases, provided appropriate measures are taken to minimize risks. Prior to use of a DNA vaccine in children or newborns, the product should be tested for safety and immunogenicity in adults, and appropriate nonclinical models, e.g. with juvenile animals, should be considered regarding toxicity and induction of immunological tolerance.

2.8 Final general recommendations for safety evaluation of DNA vaccine candidates

A generic protocol is not provided, but general recommendations are described below:

a. The choice of animal model should be appropriate for the product and clinical indication. Often rabbits are used for parenteral vaccine toxicity because their muscle mass may receive a volume equivalent to a full human clinical dose (e.g., 0.5 mL).
b. High dose should be at least 1 - 10 times the actual highest planned clinical dose; sometimes preferably not scaled on weight or body area.
c. To determine if the observed effects are dose-related (and to potentially identify an equivalent to a No-Observed-Adverse-Effect Level), 2 or 3 concentrations, to cover the range of proposed clinical doses, in addition to a vehicle and/or adjuvant control, should be used. At a minimum, the highest proposed human dose should be tested.
d. Number of proposed clinical inoculations plus one.
e. The period of study varies, depending on the frequency of dose administration (episodic, not daily), which may be abbreviated compared to the proposed clinical dosing schedule. The duration of the GLP safety studies is dependent on the study design. Tissue samples should be processed and data analyzed after intermediate and terminal sacrifice.
f. Timepoints for sacrifice: 1-3 days post-last inoculation; 2-4 weeks post-last inoculation (recovery).
g. A minimum of 5 animals per gender per dose should be included for each time point of sacrifice – this number may vary depending on animal model chosen.
h. Same route of administration as the proposed clinical route (with same delivery device, whenever possible).
i. Minimal endpoints examined should include:
    - Daily clinical observations
    - Weekly physical examinations
    - Evaluation of injection site(s) for irritation (daily in the post-dose week) and histopathology
    - Weekly body weights assessment
    - Food and water consumption, body temperatures (daily in the week following inoculations)
    - Ophthalmologic observations (pre-dosing and prior to sacrifice)
    - Clinical pathology at regular intervals for hematology, serum chemistry, serology, urinalysis measurements
    - Gross observations and organ weights at necropsy
    - Histopathology evaluation to include a select tissue list, especially the immune function organs (e.g., lymph nodes), other highly perfused organs, and the genital organs in the control and high-dose animals and target tissues in the remaining groups. Depending on the route of inoculation, additional organs may need to be examined. (Full tissue collection and preservation should be performed even when only a select list is examined histopathologically)
    - Relevant immunogenicity (humoral and/or cell mediated immune responses) studies
    - Additional endpoints may be included to address therapeutic-specific concerns. Here, specialized studies to examine genetic toxicology (e.g., biodistribution) are strongly recommended. These are studies that may incorporate the use of assays that do not (yet) meet good laboratory practices standards. General recommendations include: tissue distribution studies, integration studies in tissues where the DNA vaccine remains at doses higher than those recommended guidances, immunotoxicity studies if repeated doses are planned in the clinical evaluation.

Biodistribution studies may be waived for DNA vaccines produced by inserting a novel gene into a plasmid vector previously documented to have an acceptable biodistribution/integration profile. Biodistribution studies will still be necessary for DNA vaccines utilizing novel vectors, formulations, methods of delivery, routes of administration, or any other modifications expected to significantly impact cellular uptake and/or biodistribution. In every case, the decision should be consulted with the regulatory authorities. It is recommendable that manufacturers provide the complete sequence of the plasmid before initiating phase 1 clinical studies. Additional studies investigating multiple coding regions within the construct using multiplex PCR, confirming the integrity of extracted genomic DNA using housekeeping or constitutively expressed genes, carcinogenesis or tumorigenesis studies may be required if the vaccine is demonstrated to be integrated in tissues.

Consideration must be given to the possibility that the in vivo synthesized antigen may exhibit unwanted biological activity. If necessary, appropriate steps must be taken, e.g. by deletion mutagenesis, to eliminate this activity while retaining the desired immune response. If other gene constructs are included in the plasmid, such as antibiotic resistance genes for manufacturing reasons, then the possibility of expression of such gene sequences in mammalian cells or in micro-organisms which are potentially pathogenic, and the possible clinical consequences of such expression, should be considered.

When more than one type of vaccine is used in a sequential immunization protocol, if information supporting the safety and tolerability of the dose, schedule, and route of administration of each component proposed for use in the heterologous prime-boost regimen exist and data are deemed adequate to characterize the potential risks of the prime-boost regimen to study participants, additional toxicology studies may not be necessary. However, this information should be submitted for consideration to the regulatory authorities that will evaluate the need for additional toxicology information to support the clinical plans (Guidance for Industry Considerations for Plasmid DNA Vaccines for Infectious Disease Indications, 2007).

If modifications to the manufacturing process or the DNA product are made during the development programme, the potential impact on the product should be considered. Modifications of the genetic sequence, the use of alternative promoter/enhancer sequences, or other changes to the product, may require additional non-clinical safety evaluation. Equally, if aspects related to the immunization protocol like the route of administration are changed, then additional non-clinical test should be done to assess the impact of these modifications. The scientific rationale for the approach taken should be provided (Guidance for Industry Considerations for Plasmid DNA Vaccines for Infectious Disease Indications, 2007).

The risk/benefit evaluation for a product is related to the actual product and its intended use. For example, a prophylactic DNA vaccine for use in healthy children will have a different risk/benefit ratio compared to a therapeutic DNA vaccine against cancer or a persistent pathogen like HCV, for which there is no other available treatment or the efficacy of therapy is limited. Thus, for these and other reasons, it is likely that a flexible approach will be necessary for the non-clinical safety evaluation of DNA vaccines.

3. Conclusions

DNA vaccination is a continuously evolving and exciting field with many challenges to face. Methodological and regulatory frames are also developing every day. One important issue for a promising future in this vaccination strategy is to demonstrate efficacy in humans in a safe context. In this scenario, the pre-clinical protocols are very relevant and should be based on the design of the proposed clinical assessment. General regulatory frames rule the administration of exogenous substances, but given the nature and proposed mechanism of action for DNA vaccines additional specific considerations should be taken into account. Safety evaluation of DNA vaccines against infectious diseases should be carried out considering the particular characteristics of the disease and the causal pathogen, including the expected use, preventive or therapeutic, and target population, in a case by case approach. Fortunately, no major adverse events have been observed so far after DNA immunization in humans on clinical trials. The establishment of strong tests for releasing the product is very relevant in lots consistency and reproducibility of results at both pre-clinical and clinical level. New frontiers are opening and attention should be given to novel preparations including original adjuvants/immunostimulatory molecules or employing modern delivery vehicles for DNA vaccines, as well as the long-term pharmaco-vigilance.

4. Acknowledgments

Authors would like to thank Liz Alvarez-Lajonchere, Dioslaida Urquiza, Jeny Marante, Ariel Vina, Maylin Pupo, Lizet Aldana, Yordanka Soria, Juan Romero, Roberto Madrigal, Leticia Martinez, Miladys Limonta, Marbelis Linares, Dinorah Torres, Gabriel Marquez, Marta Pupo, Eduardo Martínez, Verena Muzio, Gerardo Guillén, Idania Gonzalez, Gillian Martínez, Ivis Guerra and Angel Pérez for the contribution to this work.

5. References

Acosta-Rivero, N., Aguilera, Y., Falcon, V., Poutou, J., Musacchio, A. & Alvarez-Lajonchere, L. (2006) Ultrastructural and immunological characterization of hepatitis C core protein-dna plasmid complexes. *Am. J. Immunol.* Vol 2, pp. 67–72.

Alvarez-Lajonchere, L. & Dueñas-Carrera, S. (2009). Advances in DNA immunization against hepatitis C virus infection: Opportunities and challenges. *Hum. Vaccin.* Vol 5, pp. 568-571.

Alvarez-Lajonchere, L., Shoukry, N.H., Grá, B., Amador-Cañizares, Y., Helle, F., Bédard, N., Guerra, I., Drouin, C., Dubuisson, J., González-Horta, E.E., Martínez, G., Marante, J., Cinza, Z., Castellanos, M., Dueñas-Carrera, S. (2009). Immunogenicity of CIGB-230, a therapeutic DNA vaccine preparation, in HCV-chronically infected individuals in a Phase I clinical trial. *J. Viral Hepat.* Vol 16, pp. 156-167.

Alvarez-Lajonchere, L., Gonzalez, M., Alvarez-Obregon, J.C., Guerra, I., Viña, A., Acosta-Rivero, N., Musacchio, A., Morales, J. & Dueñas-Carrera, S. (2006). Hepatitis C virus (HCV) core protein enhances the immunogenicity of a co-delivered DNA vaccine encoding HCV structural antigens in mice. *Biotechnol. Appl. Biochem.* Vol 44, pp. 9-17.

Armengol, G., Ruiz, L.M. & Orduz, S. (2004). The injection of plasmid DNA in mouse muscle results in lifetime persistence of DNA, gene expression, and humoral response. *Mol. Biotechnol.* Vol 27, pp. 109-118.

Bacardí, D., Amador-Cañizares, Y., Cosme, K., Urquiza, D., Suárez, J., Marante, J., Viña, A., Vázquez, A., Concepción, J., Pupo, M., Aldana, L., Soria, Y., Romero, J., Madrigal, R., Martínez, L., Hernández, L., González, I. & Dueñas-Carrera, S. 2009. Toxicology and biodistribution study of CIGB-230, a DNA vaccine against hepatitis C virus. Hum. Exp. Toxicol. Vol 2, pp.479-491.

Buckland, B.C. (2005) The process development challenge for a new vaccine. *Nat. Med.* Vol 11, pp. S16 - S19.

Bureau, M.F., Naimi, S., Torero, I.R., Seguin, J., Georger, C. & Arnould, E. (2004). Intramuscular plasmid DNA electrotransfer: biodistribution and degradation. *Biochim. Biophys. Acta.* Vol 1676, pp. 138–148.

Castellanos, M., Cinza, Z., Dorta, Z., Veliz, G., Vega, H., Lorenzo, I., Ojeda, S., Dueñas-Carrera, S., Alvarez-Lajonchere, L., Martínez, G., Ferrer, E., Limonta, M., Linares, M., Ruiz, O., Acevedo, B., Torres, D., Márquez, G., Herrera, L. & Arús, E. (2010) Immunization with a DNA vaccine candidate in chronic hepatitis C patients is safe, well tolerated and does not impair immune response induction after anti-hepatitis B vaccination. *J. Gene Med.* Vol 12, pp. 107-116.

Chan, P.K. & Hayes, A.W. (2001). Acute Toxicity and Eye Irritancy. In: *Principles and Methods of Toxicology.* Fourth Edition, edited by A. Wallace Hayes, pp. 853-915, Raven Press, Ltd., New York.

Coelho-Castelo, A.A., Trombone, A.P., Rosada, R.S., Santos, Jr., R.R., Bonato, V.L & Sartori, A. (2006). Tissue distribution of a plasmid DNA encoding Hsp65 gene is dependent on the dose administered through intramuscular delivery. *Genet. Vaccines Ther.* Vol 4, pp. 1.

Contrera, J.F., Aub, D., Barbehenn, E., Belair, E., Chen, C., Evoniuk, G., Mainigi, K., Mielach, F., Sancilio, L. (1993). A retrospective comparison of the results of 6 and 12 month non-rodent toxicity studies. *Adverse Drug React Toxicol Rev.* Vol 12, pp. 63-76.

Dean, J.H., Hincks, J.R. & Remandet, B. (1998). Immunotoxicology assessment in the pharmaceutical industry. *Toxicol. Lett.* Vol 102-103, pp. 247-255.

Food and Drug Administration (FDA). Center for Drug evaluation and Research (CDER). (1996). Guidance for industry. Single Dose Acute Toxicity Testig for Pharmaceuticals.

Ghany, M.G., Strader, D.B., Thomas, D.L. & Seeff, L.B. (2009). Diagnosis, management, and treatment of hepatitis C: an update. *Hepatology.* Vol 49, pp. 1335-1374.

Glenting J & Wessels S. (2005). Ensuring safety of DNA vaccines. *Microb. Cell Fact.* Vol 4, pp. 26.

Good manufacturing practices for biological products. (1992). In: *WHO Expert Committee on Biological Standardization.* Forty-second report. Geneva, World Health Organization, Annex 1 (WHO Technical Report Series, No. 822).

Good manufacturing practices for pharmaceutical products. (2003). In: *WHO Expert Committee on Specifications for Pharmaceutical Preparations.* Thirty-seventh report. Geneva, World Health Organization, Annex 4 (WHO Technical Report Series, No. 908).

Granham, C.E. (1987) Overview: the industry position. In: *Preclinical safety of Biotecnology Products Intended for human use.* edited by C.E. Graham Alan R. pp 183-187. Liss, New York.

Greaves, P. (2000). Histopathology of Preclinical Toxicity Studies. Interpretation and relevance in Grug Safety Evaluation. Second Edition. ELSEVIER.

U.S. Department of Health and Human Services, Food and Drug Administration, Center for Biologics Evaluation and Research. (2007). Guidance for Industry Considerations for Plasmid DNA Vaccines for Infectious Disease Indications.

Guidelines for assuring the quality and nonclinical safety evaluation of DNA vaccines. (2005). In: *WHO Expert Committee on Biological Standardization.* (WHO Technical Report Series, No. 941).

Guidelines for assuring the quality of DNA vaccines. (1998). In: *WHO Expert Committee on Biological Standardization.* Forty-seventy report, Geneva, World Health Organization, Annex 3 (WHO Technical Report Series, No. 878).

Guidelines on clinical evaluation of vaccines: regulatory expectations. (2004). In: *WHO Expert Committee on Biological Standardization.* Fifty-second report. Geneva, World Health Organization, Annex 1 (WHO Technical Report Series, No. 924).

Guidelines on nonclinical evaluation of vaccines. (2006). In: *WHO Expert Committee on Biological Standardization.* Geneva, World Health Organization, Annex 1 (WHO Technical Report Series, No. 932).

Hastings, K. (2002). Implications of the new FDA/CDER immunotoxicology guidance for drugs. *Int. Immunopharmacol.* Vol 2, pp. 1613-1618.

Hohlweg, U. & Doerfler, W. (2001). On the fate of plant or other foreign genes upon the uptake in food or after intramuscular injection in mice. *Mol. Genet. Genomics*. Vol 265, pp. 225-233.

ICH. (1995). Need for Carcinogenicity Studies Pharmaceuticals, Topic S1A, Step 5, ICH Harmonized Tripartite Guideline, International Conference in Harmonization of Technical Requirements for Registration of Pharmaceuticals for Human Use, Geneva, Switzerland.

ICH. (1996). Detection of Toxicity to Reproduction from Medicinal Products, Topic S5A, Step 5, ICH Harmonized Tripartite Guideline, International Conference in Harmonization of Technical Requirements for Registration of Pharmaceuticals for Human Use, Geneva, Switzerland

ICH. (1996). Reproductive Toxicity: Male Fertility Studies, Topic S5B, Step 5, ICH Harmonized Tripartite Guideline, International Conference in Harmonization of Technical Requirements for Registration of Pharmaceuticals for Human Use, Geneva, Switzerland.

ICH. (1997). Preclinical safety Evaluation of Biotechnology-Derived Pharmaceuticals, Topic S6, Step 5, ICH Harmonized Tripartite Guideline, International Conference in Harmonization of Technical Requirements for Registration of Pharmaceuticals for Human Use, Geneva, Switzerland.

ICH M3 (M). (2000). No-clinical safety studies for the conduct of Human clinical trials for pharmaceuticals (modification of CPMP/ICH/286/95), EMEA.

Jeong, G.J., Byun, H.M., Kim, J.M., Yoon, H., Choi, H.G. & Kim, W.K. (2007). Biodistribution and tissue expression kinetics of plasmid DNA complexed with polyethylenimines of different molecular weight and structure. *J. Control Release.* Vol 118, pp. 118–125.

Kim, B.M., Lee, D.S., Chol, J.H., Kim, C.Y., Son, M., Suh, Y.S., Baek, K.H., Park, K.S., Sung, Y.C. & Kim, W.B. (2003). In vivo kinetics and biodistribution of a HIV-1 DNA vaccine after administration in mice. *Arch. Pharm. Res.* Vol 26, pp. 493-498.

Kobayashi, N., Kuramoto, T., Yamaoka, K., Hashida, M. & Takakura, Y. (2001). Hepatic uptake and gene expression mechanisms following intravenous administration of plasmid DNA by conventional and hydrodynamics based procedures. *J. Pharmacol. Exp. Ther.* Vol 297, pp. 853–860.

Kovarik, J. & Siegrist, C.A. (2001). The search for novel adjuvants for early life vaccinations: can "danger" motifs show us the way? *Arch. Immunol. Ther. Exp. (Warsz).* Vol 49, pp. 209-215.

Ledwith, B.J., Manam, S., Troilo, P.J., Barnum, A.B., Pauley, C.J., Griffiths, I., Ind, T.G., Harper, L.B., Beare, C.M., Bagdon, W.J. & Nichols, W.W. (2000). Plasmid DNA vaccines: Investigation of integration into host cellular DNA following intramuscular injection in mice. *Intervirology.* Vol 43, pp. 258-272.

Litvinov, S. (2009). New adjuvants for accelerated and enhanced antibody response. *Nat Meth.* Vol 6, pp. 10-11.

Loeb, W.F., Bannerman, R.M.., Rininger, B.F. & Johnson, A.J. (1978). Haematological disorders in: *Pathology of laboratory animals.* Edited by Benirschke K, Garner FM & Jones JC, Vol 1. Chap. 11. pp 889-1050. Springer vervac. New York.

Liu, M.A. (2011). DNA vaccines: an historical perspective and view to the future. *Immunol. Rev.* Vol 239, pp.62-84.

Manam, S., Ledwith, B.J., Barnum, A.B., Troilo, P.J., Pauley, C.J., Harper, L.B., Griffiths, I., Ind, T.G., Niu, Z., Denisova, L., Follmer, T.T., Pacchione, S.J., Wang, Z., Beare, C.M., Bagdon, W.J. & Nichols, W.W. (2000). Plasmid DNA vaccines: Tissue distribution and effects of DNA sequence, adjuvants and delivery method on integration into host DNA. *Intervirology.* Vol 43, pp. 273-281.

Guidelines of the quality, safety and efficacy of medical products for use. The principles governing medical products to the European Community. (1992). Non-clinical local tolerance testing of medical products. Addendum No. 2. Vol. III: 137-48.

OECD, Guidelines for testing of chemicals. (1993). Section 4: Health Effects. "Acute Oral Toxicity", No. 401. France.

Oh, Y.K., Kim, J.P., Hwang, T.S., Ko, J.J., Kim, J.M. & Yang, J.S. (2001). Nasal absorption and biodistribution of plasmid DNA: an alternative route of DNA vaccine delivery. *Vaccine.* Vol 19, pp. 4519–4525.

Pal, R., Yu, Q., Wang, S., Kalyanaraman, V.S., Nair, B.C. & Hudacik, L. (2006). Definitive toxicology and biodistribution study of a polyvalent DNA prime/protein boost human immunodeficiency virus type 1 (HIV-1) vaccine in rabbits. *Vaccine.* Vol 24, pp. 1225–1234.

Parker, S.E., Borellini, F., Wenk, M.L., Hobart, P., Hoffman, S.L., Hedstrom, R., Le, T. & Norman, J.A. (1999). Plasmid DNA malaria vaccine: Tissue distribution and safety studies in mice and rabbits. *Hum. Gene Ther.* Vol 10, pp. 741-758.

Quezada, A., Larson, J., French, M., Ponce, R., Perrard, J., Durland, R. (2004). Biodistribution and safety studies of hDel-1 plasmid-based gene therapy in mouse and rabbit models. *J. Pharm. Pharmacol.* Vol 56, pp. 177–185.

Committe for Propietary Medicinal Products. EMEA. (1998). Safety Studies for Gene Therapy Products. CPMP/SWP/112/98.

Stoll, R.E. (1987). The preclinical development of biotechnology-derived pharmaceuticals: The PMA perspective. In: *Preclinical Safety of Biotechnology products intended for human use.* Edited by C.E. Graham. pp 169-171. Alan R. Liss, New York,

Tuomela, M., Malm, M., Wallen, M., Stanescu, I., Krohn, K. & Peterson, P. (2005). Biodistribution and general safety of a naked DNA plasmid, GTU® - MultiHIV, in a rat using a quantitative PCR method. *Vaccine* Vol 23, pp. 890-896.

Wang, Z., Troilo, P.J., Wang, X., Griffiths, T.G., Pacchione, S.J., Barnum, A.B., Harper, L.B., Pauley, C.J., Niu, Z., Denisova, L., Follmer, T.T., Rizzuto, G., Ciliberto, G., Fattori, E., Monica, N.L., Manam, S. & Ledwith, B.J. (2004). Detection of integration of plasmid DNA into host genomic DNA following intramuscular injection and electroporation. *Gene Ther.* Vol 11, pp. 711-721.

Wolff, J.A., Ludtke, J.J., Acsadi, G., Williams, P. & Jani, A. (1992). Long-term persistence of plasmid DNA and foreign gene expression in mouse muscle. *Hum. Mol. Genet.* Vol 1, pp. 363-369.

15

Aluminium Phosphide Poisoning

Babak Mostafazadeh
Shahid Beheshti University of Medical Sciences,
Iran

1. Introduction

Acute aluminium phosphide poisoning is an extremely lethal poisoning. Ingestion is usually suicidal in intent, uncommonly accidental and rarely homicidal. Unfortunately the absence of a specific antidote results in very high mortality and the key to treatment lies in rapid decontamination and institution of resuscitative measures.Aluminium phosphide is a solid fumigant which has been in extensive use since the 1940s. It has rapidly become one of the most commonly used grain fumigants because of its properties which are considered to be near ideal; it is toxic to all stages of insects, highly potent, does not affect seed viability, is free from toxic residues and leaves little residue on food grains(Hackenberg, 1972).

They are formulated as compressed discs, tablets or pellets that commonly weigh 3 g and contain variable amounts of a single phosphide in combination with other substances such as ammonium carbonate. Tablets are dark brown or grayish in colour. It is freely available in the markets with the major virtues of being cheap and not leaving toxic residues. The specified fatal dose in human is 0.15-0.5 gm. Phosphides are used widely to protect grain held in stores, the holds of ships and in wagons transporting it by rail and are admixed with the grain at a predetermined rate as it is put into storage. Moisture in the air between the grains mixes with phosphide and release phosphine (hydrogen phosphide, phosphorus trihydride, PH3) which is the active pesticide. After contact with an acid, phosphine is released even more vigorous. Two kinds of acute poisoning with these substances are reported: indirect inhalation of the phosphine generated during their approved use or direct ingestion of the salts.

Pure phosphine is colorless and odorless up to toxic concentrations (200 ppm), a view accepted by the International Programme on Chemical Safety and others (Pepelko, et al, 2004; Chaudhry, 1997; IPCS, 1988; Dumas & Bond, 1974), it has an odor of garlicky or decaying fish due to the presence of substituted phosphines and diphosphines .If the former view is accepted the smell emanating from phosphide poisoned patients is probably due to contaminants in the pesticide formulations and not phosphine itself. It has been suggested that these volatile contaminants may be alkylphosphines (Fluck, 1976). For "phosphine" liberated from one pesticidal formulation of aluminium phosphide, the odor threshold was 0.01–0.02 ppm, ten times lower than that derived from the technical salt alone (Fluck, 1976).The usefulness of phosphide pesticides is now threatened by the development of resistance to them.

2. Methods

To complete this review, the terms aluminum and aluminum phosphide and phosphine were searched using the TUMS (Tehran University of Medical Science) digital library,

Medline, pubmed and Google Scholar databases. All applicable articles in English were attained. Many isolated case reports and small case series do not appear in the citation list. The ability to highlight important aspects is the only criterion for inclusion in this review.
The criteria used in the current review include below criteria: Articles were selected based on the impact of lifestyle, stress, and/or environmental factor/s predisposing aluminium phosphide poisoning exposure. Criteria for selection of the literature used included yes-no responses to the appropriateness of methodology; adequacy of subject numbers; specificity of sex and/or age of subjects, and statistically significant response rates to survey questionnaires. The time frame used was principally 1990-2011 inclusive, although articles of extreme importance from earlier decades were used where appropriate. A multifactorial overview of the factors eschewed concerning aluminium phosphide poisoning exposure was elucidated. It was supposed that collective articles detailing known factors of usage were not necessarily correlated with functionality and health. Collection of materials for the review started with the published literature or easily available academic research.

3. Epidemiology

Annually about 300 000 deaths are reported by pesticides poisoning worldwide (Eddleston & Phillips, 2004). The most reports of acute pesticide poisoning only based on hospital records admission and as a result absolutely reflect a small part of the real incidence. In Asian region about 25 million agricultural workers suffer from an episode of poisoning each year(Jeyaratnam, 1990). In "phosphine" poisonings reported from Germany, 28% were planned and mostly by eating, whereas the majority of the 65% accidental exposures were by inhalation (Lauterbach, et al, 2005). A report has also been publishedfrom the United Kingdom where the majority of 93 aluminum phosphide exposures were accidental and concerned inhalation of phosphine in agricultural locations(Bogle, 2006).

4. Ingestion of phosphides

Phosphide ingestion is a particular problem in rural India, the origin of most of the data on this topic (Rastogi, et al, 1990; Chugh, et al, 1991, 1998; Singh, 1996; Gargi, et al, 2006). The aluminium salt is most commonly involved. Indeed, in a prospective study of 559 acute poisonings admitted over 14 months to a single hospital in Harayana-Rohtak, India, no fewer than 379 (68%) involved aluminium phosphide (Siwach & Gupta, 1995). Similarly, reports to the National Poisons Centre in Delhi indicate that aluminium phosphide is the pesticide most commonly ingested by children (Gupta, et al, 2003).
Much smaller numbers or only sporadic cases of phosphide poisoning have been reported from the remainder of the world, including Australia (Nocera, et al, 2000), Denmark (Andersen, et al, 1996), France (Anger, et al, 2000), Germany (Alter, et al, 2001), Greece (Frangides & Pneumatikos, 2002), Iran (Pajoumand, et al, 2002), Jordan (Abder-Rahman, et al, 2000), Morocco (Idali, et al, 2005; Hajouji, et al, 2006; Akkaoui, et al, 2007), Nepal (Lohani, et al, 2000), Sri Lanka (Roberts, et al, 2006), Turkey (Bayazit, et al, 2000), the United Kingdom (Stewart, et al, 2003; Lawler & Thomas, 2007), Canada, the United States (Broderick & Birnbaum, 2002, Ragone, et al, 2002), the former USSR (Rimalis & Bochkarnikov, 1978), and Yugoslavia (Curcic & Dadasovic, 2001). A single death from ingestion of a falsely labeled rodenticide bait has been reported (Azoury & Levin, 1998). Phosphide rodenticides were responsible for nine out of 349 deaths in 35,580 poisoning admissions to Loghman Hakim hospital poison center in Tehran (Pajoumand, et al, 2002).

5. Occupational and environmental phosphine exposure

Occupational exposures to phosphine are uncommon and rarely severe (Sudakin, 2005) but accidental inhalation is a particular risk to those in close proximity to grain that has had a metal phosphide mixed in with it. Recurring locations include ships holds (Gregorakos, et al, 2002, Hansen & Pedersen, 2001, Vohra, et al, 2006), rail wagons (Perotta, et al 1994, Vohra, et al, 2006), grain elevators (Abder-Rahman, et al, 2000), grain stores (Brautbar & Howard, 2002, Misra, et al, 1988), and even stores in homes (Abder-Rahman, et al, 2000). Potentially lethal concentrations of the gas may develop in the head-spaces of unventilated or poorly ventilated storage containers and domestic premises (Memis, et al, 2007).

Phosphine may be released during the illicit manufacture of methamphetamine (Burgess, 2001, Willers-Russo, 1999); deaths have resulted (Willers-Russo, 1999). In another incident, a packet of aluminium phosphide in a container from abroad burst open and the sweepings placed in water causing immediate fizzing and liberation of phosphine (Kamanyire & Murray, 2003). Close proximity to a source of phosphine is not required to be at risk of toxicity as phosphine gas can travel some distance as it is heavier than air (vapor density 1.2:1). Many years ago 12 individuals in a house adjacent to a warehouse used to store aluminium phosphide developed vomiting and one died. The illnesses were attributed to phosphine (Glass, 1959). More recently exposures have been alleged after use of metal phosphides to control pests in adjacent buildings (Popp, 2002).

6. Mechanism of action

The exact mechanism of action of aluminum phosphide poisoning is still unknown, however an initial survey on different animals showed non-competitive cytochrome oxidase binding by phosphine, changes valences of haeme component of haemoglobin.Other than later articles, distinguished significant inhibition of catalase goes to hydrogen peroxide agglomeration (Price, et al, 1982), Extra-mitochondrial release of hydrogen peroxide and oxygen free radicals (Bolter & Chertuka, 1989), leading to lipid peroxidation and protein denaturation of cell membrane are reported in more recent studies (Chug, et al, 1969). Also, aluminum and phosphine (Potter, et al, 1993; Al-Azzawi, et al, 1990), inhibit cholinesterases activity . Al-Azzawi showed in vitro exposure to phosphine lead to reducing human serum cholinesterase activity; in addition he showed the amount of the inhibition is related to the duration and concentration of phosphine (Al-Azzawi, et al, 1990). On the other hand, other studies declared there is no erythrocyte cholinesterase activity reduction in humans after accidental phosphine inhalation (Heyndrickx, et al, 1976; Wilson, et al, 1980).

7. Toxicokinetics

Phosphine must be quickly and easily absorbed because of the short interval between ingestion and the appearance of systemic toxicity features. Noticeably, phosphides possibly absorbed as microscopic particles of unhydrolysed salt (Stewart, et al, 2003, Chan, et al, 1983) and permanently, in vitro, interact with free hemoglobin and hemoglobin in intact erythrocytes (rat and human) to produce a hemichrome (a methemoglobin derivative resulting from distorted protein conformation) (Chin, et al, 1992, Potter, et al, 1991). Also Heinz bodies (denatured hemoglobin aggregates) are formed when phosphide concentration in vitro increases to 1.25 ppm (Potter, et al, 1991). Few cases of phosphide poisoning showed intravascular complications as hemolysis and methemoglobinaemia, these reactions support the involvement of erythrocytes in the biotransformation of phosphine in vivo in humans (Stewart, et al, 2003).

8. Clinical features

Aluminium phosphate poisoning affects the most organs and a variety of signs and symptoms appear in patients. Early symptoms include nausea, vomiting, retrosternal and epigastric pain, dyspnea, anxious, agitation and smell of garlic (Popp, et al, 2002; Aggarwal, et al, 1999; Sood, et al, 1997). on the breath. Moreover shock and peripheral circulatory failure are mainly imperative early signs of toxicity. Mortalities in past studies have ranged from 40–77% and in one survey 55% occurred within 12 h of ingestion and 91% within 24 h (Singh, et al, 1991).

8.1 Cardiac toxicity

Cardiac toxicity comprises circulatory failure (Alter, et al, 2001) hypotension (Bayazit, et al, 2000; Ragone, et al, 2002), congestion of the heart, separation of myocardial fibres by edema, fragmentation of fibres, non-specifc vacuolation of myocytes, focal necrosis, neutrophil and eosinophil infiltration were found in autopsy (Akkaoui, et al, 2007; Sinha, et al, 2005; Chugh, et al, 1991, Katira, et al, 1990). Also, significantly increasing left ventricular dimensions (Bajaj, et al, 1988), hypokinesia of the left ventricle and septum, akinesia, ejection fractions reduction (Bhasin, et al 1991), severe hypotension, raised systemic venous pressure, normal pulmonary artery wedge pressure, inadequate systemic vasoconstriction and ECG abnormalities (ST and T-wave changes) (Kalra, et al, 1991) are other signs and symptoms.

8.2 Respiratory toxicity

Tachypnea, dyspnea, crepitations, and rhonchi were present on examination in 192 out of 418 cases (46%) of phosphide poisoning (Chugh, et al, 1991) and have been found by others (Gupta, et al, 2000). Pulmonary edema is common but it is not always clear whether it is cardiogenic or non-cardiogenic in etiology. It tends to develop 4–48 h after ingestion and the finding of a reduced arterial pressure of O_2 without an increase in pulmonary artery wedge pressure, suggested it was non-cardiogenic (Kalra, et al, 1991). Others have confidently diagnosed adult respiratory distress syndrome (Singh, et al, 1991, Bajaj, et al, 1988, Gupta, et al, 1995, Chugh, et al 1989) and non-specifed pulmonary edema (Singh, et al, 1996, Chugh, et al, 1998). The edema fluid may be protein-rich and hemorrhagic (Singh, et al, 1996).

8.3 Gastrointestinal toxicity

Hematemesis (Gupta, et al, 2000), corrosive lesions of the esophagus and stomach (Madan, et al, 2006, Tiwari, et al, 2003), vomiting, epigastric pain, severe gastric erosions, duodenal erosions, esophageal strictures tracheo-oesophageal fistulae,dysphagia (Darbari, et al, 2007). Dysphagia may be apparent as soon as 3 or 4 days after ingestion of aluminium phosphide (Madan, et al, 2006, Darbari, et al, 2007) but is more usual about 2 weeks later.

8.4 Hepatic toxicity

Transient elevations of alanine aminotransferase and aspartate aminotransferase activities are not infrequent after ingestion of metal phosphides (Frangides & Pneumatikos, 2002;

Akkaoui, et al, 2007; Bayazit, et al, 2000; Memis, et al, 2007) but jaundice secondary to liver damage (Chugh, et al, 1998) is much less common. It was present in 12 out of 92 cases (Singh, et al, 1991) and was said to be common in another series of 15 patients (Singh, et al, 1985) but confirmatory laboratory data were not provided. Jaundice was alleged to be present in 16 (52%) members of the crew of a grain freighter who inhaled phosphine after an accidental release (Wilson, et al, 1980) but, in the six tested, serum bilirubin concentrations were normal and transaminase activities only minimally disturbed, casting doubt on the clinical observation. Acute hepatic failure and encephalopathy was considered to be the cause of death in one man (Chittora, et al, 1994), while a 12-yearold girl died from a combination of acute hepatic failure and encephalopathy with renal failure (Bayazit, et al, 2000). Portal edema, congestion of the portal tract and central veins, and vacuolization of hepatocytes are the most frequent findings at autopsy (Saleki, et al, 2007).

8.5 Electrolyte and metabolic abnormalities

Hypokalemia. metabolic acidosis, mixed metabolic acidosis and respiratory alkalosis, and acute renal failure are reported frequently. Also,Hypoglycemia and hypomagnesemia have been reported in several studies (Chugh, et al, 2000; Dueñas, et al, 1999). Hypokalemia is common soon after ingestion of metal phosphides and is probably secondary to vomiting, though catecholamine release could also contribute. It is thought to be the result of impaired gluconeogenesis and glycogenolysis (Frangides & Pneumatikos, 2002) possibly secondary to adrenal gland damage and low circulating cortisol concentrations (Chugh, et al, 2000). Hyperglycemia (Abder-Rahman, 1999) appears to be rare. The main controversy relates to the existence or otherwise of disturbances of magnesium homeostasis. In 1989, prompted by reports of the empirical use of magnesium sulphate to treat phosphide toxicity, this study (Singh, et al, 1989; Singh & Sharma, 1991) demonstrated that serum magnesium concentrations were increased, possibly secondary to release from damaged cardiac myocytes and hepatocytes, and confirmed the findings in subsequent studies (Singh, et al, 1991; Singh, et al, 1990). Unfortunately, other studies have found the converse, that is serum and erythrocyte concentrations were reduced rather than increased. Chugh, et al, (1991) compared serial serum and erythrocyte magnesium concentrations in four groups of people. One comprised patients poisoned with aluminium phosphide who had resulting shock and cardiotoxicity while the second included those poisoned but without shock or cardiac features. The remaining two groups acted as controls, the first being patients in shock secondary to trauma or hemorrhage but without other features of cardiac toxicity and the second, normal volunteers. The only significant finding in admission samples was that cell and serum concentrations were lower in shocked, cardiotoxic patients (mean serum and RBC concentrations 0.9 and 3.7 mEq/L respectively compared with 1.8 and 5.2 mEq/L in volunteers). Since, first, hypomagnesemia was found in toxic shocked patients but not in those with non-toxic shock and secondly, 75% of those in the toxic/shock group had ECG changes, it was concluded that the evidence supported a causal relationship between hypomagnesemia and phosphide induced shock. Without intervention both serum and cell values returned to normal by about 24 h. The authors confirmed their findings in a later study (Chugh, et al, 1994) and thought the hypomagnesemia secondary to consumption in combating free radical stress (Chugh, et al, 1997). Hypomagnesemia has also been found in a recent single case of phosphine inhalation from aluminium phosphide (Dueñas, et al, 1999). The situation became even more complicated when, in 1994, a study (Siwach, et al, 1994) found themselves unable to agree with either. They found pre-treatment mean serum and red cell magnesium concentrations to be normal. Concentrations were increased in the brains, lungs, hearts, livers, kidneys, and stomachs of fatalities but later studies showed this to be the result of magnesium administration and not phosphide toxicity (Siwach, et al, 1995). Clearly, these studies cannot all be correct and the analytical method used to generate the results may be an important factor. The results of a study (Siwach, et al, 1994) carry particular weight because they used atomic absorption spectroscopy, a technique that is superior to the colorimetric method published in 1977 and used (Singh, et al, 1991) and the titan yellow method employed (Chugh, et al, 1991) despite it being claimed that results obtained using the former method correlated extremely well with those from atomic absorption spectroscopy (Khayam-Bashi, et al, 1977). If these studies (Siwach, et al, 1994) are considered the most reliable, there is no choice but to accept that neither hypomagnesemia nor hypermagnesemia is a feature of aluminium phosphide poisoning, though confirmation by another independent study would be welcome.

8.6 Hematological toxicity

Although phosphine causes Heinz body formulation and hemoglobin oxidation *in vitro* (Chin, et al, 1992; Potter, et al, 1991), intravascular hemolysis and methemoglobinaemia are unusual complications of phosphide poisoning in humans. Nine individuals with intravascular hemolysis after ingestion of aluminium phosphide have been identified from the literature. Three were glucose-6-phosphate dehydrogenase deficient (Srinivas, et al, 2007), including one young man who had previously developed haemolysis when given primaquine (Sood, et al, 1997). Two others had no history to suggest this possible predisposing disorder (Aggarwal, et al, 1999; Lakshmi, 2002) and in the remaining four the issue was not addressed (Chugh, et al, 1991). Intravascular hemolysis was associated with renal failure and severe metabolic acidosis to which 3 days of vomiting and diarrhea may have partly contributed (Memis, et al, 2007). In addition to hemolysis one man was found to have methemoglobinaemia of 17% 32 h post-ingestion (Lakshmi, 2002) while another developed Heinz bodies (Srinivas, et al, 2007), a further indicator of damage to hemoglobin. Rats given aluminium phosphide had methemoglobin concentrations measured at 10 and 30 min intervals. They increased simultaneously with those of malonyldialdehyde suggesting that methemoglobinaemia was secondary to increased oxygen free radical generation (Lall, et al, 2000). A study revealed that there is a significant association between blood level of methemoglobin and mortality in patients with aluminium phosphide intoxication (Mostafazadeh, et al, 2010). Disseminated intravascular coagulation was present in six out of 418 patients poisoned with aluminium phosphide (Chugh, et al, 1991).

8.7 Uncommon features

Unusual complications of phosphide ingestion include atrial infarction (Jain, et al, 1992), pleural effusion (Bayazit, et al, 2000; Suman & Savani, 1999), ascites (Bayazit, et al, 2000), skeletal muscle damage (Khosla, et al, 1988), rhabdomyolysis (Abder-Rahman, 1999), a bleeding diathesis (Gupta, et al, 1990), adrenocortical congestion, hemorrhage and necrosis (Arora, et al, 1995), pancreatitis (Sarma, et al, 1996), and renal failure (Chugh, et al, 1991; Singh, et al, 1996; Bayazit, et al, 2000; Gupta, et al, 2000). Acute pericarditis has also been reported infrequently (Wander, et al, 1990; Chugh & Malhotra, 1992) though pericardial fluid was detected by echocardiography in a third of patients in one study (Bhasin, et al, 1991). Subendocardial infarction complicated the recovery of a 16-year-old male (Kaushik, et al, 2007) and a 26-year-old woman who had recovered from aluminium phosphide ingestion suffered an intracranial hemorrhage 5 days after the event. No explanation other than the poison was found (Dave, et al, 1994).

9. Diagnosis

A positive history of ingestion is the basis of diagnosis in most cases. The presence of typical clinical features, garlicky odour from the mouth and highly variable arrhythmias in a young patient with shock and no previous history of cardiac disease points towards aluminium phosphide poisoning. Aluminium phosphide poisoning risk is low down in the following instances, When taking patient's history should be special attention to these points:
If the patient uses the expired one
If aluminum phosphide is dissolved in water before use
If the patient experiences immediate vomiting
Confirmation can be done by the Silver Nitrate Test (Chugh, et al, 1989). In this test, 5 ml of gastric aspirate and 15 ml of water are put in a flask and the mouth of the flask is covered by filter paper impregnated with silver nitrate. The flask is heated at 50°C for 15 to 20 min. If phosphine is present the filter paper turns black. For performing the test on exhaled air, the silver nitrate impregnated filter paper is placed on the mouth of the patient and the patient is asked to breath through it for 15-20 minutes, blackening of the paper indicates the presence of phosphine in breath. The sensitivity of the test is 100%. However the most specific and sensitive method for detecting the presence of PH_3 in blood/air is gas chromatography (Vins Jansen A, Thrane, 1978). For spot sampling of phosphine in air, detector tubes and bulbs are available commercially (International Programme on Chemical Safety, 1998; Leesch, 1982).

10. Laboratory investigations

Laboratory evaluation is often performed to assess the prognosis. Leucopenia indicates severe toxicity. Increased aspartate aminotransferase or alanine aminotransferase and metabolic acidosis indicate moderate to severe ingestional poisoning. Electrolyte analysis shows decreased magnesium while potassium may be increased or decreased (Chugh, et al, 1990). Measurement of plasma renin is significant as its level in blood carries a direct relationship with mortality and is raised in direct proportion to the dose of pesticide. The serum level of cortisol is usually found to be decreased in severe poisoning (Chugh, et al, 1989). Chest X-ray may reveal hilar or perihilar congestion if ARDS develops. Electrocardiogram shows various manifestations of cardiac injury (ST depression or elevation, bundle branch block, ventricular tachycardia, ventricular fibrillation) (Jain, et al, 1985; Katira, et al, 1990; Siwach, et al, 1998; Singh, et al, 1989). Wall motion abnormalities, generalised hypokinesia of the left ventricle, decreased ejection fraction and pericardial effusion can be seen in echocardiography (Chugh, 1995).

11. Prognostic markers

Development of refractory shock, acute respiratory distress syndrom, aspiration, pneumonitis, anaemia, metabolic acidosis, electrolyte imbalance, coma, severe hypoxia, gastrointestinal bleeding, and pericarditis are associated with poor prognosis. The outcome correlates best with the number of vomiting the patient gets after ingestion and the severity of hypotension the patient develops (Singh, et al, 1998) 95% of the patients die within 24 hours and the commonest cause of death in this group is arrhythmia. Death after 24 hours is due to shock, acidosis, acute respiratory distress syndrom and arrhythmia. The mortality rate is highly variable, ranging from 37-100% and can reach more than 60% even in experienced and well equipped centres.

12. Management

12.1 Decontamination

Gastric lavage is probably best avoided after ingestion of phosphides as it might increase the rate of disintegration of the pesticide and increase toxicity (Maitai, et al, 2002). To reduce the absorption of phosphine, gastric lavage with potassium permanganate (1:10,000) is done. Permanganate is used as it oxidizes PH_3 to form non-toxic phosphate. This is followed by a slurry of activated charcoal (approximately 100 gm) given through a nasogastric tube. In vitro studies suggested that vegetable oil and liquid paraffin inhibit phosphine release from phosphides (Goswami, et al, 1994) but these oils have not been tested in clinical practice. However, vomiting may make the administration of charcoal difficult. Although the administration of sodium bicarbonate via a gastric tube to decrease gastric hydrochloric acid has been proposed in the belief that hydrochloric acid assists the conversion of phosphide to phosphine, there is no experimental support for its use. Moreover, based on an understanding of the mechanisms of toxicity of metal phosphides, this strategy is unlikely to reduce morbidity and mortality. Removal of victims of phosphine inhalation from the contaminated atmosphere will have been carried out by the emergency service first on scene. Supplemental oxygen may be given if necessary but further measures for airway control are unlikely to be required.

12.2 Supportive care

Many patients will die from metal phosphide poisoning despite intensive care. Supportive measures are all that can be offered and should be implemented as required by clinical developments. The most important factor for success is resuscitation of shock and institution of supportive measures as soon as possible. Intravenous access should be established and 2-3 litres of normal saline are administered within the first 8-12 hr guided by central venous pressure (CVP) and pulmonary capillary wedge pressure (PCWP). The aim is to keep the CVP at around 12-14 cm of water (Siwach, et al, 1997). Some workers have recommended rapid infusion of saline (3-6 litres) in the initial 3 hr (Kalra, et al, 1991). Low dose dopamine (4-6 μg/kg/min) is given to keep systolic blood pressure >90 mm Hg. The other vasopressures such as norepinephrine may be usefull in critical patients. The use of high doses of glucagon may benefit in the treatment of aluminum phosphide poisoning; the likely mechanism of action is the increase of cAMP in the myocardium, effectively bypassing the β-adrenergic second messenger system. Oxygen is given for hypoxia. Acute respiratory distress syndrom requires intensive care monitoring and mechanical ventilation. The blood glucose concentration should be measured in every case and hypoglycemia corrected if found. Similarly, hypokalemia should be sought and, if clinically indicated, at least partially corrected; cardiac features have resolved in occasional patients on correction of potassium concentrations (Kochar, et al, 2000). It must be remembered, however, that the onset of acidosis, renal failure and cell damage may produce life-threatening hyperkalemia. Metabolic acidosis should be managed conventionally. Bicarbonate level less than 15 mEq/L requires bicarbonate in a dose of 50-100 mEq intravenously every 8 hour (Singh, et al, 1989).

All types of ventricular arrhythmias are seen in these patients and the management is the same as for arrhythmias in other situations (International Programme on Chemical Safety, 1998).

12.3 Magnesium supplementation

The problematic decision is whether or not supplemental magnesium should be given. If magnesium depletion does not occur such a course would appear illogical but single cases have been reported where magnesium administration appeared to terminate atrial fibrillation (Chugh, et al, 1989) and supra ventricular tachycardia and ventricular tachycardia (Chugh, et al, 1991). On the other hand, magnesium sulphate 3 g given intravenously over 30 min did not abolish very frequent ventricular ectopic beats and bigeminy though it restored a normal magnesium concentration (Dueñas, et al, 1999). Only a few studies have attempted to assess the value of magnesium sulphate in large groups of patients and their results are conflicting. In a study, 50 patients after aluminium phosphide ingestion were given high doses of magnesium and the result compared with the control group that was not treated. The result showed (42%) of those given supplemental magnesium survived compared with (40%) not so treated. In addition, treatment did not considerably improve survival at any dose (number of tablets) consumed. As you see magnesium supplementation was of no value in this study (Siwach, et al, 1994). Chugh et al. (2004) obtained opposite results in a case control study. The authors showed survival remarkably improved after each dose ingested for those patients treated by magnesium (Chugh, et al, 2004). To illuminate the potential benefit of magnesium supplementation, additional studies are necessary.

12.4 N-acetylcysteine

Different studies in rats (Hsu, et al, 2000, 2002) and humans (Chugh, et al, 1997) showed glutathione concentrations reduction after treating with N-acetylcysteine in patients with aluminium phosphide poisoning (Bogle, et al, 2006).

12.5 Pralidoxime

There is experimental and clinical evidence that phosphine (Potter, et al, 1993) and aluminium (Marquis & Lerrick, 1982, 1983) inhibit acetylcholinesterase. A study (Mittra, et al, 2001) investigated the benefit of administering atropine 1 mg/kg and pralidoxime 5 mg/kg parenterally to rats dosed with aluminium phosphide 10 mg/kg (5.55 × LD50) 5 min previously. Treatment increased the survival time by 2.5-fold in nine out of 15 animals and resulted in the survival of the six remaining animals. There were no survivors in the two control groups. Further studies are required to confirm the benefit of oximes.

13. Conclusions

Acute poisoning with metal phosphides, particularly aluminium phosphide, is a worldwide problem most commonly encountered in the Indian Sub-Continent. The clinical features have been well described though it is only recently that the mechanisms of toxicity have been more clearly understood. Poisoning from phosphides is mediated by phosphine which has been shown to rapidly perturb mitochondrial morphology, inhibit oxidative respiration, and cause a severe drop in mitochondrial membrane potential. This failure of cellular respiration is likely to be due to a mechanism other than inhibition of cytochrome C oxidase as phosphine inhibits cytochrome C oxidase activity less dramatically *in vivo* than *in vitro* and only partially inhibits cytochrome C oxidase activity in humans. Phosphine can also form the highly reactive hydroxyl radical and inhibit both catalase and peroxidase leading to lipid peroxidation. The gas or gases given of in addition to phosphine when phosphide formulations come into contact with water or acid need to be identified and their toxicity determined. The observation that both aluminium and phosphine may inhibit acetylcholinesterase activity needs to be investigated further as does the report that the administration of atropine and pralidoxime reduces morbidity and mortality in aluminium phosphide poisoning. There is conflicting evidence also on the occurrence and clinical importance of magnesium disturbances which some have described. The benefit of magnesium supplementation has still to be determined.

14. References

Abder-Rahman H. Effect of aluminium phosphide on blood glucose level. Vet Hum Toxicol 1999; 41:31-32.

Abder-Rahman HA, Battah AH, Ibraheem YM et al. Aluminum phosphide fatalities, new local experience. Med Sci Law 2000; 40:164-168.

Aggarwal P, Handa R, Wig N et al. Intravascular hemolysis in aluminium phosphide poisoning. *Am J Emerg Med* 1999; 17:488-489.

Aggarwal P, Handa R, Wig N et al. Intravascular hemolysis in aluminium phosphide poisoning. Am J Emerg Med 1999; 17:488-489.

Akkaoui M, Achour S, Abidi K et al. Reversible myocardial injury associated with aluminum phosphide poisoning. Clin Toxicol 2007; 45:728-731.

Akkaoui M, Achour S, Abidi K et al. Reversible myocardial injury associated with aluminum phosphide poisoning. *Clin Toxicol* 2007; 45:728-731.

Al-Azzawi MJ, Al-Hakkak ZS, Al-Adhami BW. In vitro inhibitory effects of phosphine on human and mouse serum cholinesterase. *Toxicol Environ Chem* 1990; 29:53-56.

Alter P, Grimm W, Maisch B. Lethal heart failure caused by aluminium phosphide poisoning. Intensive Care Med 2001; 27:327.

Alter P, Grimm W, Maisch B. Lethal heart failure caused by aluminium phosphide poisoning. *Intensive Care Med* 2001; 27:327.

Andersen TS, Holm JW, Andersen TS. Forgiftning med muldvarpegasningsmidlet aluminiumfosfid. Ugeskr Laeger 1996; 158:5308-5309.

Anger F, Paysant F, Brousse F et al. Fatal aluminum phosphide poisoning. J Anal Toxicol 2000; 24:90-92.

Arora B, Punia RS, Kalra R et al. Histopathological changes in aluminium phosphide poisoning. J Indian Med Assoc 1995; 93:380-381.

Azoury M, Levin N. Identification of zinc phosphide in a falsely labeled rodenticide bait. J Forensic Sci 1998; 43:693-695.

Bajaj R, Wasir HS, Agarwal R et al. Aluminium phosphide poisoning. Clinical toxicity and outcome in eleven intensively monitored patients. *Natl Med J India* 1988; 1:270-274.

Bajaj R, Wasir HS, Agarwal R et al. Aluminium phosphide poisoning. Clinical toxicity and outcome in eleven intensively monitored patients. Natl Med J India 1988; 1:270-274.

Bayazit AK, Noyan A, Anarat A. A child with hepatic and renal failure caused by aluminum phosphide. Nephron 2000; 86:517.

Bayazit AK, Noyan A, Anarat A. A child with hepatic and renal failure caused by aluminum phosphide. *Nephron* 2000; 86:517.

Bhasin P, Mittal HS, Mitra A. An echocardiographic study in aluminium phosphide poisoning. *J Assoc Physicians India* 1991; 39:851.

Bogle RG, Theron P, Brooks P et al. Aluminium phosphide poisoning. Emerg Med J 2006; 23:e3.

Bogle RG, Theron P, Brooks P et al. Aluminium phosphide poisoning. Emerg Med J 2006; 23:e3.

Bolter CJ, Chertuka W. Extra-mitochondrial release of H2O2 from insect, mouse liver mitochondria using respiratory inhibitor phosphine, myxothiazole and antimycin and special analysis of inhibited cytochromes. Arch Biochem Biophy 1989; 278: 73.

Brautbar N, Howard J. Phosphine toxicity: report of two cases and review of the literature. Toxicol Ind Health 2002; 18:71–75.

Broderick M, Birnbaum K. Fatal ingestion of zinc phosphide rodenticide. J Toxicol Clin Toxicol 2002; 40:684.

Burgess JL. Phosphine exposure from a methamphetamine laboratory investigation. J Toxicol Clin Toxicol 2001; 39:165–168.

Chan LT, Crowley RJ, Delliou D, Geyer R. Phosphine analysis in post mortem specimens following ingestion of aluminium phosphide. *J Anal Toxicol* 1983; 7:165-167.

Chaudhry MQ. A review of the mechanisms involved in the action of phosphine as an insecticide and phosphine resistance in stored-product insects. Pestic Sci 1997; 49:213 228.

Chin KL, Mai X, Meaklim J et al. The interaction of phosphine with haemoglobin and erythrocytes. *Xenobiotica* 1992; 22:599–607.

Chin KL, Mai X, Meaklim J et al. The interaction of phosphine with haemoglobin and erythrocytes. Xenobiotica 1992; 22:599–607.

Chittora MD, Meena SR, Gupta DK, Bhargava S. Acute hepatic failure in aluminium phosphide poisoning. J Assoc Physicians India 1994; 42:924.

Chittora MD, Meena SR, Gupta DK, Bhargava S. Acute hepatic failure in aluminium phosphide poisoning. J Assoc Physicians India 1994; 42:924.

Chug SN, Arora V, Sharma A, Chug K. Free radical scavengers and lipid peroxidation in acute aluminium phosphide poisoning. *IJMR* 1996; 104: 190.

Chugh SN, Aggarwal HK, Mahajan SK. Zinc phosphide intoxication symptoms: analysis of 20 cases. Int J Clin Pharmacol Ther 1998; 36:406–407.

Chugh SN, Chugh K, Ram S, Malhotra KC. Electrocardiographic abnormalities in aluminium phosphide poisoning with special reference to its incidence, pathogenesis, mortality and histopathology. *J Indian Med Assoc* 1991; 89:32–35.

Chugh SN, Dushyant, Ram S et al. Incidence & outcome of aluminium phosphide poisoning in a hospital study. Indian J Med Res 1991; 94:232–235.

Chugh SN, Jaggal KL, Ram S et al. Hypomagnesaemic atrial fibrillation in a case of aluminium phosphide poisoning. J Assoc Physicians India 1989; 37:548–549.

Chugh SN, Jaggal KL, Sharma A et al. Magnesium levels in acute cardiotoxicity due to aluminium phosphide poisoning. Indian J Med Res 1991; 94:437–439.

Chugh SN, Juggal KL, Sharma A, Arora B, Malhotra KC. Magnesium levels in aluminium phosphide poisoning [Abstract]. J Assoc Physicians India 1990; 38:32.

Chugh SN, Kishore K, Aggarwal N, Attri S. Hypoglycaemia in acute aluminium phosphide poisoning. *J Assoc Physicians India* 2000; 48:855–856.

Chugh SN, Kolley T, Kakkar R et al. A critical evaluation of antiperoxidant effect of intravenous magnesium in acute aluminium phosphide poisoning. Magnes Res 1997; 10:225–230.

Chugh SN, Kolley T, Kakkar R et al. A critical evaluation of antiperoxidant effect of intravenous magnesium in acute aluminium phosphide poisoning. *Magnes Res* 1997; 10:225– 230.

Chugh SN, Kumar P, Sharma A et al. Magnesium status and parenteral magnesium sulphate therapy in acute aluminium phosphide intoxication. Magnes Res 1994; 7:289–294.

Chugh SN, Malhotra KC. Acute pericarditis in aluminium phosphide poisoning. J Assoc Physicians India 1992; 40:564.

Chugh SN, Malhotra S, Kumar P, Malhotra KC. Reversion of ventricular and supraventricular tachycardia by magnesium sulphate therapy in aluminium phosphide poisoning. Report of two cases. J Assoc Physicians India 1991; 39:642–643.

Chugh SN, Ram S, Chugh K, Malhotra KC. Spot diagnosis of aluminium phosphide ingestion: an application of a simple test. J Assoc Physicians India 1989;37(3):219-20.

Chugh SN, Ram S, Mehta LK et al. Adult respiratory distress syndrome following aluminium phosphide ingestion. Report of 4 cases. J Assoc Physicians India 1989; 37:271–272.

Chugh SN, Ram S, Sharma A, Arora BB, Saini AS, Malhotra KC. Adrenocortical involvement in aluminium phosphide poisoning. Indian J Med Res 1989;90:289-94.

Chugh SN. Aluminium phosphide poisoning with special reference on its diagnosis and management[Review article]. J Med Assoc Clin Med 1995:1:20-2.

Curcic M, Dadasovic J. Pokusana I izvrsena samoubistva rodenticidima od 1968 do 2000 godine. Med Pregl 2001; 54:256–260.

Darbari A, Kumar A, Chandra G, Tandon S. Tracheo-oesophageal fistula with oesophageal stricture due to aluminium phosphide (Celphos tablet) poisoning. *J Chest Dis Allied Sci* 2007; 49:241–242.

Dave HH, Dave TH, Rakholia VG et al. Delayed hemorrhagic stroke following accidental aluminium phosphide ingestion. J Assoc Physicians India 1994; 42:78–79.

Dueñas A, Pérez-Castrillon JL, Cobos MA, Herreros V. Treatment of the cardiovascular manifestations of phosphine poisoning with trimetazidine, a new antiischemic drug. *Am J Emerg Med* 1999; 17:219–220.

Dueñas A, Pérez-Castrillon JL, Cobos MA, Herreros V. Treatment of the cardiovascular manifestations of phosphine poisoning with trimetazidine, a new antiischemic drug. Am J Emerg Med 1999; 17:219–220.

Dumas T, Bond EJ. Separation of phosphine from odour-producing impurities. J Stored Prod Res 1974; 10:67–68.

Eddleston M, Phillips MR. Self poisoning with pesticides. BMJ 2004;328:42–44.

Fluck E. The odor threshold of phosphine. J Air Pollut Control Assoc 1976; 26:795.

Frangides CY, Pneumatikos IA. Persistent severe hypoglycemia in acute zinc phosphide poisoning. Intensive Care Med 2002; 28:223.

Gargi J, Rai H, Chanana A et al. Current trend of poisoning – a hospital profile. J Indian Med Assoc 2006; 104:72–73, 94.

Glass A. Account of suspected phosphine poisoning in a submarine. J R Nav Med Serv 1959; 42:184–187.

Goswami M, Bindal M, Sen P et al. Fat and oil inhibit phosphine release from aluminium phosphide – its clinical implication. Indian J Exp Biol 1994; 32:647–649.

Gregorakos L, Sakayianni K, Harizopoulou V. Recovery from severe inhalational phosphine poisoning. Report of two cases. Clin Intensive Care 2002; 13:177–179.

Gupta MS, Malik A, Sharma VK. Cardiovascular manifestations in aluminium phosphide poisoning with special reference to echocardiographic changes. J Assoc Physicians India 1995; 43:773–774, 779–780.

Gupta MS, Mehta L, Chugh SN, Malhotra KC. Aluminium phosphide poisoning. Two cases with rare presentation. J Assoc Physicians India 1990; 38:509–510.

Gupta SK, Peshin SS, Srivastava A, Kaleekal T. A study of childhood poisoning at National Poisons Information Centre, All India Institute of Medical Sciences, New Delhi. J Occup Health 2003; 45:191–196.

Gupta V, Singh J, Doodan SS, Bali SK. Multisystem organ failure (MSOF) in aluminium phosphide (ALP) poisoning. JK Pract 2000; 7:287–288.

Hackenberg U. Chronic ingestion by rats of standard diet treated with aluminum phosphide. Toxicol Appl Pharmacol 1972;23(1):147-58.

Hajouji Idrissi M, Oualili L, Abidi K et al. Facteurs de gravité de l'intoxication aiguë au phosphure d'aluminium (Phostoxin®). Ann Fr Anesth Réanim 2006; 25:382–385.

Hansen HL, Pedersen G. Poisoning at sea: injuries caused by chemicals aboard Danish merchant ships 1988–1996. J Toxicol Clin Toxicol 2001; 39:21–26.

Heyndrickx A, Van Peteghem C, Van Den Heede M, Lauwaert R.Double fatality with children due to fumigated wheat. *Eur J Toxicol* 1976; 9:113–118.

Hsu C-H, Chi B-C, Liu M-Y et al. Phosphine-induced oxidative damage in rats: role of glutathione. *Toxicology* 2002; 179:1–8.

Hsu C-H, Han B-C, Liu M-Y et al. Phosphine-induced oxidative damage in rats: attenuation by melatonin. *Free Radic Biol Med* 2000; 28:636–642.

Idali B, Miguil M, Moutawakkil S et al. Intoxication aiguë au phostoxin. Presse Med 1995; 24:611–612.

International Programme on Chemical Safety. Environmental health criteria 73: phosphine and selected metal phosphides. Geneva: World Health Organization; 1998. [cited 2007 Sep 14]. Available from: http://www.who.int/ipcs/publications.

IPCS. Environmental health criteria 73. Phosphine and selected metal phosphides. Geneva: World Health Organization, 1988.

Jain MK, Khanijo SK, Pathak N et al. Electrocardiographic diagnosis of atrial infarction in aluminium phosphide poisoning. J Assoc Physicians India 1992; 40:692–693.

Jain SM, Bharani A, Sepaha GC, Sanghvi VC, Raman PG. Electrocardiographic changes in aluminium phosphide (ALP) poisoning [Case reports]. J Assoc Physicians India 1985;33(6):406-9.

Jeyaratnam J. Acute pesticide poisoning: A major global health problem. World Health Stat Q 1990; 43:139–144.

Kalra GS, Anand IS, Jit I et al. Aluminium phosphide poisoning: haemodynamic observations. Indian Heart J 1991; 43:175–178.

Kalra GS, Anand IS, Jit I, Bushnurmath B, Wahi PL. Aluminium phosphide poisoning: haemodynamic observations. Indian Heart J 1991;43(3):175-8.

Kamanyire R, Murray V. Occupational exposures to fumigants. J Toxicol Clin Toxicol 2003; 41:489–490.

Katira R, Elhence GP, Mehrotra ML et al. A study of aluminium phosphide (Aluminium phosphide poisoning) poisoning with special reference to electrocardiographic changes. *J Assoc Physicians India* 1990; 38: 471–473.

Katira R, Elhence GP, Mehrotra ML, Srivastava SS, Mitra A, Agarwala R, et al. A study of aluminum phosphide (AlP) poisoning with special reference to electrocardiographic changes. J Assoc Physicians India 1990;38(7):471-3.

Kaushik RM, Kaushik R, Mahajan SK. Subendocardial infarction in a young survivor of aluminium phosphide poisoning. Hum Exp Toxicol 2007; 26:457–460.

Khayam-Bashi H, Liu TZ, Walter V. Measurement of serum magnesium with a centrifugal analyzer. Clin Chem 1977; 23:289–291.

Khosla SN, Nand N, Khosla P. Aluminium phosphide poisoning. J Trop Med Hyg 1988; 91:196–198.

Kochar DK, Shubhakaran, Jain N et al. Successful management of hypokalaemia related conduction disturbances in acute aluminium phosphide poisoning. J Indian Med Assoc 2000; 98:461–462.

Lakshmi B. Methemoglobinemia with aluminum phosphide poisoning. Am J Emerg Med 2002; 20:130–132.

Lall SB, Peshin SS, Mitra S. Methemoglobinemia in aluminium phosphide poisoning in rats. Indian J Exp Biol 2000; 38:95–97.

Lauterbach M, Solak E, Kaes J et al. Epidemiology of hydrogen phosphide exposures in humans reported to the Poison Center in Mainz,Germany, 1983–2003. Clin Toxicol 2005; 43:575–581.

Lawler JM, Thomas SHL. "Off gassing" following fatal aluminium phosphide ingestion. Clin Toxicol 2007; 45:362.

Leesch JG. Accuracy of different sampling pumps and detector tube combinations to determine phosphine concentration. J Econ Entomol 1982;75:899-905.

Lohani SP, Casavant MJ, Ekins BR et al. Zinc phosphide poisoning: a retrospective study of 21 cases. J Toxicol Clin Toxicol 2000; 38:515.

Madan K, Chalamalasetty SB, Sharma M, Makharia G. Corrosive-like strictures caused by ingestion of aluminium phosphide. *Natl Med J India* 2006; 19:313–314.

Maitai CK, Njoroge DK, Abuga KO et al. Investigation of possible antidotal effects of activated charcoal, sodium bicarbonate, hydrogen peroxide and potassium permanganate in zinc phosphide poisoning. East Central Afr J Pharm Sci 2002; 5:38–41.

Marquis JK, Lerrick AJ. Noncompetitive inhibition by aluminum, scandium and yttrium of acetylcholinesterase from Electrophorus electricus. Biochem Pharmacol 1982;

Marquis JK. Aluminum inhibition of human serum cholinesterase. Bull Environ Contam Toxicol 1983; 31:164–169.

Memis D, Tokatlioglu D, Koyuncu O, Hekimoglu S. Fatal aluminium phosphide poisoning. Eur J Anaesthesiol 2007; 24:292–293.

Misra UK, Bhargava AK, Nag D et al. Occupational phosphine exposure in Indian workers. Toxicol Lett 1988; 42:257–263.

Mittra S, Peshin SS, Lall SB. Cholinesterase inhibition by aluminium phosphide poisoning in rats and effects of atropine and pralidoxime chloride. Acta Pharmacol Sin 2001; 22:37–39.

Mostafazadeh B, Pajoumand A, Farzaneh E, et al. Blood Levels of Methemoglobin in Patients with Aluminum Phosphide Poisoning and its Correlation with Patient's Outcome. J. Med. Toxicol. 2011; 7:40–43.

Nocera A, Levitin HW, Hilton JMN. Dangerous bodies: a case of fatal aluminium phosphide poisoning. Med J Aust 2000; 173:133–135.

Pajoumand A, Jalali N, Abdollahi M, Shadnia S. Survival following severe aluminium phosphide poisoning. J Pharm Pract Res 2002; 32:297–299.

Patial RK, Bansal SK, Kashyap S et al. Hypoglycaemia following zinc phosphide poisoning. J Assoc Physicians India 1990; 38:306–307.

Pepelko B, Seckar J, Harp PR et al. Worker exposure standard for phosphine gas. Risk Anal 2004; 24:1201–1213.

Popp W, Mentfewitz J, Gotz R, Voshaar T. Phosphine poisoning in a German office. Lancet 2002; 359:1574.

Popp W, Mentfewitz J, Gotz R, Voshaar T. Phosphine poisoning in a German office. *Lancet* 2002; 359:1574.

Potter WT, Garry VF, Kelly JT et al. Radiometric assay of red cell and plasma cholinesterase in pesticide appliers from Minnesota. *ToxicolAppl Pharmacol* 1993; 119:150–155.

Potter WT, Garry VF, Kelly JT et al. Radiometric assay of red cell and plasma cholinesterase in pesticide appliers from Minnesota. Toxicol Appl Pharmacol 1993; 119:150-155.31:1437–1440.

Potter WT, Rong S, Griffith J et al. Phosphine-mediated Heinz body formation and hemoglobin oxidation in human erythrocytes. *Toxicol Lett* 1991; 57:37–45.

Potter WT, Rong S, Griffith J et al. Phosphine-mediated Heinz body formation and hemoglobin oxidation in human erythrocytes. Toxicol Lett 1991; 57:37–45.

Price NR, Moles KA, Hamphires OA. Phosphine toxicity and catalase activity in susceptible and resistant strains of lesser grain borer. Comp Biochem Physiol 1982; 73: 411 - 415.

Ragone S, Bernstein J, Lew E, Weisman R. Fatal aluminum phosphide ingestion. J Toxicol Clin Toxicol 2002; 40:690.

Ragone S, Bernstein J, Lew E, Weisman R. Fatal aluminum phosphide ingestion. *J Toxicol Clin Toxicol* 2002; 40:690.

Rastogi P, Raman R, Rastogi VK. Serum cholinesterase and brain acetylcholinesterase activity in aluminium phosphide binding. Med Sci Res 1990; 18:783–784.

Rimalis BT, Bochkarnikov VV. [Acute hepatorenal insufficiency in some rare acute exogenous poisoning.]. Klin Med 1978; 56:125–128.

Roberts DM, Ranganath H, Buckley NA. Acute intentional self-poisoning with zinc phosphide. Clin Toxicol 2006; 44:465–466.

Saleki S, Ardalan FA, Javidan-Nejad A. Liver histopathology of fatal phosphine poisoning. Forensic Sci Int 2007; 166:190–193.

Sarma PSA, Narula J. Acute pancreatitis due to zinc phosphide ingestion. Postgrad Med J 1996; 72:237–238.

Singh RB, Rastogi SS, Singh DS. Cardiovascular manifestations of aluminium phosphide intoxication. J Assoc Physicians India 1989; 37:590–592.

Singh RB, Saharia RB, Sharma VK. Can aluminium phosphide poisoning cause hypermagnesaemia? A study of 121 patients. Magnes Trace Elem 1990; 9:212–218.

Singh RB, Singh RG, Singh U. Hypermagnesemia following aluminum phosphide poisoning. *Int J Clin Pharmacol Ther Toxicol* 1991; 29:82–85.

Singh RB, Singh RG, Singh U. Hypermagnesemia following aluminum phosphide poisoning. Int J Clin Pharmacol Ther Toxicol 1991; 29:82–85.

Singh S, Dilwari JB, Vashist R et al. Aluminium phosphide ingestion. Br Med J 1985; 290:1110–1111.

Singh S, Sharma BK. Aluminium phosphide poisoning. J Assoc Physicians India 1991; 39:423–424.

Singh S, Singh D, Wig N et al. Aluminum phosphide ingestion – A clinicopathologic study. J Toxicol Clin Toxicol 1996; 34:703–706.

Singh S, Singh D, Wig N, Jit I, Sharma BK. Aluminum phosphide ingestion - a clinico-pathologic study. J Toxicol Clin Toxicol 1996;34(6):703-6.

Sinha US, Kapoor AK, Singh AK et al. Histopathological changes in cases of aluminium phosphide poisoning. *Indian J Pathol Microbiol* 2005; 48:177–180.

Siwach SB, Dua A, Sharma R et al. Tissue magnesium content and histopathological changes in non-survivors of aluminium phosphide poisoning. J Assoc Physicians India 1995; 43:676–678.

Siwach SB, Gupta A. The profile of acute poisonings in Harayana- Rohtak study. J Assoc Physicians India 1995; 43:756–759.

Siwach SB, Jagdish, Katyal VK, Dhall A, Bhardwaj G. Prognostic indices in aluminium phosphide poisoning observations on acidosis & central venous pressure. J Assoc Physicians India 1997;45:693-5.

Siwach SB, Singh H, Jagdish, Katyal VK, Bhardwaj G. Cardiac arrhythmias in aluminium phosphide poisoning studied by on continuous holter and cardioscopic monitoring. J Assoc Physicians India 1998;46(7):598-601.

Siwach SB, Singh P, Ahlawat S et al. Serum and tissue magnesium content in patients of aluminium phosphide poisoning and critical evaluation of high dose magnesium sulphate therapy in reducing mortality. J Assoc Physicians India 1994; 42: 107–110.

Siwach SB, Singh P, Ahlawat S et al. Serum and tissue magnesium content in patients of aluminium phosphide poisoning and critical evaluation of high dose magnesium sulphate therapy in reducing mortality. *J Assoc Physicians India* 1994; 42:107–110.

Siwach SB, Singh P, Ahlawat S. Magnesium in aluminium phosphide poisoning - where have we erred? J Assoc Physicians India 1994; 42:193–194.

Sood AK, Mahajan A, Dua A. Intravascular haemolysis after aluminium phosphide ingestion. *J R Soc Med* 1997; 90:47–48.

Sood AK, Mahajan A, Dua A. Intravascular haemolysis after aluminium phosphide ingestion. J R Soc Med 1997; 90:47–48.

Stewart A, Whiteside C, Tyler-Jones C et al. Phosphine suicide. Chemical Incident Rep 2003; 27:23–26.

Stewart A, Whiteside C, Tyler-Jones C et al. Phosphine suicide. *Chemical Incident Rep* 2003; 27:23–26.

Sudakin DL. Occupational exposure to aluminium phosphide and phosphine gas? A suspected case report and review of the literature. Hum Exp Toxicol 2005; 24:27

Suman RL, Savani M. Pleural effusion - a rare complication of aluminium phosphide poisoning. Indian Pediatr 1999; 36:1161–1163.

Tiwari J, Lahoti B, Dubey K et al. Tracheo-oesophageal fistula - an unusual complication following celphos poisoning. *Indian J Surg* 2003; 65:442–444.

Vins Jansen A, Thrane KE. Gas chromatographic determination of PH3 in ambient air. Analysis 1978; 103:1195-8.

Vohra RB, Schwarz KA, Williams SR, Clark RF. Phosphine toxicity with echocardiographic signs in railcar stowaways. Clin Toxicol 2006; 44:719–720.

Wander GS, Arora S, Khurana SB. Acute pericarditis in aluminium phosphide poisoning. J Assoc Physicians India 1990; 38:675.

Willers-Russo LJ. Three fatalities involving phosphine gas, produced as a result of methamphetamine manufacturing. J Forensic Sci 1999; 44:647–652.

Wilson R, Lovejoy FH, Jr., Jaeger RJ, Landrigan PL. Acute phosphine poisoning aboard a grain freighter: epidemiologic, clinical and pathological findings. *JAMA* 1980; 244:148–150.

Wilson R, Lovejoy FH, Jr., Jaeger RJ, Landrigan PL. Acute phosphine poisoning aboard a grain freighter: epidemiologic, clinical and pathological findings. JAMA 1980; 244:148–150.

16

Application of a New Genotoxicity Test System with Human Hepatocyte Cell Lines to Improve the Risk Assessment in the Drug Development

Tsuneo Hashizume[1,2] and Hiroaki Oda[1]
[1]*Nagoya University,*
[2]*Takeda Pharmaceutical Company Limited,*
Japan

1. Introduction

1.1 Current situation in the development of pharmaceuticals

A typical testing scheme for a small-molecule therapeutics (outlined in Fig. 1) begins with a large number of compounds and high-throughput assays (Kramer et al., 2007). As the number of viable lead molecules is reduced, incrementally more predictive but lower throughput assays identify those leads with the most drug-like properties and optimal in vitro and in vivo efficacy. Confirmed hit compounds identified in high-throughput screens are evaluated for potency, selectivity, ADME (absorption, distribution, metabolism and excretion), physical and chemical properties, and activity in relevant animal models (Fig. 1). This testing paradigm typically delivers drug-like compounds that have promising pharmacokinetic parameters and efficacy in preclinical models within a 1–2-year cycle time. Compounds that successfully meet preclinical efficacy, ADME, pharmacokinetics and safety criteria are nominated as candidates for formal development. Historically, the move from discovery to development consisted of a discreet hand-off from the 'discovery' organization to the 'development' organization, and little preclinical safety assessment was performed on lead molecules beyond a few basic in vitro toxicity assays. As toxicity is a primary cause for compound attrition and long development (Kola & Landis, 2004), companies in the past 5–10 years have increasingly integrated safety assessment principles into earlier phases of the drug discovery process.

Also as shown in Fig.1, the costs of R & D for a drug in 2001 were of the order of US $802 million (DiMasi et al., 2003); current estimates are closer to about US $900 million; Considerably more of these costs are incurred later in the pipeline, and most of the attrition occurs during full clinical development (Phases II and III). In the other literature, it has been estimated that the average cost associated with the discovery and preclinical evaluation of a single drug candidate were US $620 million (Rawlins, 2004).

Kola and Landis researched the reason why compounds undergo attrition and how this has changed over time (Kola. & Landis, 2004). In 1991, adverse pharmacokinetic and bioavailability results were the most significant cause of attrition and accounted for ~40% of all attrition. However, in 2000 the major causes of attrition in the clinical trials were lack of efficacy (accounting for approximately 30% of failures) and safety (toxicology in preclinical development and safety in clinical development accounting for a further approximately 30%). As a result, many companies developing small-molecule therapeutics have adopted a strategy that includes the earlier incorporation of preclinical safety assessment before advancement into regulated preclinical studies.

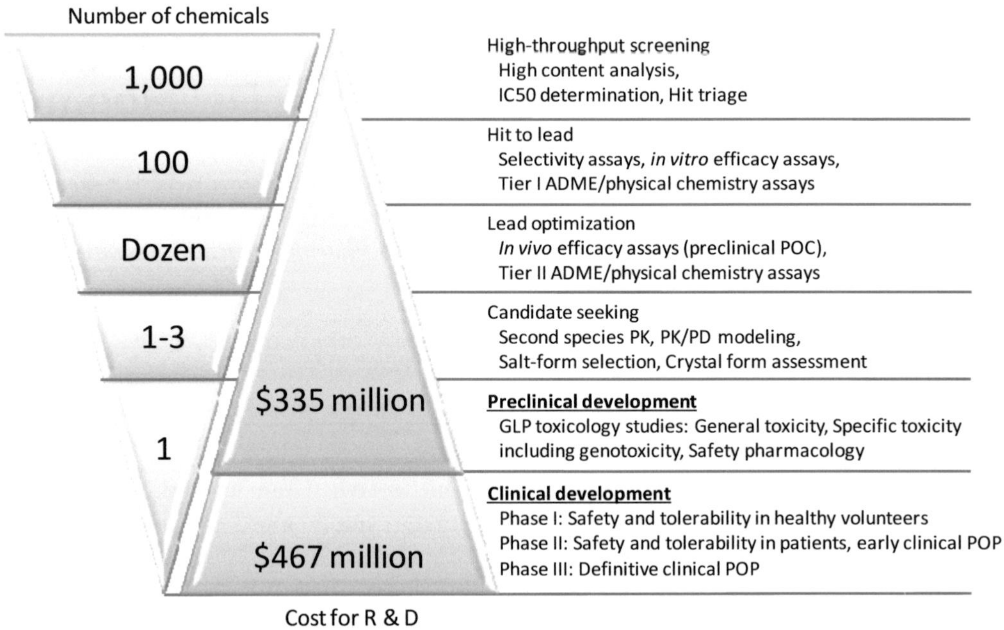

Fig. 1. A typical testing scheme in the development for a small-molecule therapeutics. PK/PD, pharmacokinetic/pharmacodynamic; POC, proof-of-concept; POP, proof-of-principle. ADME; absorption, distribution, metabolism and excretion, GLP; good laboratory practice.

1.2 Safety assessment of pharmaceutical candidates before administration to humans according to the regulatory guidance

Currently, drug companies tend to perform a fairly standard package of nonclinical studies before commencing First-In-Man (FIM) clinical trial investigations with pharmaceuticals. The non-clinical safety study recommendations for the marketing approval of a pharmaceutical usually include single and repeated dose toxicity studies, reproduction toxicity studies, genotoxicity studies, and local tolerance studies. For drugs that have special cause for concern or are intended for a long duration of use, an assessment of carcinogenic potential must be included. Other non-clinical studies include pharmacology studies for safety assessment (safety pharmacology) and pharmacokinetic (ADME) studies.

For the conventional, chemically-synthesized small molecules, such a package of studies is in agreement with international regulatory guidance as given by the International Conference on Harmonization (ICH M3-R2) (Table 1). The genotoxic potential has to be assessed comprehensively before administration to humans regardless for both chemically-synthesized small molecules and biotechnology-derived pharmaceuticals.

According to the current international guidelines on genotoxicity testing of pharmaceutical candidates (ICH S2A, S2B and M3), a standard battery of tests has to be performed. This battery generally includes (i) an in vitro test for gene mutation in bacteria; (ii) an in vitro test in mammalian cells with cytogenetic evaluation of chromosomal damage and/or a test that detects gene mutations; (iii) an in vivo test for chromosomal damage using rodent hematopoietic cells. For compounds giving negative results in all 3 of the assays, the completion of this test battery is generally considered to provide a sufficient level of safety in demonstrating the absence of genotoxic activity.

1.3 Recent achievement in the in vitro genotoxicity testing

The most widely used in vitro genotoxicity test is the Ames test (Ames et al., 1975). The relatively simplicity and low cost of the test make it a valuable screening tool for mutagens. However, DNA is naked in the prokaryote and the form of DNA is different from that in eukaryote. Thus, the test using mammalian cell lines has been developed Chromosomal alterations are quite common in malignant neoplasm, as such the detection of chromosomal abnormalities by test chemicals is considered an excellent test for the assessment of carcinogenic potential. In mammalian cell lines, most of the test systems used the same lines as used in the genotoxicity test.

An important discovery in the understanding of chemical carcinogenesis came from the investigation of the Millers who established that many carcinogens are not intrinsically carcinogenic, but require metabolic activation to be carcinogenic (Miller and Miller, 1947). They demonstrated that azo dyes covalently bind to proteins in liver, leading to the conclusion that carcinogens may bind to proteins that are critical for cell growth control (Miller and Miller, 1947). An additional investigation with other genotoxic carcinogens which requires metabolic activation confirmed that metabolism of the parent compound was necessary to produce a metabolite (activation) that was able to interact with DNA.

In standard in vitro genotoxicity testing, an activation system is included with the purpose of generating electrophilic metabolites that can react with macromolecules including nucleic acids. To address the potential role of metabolism, the induced rat liver S9 has been adopted for in vitro genotoxicity tests as an exogenous activation system for detecting promutagens (Ames et al., 1973, Paolini, 1997). Its initial choice was logical; levels of several cytochrome P450 (CYP) enzymes are elevated after induction, in particular the CYP1A subfamily of enzymes (CYP1A1 and 1A2), which are efficient catalysts of the bioactivation of polycyclic aromatic hydrocarbons and azaarenes, aromatic amines and aflatoxins. These types of compounds were some of the first known and best understood mutagens and the Aroclor 1254-induced rat S9 fraction effectively allowed for their identification as mutagens. Its choice was also logical in that it provided a reliable, robust and readily available bioactivation system at a time when human-derived systems were rare or unavailable. Also, a rodent system can be more easily standardized than an exogenous human derived system that normally would rely on human tissue samples, which are subject to significant biological variation.

1.4 Problems in the use of rat liver S9 fraction as a metabolic activation system in vitro genotoxicity testing

As mentioned in the above sections, the initial choice of rat liver S9 fraction as a metabolic activation system in the in vitro genotoxicity testing was logical. However, it can be questioned if the standard Aroclor-induced rat liver S-9 fraction represents an appropriate surrogate for the metabolic capabilities of humans for the following reasons (Ku et al., 2007; Obach and Dobo, 2008). First, it is now known that the rat and human CYP enzymes can

Menu	Purpose
General Toxicity	
Acute toxicity	To identify doses causing no adverse effect and doses causing major (life-threatening) toxicity.
(Sub) Chronic toxicity	To characterize the toxicological profile of a chemical following repeated administration.
Specific Toxicity	
Genotoxicity	To detect chemicals that induce genetic damage by various mechanisms
Reproductive and developmental toxicity	To reveal any effect of an active chemical on mammalian reproduction and development.
Carcinogenicity	To examine carcinogen that is an agent directly involved in causing cancer.
Immunotoxicology	To detect immune dysfunction resulting from exposure of an organism to a chemical
Local tolerance	To ascertain whether chemicals are tolerated at site in the body.
Safety pharmacology	To investigate the potential undesirable pharmacodynamic effects of a chemical on physiological functions in relation to exposure in the therapeutic range and above.

Table 1. Non-clinical toxicology testing. Toxicological testing is conducted on large numbers of animals of different species in an attempt to predict adverse effects that might be triggered by the drug in humans. Genotoxicity assays are mandatory regulatory studies designed to detect potential mutagens and/or carcinogens.

differ in their substrate specificities and the reactions catalyzed (Guengerich, 1997). Second, with phenobarbital/ 5,6-benzoflavone induction, although the expression levels of CYP1A and 2B enzymes are markedly elevated, others such as CYP3A are affected only in a minor way, whereas others (e.g., CYP2C11) may decrease (Guengerich et al., 1982). Third, the system is set up to favor CYP-mediated metabolism. Some phase II enzymes, such as UDP-glucuronosyltransferases (UGT), glutathione S-transferases (GST), sulfotransferase (SULT), or N-acetyl transferases, are not active in the reduced form of the nicotinamide adenine dinucleotide phosphate (NADPH)-supplemented S9 system (S9 mix) because other cofactors and additives (e.g., uridine diphosphate glucuronic acid, glutathione, acetyl-coenzyme A, etc.) would be needed (Ku et al., 2007; Obach and Dobo, 2008). This can be essential not only for reducing potential false positives (e.g., reactive electrophiles that would be rapidly quenched by conjugation in vivo before being able to cause mutation) but also for false negatives because some conjugation reactions can yield metabolites that are more reactive than their substrate (e.g., sulfation of N-hydroxy-2-acetylaminofluorene or acetylation of N-hydroxylated heterocyclic amines) (Dashwood, 2002; Ku et al., 2007). The rat liver S9 mix may represent an incomplete picture of the metabolism that can occur in vivo (Fig. 2).

To detect those genotoxic potential, some genotoxic metabolites have to be formed in the target cell by endogenous enzymes that are not represented in standard in vitro test systems. One of the major reasons is that certain types of active metabolites (including many

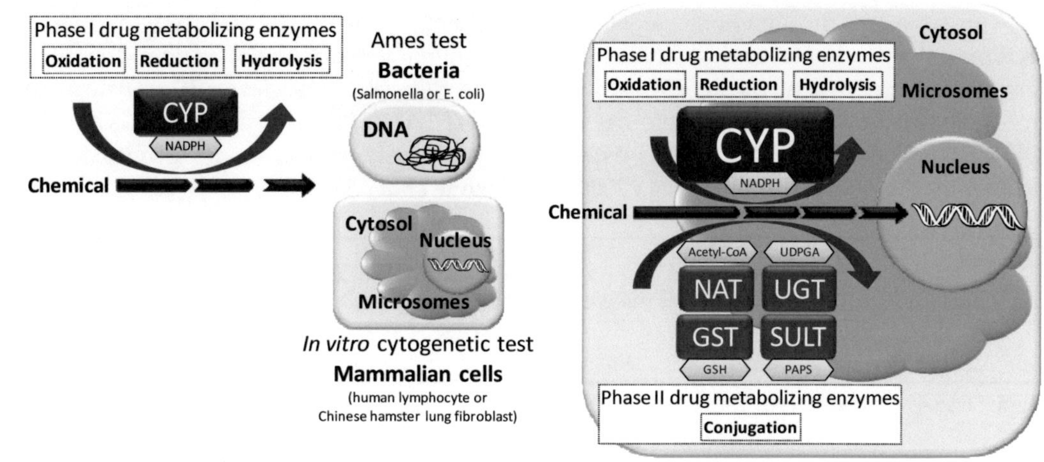

A. Rat liver S9 mix B. Human hepatocyte

Fig. 2. Detection of genotoxicity using rat liver S9 mix compared to the expression of genotoxicity occurring hepatocyte. A. The detection method of genotoxicity is currently used a rat liver S9 fraction in the *in vitro* genotoxicity testing. B. The expression of genotoxicity is occurred in the hepatocyte. It can be questioned if the standard Aroclor-induced rat liver S-9 fraction represents an appropriate surrogate for the metabolic capabilities of humans. However, in human hepatocyte, the genotoxicity was expressed through the comprehensive metabolic pathway including phase I and phase II drug-metabolizing enzymes. Thus human hepatocyte can be a good genotoxicity test system reflecting human metabolism. In addition, human hepatocyte has complete metabolism consisting oxidation, reduction, hydrolysis and conjugation, whereas rat liver S9 mix is set up to favor CYP-mediated metabolism and the other enzymes present in the system that could be responsible for detoxification of reactive intermediates are not supplemented with the appropriate cofactors (e.g., UGT, GST, methyl transfereases, etc), thus potentially providing an unrealistic metabolic profile.

short-life phase-2 metabolites) will not penetrate cell membranes sufficiently. If these types of metabolites are generated extracellularly, most in vitro genotoxicity testing showed negative results since the access to nuclear DNA was difficult. Another reason is that the diffusion pathways are longer for externally generated active metabolites resulting in more opportunities for alternative chemical reactions (e.g. with components of S9 or cell membranes) than for metabolites formed in the target cell. Electrophilic metabolites of a chemical bind to serum or S9 proteins (forming protein adducts) and this reduces the rate of binding to DNA to form DNA adducts.

Therefore it is considered that the use of genetically engineered cells is the most reliable remedy to avoid the shortcomings of the extracellular metabolic activation systems such as human S9 and recombinant human CYPs (Fig. 3). To be useful tools for the prediction of drug metabolism and toxicity in the human liver, Yoshitomi et al. established a series of HepG2 transformants expressing the cytochromes 1A1, 1A2, 2A6, 2B6, 2C8, 2C9, 2C19, 2D6, 2E1 and 3A4 with the apparent Vmax values for characteristic substrates (Table 2) in a previous work (Yoshitomi et al., 2001). Since most human drug metabolism is catalyzed by CYP1A2, 2C8, 2C9, 2C19, 2D6, 2E1 and 3A4, this HepG2 transformant system would be more suitable for the genotoxic assessment of chemicals than the induced rat liver S9 fraction in the routine screening when considering human hepatic metabolism in the future. Therefore in the present thesis, we explored the usefulness of a series of 10 transformants expressing major human CYP isoforms such as CYP1A1, 1A2, 2A6, 2B6, 2C8, 2C9, 2C19, 2D6, 2E1 and 3A4 in HepG2 cells established previously to assess the genotoxicity of metabolites (Fig.3) (Hashizume et al., 2009; Hashizume et al., 2010).

Name of transformant	Expressed CYP isoform	Catalytic reaction measured	Kinetic analysis		
			Transformant *K*m (μM)	Human liver microsomes *K*m (μM)[a]	Transformant *V*max (ρmol/min/mg)
Hepc/1A1.4	CYP1A1	7-Ethoxyresorufin *O*-deethylation	0.25	0.19	56
Hepc/1A2.9	CYP1A2	7-Ethoxyresorufin *O*-deethylation	0.72	0.39	2
Hepc/2A6L.14	CYP2A6	Coumarin 7-hydroxylation	5.1	2.3	812 000
Hepc/2B6.68	CYP2B6	7-Ethoxycoumarin *O*-deethylation	81	–	80 000
Hepc/2C8.46	CYP2C8	Taxol 6-hydroxylation	7.4	24	9400
Hepc/2C9.1	CYP2C9	Tolbutamide 4-hydroxylation	45	120	25 000
Hepc/2C19.12	CYP2C19	(S)-Mephenytoin 4'-hydroxylation	8.3	16	140 000
Hepc/2D6.39	CYP2D6	Bufuralol 1'-hydroxylation	17	40	14
Hepc/2E1.3-8	CYP2E1	p-Nitrophenol hydroxylation	88	30	120
Hepc/3A4.2-30	CYP3A4	Testosterone 6β-hydroxylation	96	89	71

Table 2. Characteristics of a series of 10 transformants expressing major human CYP isoforms such as CYP1A1, 1A2, 2A6, 2B6, 2C8, 2C9, 2C19, 2D6, 2E1 and 3A4 in HepG2 cells (Yoshitomi et al., 2001). a). Iwata et al., 1998.

2. Advantages of HepG2 transformants expressing a series of human CYP isoforms in the in vitro genotoxicity testing

The need for metabolism, especially CYP-mediated one, for in vitro genotoxicity testing has been recognized for many years. Most target cells for genotoxicity assays lack sufficient CYP to activate many promutagens. Therefore, extracellular systems are commonly utilized to provide metabolism. The rat liver S9 fraction contains multiple CYPs and have been used with many target cell types in genotoxicity testing. However, this metabolic activation system suffers from certain limitations; (1) generation of reactive metabolites outside of the target cell, (2) requirement of high exposure concentration to compensate for short exposure times and (3) differences in metabolism compared to intact tissues. To overcome these limitations, the use of genetically engineered stable cell lines expressing CYPs has studied.

The liver is the tissue containing the greatest concentrations of drug-metabolizing enzymes, such as the CYP enzyme family, among many others. In human liver, about 70% of the total CYP could be accounted for by CYP1A2, 2A6, 2B6, 2C, 2D6, 2E1 and 3A proteins (Rendic and Guengerich, 1997). In the extrahepatic organs such as lungs and kidneys, CYP1A1 is present. CYPs catalyze to form toxic reactive intermediates from many chemicals. As it is well known that there are significant quantitative and qualitative differences between laboratory animals and humans in their CYP subtypes, it is necessary to use human CYP isoforms to predict the metabolism and toxicity of chemicals in humans.

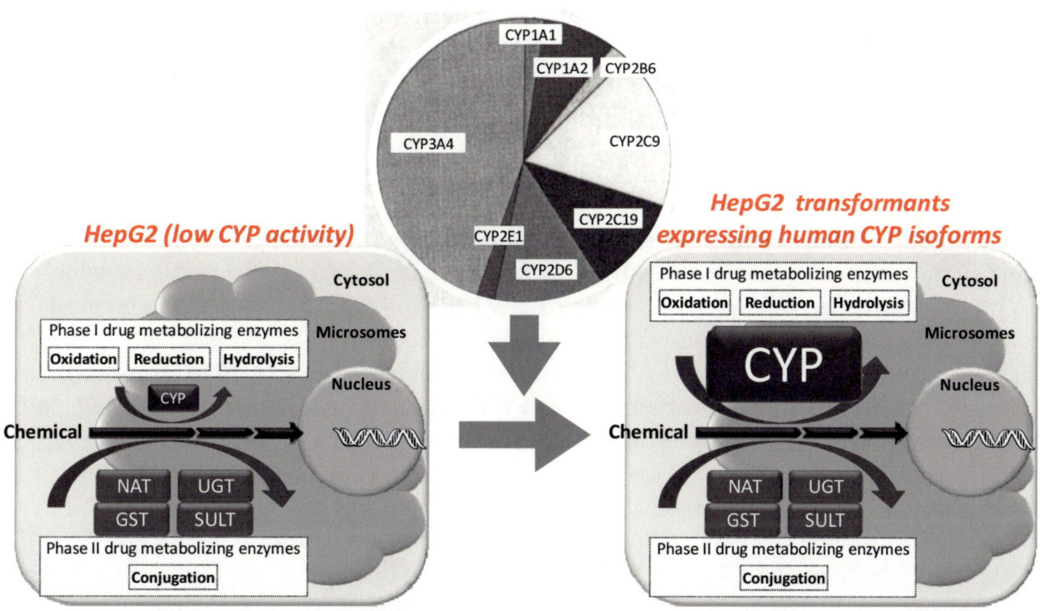

Fig. 3. HepG2 transformants expressing human CYP isoforms relating drug metabolism. The pie chart shows the contribution of each CYP isoform to the human drug metabolism (Lewis, 2004). It has been concerned about the low CYP activities in HepG2 cells, so we established the HepG2 transformant system expressing a series of human CYP isoforms.

In vitro systems, particularly those derived from liver, are a commonly applied tool to gain a better understanding of the metabolism of drugs and other xenobiotics. Also in genotoxicity, a number of publications are discussed which are relevant for the use of human derived liver cell lines. One of the most promising lines is the human HepG2 cell line, originally isolated by Aden et al. in 1972 from a primary hepatoblastoma of an 11-year-old Argentine boy. This cell line retains many of the specialized functions normally lost by primary hepatocytes in culture such as secretion of the major plasma proteins. Since several publications alerted that HepG2 lacks a few drug-metabolizing enzymes such as CYP2E1 and 1A2, transfectants constitutively expressing these enzymes have been constructed. Cederbaum and coworkers developed a line, which possesses CYP2E1 activity and used it in a number of mechanistic studies (for review see Kessova and Cederbaum, 2003).

In our previous study, Yoshitomi et al. has established a series of HepG2 transformants expressing the CYP1A1, 1A2, 2A6, 2B6, 2C8, 2C9, 2C19, 2D6, 2E1 and 3A4 (Yoshitomi et al., 2001). Since most human drug metabolism is catalyzed by CYP1A2, 2C8, 2C9, 2C19, 2D6, 2E1 and P3A4, this HepG2 transformant system would be more suitable for the genotoxic assessment of chemicals than the induced rat liver S9 fraction in the routine screening when considering human hepatic metabolism in the future.

Therefore, we examined the advantages of HepG2 transformants expressing a series of human CYP isoforms as a better alternative for metabolic activation system in the in vitro genotoxicity testing. In section 2.1, the sensitivity of this system to detect genotoxicity requiring CYP activation was confirmed in the in vitro micronucleus (MN) tests using well-studied model chemicals. In section 2.2, this system allowed us to investigate the genotoxicity of model chemicals for which the contributing CYP isoforms, especially those mediated by CYP1A2 or 3A4 which is known to metabolize many drugs in humans, have not yet been identified. In section 2.3, the relevance of the interaction between phase I and phase II drug-metabolizing enzymes, e.g., UGT, GST, and SULT, in the test system was demonstrated in a MN test of tamoxifen or safrole, which has been reported to be metabolized by enzymes of both phases.

2.1 Basic characteristics of the HepG2 transformants on genotoxic assessment and confirmation of their sensitivity with model chemicals requiring CYP activation

HepG2 transformants were checked for their response to known chemicals in which the CYP isoforms responsible for which genotoxicity has been reported. As model chemicals, we selected BP, DMBA, CP and ifosfamide. In BP metabolism, CYP1A1 showed clearly the highest activity among the hepatic CYP isoforms reported (Fig. 4 A). Significant formation of some metabolites was also observed with CYP1A2 and 3A4 (Bauer et al., 1995). In the DMBA metabolism (Fig. 4 B), it had been shown that CYP1A1 had clearly the highest activity among the hepatic CYP isoforms (Shimada and Fujii-Kuriyama, 2004; Shou et al., 1996) and that significant formation of some metabolites was also observed with CYP1A2, 2B6 and 2C9 (Shou et al., 1996). CP is efficiently metabolized by CYP2B6, 2C9 and 3A4 (Jing et al., 2006, Chang et al., 1993)(Fig. 4 C). Ifosfamide had been demonstrated to be efficiently metabolized by CYP2B6 and 3A4 (Chang et al., 1993; Jing et al., 2006)(Fig. 4 D).

Firstly, BP treatment produced MN induction in the transformants expressing CYP1A1, CYP1A2 and CYP3A4 (Fig. 5 A). These CYP isoforms were reported to be responsible for BP activation (Bauer et al., 1995). Secondly, MN induction by DMBA in a HepG2 transformant expressing CYP1A1 was significantly higher than those in HepG2 and Hepc-Mock cells (Fig. 5 B). CYP1A1 is known to be the most active among the CYP isoforms to metabolize DMBA (Shou et al., 1996). Thirdly, CP treatment caused MN induction in the transformants expressing CYP1A2, 2B6, 2C9 and 3A4 (Fig. 5 C). CYP2B6, 2C9 and 3A4 are reported to be involved the metabolic activation of CP (Jing et al., 2006; Chang et al., 1993). Finally, in the treatment with ifosfamide, significant MN inductions were found in the transformants expressing CYP1A1, 2C9, 2C19, 2D6 and 3A4 (Fig. 5 D). Ifosfamide had been demonstrated to be efficiently metabolized by CYP2B6 and 3A4 (Chang et al., 1993; Jing et al., 2006). These results showed HepG2 transformants system have the appropriate sensitivity to detect genotoxicity requiring CYP activation tests using well-studied model chemicals.

In addition, DMBA treatment unexpectedly produced MN induction in some transformants expressing CYP2C9, 2D6 and 3A4 (Fig. 4 B). However, it was reported that CYP2C9 was capable of metabolizing DMBA while CYP2D6 and 3A4 exhibited relatively low metabolic activity to DMBA (Shou et al., 1996). Similarly, significant MN inductions by ifosfamide were found in the transformants expressing CYP1A1, 2C9, 2C19, 2D6 and 3A4 (Fig. 4 D). Ifosfamide is mainly metabolized by CYP2B6 and 3A4 (Chang et al., 1993; Jing et al., 2006). CYP1A1 and 2C19 are relatively minor CYP isoforms to DMBA metabolic activation, but the involvement in the genotoxicity of ifosfamide metabolite of these CYP isoforms were demonstrated in the present study (Fig. 4 D).

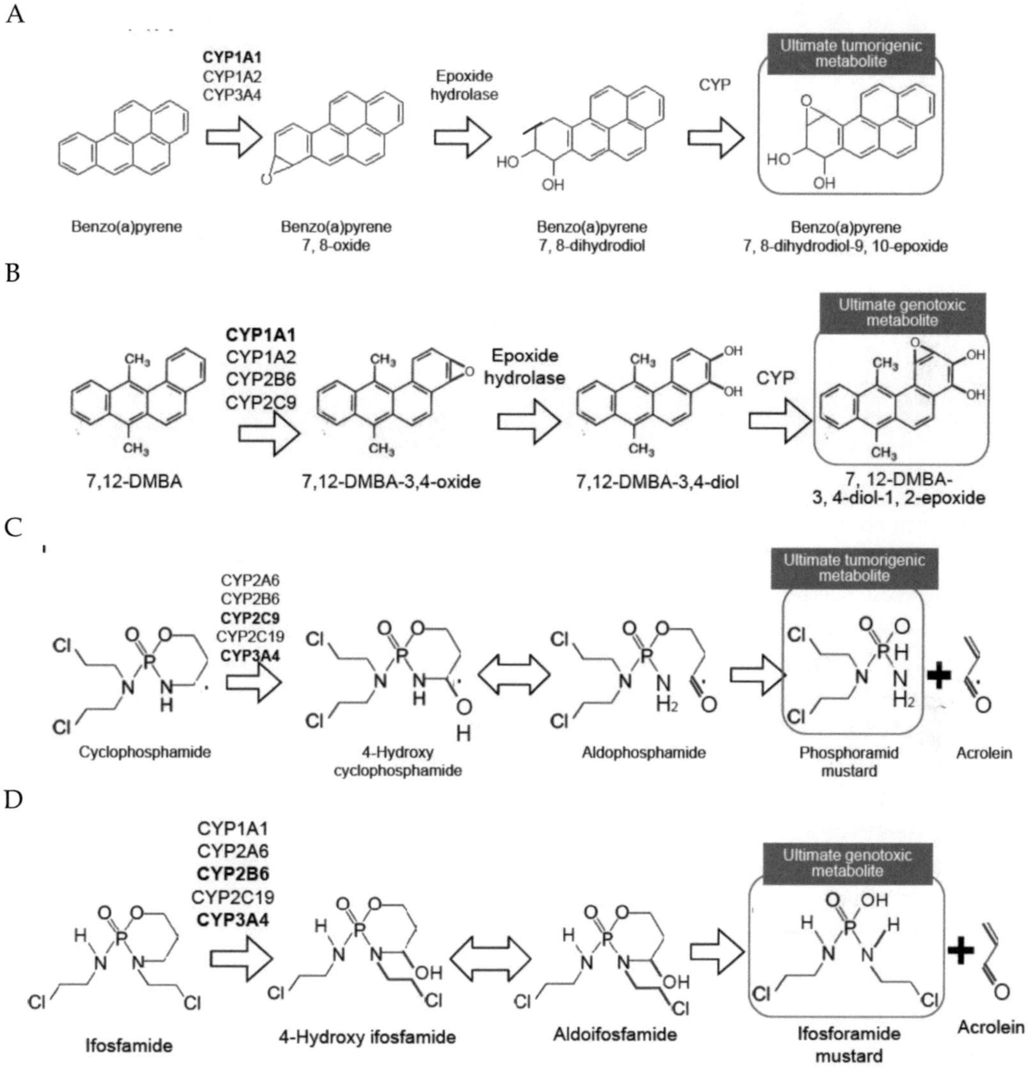

Fig. 4. Metabolic activation pathway of BP (A), DMBA (B), CP (C) and ifosfamide (D). A). BP is mainly metabolized by CYP1A1 to produce the benzo(a)pyrene 7, 8-oxide. B). DMBA (7, 12-DMBA) is mainly metabolized by CYP1A1 to produce the 7, 12-DMBA-3, 4-oxide. C). Cyclophosphamide (CP) is mainly metabolized by CYP2C9 and 3A4 to produce the 4-hydroxy cyclophosphamide. D). Ifosfamide is mainly metabolized by CYP2B6 and 3A4 to produce the 4-hydroxy ifosfamide.

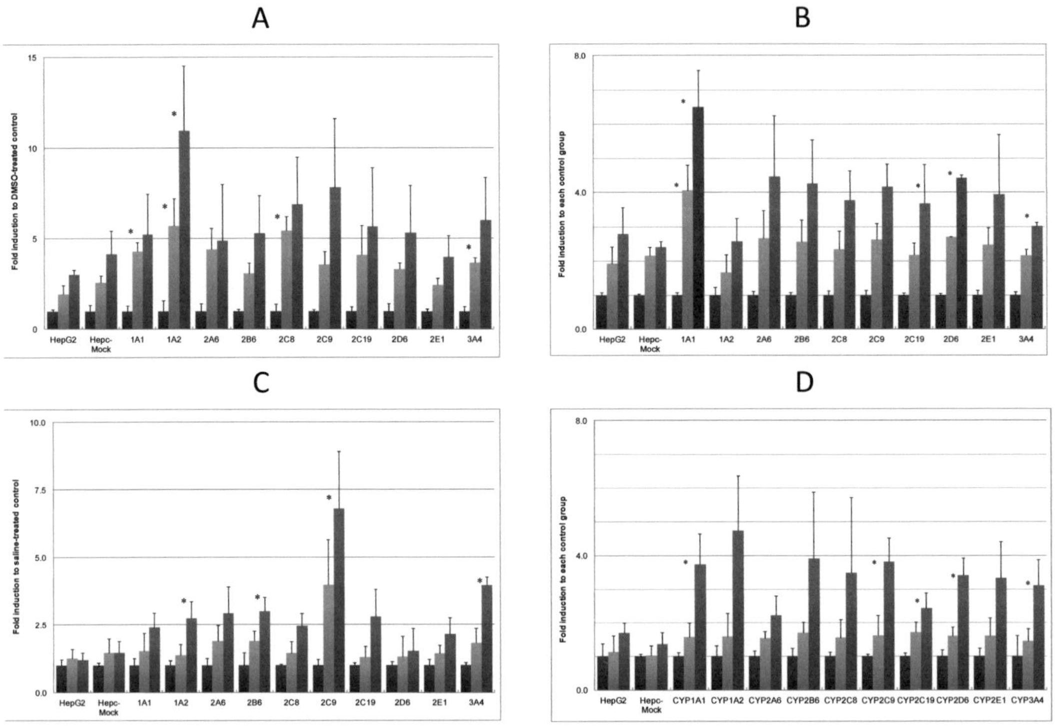

Fig. 5. Micronucleus induction of BP (A), DMBA (B), CP (C) and ifosfamide (D) by expression of CYP1A1, 1A2, 2A6, 2B6, 2C8, 2C9, 2C19, 2D6, 2E1 and 3A4. A). The cells (1×10^5 cells) were seeded onto a 24-well plate for 24 h and then treated with 0.5% DMSO (heavy gray bars), 200 ng/ml (light gray bars) or 400 ng/ml (medium gray bars) BP. B). The cells (1×10^5 cells) were seeded onto a 24-well plate for 24 h and then treated with 0.5% DMSO (heavy gray bars), 78 ng/ml (light gray bars) or 156 ng/ml (medium bars) DMBA. C). The cells (1×10^5 cells) were seeded onto a 24-well plate for 24 h and then treated with 0.5% saline (heavy gray bars), 1 mg/ml (light gray bars) or 2 mg/ml (medium gray bars) CP. D). The cells (1×10^5 cells) were seeded onto a 24-well plate for 24 h and then treated with 0.5% saline (heavy gray bars), 500 μg/ml (light gray bars) or 1000 μg/ml (medium gray bars) ifosfamide. Values were normalized with the mean DMSO- or saline-treated control value of 3 experiments for each transformant. Each bar represents the mean ± S.D. Data were tested using Student's t-test when the variance was homogeneous or Aspin & Welch t test when the variance was heterogeneous (*$P<0.05$, compared with Hepc-Mock).

Based on the results in section 2.1, it was showed that genotoxic metabolites could be produced by not only the most active CYP isoform but also by other less active CYPs and that this transformant system could detect the genotoxic potential of chemicals requiring CYP activation not tested routinely in the early stage of drug development.

One of major advantages of our system is the variety of human CYP isoforms. When considering replacement of the rat induced liver S9 fraction, increasing the number of the principal CYP isoforms would be desirable in order to cover the diverse CYP activities. As mentioned in the general introduction, our HepG2 system includes CYP1A1, 1A2, 2A6, 2B6,

2C8, 2C9, 2C19, 2D6, 2E1 and 3A4. Seven CYP isoforms (1A1, 1A2, 2C9, 2C19, 2D6, 2E1 and 3A4) account for 95% of this activity and with 3A4 responsible for over 65% of the metabolism of current therapeutic agents. During phase I metabolism in humans, 90% of all drugs are oxidized by CYP isoforms with different substrate selectivities. Thus, our HepG2 transformant system seems to cover most human drug metabolism mediated by human CYP isoforms but not by rat ones. Based on the results obtained in section 2.1, it was demonstrated that our HepG2 transformant system has an appropriate sensitivity for well-studied chemicals which requires CYP activation for their genotoxicity.

For assessing the genotoxicity of chemicals with human metabolism, our HepG2 transformant system has more appropriate characteristics than other established cell lines used in toxicological testing and reviewed by Sawada and Kamataki (Sawada and Kamataki, 1998). Our HepG2 transformants are derived from hepatocyte that possesses other factors necessary for the function of CYP. Generally, the reactions catalyzed by CYP molecules require the presence of NADPH-CYP reductase and cytochrome b5 to support some CYP-mediated reactions. HepG2 has been shown to have NADPH-CYP reductase activity and cytochrome b5, although the levels are lower than those of human liver (Waxman et al., 1991; Patten et al., 1992). Therefore, our HepG2 transformant system does not need co-expression of reductase and/or cytochrome b5 with CYP enzymes.

2.2 An exploration using HepG2 transformant to identify the CYP isoforms contributing to the genotoxicity by novel chemicals

Given the multiplicity of CYP isoforms and the importance of other enzymes (hydrolases, transferase, etc.) in the metabolism of chemicals, there are two possible approaches to engineering cell lines. The introduction of single enzymes allows simple controlled mechanistic studies of the role of an individual enzyme in the metabolic activation of chemicals. Such system can also be viewed as the replacement of the laborious CYP purification/reconstitution analyses with a panel of engineered cells. However, to specify CYP isoform(s) involved in the activation of a certain chemical of unknown metabolism, a set of cell lines individually expressing the different CYP isoforms is needed. A series of HepG2 transformants expressing major 10 human CYP isoforms is a valuable tool, since most human hepatic drug metabolism is catalyzed by these expressing CYP isoforms.

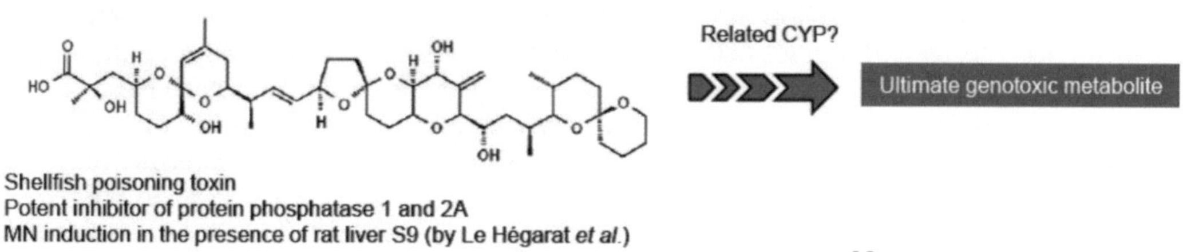

Fig. 6. Chemical structure and significant biological features of okadaic acid. This chemical is a shellfish poisoning toxin and known as a potent phosphatase 1 and 2A. This chemical was reported to be induced micronucleus in the presence of rat liver S9 mix (Hégarat et al., 2004).

In this section, the following possibility was elucidated that the set of transformants can be used for screening for the genotoxicity of newly developed pharmaceutical candidates of unknown metabolism in human in vivo. As model chemicals, we selected okadaic acid (OA) and β-endosulfan.

Hégarat et al. found that OA enhanced formation of MN in the presence of a metabolic activation system (Hégarat et al., 2004), although the CYP isoforms involved in the MN induction were not reported. Thus we selected OA as a model chemical to evaluate the ability of our system to investigate which CYP isoform is involved in producing unknown genotoxic metabolites.

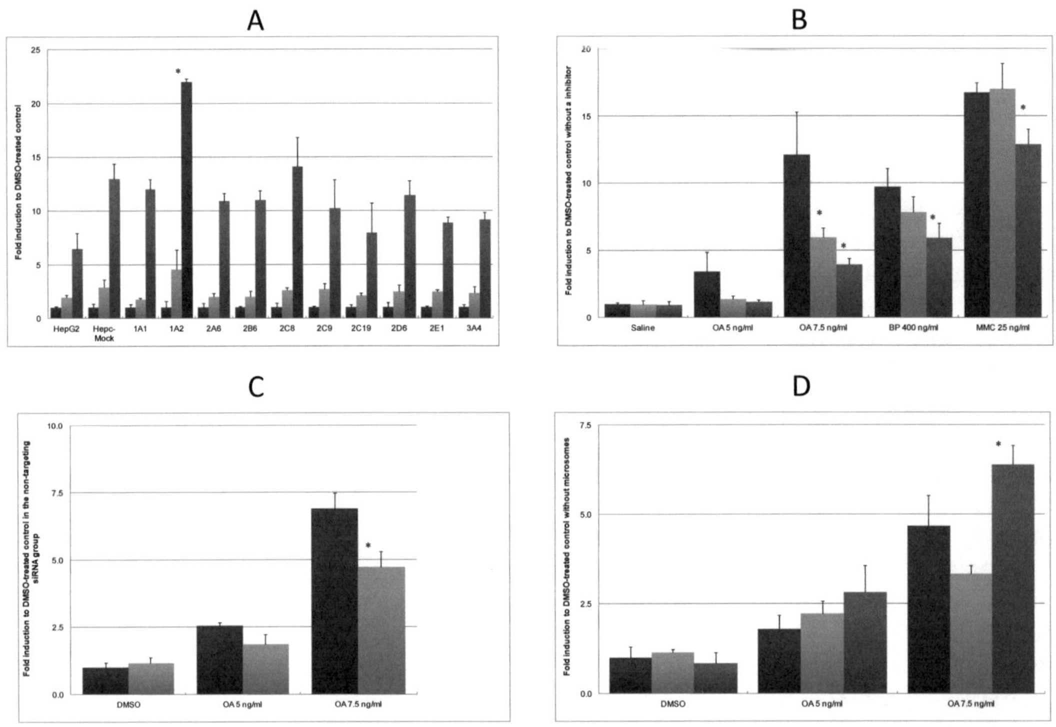

Fig. 7. Micronucleus induction of OA. A). Micronucleus induction of OA by expression of CYP1A1, 1A2, 2A6, 2B6, 2C8, 2C9, 2C19, 2D6, 2E1 and 3A4. The cells (1×10^5 cells) were seeded onto a 24-well plate for 24 h, and then treated with 0.5% DMSO (heavy gray bars), 5 ng/ml (light gray bars) or 10 ng/ml (medium gray bars) OA. After 48 h, the cells were collected and sampled. One thousand interphase cells per each treatment were scored and the incidence of cells with micronuclei was calculated. Values were normalized with the mean DMSO-treated control value of 3 experiments in each transformant. Each bar represents the mean ± S.D. of 3 experiments. Data were tested using Student's t-test (*$P<0.05$, compared with Hepc-Mock). B). Effects of furafylline, a CYP1A2 specific inhibitor for micronucleus induction by various chemicals in the transformant expressing CYP1A2. The cells (1×10^5 cells) were seeded onto a 24-well plate for 24 h, and then treated with 0.5% DMSO, 5 or 7.5 ng/ml OA, 400 ng/ml BP and 25 ng/ml MMC in the absence (heavy gray bars) or presence of 5 µM (lihgt gray bars) or 50 µM (medium gray bars) furafylline. Values were normalized with the mean DMSO-treated control value without an inhibition of three experiments in each transformant. Each bar represents the mean ± S.D. of 3 experiments. Data were tested using Student's t-test (*$P<0.05$, compared with no inhibition). C). Effects of siRNA to CYP1A2 on micronucleus induction by OA in the transformant expressing CYP1A2. The cells (1×10^5 cells) were seeded onto a 24-well plate for 24 h in the presence of 50 nM siRNA for non-targeting (heavy gray bars) or CYP1A2 (light gray bars). Medium was

changed with a fresh one containing 0.5% DMSO, 5 and 7.5 ng/ml OA. After 48 h, the cells were collected and sampled. Values were normalized with the mean DMSO-treated control value without siRNA of three experiments in each transformant. Each bar represents the mean ± S.D. of 3 experiments. Data were tested using Student's t-test (*P<0.05, compared with non-targeting siRNA). D). Effects of external metabolic activation system for CYP1A2 on micronucleus induction by okadaic acid in Hepc. The cells (1×10^5 cells) were seeded onto a 24-well plate for 24 h, and then treated with 0.5% DMSO, 5 or 7.5 ng/ml OA in the absence (heavy gray bars) or presence of Insect Cell Control SupersomesTM (light gray bars) or Human CYP1A2 Supersomes™ (medium gray bars). Values were normalized with the mean DMSO-treated control value without microsomes of 3 experiments in each transformant. Each bar represents the mean ± S.D. of 3 experiments. Data were tested using Student's t-test (*P<0.05, compared with the control microsomes).

OA significantly increased the fold induction of MN in the transformant expressing CYP1A2 compared with that obtained in Hepc-Mock (Fig. 7 A). Furthermore, inhibitory effects of a specific inhibitor of CYP1A2 and siRNA to CYP1A2 on MN induction by OA were shown (Figs.7 B and 7 C, respectively). Moreover, co-treatment with OA and microsomes expressing CYP1A2 showed MN induction in Hepc-Mock cells (Fig. 7 D). These results indicated that MN induction by OA could be associated with the presence of CYP1A2 activity, suggesting that CYP1A2 is involved in the genotoxic activation of OA.

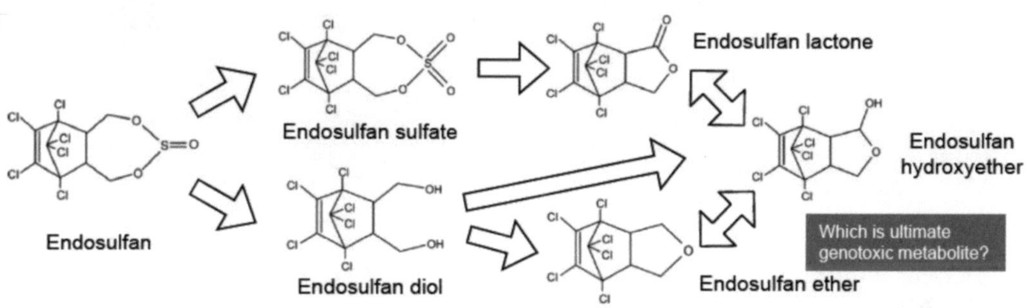

Fig. 8. Proposed metabolic pathway of β-endosulfan. In mammalian systems, β-endosulfan is metabolized to endosulfan sulfate, which is the most persistent metabolite, and also to endosulfan diol, which is further metabolized to endosulfan ether, hydroxyether, and lactone [WHO, 1999].

β-Endosulfan, shown in Fig. 8, is also reported to induce MN in HepG2 cells, suggesting that CYP activation might be involved in the MN induction (Lu et al., 2000); however the contributing CYP isoform to induce MN has not yet been investigated, to the best of our knowledge. Therefore we examined whether a series of HepG2 transformants could identify the CYP isoform contributing to the MN induction by β-endosulfan as a model chemical.
β-Endosulfan significantly increased the fold induction of MN in the transformant expressing CYP3A4 compared with that obtained with the transformant Mepc-Mock (Fig. 8 A). Furthermore, inhibitory effects of a specific inhibitor of CYP3A4 and of siRNA to CYP3A4 on MN induction by β-endosulfan were shown (Figs. 8 B and 8 C, respectively). The activity of CYP3A4 in the transformant using the luminogenic substrate demonstrated that these inhibitory conditions decreased the activity to approximately 10% compared to control level. These results indicated that MN induction by β-endosulfan could be

associated with the presence of CYP3A4 activity and suggested that CYP3A4 is involved in producing the genotoxic metabolites of β-endosulfan.

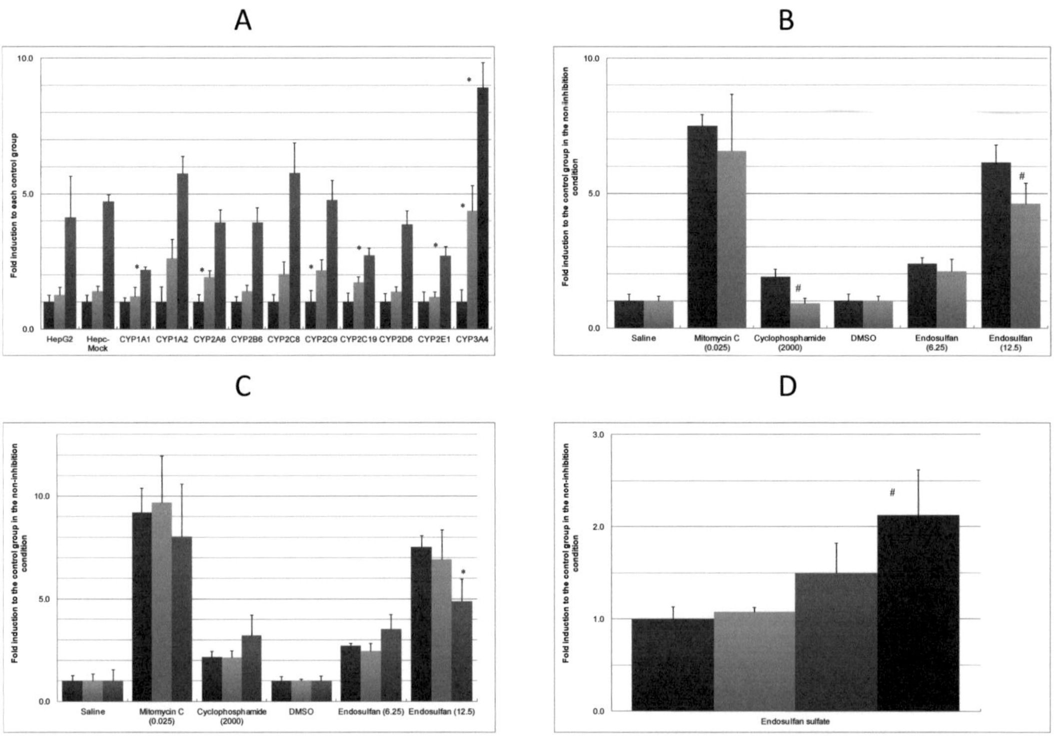

Fig. 9. Micronucleus induction of β-endosulfan by CYP3A4-mediated activation. a). A micronucleus induction of β-endosulfan by expression of CYP1A1, 1A2, 2A6, 2B6, 2C8, 2C9, 2C19, 2D6, 2E1 and 3A4. The cells (1×10^5 cells) were seeded onto a 24-well plate for 24 h, and then treated with 0.5% DMSO (heavy gray bars), 6.25 μg/ml (light gray bars) or 12.5 μg/ml (medium gray bars) β-endosulfan. b). Effects of ketoconazole, a CYP3A4 specific inhibitor for micronucleus induction by various chemicals in the transformant expressing CYP3A4. The cells (1×10^5 cells) were seeded onto a 24-well plate for 24 h, and then treated with 0.5% saline, 100 ng/ml mitomycin C, 1000 μg/ml cyclophosphamide, 0.5% DMSO, 6.25 or 12.5 μg/ml β-endosulfan in the absence (heavy gray bars) or presence (light gray bars) of 1 μM ketoconazole. c). Effects of siRNA to CYP3A4 on micronucleus induction by various chemicals in the transformant expressing CYP3A4. The cells (1×10^5 cells) were seeded onto a 24-well plate for 8 h in absence (heavy gray bars) or the presence of 50 nM siRNA for Negative control (light gray bars) or CYP3A4 (medium gray bars). d). Micronucleus induction of endosulfan sulfate in Hepc-Mock, the transformant expressing an empty vector only. The cells (1×10^5 cells) were seeded onto a 24-well plate for 24 h and then treated with 0.5% DMSO (heavy gray bars), 8 μg/ml, (light gray bars), 10 μg/ml (medium gray bars) or 12.5 μg/ml (solid bars) endosulfan sulfate. Statistical analysis was done in the same procedure as Fig. E, except for the Student's t- test (#$P<0.05$, compared with the DMSO-treated control group) in Fig. F d).

Lee et al. reported that β-endosulfan is metabolized by CYP3A4 based on the results in the study with CYP isoform-selective inhibitor in human liver microsomes and with the incubation study of cDNA-expressed enzymes (Lee et al., 2006). They have also reported that human liver microsome incubation of β-endosulfan in the presence of NADPH resulted in the formation of endosulfan sulfate (Lee et al., 2006). Based on these reports, we examined the genotoxicity of endosulfan sulfate in the Hepc-Mock cells in order to investigate whether this sulfate is the metabolite that induces MN in the β-endosulfan-treated transformant expressing CYP3A4. As shown in Fig. Fd, endosulfan sulfate induced MN with statistical significance at 12.5 μg/ml. This result demonstrated that endosulfan sulfate was the genotoxic metabolite and that this metabolite was formed by CYP3A4 in the transformant treated with β-endosulfan.

Based on the results obtained in the OA and β-endosulfan treatments, it was clearly demonstrated that the HepG2 transformant system was able to identify the CYP isoform relating to the genotoxicity of chemical metabolite(s) and was useful to elucidate the genotoxicity of a new chemical or a drug candidate in the presence of the metabolic activation system.

More effort as for CYP induction is necessary, but the results obtained in the present study demonstrated the availability of these transformants expressing human CYP to elucidate the genotoxic potential of the chemicals that require metabolic activation to create risk to humans. In order to validate these transformants, an additional study is in progress with more chemicals that have been well studied in the metabolic activation or inactivation by CYP enzymes.

These results clearly demonstrated that the HepG2 transformant system was able to identify the CYP isoform related to the genotoxicity of chemical metabolite(s) and was useful to elucidate the genotoxicity of a new chemical or a drug candidate in the presence of the metabolic activation system.

2.3 Genotoxic assessment of chemicals metabolized by phase I and phase II drug-metabolizing enzymes

As mentioned in the Introduction section, to detect chemicals which require bioactivation to electrophiles to exhibit a genotoxic and carcinogenic response, the standard in vitro genotoxicity testing also include incubation of the test chemicals with liver microsomal or S9 fractions, as activation systems so that chemically stable xenobiotics can be converted to reactive electrophiles (Malling, 1971; Ames et al., 1973; Levin et al., 1984). However, it is possible that the Aroclor induced rat liver S9 system is not the most appropriate metabolite generation system for detecting drugs that may pose a carcinogenic hazard to humans. This is because the system is set up to favor CYP-mediated metabolism and the other enzymes present in the system that could be responsible for detoxication of reactive intermediates are not supplemented with the appropriate cofactors (e.g., UGT, GST, methyl transferases, etc), thus potentially providing an unrealistic metabolic profile. In a recent work by Obach and Dobo, it was revealed that many human in vivo metabolites arise via conjugation reactions with the limited 16 drugs (Obach and Dobo, 2008). This can be important not only for reducing potential false positives (e.g., reactive electrophiles that would be rapidly quenched by conjugation in vivo before being able to cause mutation) but can also be important for false negatives because some conjugation reactions can yield metabolites that are more reactive than their substrate (e.g., sulfation of aliphatic alcohols or glucuronidation of carboxylic acids; [Glatt et al., 1998; Sallustio et al., 2006]).

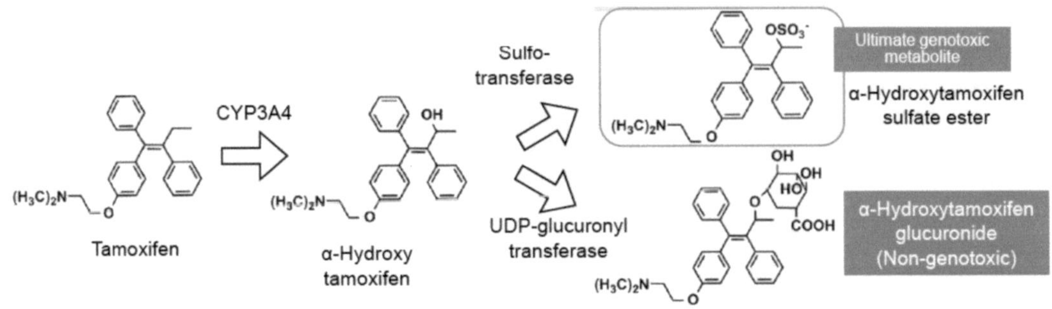

Fig. 10. Metabolic activation and inactivation pathways of tamoxifen.

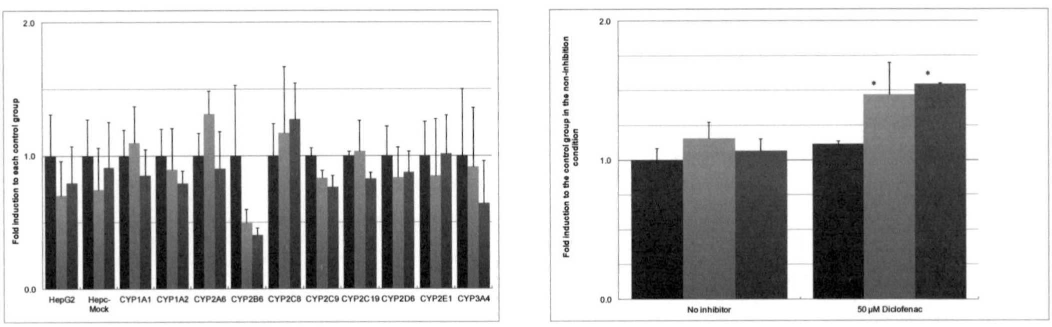

A B

Fig. 11. Micronucleus induction of tamoxifen by expression of CYP1A1, 1A2, 2A6, 2B6, 2C8, 2C9, 2C19, 2D6, 2E1 and 3A4 (A), and effects of a phase II inhibitro on micronucleus indcution by tamoxifen (B). A). The cells (1×10^5 cells) were seeded onto a 24-well plate for 24 h, and then treated with 0.5% DMSO (heavy gray bars), 1 μg/ml (light gray bars) or 2 μg/ml (medium gray bars) tamoxifen. No statistically significant increase was observed when compared with both Hepc-Mock and HepG2. B). The transformant cells expressing CYP3A4 (1×10^5 cells) were seeded onto a 24-well plate for 24 h, and then treated with 0.5% DMSO (heavy gray bars), 2 μg/ml (light gray bars) or 3 μg/ml (medium gray bars) tamoxifen in the absence or presence of 50 μM diclofenac, a UGT inhibitor.

In order to evaluate the relevance of the interaction between phase I and phase II drug-metabolizing enzymes in the test system, the transformants were treated with tamoxifen as shown in Fig. 10. Tamoxifen is reported to be metabolized by CYP3A4 to α-hydroxytamoxifen and further metabolized by SULT to α-hydroxytamoxifen sulfate ester as the putative reactive intermediate (Brown, 2009; White, 2003; Zhao et al., 2009). This intermediate reacts with the exocyclic amino group of guanines (the major reaction) and adenines (a minor reaction) in DNA (Osborne et al., 1996). UGT plays a detoxification role through the glucuronidation of α-hydroxytamoxifen (Brown, 2009; White, 2003; Zhao et al., 2009).

As shown in Fig. 11 A, tamoxifen did not significantly induce MN at any concentration tested in any transformant. At much higher concentrations of each chemical, the frequencies of the micronuclei were decreased (data not shown), suggesting that the tested concentrations were appropriate to evaluate MN induction. Then to investigate the involvement of the detoxification pathway by UGT in the metabolism of tamoxifen, we tested the effect of UGT inhibitor on the MN induction by tamoxifen. A small but significant increase in MN by tamoxifen was observed in the presence of the UGT inhibitor, diclofenac, in the transformants expressing CYP3A4 which contribute to the metabolic activation of tamoxifen to α-hydroxytamoxifen (Fig. 11 B). This result indicated that the CYP3A4-metabolite, α-hydroxy-tamoxifen, was further metabolized by UGT to a genotoxically inactive substance.

Another example is safrole. Safrole is reported to be hydroxylated predominantly by CYP2A6, 2C9, 2D6 or 2E1 and further metabolized by SULT to 1′-sulfooxysafrole (Andrew and Brian, 2007; Rietjens et al., 2005)(Fig. 12). This intermediate forms the electrophilic carbocation of safrole, suggesting the production of DNA adduct (Rietjens et al., 2005). On the other hand, the safrole-2′, 3′-oxide formed from the parent safrole by epoxide hydrolases or 1′-hydroxysafrole-2′, 3′-oxide from 1′-hydroxysaforle are reported to be detoxified by GST (Rietjens et al., 2005).

As shown in Fig. 13 A, safrole did not significantly induce MN at any concentration tested in any transformant. At much higher concentrations of each chemical, the frequencies of the micronuclei were decreased (data not shown), suggesting that the tested concentrations were appropriate to evaluate MN induction. Then to investigate the involvement of the detoxification pathway by GST in the metabolism of safrole, we tested the effect of GST inhibitor on the MN induction by safrole. Significant increases were seen in the presence of the GST inhibitor, ethacrynic acid, in the transformants expressing CYP2D6 responsible for the genotoxic activation of safrole to 1′-hydroxysafrole (Fig. 13 B). This result suggested that CYP2D6-mediated metabolite, 1′-hydroxysafrole, was further metabolized by GST not exerting its genotoxicity in the metabolic pathway.

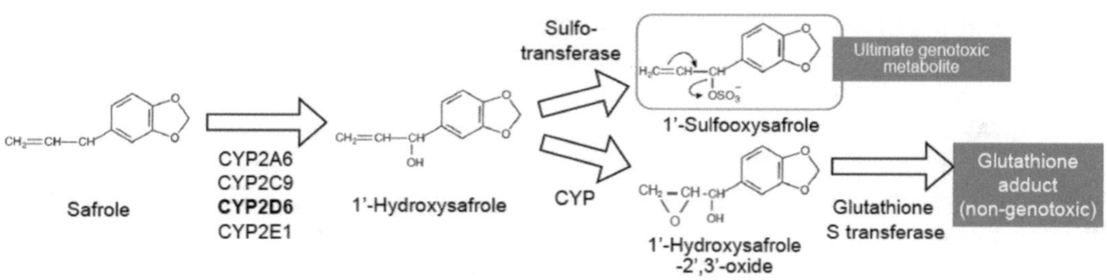

Fig. 12. Metabolic activation and inactivation pathways of safrole.

The results for tamoxifen and safrole clearly demonstrated that interaction between the phase I and II drug-metabolizing enzymes was crucial to assess the genotoxicity of chemicals in the presence of a metabolic activation system. The interplay between the phase I and II enzymes is lacking in the NADPH-supplemented rat liver S9 system due to an absence of co-factor necessary for several phase II enzymes such as UGT or GST. Furthermore, the reactive intermediates have to be formed in the target cell because some conjugates have poor membrane permeability. These results raise the possibility that the induced rat liver S9 system may generate mutagenic metabolites of no relevance, or worse even may not generate a mutagenic metabolite that would be generated by human enzymes. Therefore, a set of HepG2 transformants is a superior test system for mimicking the metabolism occurring in the human liver and the use of this system can potentially provide more relevant data than current genotoxicity tests.

Drug metabolism is generally regarded as proceeding via 2 stages, phase I and phase II. The induced rat liver S9 fraction as an exogenous metabolic activation system is supplemented with only NADPH for CYP-mediated metabolism. The appropriate cofactors for phase II drug-metabolizing enzymes (e.g. UGT, GST, SULT and NAT) are absent. This means these phase II enzymes are not active in the rat liver S9 fraction and that this leads not only for potential false positives (e.g., reactive electrophiles that would be rapidly quenched by conjugation in vivo before being able to cause mutation) but also for false negatives because some conjugation reactions can yield metabolites that are more reactive than their substrate (Dashwood, 2002; Ku et al., 2007). In other words, the use of an S9 system with NADPH may represent an incomplete picture of the metabolism that can occur in vivo. In particular, it is well-studied that SULTs are able to sequester some proximate mutagens through the

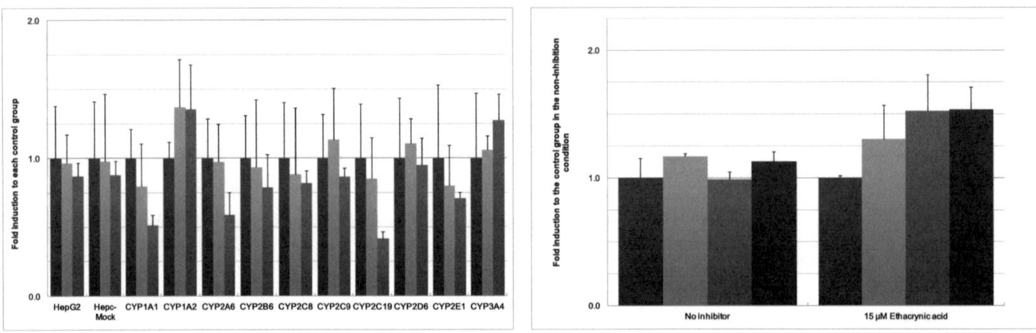

A B

Fig. 13. Micronucleus induction of safrole by expression of CYP1A1, 1A2, 2A6, 2B6, 2C8, 2C9, 2C19, 2D6, 2E1 and 3A4 (a), and effects of a phase II inhibitro on micronucleus indcution by safrole (b). a). The cells (1×10^5 cells) were seeded onto a 24-well plate for 24 h, and then treated with 0.5% DMSO (heavy gray bars), 83.3 μg/ml (light gray bars) or 125 μg/ml (medium gray bars) safrole. No statistically significant increase was observed when compared with both Hepc-Mock and HepG2. b). The transformant cells expressing CYP2D6 (1×10^5 cells) were seeded onto a 24-well plate for 24 h and then treated with 0.5% DMSO (heavy gray bars), 41.7 μg/ml (light gray bars), 62.5 μg/ml (medium gray bars) or 83.3 μg/ml (solid bars) safrole in the absence or presence of 15 μM ethacrynic acid, a GST inhibitor.

transfer of a sulfuryl group. However are these are also not active in the standard testing system because the necessary cofactor, 3'-phosphoadenosine-5'-phosphosulfate, is not added (Glatt, 2000; Glatt, 2005). From the study by Obach and Dobo using 16 drugs commonly used, not all metabolites observed as significant in humans in vivo are generated in the system using rat or human S9 fractions (Obach and Dobo, 2008).. Furthermore, they reported that a metabolite observed in humans in vivo was only seen in the rat S9 system and not the human S9 system in a few cases, (Obach and Dobo, 2008). Many human in vivo metabolites arise via conjugation reactions, which will not be observed in the in vitro S9 system as presently supplemented in standard in vitro genotoxicity tests. In addition, with regard to similarity to in vivo metabolite profiles, the results of the in vitro testing presented in the literature by Obach and Dobo clearly demonstrate a limitation of both systems, in that both human and rat S9 predominantly generate metabolites that are the result of one to two metabolic reactions (>90%).

The induced rat liver S9 fraction has another limitation. To be detected as mutagens, some genotoxic metabolites have to be formed within the target cell by enzymes that are not represented in standard in vitro test systems. SULT-dependent activations are not uncommon. Using genetically modified target cells, activation by SULTs has been demonstrated for more than 100 chemicals, including various carcinogens (such as tamoxifen, cyproterone acetate, safrole, nitrofen and some nitrotoluenes) that are missed in conventional test systems (Glatt 2000, Glatt 2005, Glatt and Meinl, 2005). Depending on the compound, varying SULT forms were required for the activation. Like N-sulfooxy-2-acetylaminofluorene, several other sulfo conjugates [e.g. furfuryl sulfate and 1-(L-sulfooxyethyl) pyrene] had to be formed within the target for a positive test result. Other reactive sulfo conjugates undergo spontaneous substitution reactions with components of the culture medium, such as chloride anions, leading to the formation of secondary, membrane-penetrating active species (Glatt et al., 1990). Moreover, cDNA-mediated expression of organic anion transporters in target cells enhanced the genotoxic effects of some reactive sulfuric acid esters externally added (Bakhiya et al., 2006). Such uptake mechanisms might play a role in the organotropism of reactive species, but should not be relied on when testing new compounds.

Other conjugating enzymes (some UGTs, GSTs and NATs) have also been expressed in target cells. The activation of promutagens by UGTs in such models has not yet been reported (and not been studied). However, co-expression of human UGT1A1 provided protection against the mutagenicity and cytotoxicity of PhIP in CHO-derived cells engineered for expression of CYP1A2 (Malfatti et al., 2005). Human GST T1, expressed in Salmonella typhimurium, strongly enhanced the mutagenicity of various dihalogenated alkanes as well as diepoxybutane (Thier et al., 1996). The activation of some of these agents could also be demonstrated using external GSH-conjugating systems (Rannug et al., 1978), but the extent of the uptake and its dependence on the structures of the reactive GSH conjugates are largely unexplored. Heterologous expression of GSTs in mammalian cells conferred resistance against various alkylating agents; in some cases, this protection was enhanced by, or was even strictly dependent on, the co-expression of an export pump (MRP-1 or MRP-2) (Smitherman et al., 2004). The expression of endogenous acetyltransferases in Salmonella may be a reason for the high mutagenic activity observed in the Ames test with many amino- and nitro-arenes, whose final activation step is often an O-acetylation. Salmonella strains are available in which O-acetyltransferase has been replaced by a mammalian NAT (Glatt and Meinl 2005, Grant et al., 1992), which differ in substrate specificity. Thus, various aromatic hydroxamic acids are activated to mutagens by human NATs, but not by OAT. Such differences may often lead to misleading results when the standard bacterial strains are used. Unlike typical phase II metabolites, acetyl conjugates are uncharged. Nevertheless the site of their formation can strongly affect the outcome of mutagenicity experiments. Thus, PhIP shows much higher mutagenicity in S. typhimurium TA98 compared to an O-acetyltransferase-deficient variant of this strain; however, purified O-acetyltransferase in the presence of its cofactor acetyl-CoA had drastically reduced its bacterial mutagenicity (although it strongly enhanced the covalent binding to naked DNA) (Saito et al., 1985). Various standard mammalian target cells, including most sublines of V79 cells, do not express any endogenous NAT. Heterologous expression of human NATs in these cells strongly enhanced the genotoxic effects of many amino- and nitro-arenes (Glatt, 2005; Glatt, 2006). For example, induction of gene mutations by 3-nitrobenzanthrone required 100 times lower substrate concentrations in NAT2-expressing compared to control V79 cells. The isomer, 2-nitrobenzanthrone, was mutagenic in cells engineered for

expression of human SULT1A1, but not in control cells. 2-Amino-3-methylimidazo[4,5-f]-quinoline induced gene mutations in V79 cells co-expressing human NAT2 or NAT1 together with human CYP1A2, even at a concentration of 0.01 and 1 µM, respectively, but was inactive (even at 30 µM) in cells expressing only CYP1A2 (Glatt, 2005; Glatt, 2006).
Genotoxicity is a branch of the field of toxicology that assesses the effects of chemicals on DNA or genetic processes of living cells. Such effects can be accessed directly by measuring the interaction of chemicals with DNA or more indirectly through the production of gene mutation or chromosome alterations. The observations of these consequences in the genotoxicity tests suggest the carcinogenic concern of a chemical. Thus it is important to improve the genotoxicity test system to evaluate accurately based on the in vivo situation in human as much as possible. In the present research, I tried to imitate human metabolism by using human hepatocyte cell line expressing human CYP enzymes. My results indicated that metabolism focused only on CYP was not sufficient to evaluate the genotoxicity of the chemicals such as tamoxifen and safrole. A comprehensive metabolic pathway not only by phase I drug-metabolizing enzymes but also by phase II enzymes would be needed for the accurate assessment of genotoxicity. Moreover, other cellular defense systems (i.e., antioxidant system, GSH or ascorbic acid, and DNA repair system) are involved in the expression of genotoxicity by a chemical. Despite the proof that most chemical carcinogens undergo metabolic conversion into DNA-reactive intermediates, some compounds do not bind to DNA and are not mutagenic, yet they are carcinogenic in animal models and possibly also in humans. These non-genotoxic mechanisms such as induction of inflammation, immunosuppression, formation of reactive oxygen species, activation of receptors such as arylhydrocarbon receptor or estrogen receptor, and epigenetic silencing. Therefore ,another approach based on the non-genotoxic mechanism is necessary to predict the carcinogenic action from a certain chemical. Together, these genotoxic and non-genotoxic mechanisms can alter signal-transduction pathways that finally result in hypermutability, genomic instability, loss of proliferation control, and resistance to apoptosis – some of the characteristic features of cancer cells. In this regard, we need to learn much more about the role and interplay of susceptibility and resistance function targeted by human carcinogens or involved in modulating human responses to carcinogenic chemicals.

3. Future considerations

Genotoxicity is a branch of the field of toxicology that assesses the effects of chemicals on DNA or genetic processes of living cells. Such effects can be accessed directly by measuring the interaction of chemicals with DNA or more indirectly through the production of gene mutation or chromosome alterations. The observations of these consequences in the genotoxicity tests suggest the carcinogenic concern of a chemical. Thus it is important to improve the genotoxicity test system to evaluate accurately based on the in vivo situation in human as much as possible. In the present research, I tried to imitate human metabolism by using human hepatocyte cell line expressing human CYP enzymes. My results indicated that metabolism focused only on CYP was not sufficient to evaluate the genotoxicity of the chemicals such as tamoxifen and safrole. A comprehensive metabolic pathway not only by phase I drug-metabolizing enzymes but also by phase II enzymes would be needed for the accurate assessment of genotoxicity. Moreover, other cellular defense systems (i.e., antioxidant system, GSH or ascorbic acid, and DNA repair system) are involved in the expression of genotoxicity by a chemical. Despite the proof that most chemical carcinogens undergo metabolic conversion into DNA-reactive intermediates, some compounds do not bind to DNA and are not mutagenic, yet they are carcinogenic in animal models and possibly also in humans. These non-genotoxic mechanisms such as induction of inflammation, immunosuppression, formation of reactive oxygen species, activation of receptors such as arylhydrocarbon receptor or estrogen receptor, and epigenetic silencing. Therefore ,another approach based on the non-genotoxic mechanism is necessary to predict the carcinogenic action from a certain chemical. Together, these genotoxic and non-genotoxic mechanisms can alter signal-transduction pathways that finally result in hypermutability, genomic instability, loss of proliferation control, and resistance to apoptosis – some of the characteristic features of cancer cells. In this regard, we need to learn much more about the role and interplay of susceptibility and resistance function targeted by human carcinogens or involved in modulating human responses to carcinogenic chemicals.

4. Summary and conclusion

Many carcinogens are known to be procarcinogens and require metabolic activation to exert their genotoxicity through the formation of reactive intermediates. Therefore, for hazard identification on the genotoxic potential of drug candidate and its metabolites, S9 fraction prepared from the livers of rats pretreated with phenobarbital and 5,6-benzoflavone or with Aroclor 1254 to induce drug-metabolizing enzyme activity must be used in the in vitro genotoxicity testing. However, it is frequently questioned as to whether such an in vitro metabolite generation system is the most relevant for human risk, or whether the assay would be better served by using a human-derived in vitro system. In the present study, we examined the advantages of HepG2 transformants expressing a series of human CYP isoforms as a better alternative for metabolic activation system in the in vitro genotoxicity testing.

In section 2.1, the sensitivity of this system to detect genotoxicity requiring CYP activation was confirmed in the in vitro micronucleus tests using well-studied model chemicals. These results showed HepG2 transformants system have the appropriate sensitivity to detect genotoxicity requiring CYP activation tests using well-studied model chemicals. In addition, based on results obtained in the DMBA and ifosfamide treatments, HepG2 transformant system showed that genotoxic metabolites would be produced by not only the most active CYP isoform but also by other less active CYPs.

In chapter 2.2, this system allowed us to investigate the genotoxicity of model chemicals for which the contributing CYP isoforms, especially those mediated by CYP1A2 or 3A4 which is known to metabolize many drugs in humans, have not yet been identified. Based on the results obtained in the okadaic acid and β-endosulfan treatments, it was clearly demonstrated that the HepG2 transformant system was able to identify the CYP isoform relating to the genotoxicity of chemical metabolite(s) and was useful to elucidate the genotoxicity of a new chemical or a drug candidate in the presence of the metabolic activation system.

In chapter 2.3, the relevance of the interaction between phase I and phase II drug-metabolizing enzymes, e.g., UGT, GST, and SULT, in the test system was demonstrated in a MN test of tamoxifen or safrole, which has been reported to be metabolized by enzymes of both phases. Based on the results for tamoxifen and safrole, it was clearly demonstrated that the interaction between the phase I and phase II drug-metabolizing enzymes was crucial to

assess the genotoxicity of chemicals in the presence of a metabolic activation system. Therefore, a set of HepG2 transformants is a superior test system for mimicking the metabolism occurring in the human liver and the use of this system can potentially provide more relevant data than current genotoxicity tests.
In conclusion, we have demonstrated the benefits of a newly established HepG2 transformants expressing a series of human CYP isoforms for in vitro genotoxicity testing that reflects the comprehensive metabolic pathways including not only human CYP isoforms but also the phase II drug-metabolizing enzymes.

5. References

Ames, B. N.; Durston, W. E.; Yamasaki, E. & Lee, F. D. (1973). Carcinogens as mutagens: a simple test system combining liver homogenates for activation and bacteria for detection, *Proc. Natl. Acad. Sci.* 70: 2281-2285.

Andrew, P. & Brian, W. O. (2007). 6. Biotransformation of xenobiotics. In Casarett and Doull's Toxicology, The basic science of poisons (Cartis D Klaassen ed.), 7th ed., The McGraw-Hill Companies, Inc. Columbus, Ohio, pp. 161-304.

Bakhiya, N., Stephani, M., Bahn, A., Ugele, B.; Seidel, A.; Burckhardt, G. & Glatt,H. (2006) Uptake of chemically reactive, DNA-damaging sulfuric acid esters into renal cells by human organic anion transporters, *J. Am. Soc. Nephrol.* 17: 1414-1421.

Bauer, E.; Guo, Z.; Ueng, Y. F.; Bell, L. C.; Zeldin, D. & Guengerich, F. P. (1995) Oxidation of benzo[a]pyrene by recombinant human cytochrome P450 enzymes. *Chem. Res. Toxicol.* 8: 136-142.

Brown, K. (2009). Is tamoxifen a genotoxic carcinogen in women? *Mutagenesis* 24: 391-404.

Chang, T. K. H.; Weber, G. F., Crespi; C. L. & Waxman, D. J. (1993). Differential activation of cyclophosphamide and ifosphamide by cytochromes P-450 2B and 3A in human liver microsomes, *Cancer Res.* 53: 5629-5637.

Dashwood, R. H. (2002). Modulation of heterocyclic amine-induced mutagenicity and carcinogenicity: an 'A-to-Z' guide to chemopreventive agents, promoters, and transgenic models. *Mutat. Res.* 511: 89-112.

DiMasi, J. A.; Hansen, R. W. & Grabowski, H. G. (2003) The price of innovation: new estimates of drug development costs. *J. Health Econ.* 22: 151-185.

Glatt, H.; Henschler, R.; Phillips, D. H.; Blake, J. W.; Steinberg, P.; Seidel, A. & Oesch, F. (1990) Sulfotransferase-mediated chlorination of 1-hydroxymethylpyrene to a mutagen capable of penetrating indicator cells, *Environ. Health Perspect.* 88: 43-48.

Glatt H., Bartsch I., Christoph S., Coughtrie M. W. H., Falany C. N., Hagen M., Landsiedel R., Pabel U., Phillips D. H., Seidel A., Yamazoe Y. (1998). Sulfotransferase-mediated activation of mutagens studied using heterologousexpression systems. Chem. Biol. Interact. 109, 195-219.

Glatt, H. (2000) Sulfotransferases in the bioactivation of xenobiotics, *Chem. Biol. Interact.* 129: 141-170.

Glatt, H. (2005) Activation and inactivation of carcinogens by human sulfotransferases, in: G.M. Pacifici, M.W.H. Coughtrie (Eds.), *Human Cytosolic Sulfotransferases*, Taylor & Francis, London, pp. 281-306.

Glatt, H. & Meinl, W. (2005) Sulfotransferases and acetyltransferases in mutagenicity testing: technical aspects, *Meth. Enzymol.* 400: 230-249.

Glatt, H. (2006) Metabolic factors affecting the mutagenicity of heterocyclic amines, in: K. Skog, J. Alexander (Eds.), *Acrylamide and Other Health Hazardous Compounds in Heat-treated Foods*, Woodhead Publishing, Cambridge, pp. 358-404.

Grant, D. M.; Josephy, P. D; Lord, H. L. & Morrison, L. D. (1992) Salmonella typhimurium strains expressing human arylamine N-acetyltransferases: metabolism and mutagenic activation of aromatic amines, *Cancer Res.* 52: 3961-3964.

Guengerich, F. P.; Dannan, G. A. & Wright, S. T. (1982). Purification and characterization of liver microsomal cytochromes P-450: electrophoretic, spectral, catalytic, and immunochemical properties and inducibility of eight isozymes isolated from rats treated with phenobarbital or β-naphthoflavone, *Biochemistry* 21: 6019-6030.

Guengerich, F. P. (1997). Comparisons of catalytic selectivity of cytochrome P450 subfamily enzymes from different species, *Chem. Biol. Interact.* 106: 161-182.

Guengerich, F. P. (2001) Common and uncommon cytochrome P450 reactions related to metabolism and chemical toxicity, *Chem. Res. Toxicol.* 14: 611-650.

Hashizume, T., Yoshitomi, S., Asahi, S., Matsumura, S., Chatani, F. & Oda, H. (2009). In vitro micronucleus test in HepG2 transformants expressing a series of human cytochrome P450 isoforms with chemicals requiring metabolic activation, *Mutat. Res.* 677: 1-7.

Hashizume, T., Yoshitomi, S., Asahi, S., Uematsu, R., Matsumura, S., Chatani, F., Oda, H. (2010). Advantages of human hepatocyte-derived transformants expressing a series of human cytochrome p450 isoforms for genotoxicity examination., *Toxicol. Sci.* 116: 488-497.

Le Hégarat, L.; Fessard, V.; Poul, J. M.; Dragacci, S. & Sanders, P. (2004) Marine toxin okadaic acid induces aneuploidy in CHO-K1 cells in presence of rat liver postmitochondrial fraction, revealed by cytokinesis-block micronucleus assay coupled to FISH, *Environ. Toxicol.* 19: 123-128.

Levin, D. E.; Hollstein, M.; Christman, M. F. & Ames, B. N. (1984). Detection of oxidative mutagens with a new Salmonella tester strain (TA102). *Methods Enzymol.* 105: 249-254.

ICH, M3-R2. (2006) Final Concept Paper M3(R2): Revision of the ICH Guideline on Non-Clinical Safety Studies for the Conduct of Human Clinical Trials for Pharmaceuticals. Available at: www.ich.org.

ICH S2A. (1997). Genotoxicity: Specific aspects of regulatory genotoxicity tests for pharmaceuticals. Available at: www.ich.org.

ICH S2B. (1997). Genotoxicity: A standard battery for genotoxicity testing of pharmaceuticals. Available at: www.ich.org.

Iwata, H.; Fujita, K.; Kushida, H.; Susuki, A.; Konno; Y., Nakamura; K., Fujino & A., Kamataki, T. (1988). High catalytic activity of human NADPH-cytochrome P450 reductase in Escherichia coli., *Biochem. Pharmacol.* 55: 1315-1325.

Jing, Z.; Quan, T. & Shu-Feng. Z. (2006). Clinical pharmacology of cyclophosphamide and ifosfamide, *Curr. Drug Ther.* 1: 55-84.

Kessova, I. & Cederbaum, A. I. (2003) CYP2E1: biochemistry, toxicology, regulation and function in ethanol-induced liver injury. *Curr. Mol. Med.* 3: 509-518.

Kola, I. & Landis, J. (2004) Can the pharmaceutical industry reduce attrition rates? *Nat. Rev. Drug Discov.* 3: 711-715.

Kramer, J. A.; Sagartz, J. E. & Morris, D. L. (2007) The application of discovery toxicology and pathology towards the design of safer pharmaceutical lead candidates. *Nat. Rev. Drug Discov.* 6: 636-649.

Ku, W. W.; Bigger, A.; Brambilla, G.; Glatt, H.; Gocke, E.; Guzzie, P. J.; Hakura, A.; Honma, M.; Martus, H. J.; Obach, R. S. & Roberts, S. Strategy Expert Group, IWGT, (2007). Strategy for genotoxicity testing-Metabolic considerations, *Mutat. Res.* 627: 59-77.

Lee, H. K.; Moon, J. K.; Chang, C. H.; Choi, H.; Park, H. W.; Park, B. S.; Lee, H. S.; Hwang, E. C.; Lee, Y. D.; Liu, K. H. & Kim, J. H. (2006). Stereoselective metabolism of endosulfan by human liver microsomes and human cytochrome P450 isoforms. *Drug Metab. Dispos.* 34: 1090-1095.

Lu, Y.; Morimoto, K.; Takeshita, T.; Takeuchi, T. & Saito, T. (2000). Genotoxic effects of α-endosulfan and β-endosulfan on human HepG2 cells, *Environ. Health Perspect.* 108: 559-561.

Lewis, D. F. V. (2004). 57 varieties: the human cytochromes P450, *Pharcogenomics* 5: 305-318.

Malling, H. V. (1971) Dimethylnitrosamine: Formation of mutagenic compounds by interaction with mouse liver microsomes. *Mutat Res.* 13: 425-429.

Miller, E. C. & Miller, J. A. (1947) The presence and significance of bound amino azodyes in the livers of rats fed p-dimethylaminoazobenzene. *Cancer Res.* 7: 468-480.

Obach, R. S. & Dobo K. L. (2008). Comparison of metabolite profiles generated in Aroclor-induced rat liver and human liver subcellular fractions: considerations for in vitro genotoxicity hazard assessment, *Environ. Mol. Mutagen.* 49: 631-641.

Osborne, M. R.; Hewer, A.; Hardcastle, I. R.; Carmichael, P. L. & Phillips, D. H. (1996) Identification of the major tamoxifen-deoxyguanosine adduct formed in the liver DNA of rats treated with tamoxifen, *Cancer Res.* 56: 66-71.

Paolini, M. & Cantelli-Forti, G. (1997). On the metabolizing systems for short-term genotoxicity assays: a review, *Mutat. Res.* 387: 17-34.

Patten, C. J.; Ishizaki, H.; Aoyama, T.; Lee, M.; Ning, S. M.; Huang, W.; Gonzalez, F. J. & Yang C. S., (1992) Catalytic properties of the human cytochrome P450 2E1 produced by cDNA expression in mammalian cells. Arch. *Biochem. Biophys.* 299: 163-171.

Rannug, U.; Sundvall, A. & Ramel, C. (1978) The mutagenic effect of 1,2-dichloroethane on Salmonella typhimurium. I. Activation through conjugation with glutathion in vitro, Chem. *Biol. Interact.* 20: 1-16.

Rawlins, M. D. (2004) Cutting the cost of drug development. *Nat. Rev. Drug Discov.* 3: 360-364.

Rendic, S. & Guengerich, F. P. (1997) Human cytochrome P450 enzymes, a status report summarizing their reactions, substrates, inducers and inhibitors. *Drug Metab. Rev.* 29: 413-580.

Rietjens, I. M. C. M.; Boersma, M. G.; Van Der Woude H.; Jeurissen, S. M. F.; Schutte, M. E. & Alink, G. M. (2005). Flavonoids and alkenylbenzenes: Mechanisms of mutagenic action and carcinogenic risk, *Mutat. Res.* 574: 124-138.

Saito, K.; Shinohara, A.; Kamataki, T. & Kato, R. (1985) Metabolic activation of mutagenic N-hydroxyarylamines by O-acetyltransferase in Salmonella typhimurium TA98, *Arch. Biochem. Biophys.* 239: 286–295.

Sallustio, B. C.; DeGraaf, Y. C.; Weekley, J. S. & Burcham, P. C. (2006). Bioactivation of carboxylic acid compounds by UDP-glucuronosyltransferases to DNA-damaging intermediates: Role of glycoxidation and oxidative stress in genotoxicity. *Chem. Res. Toxicol.* 19: 683-691.

Sawada, M. & Kamataki, T. (1998) Genetically engineered cells stably expressing cytochrome P450 and their application to mutagen assays, *Mutat. Res.* 411: 19-43.

Shimada, T. & Fujii-Kuriyama, Y. (2004). Metabolic activation of polycyclic aromatic hydrocarbons to carcinogens by cytochromes P450 1A1 and 1B1. *Gann Monographs on Cancer Research* 52: 109-124.

Shou, M.; Korzekwa, K. R.; Krausz, K. W.; Buters, J. T. M.; Grogan, J.; Goldfarb, I.; Hardwick, J. P.; Gonzalez, F. J. & Gelboin, H. V. (1996) Specificity of cDNA-expressed human and rodent cytochrome P450s in the oxidative metabolism of the potent carcinogen 7,12-dimethylbenz[a]anthracene. *Mol. Carcinog.* 17: 241-249.

Smitherman, P. K.; Townsend, A. J.; Kute, T. E. & Morrow, C. S., (2004) Role of multidrug resistance protein 2 (MRP2, ABCC2) in alkylating agent detoxification: MRP2 potentiates glutathione S-transferase A1-1-mediated resistance to chlorambucil cytotoxicity, *J. Pharmacol. Exp. Ther.* 308: 260-267.

Thier, R.; Pemble, S. E.; Kramer, H.; Taylor, J. B.; Guengerich, F. P &, Ketterer, B. (1996) Human glutathione S-transferase T1-1 enhances mutagenicity of 1,2-dibromoethane, dibromomethane and 1,2,3,4-diepoxybutane in Salmonella typhimurium, Carcinogenesis 17: 163-166.

Uchaipichat, V.; Mackenzie, P. I.; Guo, X. H.; Gardner-Stephen, D.; Galetin, A.; Houston, J. B. and Miners, J. O. (2004). Human UDP-glucuronosyl- transferases: Isoform selectivity and kinetics of 4-methylumbelliferone and 1-naphthol glucuronidation, effects of organic solvents, and inhibition by diclofenac and probenecid, *Drug Metab. Dispos.* 32: 413-423.

Waxman D. J., Lapenson D. P., Aoyama T., Gelboin H. V., Gonzalez F. J., Korzekwa K. (1991) Steroid hormone hydroxylase specificities of eleven cDNA- expressed human cytochrome P450s. Arch. Biochem. Biophys. 290, 160-166.

White, I. N. H. (2003). Tamoxifen: Is it safe? comparison of activation and detoxication mechanisms in rodents and in humans. *Curr. Drug Metab.* 4: 223-239.

Williams, J. A.; Hyland, R.; Jones, B. C.; Smith, D. A.; Hurst, S.; Goosen, T. C.; Peterkin, V.; Koup, J. R.; Ball, S. E. (2004) Drug-drug interactions for UDP-glucuronosyl-trasnferase substrates: a pharmacokinetic explanation for typically observed low exposure (AUCi/AUC) ratios. *Drug Metab. Dispos.* 32: 1201-1208.

World Health Organization (WHO). (1999). Pesticide residues in food - 1998 evaluations. II. Toxicological. WHO/PCS/99.18 (nos 943-956 on INCHEM).

Yoshitomi, S.; Ikemoto, K.; Takahashi, J.; Miki, H.; Namba, M. & Asahi, S. (2001). Establishment of the transformants expressing human cytochrome P450 subtypes in HepG2, and their applications on drug metabolism and toxicology, *Toxicol. In Vitro.* 15: 245-256.

Zhao, L.; Krishnan, S.; Zhang, Y.; Schenkman, J. B. & Rusling, J. F. (2009). Differences in metabolite-mediated toxicity of tamoxifen in rodents versus humans elucidated with DNA/microsome electro-optical arrays and nanoreactors, *Chem. Res. Toxicol.* 22: 341-347.

17

Genotoxic Impurities in Pharmaceuticals

Abolghasem Jouyban[1] and Hamed Parsa[2]
[1]*Drug Applied Research Center and Faculty of Pharmacy,*
[2]*Tuberculosis and Lung Disease Research Center,*
Tabriz University of Medical Sciences, Tabriz,
Iran

1. Introduction

Genotoxic compounds induce genetic mutations and/or chromosomal rearrangements and can therefore act as carcinogenic compounds (McGovern and Jacobson-Kram, 2006). These compounds cause damage to DNA by different mechanisms such as alkylation or other interactions that can lead to mutation of the genetic codes. In general, chemists employ the terms "genotoxic" and "mutagenic" synonymously; however, there is a subtle distinction. Genotoxicity pertains to all types of DNA damage (including mutagenicity), whereas mutagenicity pertains specifically to mutation induction at the gene and chromosome levels. Thus, the term "genotoxic" is applied to agents that interact with DNA and/or its associated cellular components (e.g. the spindle apparatus) or enzymes (e.g. topoisomerases) (Dearfield *et al.*, 2002; Robinson, 2010). Irrespective of the mechanism by which cancer is induced, it is now well agreed that it involves a change in the integrity or expression of genomic DNA. The majority of chemical carcinogens are capable of causing DNA damage, i.e., are "genotoxic" (Ashby, 1990). Moreover, a genotoxic compound also carries with it the carcinogenic effect which causes additional concern from the safety viewpoint.
Drug substances and their relative compounds such as impurities constitute an important group of genotoxic compounds. Thus, these compounds pose an additive concern to clinical subjects and patients (Müller *et al.*, 2006). Considering the importance of this problem, the challenge for regulatory agencies is to form guidelines and standards for the identification and control of genotoxic compounds and their impurities especially in pharmaceuticals. In this article, genotoxicity profiles of the main group of genotoxic compounds are discussed. The article throws light on the challenges in analyzing and predicting for these groups and also deals with the different management problems of genotoxic impurities in pharmaceuticals.

2. Guidelines

2.1 ICH guidelines

The International Conference on Harmonization (ICH) of Technical Requirements for Registration of Pharmaceuticals for Human Use project represents the main group of guidelines with topics such as "Quality" topics and "Safety" topics. Quality topics relate to chemical and pharmaceutical quality assurance (stability testing, impurity testing, etc.) and safety topics deal with *in vitro* and *in vivo* pre-clinical studies (carcinogenicity testing, genotoxicity testing, etc.) (ICH, 2008).

The ICH initially published guidelines on impurities of drug substances and pharmaceutical products in the late 1990s. In the guidelines, genotoxicity tests have been defined as *in vitro* and *in vivo* tests designed for detecting compounds that induce genetic damage directly or indirectly (International Conference on Harmonization, 1997). The ICH quality guidelines Q3A(R) and Q3B(R) respectively address the topics of control of impurities in drug substances and degradants in pharmaceutical products, while the Q3C guideline deals with the residual solvents. However, several important issues have not been addressed in the guidelines, for example, the acceptable levels of impurities in drugs during development as well as the control of genotoxic impurities. Table 1 illustrates a series of thresholds described in ICH Q3A(R) that trigger reporting, identification, and qualification requirements. Subsequently, Table 2 depicts the thresholds for reporting, identification, and qualification of impurities in new drug products (ICH, 2006; Jacobson-Kram and McGovern, 2007). In addition, two options for standard test battery for genotoxicity are available in the ICH S2 (R1) guideline (ICH, 2008):

Thresholds	Maximum daily dose	
	≤2 g/day	>2 g/day
Reporting threshold	0.05%	0.03%
Identification threshold	0.10% or 1.0 mg per day intake (whichever is lower)	0.05%
Qualification threshold	0.15% or 1.0 mg per day intake (whichever is lower)	0.05%

Table 1. Threshold for APIs

Option 1

i. A test for gene mutation in bacteria;

ii. A cytogenetic test for chromosomal damage (the *in vitro* metaphase chromosome aberration test or *in vitro* micronucleus test), or an *in vitro* mouse lymphoma *tk* gene mutation assay;

iii. An *in vivo* test for genotoxicity, generally a test for chromosomal damage using rodent hematopoietic cells, either for micronuclei or for chromosomal aberrations in metaphase cells.

Option 2

i. A test for gene mutation in bacteria;

ii. An *in vivo* assessment of genotoxicity with two tissues, usually an assay for micronuclei using rodent hematopoietic cells and a second *in vivo* assay.

As stated by the ICH safety guidelines (S2A and S2B), "for compounds giving negative results, the completion of 3-test battery, perform and evaluate in accordance with current recommendations, will usually provide a sufficient level of safety to demonstrate the absence of genotoxic activity." Thus, any compound that produces a positive result in one or more assays in the standard battery has historically been regarded as genotoxic, which may require further testing for risk assessment (Müller *et al.*, 2006).

Maximum Daily Dose[1]	Reporting Thresholds[2,3]	Identification Thresholds[2,3]	Qualification Thresholds[2,3]
≤ 1 mg		1.0% or 5 μg TDI whichever is lower	
1 - 10 mg		0.5% or 20 μg TDI whichever is lower	
10 - 100 mg			0.5% or 200 μg TDI whichever is lower
<10 mg			1.0% or 50 μg TDI whichever is lower
> 10 mg - 2 g		0.2% or 2 mg TDI whichever is lower	
> 100 mg - 2 g			0.2% or 3 mg TDI whichever is lower
≤1 g	0.1 %		
> 1 g	0.05 %		
> 2 g		0.1%	
> 2 g			0.15%

[1] The amount of drug substance administered per day
[2]Thresholds for degradation products are expressed either as a percentage of the drug substance or as a total daily intake (TDI) of the degradation product. Lower thresholds can be appropriate if the degradation product is unusually toxic.
[3]Higher thresholds should be scientifically justified.

Table 2. Thresholds for degradation products in new drug products (Jacobson-Kram and McGovern, 2007)

2.2 EMEA guideline

The European Medicines Agency (EMEA) guideline describes a general framework and practical approaches on how to deal with genotoxic impurities in new active substances. According to the guideline "The toxicological assessment of genotoxic impurities and the determination of acceptable limits for such impurities in active substances is a difficult issue and not addressed in sufficient detail in the existing ICH Q3X guidance". In addition, the EMEA guideline proposed a toxicological concern (TTC) threshold value of 1.5 μg/day intake of a genotoxic impurity which is considered to be associated with an acceptable risk (excess cancer risk of <1 in 100,000 over a lifetime) in most pharmaceuticals. Based on the TTC value, a permitted level of an active substance can be calculated concerning the expected daily dose. Higher limits might be justified under certain conditions such as short-term exposure periods (European Medicines Agency/ Committee for Medicinal Products (CHMP) for Human Use, 2006). In the context of this guideline, the classification of a compound (impurity) as genotoxic in general indicates that there are positive findings in established *in vitro* or *in vivo* genotoxicity tests with the focus on DNA reactive substances that have a potential for direct DNA damage. In the absence of such information, *in vitro* genotoxics are usually considered as presumptive *in vivo* mutagens and carcinogens (EMEA/CHMP, 2006).

Based on the importance of the mechanism of action and the dose-response relationship in the assessment of genotoxic compounds, the EMEA guideline presents two classes of genotoxic compounds:

1. Genotoxic compounds with sufficient (experimental) evidence for a threshold-related mechanism,
2. Genotoxic compounds without sufficient (experimental) evidence for a threshold-related mechanism.

Those genotoxic compounds with sufficient evidence would be regulated according to the procedure as outlined for class 2 solvents in the "Q3C Note for Guidance on Impurities: Residual Solvents". For genotoxic compounds without sufficient evidence for a threshold-related mechanism, the guideline proposes a policy of controlling levels to "as low as reasonably practicable" (ALARP) principle, where avoiding is not possible.

On the other hand, this guideline provides no advice on acceptable TTCs for drugs during development, especially for trials of short duration (Jacobson-Kram and McGovern, 2007).

The pharmaceutical research and manufacturing association (PhRMA) has established a procedure for the testing, classification, qualification, toxicological risk assessment, and control of impurities processing genotoxic potential in pharmaceutical products. As most medicines are given for a limited period of time, this procedure proposes a staged TTC to adjust the limits for shorter exposure time during clinical trials (Table 3). Thus, the staged TTC can be used for genotoxic compounds having genotoxicity data that are normally not suitable for a quantitative risk assessment (Muller *et al.*, 2006).

	Duration of clinical trial exposure				
	≤ 1 month	> 1-3 month	> 3-6 month	>6-12 month	>12 month
Allowable Daily Intake (μg/day) for all phases of development	120	60	20	10	1.5
Alternative maximum level of allowable impurity based on percentage of impurity in API	0.5%	0.5%	0.5%	0.5%	0.5%

Table 3. PhRMA genotoxic impurity task force proposal – allowable daily intake (μg/day) for genotoxic impurities during clinical development using the staged TTC approach

3. Genotoxic impurities (GIs)

3.1 Sulfonates

Sulfonate salts (Figure 1) are the most frequently used compounds in pharmaceutical developments. Salt formation is a useful technique for optimizing the physicochemical processing (formulation), biopharmaceutical or therapeutic properties of active pharmaceutical ingredients (APIs), and sulfonate salts are widely used for this purpose (Elder and Snodin, 2009). In addition to the advantages of processing, sulfonate salts possess some advantages over other salts such as producing higher melting point of the sulfonated API. This helps to enhance the stability and provide good solubility and may have certain *in vivo* advantages as well. For instance, in contrast to other salts of strong acids, mesylates do not have a tendency to form hydrates, which makes them an attractive salt form for secondary processing, especially wet granulation. Another benefit of these salts is their high melting point because APIs with low melting points often exhibit plastic deformation during processing which can cause both caking and aggregation. Typically, an increase in the melting point has an adverse effect on aqueous solubility owing to an increase in the crystal lattice energies. Sulfonic acid salts tend to be an exception to this rule, since they exhibit both high melting points as well as good solubility. In addition, as mentioned in the literature, the high solubility and high surface area of haloperidol mesylate result in enhanced dissolution rates (<2 min in pH 2 simulated gastric media), which are more rapid than the competing common ion formation (Elder and Snodin, 2009; Elder *et al.*, 2010a).

On the other hand, sulfonic acids can react with low molecular weight alcohols such as methanol, ethanol, or isopropanol to form the corresponding sulfonate esters. In general, sulfonic acid esters are considered as potential alkylating agents that may exert genotoxic effects in bacterial and mammalian cell systems and possibly carcinogenic effects *in vivo*; thus, these compounds have raised safety concerns in recent times (Snodin, 2006; Teasdale *et al.*, 2009).

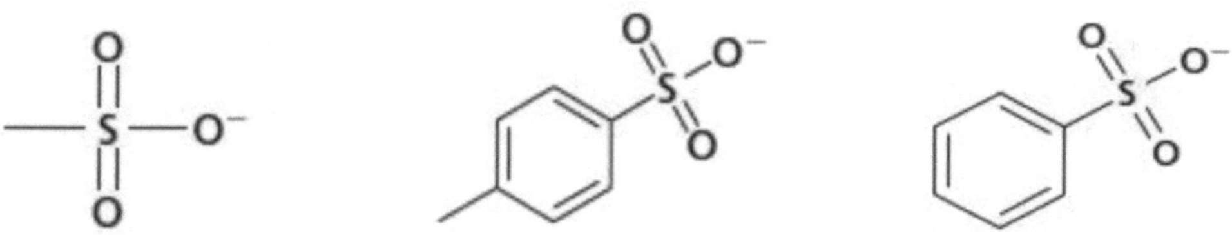

Mesyla Tosylate Besylate

Fig. 1. Structures of common sulfonate salts

3.1.1 Genotoxicity profile

Sulfonate impurities comprise the most investigated group of genotoxic impurities (GIs). Initially in 2007, sulfonate impurities raised major concern when over a period of three months (March to May 2007), several thousand HIV patients in Europe were exposed to Viracept^R (nelfinavir mesylate) tablets containing the contaminant ethyl methane sulfonate (EMS). However, the available *in vitro* and animal data indicated that the levels at which HIV patients were exposed to EMS (maximal dose of 0.055 mg/kg/d) did not induce any risk; nevertheless, any further level was of significant concern to their safety (Elder and Snodin, 2009). Since 2007 other drugs have been reported for contamination by sulfonate impurities, such as alkyl benzene sulfonates in amlodipine besylate (Raman *et al.*, 2008), dimethyl sulfate (DMS) in pazopanib hydrochloride (Liu *et al.*, 2009), EMS and methyl methane sulfonate (MMS) in imatinib mesylate (Ramakrishna *et al.*, 2008), EMS in zugrastat (Schülé *et al.*, 2010), alkyl sulfonates in flouroaryl-amine (Cimarosti *et al.*, 2010), and ethyl besylate in UK-369,003-26, a novel PDE5 inhibitor (Hajikarimian *et al.*, 2010).

EMS is a well-established genotoxic agent in this group which reacts with DNA producing alkylated (specifically ethylated) nucleotides. MMS, an analog of EMS, is a genotoxic compound both *in vitro* and *in vivo*. The international agency for research on cancer (IARC) has classified EMS and MMS in group 2B and 2A, respectively (Snodin, 2006; Gocke *et al.*, 2009a).

Gocke *et al.* (2009a) reviewed both *in vivo* and *in vitro* genotoxicity, carcinogenicity, general toxicity, and the effects on reproductive and embryo fetal development of EMS. They reported that the genotoxic effects induced by EMS were observed in viruses/phages, bacteria, fungi, plant, insect, and mammalian cells. In another study, the induction of gene mutations at the hprt locus and the induction of chromosomal damage were examined as evidenced by the formation of micronuclei in human lymphoblastoid cells. It was found that the lowest dose inducing a positive response was 1.40 µg/ml, and a no observed effect level (NOEL) could be defined at 1.2 µg/ml. Also, no toxicity was observed at doses up to 2.5 µg/plate. This observation is in strong contrast to the largely linear dose–response observed in the previous studies. As a result of *in vivo* assays for the induction of DNA damage, EMS is distributed rather uniformly over the body and induces similar levels of DNA damage in the various organs. Also, EMS is clastogenic in all test systems. The minimal dose of EMS applied in these studies was either 50 mg/kg or 100 mg/kg. In the majority of studies the dose–response relationships appeared sub linear and a threshold below 50 mg/kg appeared possible. Gocke *et al.* (2009a) demonstrated that EMS in various gene mutation tests such as induction of hprt, lacZ, and dlb-1 mutations in mice was mutagenic. The carcinogenicity of EMS was confirmed in several animal models. In another study, three methanesulfonates and three benzenesulfonates were tested by micronucleus and Yeast deletion recombination (DEL) assays. It was observed that all six substances produced positive responses in the tests (Sobol *et al.*, 2007).

3.2 Alkyl halides and esters

Owing to their electrophilic nature, alkylating agents can introduce lesions at nucleophilic centers of DNA. Drug salt formation includes strong acid/base interactions in the presence of alcohols, and can form impurities such as alkyl halides. As salt formation is a common method in drug formulation processes, alkyl halides exist as impurities in several drugs (Sobol *et al.*, 2007; Elder *et al.*, 2008a).

3.2.1 Genotoxicity profile

The nucleophilic attack mechanisms of alkylating compounds determine their reactivity against DNA. The SN1 mechanism leads to *O*-alkylation (*O-6*-methylguanine) which is mutagenic but not clastogenic, whereas the SN2 mechanism leads to N-methylation which is clastogenic and not mutagenic. In this group, it seems that bromo compounds are more reactive as compared to chloro compounds (Sobol *et al.*, 2007; Snodin, 2010).

Various tests have been performed to study DNA damage and mutation in alkyl halides. In the Ames test, it was found that most alkyl halides, especially bromides, are Ames positive except 1-chloropropane, 1-chlorobutane, and neopentyl bromide. As chloro- and bromobenzene are not alkylating agents, these compounds are Ames-negative. In Yeast deletion recombination (DEL) and micronucleus assays, alkyl chlorides such as *n*-propyl chloride are found to be negative (Sobol *et al.*, 2007; Snodin, 2010).

It was observed that alkyl chlorides in the NBP [4-(*p* nitrobenzyl) pyridine] alkylation assay are not reactive and that allyl chloride has minimal activity. Although benzyl chloride is more active than other chloro compounds, ethyl, propyl, or butyl bromides have at least 1/40 MMS activity; however, allyl bromide appears to be more active (around one-eighth of the activity of MMS) (Sobol *et al.*, 2007).

As indicated by the *in vivo* test in rodent bioassay, these compounds are either non-carcinogens (1- chlorobutane, bromomethane) or low-potency carcinogens (chloroethane, bromoethane). According to *in vivo* tests, chloroethane and alkyl bromides seem to be non-genotoxic carcinogens rather than genotoxic carcinogens. Based on the available data, the United States environmental protection agency (USEPA), considers tert-butyl chloride to be a group D compound or "not classifiable as to human carcinogenicity" (Bercu *et al.*, 2009; Snodin, 2010).

3.3 Hydrazines

Hydrazine is used as a medicine or as a starting compound for synthesizing some medicines. Hydrazine and some of its *N*-alkyl, *N*-aryl, and *N*-acyl analogues have been subjected to extensive toxicological evaluations. Hydrazines, hydrazides, and hydrazones have structural alerts for genotoxic potential and the metabolism increases their effects. Hydrazines adduct with DNA and the mechanism of adduction could include the formation of methyldiazanium ions or methyl free radicals. In addition, it seems that hydrazine reacts with endogenous formaldehyde to produce formaldehyde hydrazone. Subsequent to some other reactions, alkylating compounds like diazomethane as the genotoxic moiety are produced (Bercu *et al.*, 2009; Snodin, 2010).

3.3.1 Genotoxicity profile

In vitro studies have shown genotoxic effects for three hydrazine derivatives (hydrazines, hydrazides, and hydrazones). These compounds induce gene mutations in human teratoma cells, mouse lymphoma cells, and in several strains of bacteria. Hydralazine (1-hydrazinylphthalazine) and its hydrochloride salt are Ames-positive. In another study, 20 hydrazine-derivatives were found to induce a direct DNA damage in *Escherichia coli* and 16 of them (80%) were Ames positive as well (Flora *et al.*, 1984; Agency for Toxic Substance and Disease Registry, 1997; Snodin, 2010).

Although it was seen that hydrazine did not induce unscheduled DNA synthesis in mouse sperm cells, *in vivo* studies on the genotoxicity of hydrazines have largely produced positive results. In addition, it was observed that 1, 2-dimethylhydrazine failed to induce micronuclei in rat bone marrow cells, while this effect had been observed in mouse bone marrow cells (Agency for Toxic Substance and Disease Registry, 1997).

The non-carcinogenic effects of hydrazine were also evaluated; however, it was found that hydrazine, methyl hydrazine, 1,1- and 1,2-dimethylhydrazine, and other analogues are carcinogenic in rodents and possibly in human. In addition, it was seen that hydrazine derivatives like hydralazine and its hydrochloride salt were tumorigenic in rodents. It should be mentioned that the clinical use of hydralazine hydrochloride for several years has shown no evidence for carcinogenicity (Flora *et al.*, 1984; Bercu *et al.*, 2009; Snodin, 2010).

3.4 Epoxides

Epoxides are considered as electrophilic compounds owing to the strained epoxide ring. These alkylating agents directly react with DNA. Alkene oxides are more reactive than arene oxides and symmetrically substituted epoxides are less reactive than asymmetrically substituted compounds. Some examples for APIs with epoxide impurities are betamethasone acetate, atenolol, and some herbal remedies. Carbamazepine, cyproheptadine, and protriptyline have stable epoxide metabolites. In addition, phenytoin,

lamotrigine, amitryptiline, and diclofenac tend to form reactive arene oxide metabolic intermediates (Flora *et al.*, 1984; Elder *et al.*, 2010b; Snodin, 2010).
The metabolism of epoxides mainly involves epoxide hydrolase (EH) and glutathione *S*-transferase (GST), which leads to either detoxification or production of epoxides. These pathways play a key role in the genotoxic action of epoxides (Snodin, 2010).

3.4.1 Genotoxicity profile

As indicated in *in vitro* studies, epoxides are genotoxic in bacterial reverse mutation assays; however, other studies have shown different results. Hude *et al.* (1990) reported that 12/51 epoxides were nongenotoxic in the Ames *Salmonella* assay. In this study, 51 epoxides were assessed with the SOS-Chromo test using *Escherichia coli* PQ37 followed by a comparison with the results of the Ames test. All compounds were tested with and without S9 mixture up to cytotoxicity. In tests without S9 mixture the SOS-repair induction of each experiment was controlled by the response to 4-nitroquinoline-N-oxide, and in tests with S9 mixture, it was controlled with benzo[a]pyrene. In the Ames test, 20 epoxides were tested for mutagenic activity with the *Salmonella typhimurium* strains TA100, TA1535, TA98, and TA1537. By comparing the results of the Ames test and the SOS-Chromo test, it was found that among 51 epoxide-bearing chemicals 39 induced base-pair mutations in at least one Salmonella strain.
Wade *et al.* (1978) studied the mutagenicity of 17 aliphatic epoxides using the specially constructed mutants of *Salmonella typhimurium* that were developed by Ames. It was found that all the compounds in the study, with the exception of 2-methyl-3,3,3-trichloropropylene oxide, *cis-stilbene* oxide, and cyclohexene oxide that were mutagenic in strain TA100 were also mutagenic, but-with reduced sensitivity, in the second strain TA1535. However, none of the epoxides in this study were found to be mutagenic in strains TA1537 and TA98 which detect frame-shift mutagens. The results indicate that the monosubstituted epoxides are the most potent mutagens and that the addition of a single methyl group to the oxirane ring could reduce or eliminate mutagenicity.
Glatt *et al.* (1983) investigated 35 epoxides for mutagenicity, using reversion of his-*Salmonella typhimurium* TA98 and TA100 as the biological end-point. The results obtained were negative with the antibiotics oleandomycin, anticapsin and asperlin, the cardiotonic drug resibufogenin, the widely used parasympatholytic drugs butylscopolamine and scopolamine, the sedatives valtratum, didovaltratum and acevaltratum, the tranquilizer oxanamide as well as the drug metabolites carbamazepine 10,11-oxide and diethylstilbestrol α and β oxide. It was found that among the drugs and drug metabolites, only the cytostatic ethoglucide was markedly mutagenic. Three barbiturate epoxides showed very weak mutagenicity only at extremely high concentrations such that the effects were probably of low practical relevance.
Later, the role of metabolism was also examined. For example, *in vitro* studies in rat-liver S9 fractions which contain both microsomal and cytosolic detoxifying enzymes, such as EH and GST showed a decrease of bacterial genotoxicity (Flora *et al.*, 1984).
In vivo rodent bioassays on epoxides are not always positive and several epoxides are carcinogenic only at the point of administration. For example, it was found that when given by oral gavage, both ethylene oxide and propylene oxide caused late-onset tumors only in the rat fore-stomach. Again, when administered by inhalation, propylene oxide is a nasal carcinogen. On the other hand, *in vivo* studies in rat have shown that carbamazepine-10, 11-

epoxide have the potential to initiate cellular damage if not adequately detoxified via conjugation with glutathione (Snodin, 2010).

It was observed that owing to the role of metabolism, epoxides that are formed *in vivo*, such as those generated by epoxidation of alkenes and arenes, have a greater potential to cause adverse effects than preformed epoxides. This is because they are often produced at close proximity to their site of action and can thus reach their target quite readily. Therefore, this mechanism can explain the limited evidence of animal carcinogenicity tests for some epoxide compounds (Flora *et al.*, 1984).

3.5 Aromatic compounds

Aromatic compounds involve various impurities; some impurities, such as fentanyl impurities, tremogenic impurities, p-nitrophenol (PNP) that have aromatic structure and aromatic amines will be discussed in this section.

3.5.1 Aromatic amines

Primary and secondary aromatic amines (generally after metabolism) generate an electrophilic species and thus produce a positive result in the Ames test when S9 mixture exists. 2, 4-Diaminotoluene, 2, 4-diaminoethylbenzene and a few amines containing a nitro-group are direct mutagens. According to the *in vivo* carcinogenicity test, Ames positive compounds produce positive results, although *p*-anisidine and *p*-chloroaniline are noncarcinogenic in rodent bioassays (Snodin, 2010).

3.5.2 p-Nitrophenol

This synthetic chemical possesses fungicidal activity and is used as a starting material for the synthesis of some drugs. PNP and other substituted nitro benzenes after reduction produce arylhydroxylamines or hydroxamic esters which contain electrophilic nitrogen atoms. Thus, the electrophilic atoms might show genotoxic property for these compounds (Eichenbaum *et al.*, 2009).

It should be mentioned that negative results were obtained for Ames tests with the various strains of *Salmonella typhimurium* in the absence and presence of metabolic activation with rat liver S9. Another *in vitro* test, the hprt mutation test in Chinese hamster ovary (CHO) cells presented the same result as the Ames test for PNP. However, it was seen that PNP could induce chromosomal aberrations in mammalian cells, particularly in the presence of metabolic activation. Also, PNP was negative in the bone marrow micronucleus assay in mice at doses ranging from little toxicity to the maximum tolerated dose. In addition, PNP was cytotoxic to the bone marrow of male mice at tested doses (Eichenbaum *et al.*, 2009).

3.5.3 Fentanyl impurities

The forced degradation of fentanyl produced seven aromatic degradants. Among these, propionanilide (PRP), N-phenyl-1-(2-phenylethyl)-piperidin-4-amine (PPA), 1-phenethyl-1H-pyridin-2-one (1-PPO), fentanyl N-oxide, and 1-styryl-1H-pyridin-2-one (1-SPO) possibly indicate safety concerns. PPA was suggested as a potential genotoxic compound and the DNA damage in unscheduled DNA synthesis (UDS); the results were positive for PRP when *in vitro* rat hepatocytes were checked. In the ACD/Tox suite, 1-PPO and 1-SPO were identified as Ames hazards. These compounds were also predicted to have higher probabilities of being Ames positive (Garg *et al.*, 2010).

3.5.4 Tremogenic impurities

Tremogenic impurities comprise another sub-class of highly toxic impurities in APIs. Two pharmacopoeial APIs are known to have the potential to be contaminated with tremogenic impurities; pethidine and paroxetine (3-[(1, 3-benzodioxol-5-yloxy) methyl]-4-(4-fluorophenyl) piperidine). Pethidine can contain trace amounts of 1-methyl-4- phenyl-1, 2, 3, 6-tetrahydropyridine (MPTP) derived from the hydrolytic degradation of side chain. 4-(4-Fluorophenyl)-1-methyl-1,2,3,6-tetrahydropyridine (FMTP) can be a potential reactant/intermediate in the synthesis of paroxetine. Owing to their toxicity to cells in the *Substantia nigra,* these highly potent impurities can induce Parkinsonism in humans. Thus, these compounds are known toxic impurities; however their genotoxicity remains unclear (Borman *et al.,* 2008).

3.6 β-lactam related impurities

The following two impurities relate to the well known antibiotics cefotaxime and piperacillin.

3.6.1 Dimeric impurity of cefotaxime

The manufacturing and storage processes of cefotaxime produce various impurities such as dimeric impurity (Figure 2).

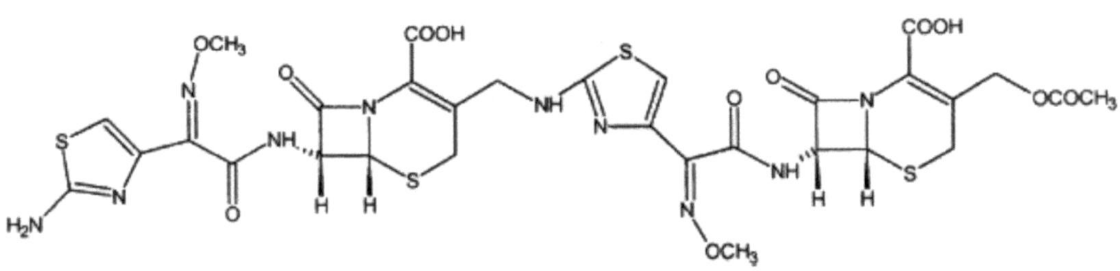

Fig. 2. Structure of the dimeric impurity of cefotaxime

The results of the mutagenesis assay indicate that the dimeric impurity is nonmutagenic to any test strains used in the presence and absence of S9 fraction. The results of the *in vitro* chromosomal assay show some chromosomal aberrations in cultured mammalian cells up to the maximum recommended concentration of 45 mg per culture, and no clastogenicity in mammalian cells *in vitro* (Agarwal *et al.,* 2004).

3.6.2 Piperacillin impurity-A

The piperacillin impurity-A is a prominent degradation product of piperacillin that appears during manufacturing and storage processes (Figure 3).

In all the strains of *S. typhimurium;* TA 97a, TA 98, TA 100, TA 102, and TA 1535, piperacillin impurity in the presence and absence of metabolic activation was found to be non-mutagenic. Also, *in vitro* chromosomal aberration assay did not reveal any significant alterations. It is found that piperacillin impurity-A up to 5 mg/ml is nonclastogenic to CHO cell lines in the presence and absence of metabolic activation (Vijayan *et al.,* 2007).

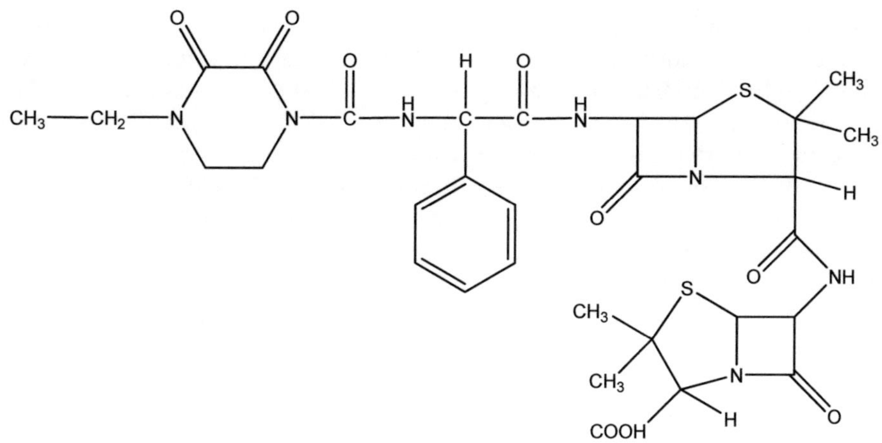

Fig. 3. Structure of piperacillin impurity-A

4. Analytical approaches

As discussed above, GIs possess unwanted effects and their contamination levels should be controlled. To achieve this, pharmaceutical R&D should employ robust and sensitive analytical methods for supporting drug development and monitoring the levels of GIs. In addition, analytical methods that are capable of measuring trace GIs must be employed to monitor the outcome of GIs during chemical synthesis. In recent years, manufacturers have developed sensitive methods for analyzing various GIs. In this context, conventional HPLC/UV methods are the first option for GIs analysis; however, these methods are often inadequate for the accurate determination of analytes at trace levels, depending on the properties of the analytes and sample matrices. Some of the challenges in the analytical determination of GIs in pharmaceuticals at trace levels include the diverse structural types of GIs, the unstable or chemically reactive nature of GIs, and an extremely high level of API as contaminant (Bai *et al.*, 2010; Liu *et al.*, 2010).

4.1 HPLC methods

In general, non-volatile GIs are analyzed by HPLC separation techniques, among which reversed phase HPLC (RPLC) is the most widely used separation mode (Elder *et al.*, 2008a; Liu *et al.*, 2010). A simple isocratic RPLC method has been employed for the determination of four genotoxic alkyl benzenesulfonates (ABSs) viz. methyl, ethyl, *n*-propyl, and *iso*propyl benzenesulfonates (MBS, EBS, NPBS, and IPBS) in amlodipine besylate (ADB). The RPLC is also applicable for sulfonate impurities with phenyl moiety such as methyl (MTs), ethyl (ETs) and *iso*propyl tosylates (ITs), methyl (MBs), ethyl (EBs), butyl (BBs) and isopropyl besylates (IBs) (Raman *et al.*, 2008).

Epoxides/hydroperoxides were analyzed using HPLC, and simple RPLC methods employing direct analysis (no sample preparation) were used for some of them. Yasueda *et al.* (2004) described an HPLC method for the determination of loteprednol impurities including a minor photolytic epoxide degradation product. Lacroix *et al.* (1992) reported an HPLC method for the determination of related substances, including the epoxide impurity of nadalol. A rapid resolution HPLC method was used for separating and quantifying the related impurities of atorvastatin, including two epoxide impurities atorvastatin epoxy dihydroxy and atorvastatin epoxy diketone. The limit of detection (LOD) and limit of quantitation (LOQ) for atorvastatin epoxy dihydroxy and atorvastatin epoxy diketone were 0.025 and 0.075 g/ml, and 0.026 and 0.077 g/ml, respectively (Petkovska *et al.*, 2008). Kong *et al.* (2001) determined two epoxide terpenoid impurities (actein and 27-deoxyactein) in a traditional Chinese herbal preparation (*Cimicifuga foetida* L.). Subsequently, they compared the HPLC results with evaporative light scattering detection (ELSD) with UV detection and found that the ELSD was significantly more sensitive. Sample pretreatment was performed prior to analysis owing to the complexity of the matrix. For the two epoxides the on-column sensitivity using UV detection was found to be 606 and 880 ng, respectively, whereas the sensitivity using ELSD was 40 and 33 ng, respectively. Using the optimized extraction procedure (methanol/water, 80/20 v/v) the levels of the two analytes were detected to be 3.44±0.02% and 1.42±0.01%, respectively.

A more common method for the analysis of alkylating impurities is by RPLC and MS detection; however, HPLC/UV methods are also carried out successfully for alkylating impurities. Valvo *et al.* (1997) reported an HPLC/UV method for the separation of 13 impurities of verapamil; this method is claimed to be superior to both the existing pharmacopoeial methods for verapamil. Using this method, the LOD and LOQ were found to be 0.01% (0.05 μg/ml) and 0.02% (1.0 μg/ml), respectively. Also, the method was found to be sensitive to pH and mobile phase composition; however, it was in contrast to the findings of previous studies insensitive to stationary phase changes.

Hydrophilic interaction liquid chromatography (HILIC) seems complementary to RPLC for the retention and separation of small molecule polar analytes, and has thus gained increasing attention recently. Good retention can be achieved for more polar analytes, which is not possible on RPLC columns. In the hydrazine group, the HILIC method was used in addition to the HPLC/UV and HPLC/MS methods (Elder *et al.*, 2010c; Liu *et al.*, 2010). An Indian research group reported the development and validation of a stability indicating HPLC method for the determination of the anti-tuberculosis drug, rizatriptan, and its degradation products, including a hydrazone impurity (Rao *et al.*, 2006). Hmelnickis *et al.* (2008) used an HILIC method with different polar stationary phases (silica, cyano, amino, and the zwitterionic sulfobetaine) to separate six polar impurities, including 1,1,1-trimethylhydrazinium bromide, and demonstrated that HILIC was a useful alternative to reverse phase or ion chromatography (IC). Elder *et al.* (2010c) reported a table summarizing the various HPLC methods that were used in the literature for a wide range of drugs (Table 4).

Active Potential Ingredient (API)	**Impurities**	**Method details**
Allopurinol	Hydrazine	Derivatization using benzaldehyde, followed by LLE. HPLC with a 5 μm cyanosilyl stationary phase (R type) at 30 °C. Mobile phase: 2-propanol/hexane (5/95, v/v). Flow rate 1. 5 ml/min; detection at 310 nm.
API (general method)	Hydrazine	HPLC with (1) 5 μm ZIC HILIC (SeQuant), (2) 5 μm Develosil 100 Diol-5(Nomura), (3) 5 μm TSK-Gel Amide-80 (Tosoh Bioscience) and (4) 5 μm Zorbax NH_2 (Agilent) at different column temperatures (10–60 °C). Mobile phase: TFA/water/ethanol (0.1/30/70, v/v). Flow rate 0.4 ml/min; CLND detection.

Active Potential Ingredient (API)	Impurities	Method details
API (general method)	Hydrazine	(1) Derivatization using benzaldehyde. HPLC with no operating conditions reported. (2) LSE, followed by derivatization using benzaldehyde at lower temperatures. HPLC with no operating conditions reported. Detection at 190 nm.
Azelastine	Impurity A: benzohydrazide, impurity B: 1-benzoyl-2-[(4RS)-1-methylhexahydro-1Hazepin-4yl] diazane	HPLC with a 10µm cyanosilyl stationary phase (R) at 30°C. Mobile phase: pH 3.0 phosphate buffer and sodium octane sulphonic acid in water/acetonitrile (740/260, v/v). Flow rate 2.0 ml/min; detection at 210 nm.
Aryl hydrazones	E-Aryl hydrazones	HPLC with a 5 µm ODS stationary phase (Merck LiChrospher) at 25°C. Mobile phase: 1mM pH 6.0 phosphate buffer with 2 mM EDTA and methanol (40/60, v/v). Flow rate 1.0 ml/min; detection at 200–400 nm (DAD). HPLC with a 5 µm phenyl hexyl stationary phase (Phenomenex Luna) at 25 °C. Mobile phase: water and acetonitrile (50/50, v/v). Flow rate 0.3 ml/min. Positive and negative ion mode ESI with ion trap analyzer in SIM mode (M + H ion). Range 50–1000 m/z. Voltage 4 kV, capillary temperature 250 °C.
Carbidopa	Hydrazine	Derivatization using benzaldehyde, followed by LLE. HPLC with a 5µm ODS stationary phase (Altima C18 or Hypersil ODS). Mobile phase: aqueous 0.03% EDTA and acetonitrile (300/700, v/v). Flow rate 1.0 ml/min; detection at 305 nm.
Celecoxib	Intermediate I: 4-hydrazine benzene sulphonamide	HPLC with a 4 µm ODS stationary phase (NovapaK C18). Mobile phase: pH 4.8 10mM phosphate buffer and acetonitrile (450/550, v/v). Flow rate 1.0 ml/min; detection at 252 nm.
Copovidone	Hydrazine	Derivatization using benzaldehyde, followed by LLE. HPLC with a 5µm ODS stationary phase (Altima C18 or Hypersil ODS). Mobile phase: aqueous 0.03% EDTA and acetonitrile (300/700, v/v). Flow rate 1.0 ml/min; detection at 305 nm.
Dihydralazine sulphate	Hydrazine (impurity B)	Derivatization using benzaldehyde, followed by LLE. HPLC with a 5µm ODS stationary phase (R type). Mobile phase: aqueous 0.03% EDTA and acetonitrile (300/700, v/v). Flow rate 1.0 ml/min; detection at 305 nm.

Active Potential Ingredient (API)	Impurities	Method details
Ebifuramin	Impurity III: (+)-5-morpholino methyl-3-(5-nitrofurfurylidene amino)-oxazolidin-2-one	HPLC with a 5μm ODS stationary phase (Hypersil ODS). Mobile phase: acetonitrile/THF/pH 2.6 10mM dibutyl aminephosphate (15/5/80, v/v/v). Flow rate 1.5 ml/min; detection at 254 nm.
Hydralazine	Hydrazine	Derivatization using benzaldehyde, followed by LLE. HPLC with a 5 μm ODS stationary phase (Altima C18 or Hypersil ODS). Mobile phase aqueous 0.03% EDTA and acetonitrile (300/700, v/v). Flow rate 1.0 ml/min; detection at 305 nm.
Hydralazine tablets	Hydralazine hydrazone	HPLC with a 10μm ODS stationary phase (Waters μBondapak) at room temperature. Mobile phase: acetonitrile/5 mM SDS/phosphoric acid (150/850/0.45, v/v/v). Flow rate 2.0 ml/min; detection at 220 nm.
Isoniazid	Impurity I: 1-nicotinyl-2- lactosyl hydrazine	HPLC with a 10 μm cyanopropyl stationary phase and a mobile phase consisting of a mixture of pH 3.5 10 mM acetate buffer and acetonitrile (95/5, v/v). Flow rate and detection wavelength not specified.
Isoniazid	Hydrazine (I), isonictonic acid-N´-(pyridyl-4-carbonyl) hydrazide (II), isonictonic acid-pyridine-4-ylmethylene hydrazide (III), isonictonic acid ethylidene hydrazide) (IV)	HPLC with a 5μm ODS stationary phase (Zorbax XDB Eclipse C18). Mobile phase water and acetonitrile (960/40, v/v). Flow rate 0.5 ml/min; detection at 252 nm.
Isoniazid	Hydrazine	HPLC-MS using negative electrospray ionization ESI with a Bruker Daltonics ToF. TLC with a silica gel F_{254} TLC plate with a water/acetone/methanol/ethylacetate (10/20/20/50, v/v) mobile phase. Visualization using dimethyl aminobenzaldehyde solution; examination under daylight.
Mildronate	Impurity 2: 1,1,1-trimethyl hydrazinium bromide	HILIC with a 3 μm silica stationary phase (Atlantis HILIC silica, Alltima HP silica, and Spherisorb silica), 5 μm cyano stationary phase (Discovery cyano), 3 μm amino stationary phase (Hypersil APS-1), and 5 μm sulfobetaine stationary phase (ZIC-HILIC) at 30 °C. Mobile phase acetonitrile and 0.1% formic acid in water. Flow rate 0.2 ml/min with positive ion mode ESI detection at 20–35 kV using a triple quadra pole MS.

Active Potential Ingredient (API)	Impurities	Method details
Nitrofural, nitrofurazone and nitrofuroxazide	Hydrazine	Derivatization using benzaldehyde, followed by LLE. HPLC with a 5μm ODS stationary phase (Altima C18 or Hypersil ODS). Mobile phase aqueous 0.03% EDTA and acetonitrile (300/700, v/v). Flow rate 1.0 ml/min; detection at 305 nm.
Nitrofurazone	Impurity A: Bis-[(5-nitrofuran-2- yl) methylene] diazane	HPLC with a 5 μm ODS stationary phase (R type). Mobile phase acetonitrile/water (400/600, v/v). Flow rate 1.0 ml/min; detection at 310 nm.
Povidone	Hydrazine	Derivatization using benzaldehyde, followed by LLE. HPLC with a 5 μm ODS stationary phase (Altima C18, Hypersil ODS). Mobile phase aqueous 0.03% EDTA and acetonitrile (300/700, v/v). Flow rate 1.0 ml/min; detection at 305 nm.
Pyridoxal isonicotinoyl hydrazone	Hydrazine, isoniazid	HPLC with 5 μm ODS (Nucleosil C18) and an isocratic mobile phase consisting of a mixture of methanol (A) and pH 3.0 10 mM phosphate buffer containing 5 mM 1-heptane sulphonic acid and 2 mM EDTA (B) in a ratio of 49/51, v/v. Flow rate 0.9 ml/min; detection at 297 and 254 nm.
Rifampicin	Hydrazones: rifampicin quinone and 25-desacetyl rifampicin	HPTLC with a silica gel 60 TLC plate (Merck) with a chloroform/methanol/water (80/20/2.5, v/v/v) mobile phase. Examined using Scanner II (Camag) at 330nm for 25-desacetyl rifampicin and 490 nm for rifampicin quinone.
Rifampicin	Hydrazones: rifampicin quinone	HPLC with 10 μm silyl and 10μm nitrile stationary phases (Micro Pak Si-10 and MicroPak CN, respectively) and anisocratic mobile phase consisting of a mixture of chloroform and methanol of varying proportions. Flow rate 0.2–0.7 ml/min; detection at 334 nm.
Rifampicin	Hydrazones: rifampicin quinone, 25-desacetyl-21-acetyl-rifampicin, 25-desacetyl-23-acetyl-rifampicin	HPLC with direct injection (DI) onto a 3 μm ODS stationary phase (Hypersil ODS) at 25 °C and an isocratic mobile phase consisting of a mixture of pH 7.4 50 mM phosphate buffer and acetonitrile (64/36, v/v). Flow rate 1.4 ml/min; detection at 240 nm. Alternatively, a 10 μm ODS stationary phase (Hypersil ODS)
Rifampicin, isoniazid, pyrazinamide FDC	Hydrazones: rifampicin quinone, desacetyl rifampicin, isonicotinyl hydrazone	HPLC with a 5 μm L1 ODS stationary phase at 25 °C and a gradient mobile phase consisting of varying mixtures of mobile phase A (pH 6.8 phosphate buffer/acetonitrile, 96/4, v/v) and mobile phase B (pH 6.8 phosphate buffer/acetonitrile, 45/55, v/v or 55/45, v/v). Flow rate 1.5 or 1.0 ml/min; detection at 238 nm. Three L1 columns were evaluated: 1: Zorbax XDB, 2: Shim-pak CLC ODS and 3. Nucleosil EC 120-5.

Active Potential Ingredient (API)	Impurities	Method details
Rizatriptan	Impurity I: 1-(4-hydrazinophenyl) methyl-1,2,3-triazole	HPLC with a 5 μm nitrile stationary phase (Zorbax SB-CN) at 25 °C and a gradient mobile phase consisting of varying mixtures of pH 3.4 10 mM phosphate buffer, acetonitrile, and methanol. Flow rate 1.0 ml/min; detection at 225 nm.
Vindesine sulphate	Impurity C (desacetyl vinblastine hydrazide)	HPLC with a 5 μm ODS stationary phase (R type) and a gradient mobile phase consisting of varying mixtures of pH 7.5 diethyl aminephosphate buffer and methanol. Flow rate 2.0 ml/min; detection at 270 nm.

Table 4. Various HPLC methods used for a wide range of drugs; Abbreviations: DAD: diode array detection; EC: electrochemical detection; ESI: electrospray ionization; FDC: Fixed Dose Combination; HILIC: hydrophobic interaction liquid chromatography; LLE: liquid liquid extraction; LSE: liquid solid extraction; MS: mass spectroscopy; ODS: octadecyl silyl; SDS: sodium dodecyl sulphate; SIM: single ion monitoring; ToF: time of flight (Elder *et al.*, 2010c).

The use of water as sample diluent could pose a limitation for this separation technique, especially when high water content is required for dissolving the drug substance or the formulated drug product (Liu *et al.*, 2010).

4.2 GC methods

GC methods are commonly used for the analysis of several volatile small molecule GIs. Some examples include the liquid injection technique and the headspace sampling technique. Liquid injection is prone to contamination in which injection of a large amount of non-volatile API can accumulate in the injector liner or on the head of the GC column, which can cause a sudden deterioration in method performance. Headspace injection, on the other hand, is desirable because it minimizes potential contamination of the injector or column by avoiding the introduction of a large quantity of API (Liu *et al.*, 2010).

David *et al.* (2010) proposed a method selection chart (Figure 4) containing GC or LC methods, both in combination with a single quadrupole mass spectrometer as detector. These methods applied for a wide range of analytes including sulphonates, alkyl halides, and epoxides.

Nassar *et al.* (2009) developed a GC/MS method for residual levels of EMS in a mesylate salt of an API crystallized from ethanol. The method was capable of detecting EMS down to levels of 50-200 ppb. Subsequently, extraction techniques were developed for eliminating or reducing matrix related interference. Thus, Colon and Richoll (2005) surveyed liquid–liquid extraction (LLE), liquid phase micro-extraction (LPME), solid phase extraction (SPE), and solid phase micro-extraction (SPME) coupled with GC/MS and single ion-monitoring (SIM). Using these approaches, they developed limit tests (5 ppm) for some alkyl aryl esters of sulfonic acids.

Similar attempts were made for reducing or eliminating the matrix effect for alkylating agents as well. In all these procedures, a specific physical property of the analyte not shared by the matrix was utilized, e.g. low boiling point and/or in the presence of halide atom (Elder *et al.*, 2008a).

GC methods were rarely used for the analysis of epoxides/hydroperoxides, as compared to other impurities, owing to the size of molecule and the volatility properties within this group (Elder et al., 2010b). Klick (1995) used a GC method for the determination of residual levels of a chlorohydrin and the corresponding epoxide impurities in almokalant. Other literatures give an account of GC–MS methods for the analysis of volatile components in traditional Chinese herbal medicines (Yu *et al.*, 2007; Guo *et al.*, 2003).

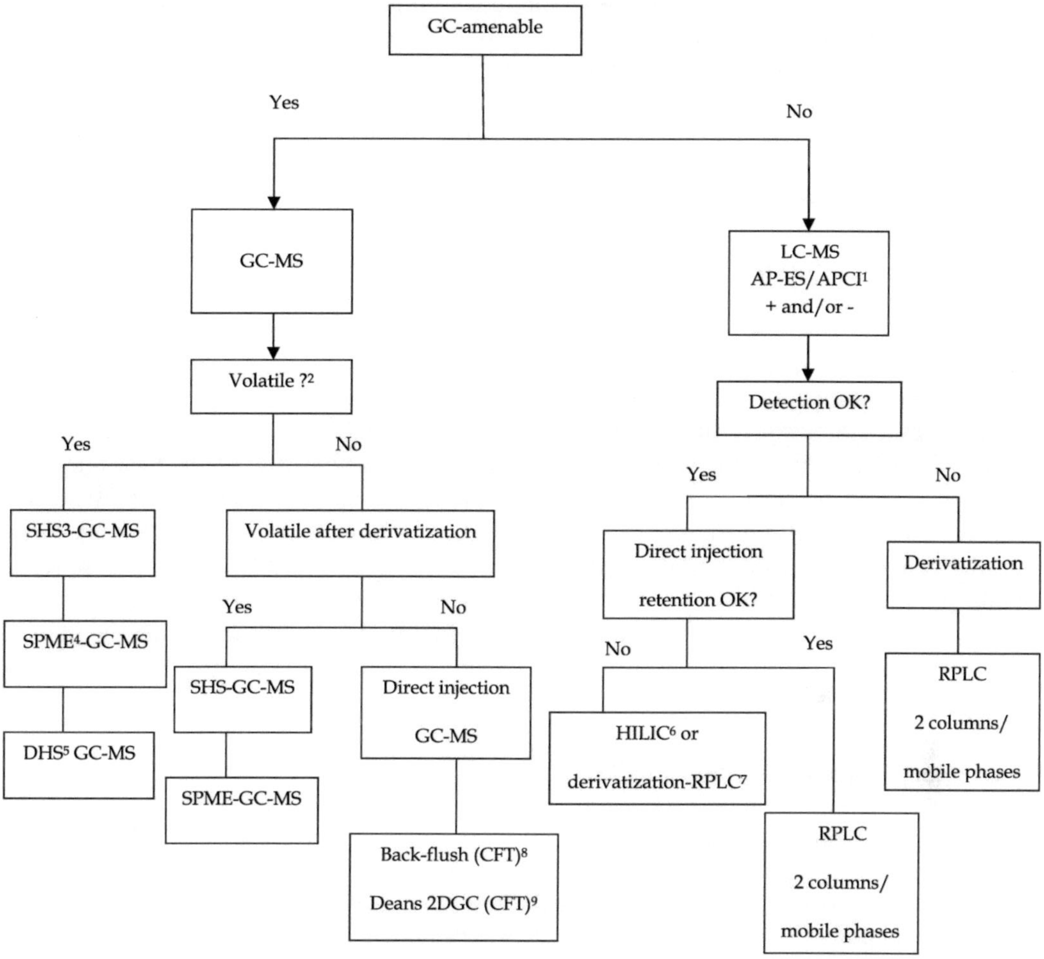

Fig. 4. Method selection chart for analyzing genotoxic impurities with GC/LC; [1]AP-ES/APCI: atmospheric pressure electrospray ionization/ atmospheric pressure chemical ionization; [2] If the analyte has sufficient vapor pressure in water or other low volatile solvent; [3] SHS: static headspace; [4] SPME: solid-phase micro-extraction; [5] DHS: dynamic headspace; [6] HILIC: hydrophobic interaction liquid chromatography; [7] derivatization-RPLC: reversed phase HPLC with precolumn derivatization; [8] Back-flush (CFT): capillary flow technology based back-flushing; [9] Deans 2DGC (CFT): capillary flow technology based two-dimensional GC (Figure is reproduced from David *et al.*, 2010).

For the hydrazine group the normal flame ionization detection (FID) in GC analysis is not appropriate because these compounds possess no carbon atoms (Elder *et al.*, 2010c). A GC procedure involving the formation of a benzalazine derivative was developed for monitoring the residual levels of hydrazine in hydralazine and isoniazid APIs, tablets, combined tablets, syrups, and injectable products in which nitrogen selective detection was used (Matsui *et al.*, 1983).

In addition, Carlin *et al.* (1998) adapted a previously published method for monitoring a benzalazine derivative using GC with electron capture (EC) detection. The LOQ was 10 ppm and the method was linear over the range of 10-100 ppm. The inter-day residual standard deviation (RSD) based on six measurements at analyte levels of 10 ppm was 15%; however, this improved slightly at increased analyte concentrations of 25 and 100 ppm, to 9.5% and 11.3%, respectively.

Nevertheless, non-volatile API does not partition into the headspace and therefore does not enter the GC system; as a result, headspace injection becomes the preferred choice whenever possible (Liu *et al.*, 2010).

4.3 TLC/HPTLC methods

In general practice, thin layer chromatography (TLC) is not preferred for the accurate determination of very low residual analyte level. However, this technique is still used for the determination of related substances in the pharmacopoeial monographs for amiodarone, bromazepam, carmustine, ifosamide, indoramin, and tolnaftate (Elder *et al.*, 2008).

Nevertheless, there are several examples of its use in association with determining levels of the epoxyl alkaloid, including scopolamine in extracts of *Datura stramonium*. Sass and Stutz (1981) used TLC to determine residual sulfur and nitrogen mustards (beta haloethyl compounds) in a variety of substrates in which the sensitivities in the microgram range were typically achievable. High performance thin layer chromatography (HPTLC) was used for monitoring the degradation products of rifampicin, including the hydrazones (25-desacetyl rifampicin (DAR)) and rifampicin quinone (RQU). Finally, it was concluded that the method is suitable for routine quality control and stability analyses, especially in the developing world (Jindal *et al.* 1994).

4.4 Capillary electrophoresis methods

Jouyban and Kenndler (2008) reviewed the applicability of capillary electrophoresis (CE) methods for the analysis of pharmaceutical impurities. In addition, they discussed the applications of these methods in various groups of compounds such as chemotherapeutic agents, central nervous system (CNS) drugs, histamine receptor and cardiovascular drugs.

The main advantage of CE techniques is their selectivity; thus, they are suitable for the analysis of complex herbal products. Bempong *et al.* (1993) reported the separation of 13-cis and all-trans retinoic acid and their photo-degradation products (including all-trans-5, 6-epoxy retinoic acid, 13-cis-5, 6-epoxy retinoic acid) using both capillary zone electrophoresis (CZE) and micellar electrokinetic chromatography (MEKC) methods. A Chinese research group reported the development of CE methods for the simultaneous determination of some hydrazine related impurities (Liu *et al.*, 1996).

Hansen and Sheribah (2005) evaluated a series of electrically driven separation techniques: CZE, MEKC, and microemulsion electrokinetic chromatography (MEEKC) for the determination of residual alkylating impurities in bromazepam API. However, the poor sensitivity of the techniques posed a problem even when specialized detection cells (e.g. bubble or Z-cells) were used. Mahuzier *et al.* (2001) demonstrated the poor sensitivity of CE based methods, in comparison to other separation methods. The problem of limited sensitivity of CE methods can be solved either by the use of detection methods with sensitivity higher than UV absorption or by pre-concentration of the analytes (Jouyban and Kenndler, 2008).

4.5 Enhancing methods

Alternatively, the structure of the molecule as well as its properties can be altered to enhance detectability which in turn will help to achieve the desired sensitivity. This is especially true for GIs that lack structural features for sensitive detection (Bai *et al.*, 2010; Liu *et al.*, 2010). A number of general approaches could be considered, some of which are explained below:

4.5.1 Chemical derivatization

This method is generally used for stabilizing reactive GIs and for introducing a detection specific moiety for enhanced detection, i.e. chromophore for UV. Also, this method sometimes produces a single compound for several GIs; thus, it becomes non-specific which can be considered as an advantage in determining a group of structurally related compounds (Liu *et al.*, 2010). Bai *et al.* (2010) introduced a chemical derivatization method for analyzing two alkyl halides and one epoxide. The objective of the three derivatization reactions is to generate a strong basic center by introducing an amine functional group. All three derivatization products are good candidates for electrospray ionization (ESI)-MS owing to the high proton affinity or the permanent charge.

4.5.2 Coordination ion spray-MS

Owing to their structural features, several analytes are not amenable to atmospheric pressure ionization methods, such as the ESI method. Alkali metal ions such as Li^+, Na^+, and K^+ can form complexes with some organic molecules in the gas phase; this fact could be used as a solution for the analytes subjected previously (Liu *et al.*, 2010).

4.5.3 Matrix deactivation

The matrix deactivation approach is a chemical approach to stabilize unstable/reactive analytes. It is based upon the hypothesis that the instability of certain GIs at trace level is caused by the reaction between the analytes and reactive species in the sample matrix. Thus, controlling the reactivity of the reactive species in the sample matrix would stabilize the unstable/reactive GI analytes (Liu *et al.*, 2010).

As an example the alkylators are reactive unknown impurities which possess mainly nucleophilic characteristics. Their reactivity can be attenuated by either protonation or scavenging approaches. Sun *et al.* (2010) reported a matrix deactivation methodology for improving the stability of unstable and reactive GIs for their trace analysis. This approach appears to be commonly applicable to techniques like direct GC–MS and LC–MS analyses, or coupled with chemical derivatization as well.

5. Genotoxicity prediction

The concept of using structural alerts to predict potential genotoxic activity for identified impurities is now well established; however, the concordance between such alerts and biologically relevant genotoxic potential (in the context of genotoxic impurities) could be highly imperfect. Structural alerts are defined as molecular functionalities (structural features) that are known to cause toxicity, and their presence in a molecular structure alerts the investigator to the potential toxicities of the test chemical. Nevertheless, the assumption that any impurity with a structural alert is potentially DNA-reactive and thus subject to the default TTC limit may often lead to unnecessary restrictive limits. From a resource and time table viewpoint of a new drug production, the experimental determination of genotoxicity is not feasible for millions of drug candidates in the pharmaceutical industry. Thus, compounds identified as potential hazards by *in silico* methods would be high priority candidates for confirmatory laboratory testing (Kruhlak *et al.*, 2007; Snodin, 2010).

In silico toxicology is the application of computer technologies to analyze existing data, model, and predict the toxicological activity of a substance. In sequence, toxicologically based QSARs are mathematical equations used as a predictive technique to estimate the toxicity of new chemicals based upon a model of a training set of chemicals with known activity and a defined chemical space (Valerio, 2009).

Ashby and Tennant (1991) reported some correlations of electrophilicity with DNA reactivity (assessed by Ames-testing data) for about 300 chemicals and elucidated the concept of structural alerts for genotoxic activity in the 1980s/1990s. Using a database of >4000 compounds, Sawatari *et al.* (2001) determined correlations between 44 substructures and bacterial mutagenicity data. A high proportion of genotoxic compounds were found for electrophilic reagents such as epoxides (63 %), aromatic nitro compounds (49 %), and primary alkyl monohalides (46 %). In a retrospective analysis of starting materials and intermediates involved in API syntheses, the most common structurally alerting groups were found to be aromatic amines, aromatic nitros, alkylating agents and Michael acceptors (Snodin, 2010).

One of the strengths of QSAR models is that they contribute to a mechanistic understanding of the activity, and, at the same time, they constitute practical tools to predict the activity of further, untested chemicals solely based on chemical structure (Benigni *et al.*, 2005). Another strength of QSAR models is that they are strictly data-driven, and are not based on a prior hypotheses. On the other hand, high-quality experimental data must be used to build the training data set. As error (e.g. incorrect molecular structure or erroneous data from toxicology studies of a chemical) is introduced into the model, amplification of that error is generated and represented in the prediction (Benigni *et al.*, 2005; Valerio, 2009).

Cunningham *et al.* (1998) investigated a SAR analysis of the mouse subset of the carcinogenic potency database (CPDB) which also included chemicals tested by the US national toxicology program (NTP). This database consisted of 627 chemicals tested in mice for carcinogenic activity with the tumorigenicity data being standardized and reported as TD_{50} values. In addition, MULTICASE software (www.multicase.com) was used to identify several structural features that are not explained by an electrophilic mechanism and which may be indicative of non-genotoxic chemicals or mechanisms involved in carcinogenesis other than mutations. The prediction capabilities of the system for identifying carcinogens and noncarcinogens were 70 % and 78 % for a modified validation set.

Tafazoli *et al.* (1998) used the micronucleus (MN) test and the alkaline single cell gel electrophoresis (Comet) assay for analyzing potential mutagenicity, genotoxicty, and cytotoxicity of five chlorinated hydrocarbons. Using the generated data as well as the data of another five related chemicals that were investigated previously, a QSAR analysis was performed and the results indicated that LB_{C_Cl} (longest carbon-chlorine bond length), MR (molar refractivity), and E_{LUMO} (energy of the lowest unoccupied molecular orbital, indicating electrophilicity) were the most significant factors to be considered for discriminating between genotoxins and nongenotoxins.

Benigni *et al.* (2005) showed that the QSAR models could correctly predict-- based only on the knowledge of the chemical structure--the genotoxicity of simple and unsaturated aldehydes. The active and inactive compounds were separated based on the hydrophobicity (log P) and bulkiness (MR) properties.

Bercu *et al.* (2010) used *in silico* tools to predict the cancer potency (TD_{50}) of a compound based on its structure. SAR models (classification/regression) were developed from the carcinogenicity potency database using MULTICASE and VISDOM (a Lilly Inc. in-house software).

It is commonly accepted that the carcinogenicity of chemicals is owing to their genotoxicity and, in fact, the mutation and carcinogenesis data are practically coincident. Thus, the two endpoints were collapsed into one "genotoxicity" classification, in which QSAR analysis was applied. Now the question remains as to how to predict non-genotoxic carcinogenicity. In fact, it cannot be well approached until some mechanistic understanding of non-genotoxic carcinogenesis is achieved. At this time, this approach is unable to grasp the structural features of non-genotoxic carcinogens (Ashby, 1990; Cunningham *et al.*, 1998; Benigni *et al.*, 2005).

The other limitation to currently available QSARs is the lack of models for organometallics, complex mixtures (e.g. herbal extracts), and high molecular weight compounds such as polymers (Valerio, 2009). However, the QSAR predictive software offers a rapid, reliable, and cost effective method of identifying the potential risk of chemicals that are well represented in QSAR training data sets, even when experimental data are limited or lacking (Kruhlak *et al.*, 2007). These models should be further developed/validated by employing new mechanistic findings and using newly reported experimental data.

6. Conclusion

Since 2007, following the EMEA suspension of the marketing authorization of viracept (nelfinavir mesylate), genotoxic impurities have become a common issue for health concerns. Thus, regulatory agencies have made several attempts to construct a systematic method for controlling and analyzing GIs. However, several points must be considered for achieving a general view on the regulation of GIs.

One of the main problems is the very conservative limit regulated by agencies (1.5 μg/day). Bercu *et al.* (2009) calculated the permissible daily exposure (PDE) for EMS, which was the first GI of concern in 2007, as 0.104 mg/day. This value was found to be about 70-fold higher than the TTC level of 1.5 μg/day currently applied to EMS based on the generic linear back extrapolation model for genotoxins acting via non-threshold mechanisms. Other literatures highlighted this conservative limit as well (Gocke *et al.*, 2009b; Elder *et al.*, 2010a; Snodin, 2010). In addition, Gocke *et al.* (2009b) reported that the accidental exposure of viracept patients did not result in an increased likelihood for adverse genotoxic, teratogenic or cancerogenic effects.

In addition to the challenge of setting a more pragmatic limit for GIs, the development of extremely sensitive and robust analytical methods that can adequately monitor GIs at very low levels is very difficult. Also, the pharmaceutical industry has no long-term experience in the use of these methodologies within the factory setting. Thus, analysts make attempts to determine a way for analyzing various GIs by using unique robust methods as far as possible. In this way, simple HPLC/UV or GC/FID methods are usually performed at the first stage, while more complicated LC/MS or LC/MS/MS methods are used as alternatives (Dobo *et al.*, 2006; Elder *et al.*, 2008b; Liu *et al.*, 2010).

Teasdale *et al.* (2009) studied the formation of sulfonate esters as a mechanistic view, and showed that when a slight excess of base is present, there is no discernible reaction rate to form the sulfonate ester and no mechanistic pathway to their formation. From this point of view, the formation of GIs and suspicious substances in the API syntheses can be easily avoided, and therefore this is the preferred option (Robinson, 2010).

Finally, it can be mentioned that in such a situation, *in silico* approaches can prove to be a more effective solution in terms of time and cost for screening genotoxic compounds. As subjected by Luis and Valerio (2009), high-quality experimental data must be used. In addition, for non-genotoxic carcinogens, QSAR studies can provide a better understanding about the mechanism of carcinogenesis of these compounds. The in silico methods used in agencies have not been specified yet; however, by overcoming the limits these can become an innate part of regulatory systems.

7. Acknowledgment

This work is dedicated to Professor Hassan Mohseni, Tabriz University of Medical Sciences, Tabriz, Iran, for his enduring efforts in training toxicology in Iran.

8. References

Agency for Toxic Substance and Disease Registry. (1997). Toxicological profile for hydrazines, In: *Agency for Toxic Substances and Disease Registery,* 11 Feb, 2011, Available from: <http://www.atsdr.cdc.gov/toxprofiles/tp100.html.>

Agarwal, S. K., Bhatnagar, U. & Rajesh, N. (2004). Acute and genotoxic profile of a dimeric impurity of cefotaxime. *International Journal of Toxicology,*Vol.23, pp. 41-45.

Ashby, J. (1990). Determination of the genotoxic status of a chemical. *Mutation Research,*Vol. 248, pp. 221-231.

Ashby, J. & Tennant, R. W. (1991). Definitive relationships among chemical structure, carcinogenicity and mutagenicity for 301 chemicals tested by the U.S. NTP. *Mutation Research,* Vol. 257, pp. 229-306.

Bai, L., Sun, M., An, J., Liu, D. Q., Chen, T. K. & Kord, A. S. (2010). Enhancing the detection sensitivity of trace analysis of pharmaceutical genotoxic impurities by chemical derivatization and coordination ion spray-mass spectrometry. *Journal of Chromatography A,*Vol. 1217, pp. 302-306.

Bempong, D. K., Honigberg, I. L. & Meltzero, N. M. (1993). Separation of 13-cis and all-trans retinoic acid and their photodegradation products using capillary zone electrophoresis and micellar electrokinetic chromatography (MEC). *Journal of Pharmaceutical and Biomedical Analysis,* Vol. 11, No. 9, pp. 829-833.

Benigni, R., Conti, L., Crebelli, R., Rodomonte, A. & Vari, M. R. (2005). Simple and a,b-unsaturated aldehydes: correct prediction of genotoxic activity through structure-activity relationship models. *Environmental and Molecular Mutagenesis,* Vol. 46, pp. 268-280.

Bercu, J. P., Morton, S. M., Deahl, J. T., Gombar, V. K., Callis, C. M. & Van Lier, R. B. L. (2010). In silico approaches to predicting cancer potency for risk assessment of genotoxic impurities in drug substances. *Regulatory Toxicology and Pharmacology,* Vol. 57, pp. 300-306.

Bercu, J. P., Dobo, K. L., Gocke E. & McGovern, T. J. (2009). Overview of genotoxic impurities in pharmaceutical development. *International Journal of Toxicology,* Vol. 28, pp. 468-478.

Borman, P. J., Chatfield, M. J., Crowley, E. L., Eckers, C., Elder, D. P., Francey, S. W., Laures, A. M. F. & Wolf, J. C. (2008). Development, validation and transfer into a factory environment of a liquid chromatography tandem mass spectrometry assay for the highly neurotoxic impurity FMTP (4-(4 fluorophenyl)-1-methyl-1,2,3,6-tetrahydropyridine) in paroxetine active pharmaceutical ingredient (API). *Journal of Pharmaceutical and Biomedical Analysis,*Vol. 48, pp. 1082–1089.

Carlin, A., Gregory, N. & Simmons, J. (1998). Stability of isoniazid in isoniazid syrup: formation of hydrazine. *Journal of Pharmaceutical and Biomedical Analysis,* Vol. 17, pp. 885–890.

Cimarosti, Z., Bravo, F., Stonestreet, P., Tinazzi, F., Vecchi, O. & Camurri, G. (2010). Application of quality by design principles to support development of a control strategy for the control of genotoxic impurities in the manufacturing process of a drug substance. *Organic Process Research and Development,* Vol. 14, pp. 993-998.

Col´on, I. & Richoll, S. M. (2005). Determination of methyl and ethyl esters of methanesulfonic, benzenesulfonic and *p*-toluenesulfonic acids in active pharmaceutical ingredients by solid-phase microextraction (SPME) coupled to GC/SIM-MS. *Journal of Pharmaceutical and Biomedical Analysis,* Vol. 39, pp. 477–485.

Cunningham, A. R., Rosenkranz, H. S., Zhang, Y. P. & Klopman, G. (1998). Identification of 'genotoxic' and 'non-genotoxic' alerts for cancer in mice: the carcinogenic potency database. *Mutation Research,* Vol. 398, pp. 1–17.

David, F., Jacq, K., Sandra, P., Baker, A. & Klee, M. S. (2010). Analysis of potential genotoxic impurities in pharmaceuticals by two-dimensional gas chromatography with Deans switching and independent column temperature control using a low-thermal-mass oven module. *Analytical and Bioanalytical Chemistry,* Vol. 396, pp. 1291-1300.

Dearfield, K. L., Cimino, M. C., McCarroll, N. E., Mauer, I. & Valcovic, L. R. (2002). Genotoxicity risk assessment: a proposed classification strategy. *Mutation Research - Genetic Toxicology and Environmental Mutagenesis,* Vol. 521, pp. 121–135.

Dobo, K. L., Greene, N., Cyr, M. O., Caron, S. & Ku, W. W. (2006). The application of structure-based assessment to support safety and chemistry diligence to manage genotoxic impurities in active pharmaceutical ingredients during drug development. *Regulatory Toxicology and Pharmacology,* Vol. 44, pp. 282-293.

Eichenbaum, G., Johnson, M., Kirkland, D., O'Neill, P., Stellar, S., Bielawne, J., DeWire, R. & Areia, D. (2009). Assessment of the genotoxic and carcinogenic risks of p-nitrophenol when it is present as an impurity in a drug product. *Regulatory Toxicology and Pharmacology,* Vol. 55, pp. 33-42.

Elder, D. P., Delaney, E., Teasdale, A., Eyley, S., Reif, V. D., Jacq, K., Facchine, K. L., Oestrich, R. S., Sandra, P. & David, F. (2010a). The utility of sulfonate salts in drug development. *Journal of Pharmaceutical Sciences*, Vol. 99, pp. 2948-2961.

Elder, D. P., Snodin D., & Teasdale, A. (2010b). Analytical approaches for the detection of epoxides and hydroperoxides in active pharmaceutical ingredients, drug products and herbals. *Journal of Pharmaceutical and Biomedical Analysis*, Vol. 51, pp. 1015-1023.

Elder, D. P., Snodin, D. & Teasdale, A. (2010c). Control and analysis of hydrazine, hydrazides and hydrazones-Genotoxic impurities in active pharmaceutical ingredients (APIs) and drug products. *Journal of Pharmaceutical and Biomedical Analysis* .

Elder, D. P. & Snodin, D. J. (2009). Drug substances presented as sulfonic acid salts: Overview of utility, safety and regulation. *Journal of Pharmacy and Pharmacology,*Vol. 61, pp. 269-278.

Elder, D. P., Lipczynski, A. M., & Teasdale, A. (2008a). Control and analysis of alkyl and benzyl halides and other related reactive organohalides as potential genotoxic impurities in active pharmaceutical ingredients (APIs). *Journal of Pharmaceutical and Biomedical Analysis*, Vol. 48, pp. 497-507.

Elder, D. P., Teasdale, A. & Lipczinsky, A. M. (2008b). Control and analysis of alkyl esters of alkyl and aryl sulfonic acids in novel active pharmaceutical ingredients (APIs). *Journal of Pharmaceutical and Biomedical Analysis,* Vol. 46, pp. 1-8.

EMEA/CHMP. (June 2006). Guideline on the limits of genotoxic impurities, In: *European Medicines Agency,* 20 January 2011, Available from: <http://www.emea.eu.int.>

Flora, S. D., Zanacchi, P., Camoirano, A., Bennicelli, C. & Badolati, G. S. (1984). Genotoxic activity and potency of 135 compounds in the Ames reversion test and in a bacterial DNA-repair test. *Mutation Research,* Vol. 133, pp. 161-198.

Garg, A., Solas, D. W., Takahashi L. H. & Cassella, J. V. (2010). Forced degradation of fentanyl: Identification and analysis of impurities and degradants. *Journal of Pharmaceutical and Biomedical Analysis,* Vol. 53, pp. 325-334.

Glatt, H., Jung, R. & Oesch, F. (1983) Bacterial mutagenicity investigation of epoxides: drugs, drug metabolites, steroids and pesticides. *Mutation Research,* Vol. 11, pp. 99-118.

Gocke, E., Bürgin, H., Müller, L. & Pfister, T. (2009a). Literature review on the genotoxicity, reproductive toxicity, and carcinogenicity of ethyl methanesulfonate. *Toxicology Letters,* Vol. 190, pp. 254-265.

Gocke, E., Müller, L. & Pfister T. (2009b). EMS in Viracept-Initial ('traditional') assessment of risk to patients based on linear dose response relations. *Toxicology Letters,* Vol. 190, pp. 266-270.

Guo, F. Q., Liang, Y. Z., Xu, C. J. & Huang, L. F. (2003). Determination of the volatile chemical constituents of Notoptergium incium by gas chromatography-mass spectrometry and iterative or non-iterative chemometrics resolution methods. *Journal of Chromatography A,* Vol. 1016, pp. 99-110.

Hajikarimian, Y., Yeo, S., Ryan, R. W., Levett, P., Stoneley, C. & Singh, P. (2010). Investigation into the formation of the genotoxic impurity ethyl besylate in the final step manufacturing process of UK-369,003-26, a novel PDE5 inhibitor. *Organic Process Research and Development,* Vol. 14, pp. 1027-1031.

Hansen S. H. & Sheribah Z.A. (2005). Comparison of CZE, MEKC, MEEKC and non-aqueous capillary electrophoresis for the determination of impurities in bromazepam. *Journal of Pharmaceutical and Biomedical Analysis,* Vol. 39, pp. 322-327.

Hmelnickis, J., Pugovics, O., Kazoka, H., Viksna, A., Susinskis, I. & Kokums, K. (2008). Application of hydrophilic interaction chromatography for simultaneous separation of six impurities of mildronate substance. *Journal of Pharmaceutical and Biomedical Analysis,* Vol. 48, pp. 649-656.

Hude, W., Seelbach, A. & Basler, A. (2010). Epoxides: Comparison of the induction of SOS repair in *Escherichia coli* PQ37 and the bacterial mutagenicity in the Ames test. *Mutation Research,* Vol. 231, pp. 205-218.

ICH. (March 2008). Guidance on genotoxicity testing and data interpretation for pharmaceuticals intended for human use S2(R1), In: I*nternational conference on harmonisation of technical requirements for registration of pharmaceuticals for human use,* accessed on 20 January 2011, Available from: <http://www.ich.org.>

ICH. (October 2006). Impurities in new drug substances Q3A(R2). In: I*nternational conference on harmonisation of technical requirements for registration of pharmaceuticals for human use,* Accesssed on 20 January 2011, Available from: <http://www.ich.org.>

ICH. (July 1997). Genotoxicity : A standard battery for genotoxicity testing of pharmaceuticals S2B. In: I*nternational conference on harmonisation of technical requirements for registration of pharmaceuticals for human use,* Accessed on 20 January 2011, Available from: <http://www.ich.org.>

Jacobson-Kram, D. & McGovern, T. (2007). Toxicological overview of impurities in pharmaceutical products. *Advanced Drug Delivery Reviews,* Vol. 59, pp. 38-42.

Jindal, K. C., Chaudhary, R. S., Gangwal, S. S., Singla, A. K. & Khanna, S. (1994). High-performance thin-layer chromatographic method for monitoring degradation products of rifampicin in drug excipient interaction studies. *Journal of Chromatography A,* Vol. 685, pp. 195-199.

Jouyban, A. & Kenndler, E. (2008). Review: Impurity analysis of pharmaceuticals using capillary electromigration methods. *Electrophoresis, Vol.* 29, pp. 3531-3551.

Klick, S. (1995). Evaluation of different injection techniques in the gas chromatographic determination of thermolabile trace impurities in a drug substance. *Journal of Pharmaceutical and Biomedical Analysis,* Vol. 13, pp. 563-566.

Kong, L., Li, X., Zou, H., Wang, H., Mao, X., Zhang, Q. & Ni, J. (2001). Analysis of terpene compounds in *Cimicifuga foetida* L. by reversed-phase high-performance liquid chromatography with evaporative light scattering detection. *Journal of Chromatography A,* Vol. 936, pp. 111-118.

Kruhlak, N. L., Contrera, J. F., Benz, R. D. & Matthews, E. J. (2007). Progress in QSAR toxicity screening of pharmaceutical impurities and other FDA regulated products. *Advanced Drug Delivery Reviews,* Vol. 59, pp. 43-55.

Lacroix, P. M., Curran, N. M. & Lovering, E. G. (1992). Nadolol: High-pressure liquid chromatographic methods for assay, racemate composition and related compounds. *Journal of Pharmaceutical & Biomedical Analysis,* Vol. 10, pp. 917-924.

Liu, D. Q., Sun, M. & Kord, A. S. (2010). Recent advances in trace analysis of pharmaceutical genotoxic impurities. *Journal of Pharmaceutical and Biomedical Analysis,* Vol. 51, pp. 999-1014.

Liu, D. Q., Chen, T. K., McGuir, M. A. & Kord, A. S. (2009). Analytical control of genotoxic impurities in the pazopanib hydrochloride manufacturing process. *Journal of Pharmaceutical and Biomedical Analysis*, Vol. 50, pp. 144-150.

Liu, J., Zhou, W., You, T., Li, F., Wang, E. & Dong, S. (1996). Detection of hydrazine, methylhydrazine, and isoniazid by capillary electrophoresis with a palladium-modified microdisk array electrode. *Analytical Chemistry*, Vol. 68, pp. 3350-3353.

Matsui, F., Robertson, D. L. & Lovering, E. G. (1983). Determination of hydrazine in pharmaceuticals 111: Hydralazine and Isoniazid Using GLC. *Journal of Pharmaceutical Sciences*, Vol. 72, pp. 948-951.

Mahuzier, P. E., Clark, B. J., Crumpton, A. J. & Altria, K. D. (2001). Quantitative microemulsion electrokinetic capillary chromatography analysis of formulated drug products. *Journal of Separation Science*, Vol. 24, pp. 784-788.

McGovern, T. & Jacobson-Kram, D. (2006). Regulation of genotoxic and carcinogenic impurities in drug substances and products. *Trends in Analytical Chemistry*, Vol. 25, pp. 790-795.

Müller, L., Mauthe, R. J., Riley, C. M. *et al.* (2006). A rationale for determining, testing, and controlling specific impurities in pharmaceuticals that possess potential for genotoxicity. *Regulatory Toxicology and Pharmacology*, Vol. 44, pp. 198-211.

Nassar, M. N., Cucolo, M. & Miller, S. A. (2009). Ethyl methanesulphonate in a parenteral formulation of BMS-214662 mesylate, a selective farnesyltransferase inhibitor: Formation and rate of hydrolysis. *Pharmaceutical Development and Thecnology*, Vol. 14, pp. 672-677.

Petkovska, R., Cornett, C. & Dimitrovska, A. (2008). Development and validation of rapid resolution RP-HPLC method for simultaneous determination of atorvastatin and related compounds by use of chemometrics. *Analytical Letters*, Vol. 41, pp. 992-1009.

Ramakrishna, K., Raman, N. V. V. S. S., Narayana Rao, K. M. V., Prasad, A.V. S. S. & Subhaschander Reddy, K. (2008). Development and validation of GC–MS method for the determination of methyl methanesulfonate and ethyl methanesulfonate in imatinib mesylate. *Journal of Pharmaceutical and Biomedical Analysis*, Vol. 46, pp. 780-783.

Raman, N. V. V. S. S., Reddy, K. R., Prasad, A.V.S.S. & Ramakrishna, K. (2008). Development and validation of RP-HPLC method for the determination of genotoxic alkyl benzenesulfonates in amlodipine besylate. *Journal of Pharmaceutical and Biomedical Analysis*, Vol. 48, pp. 227-230.

Rao, B. M., Sangaraju, S., Srinivasu, M. K., Madhavan, P., Devi, L. M., Kumar, R. P., Chandrasekhar, K. B., Arpitha, C. & Balaji, T. S. (2006). Development and validation of a specific stability indicating high performance liquid chromatographic method for rizatriptan benzoate. *Journal of Pharmaceutical and Biomedical Analysis*, Vol. 41, pp. 1146-1151.

Robinson, D. I. (2010). Control of genotoxic impurities in active pharmaceutical ingredients: A review and perspective. *Organic Process Research and Development*, Vol. 14, pp. 946-959.

Sass, S. & Stutz, M. H. (1981). Thin-layer chromatography of some sulfur and nitrogen mustards. *Journal of Chromatography A*, Vol. 213, pp. 173-176.

Sawatari, K., Nakanishi, Y. & Matsushima, T. (2001). Relationships between chemical structures and mutagenicity: a preliminary survey for a database of mutagenicity test results of new work place chemicals. *Industrial Health,* Vol. 39,pp. 341-345.

Schülé, A., Ates, C., Palacio, M., Stofferis, J., Delatinne, J.-P., Martin, B. & Lloyd, S. (2010). Monitoring and control of genotoxic impurity acetamide in the synthesis of zaurategrast sulfate. *Organic Process Research and Development,* Vol. 14, pp. 1008-1014.

Snodin, D. J. (2010). Genotoxic impurities: From structural alerts to qualification. *Organic Process Research and Development,* Vol. 14, pp. 960-976.

Snodin, D. J. (2006). Residues of genotoxic alkyl mesylates in mesylate salt drug substances: real or imaginary problems? *Regulatory Toxicology and Pharmacology,* Vol. 45, pp. 79-90.

Sobol, Z., Engel, M. E., Rubitski, E., Ku, W. W., Aubrecht, J. & Schiestl, R. H. (2007). Genotoxicity profiles of common alkyl halides and esters with alkylating activity. *Mutation Research - Genetic Toxicology and Environmental Mutagenesis,* Vol. 633, pp. 80-94.

Sun, M., Bai, L., Terfloth, G. J., Liu, D. Q. & Kord, A. S. (2010). Matrix deactivation: A general approach to improve stability of unstable and reactive pharmaceutical genotoxic impurities for trace analysis. *Journal of Pharmaceutical and Biomedical Analysis,* Vol. 52, pp. 30-36.

Tafazoli, M., Baeten, A., Geerlings, P. & Kirsch-Volders, M. (1998). *In vitro* mutagenicity and genotoxicity study of a number of short-chain chlorinated hydrocarbons using the micronucleus test and the alkaline single cell gel electrophoresis technique (Comet assay) in human lymphocytes: a structure-activity relationship (QSAR) analysis of the genotoxic and cytotoxic potential. *Mutagenes,* Vol. 13, pp. 115-126.

Teasdale, A., Eyley, S. C., Delaney, E., Jacq, K., Taylor-Worth, K., Lipczynski, A., Reif, V., Elder, D. P., Facchine, K. L., Golec, S., Oestrich, R. S., Sandra, P. & David, F. (2009). Mechanism and processing parameters affecting the formation of methyl methanesulfonate from methanol and methanesulfonic acid: an illustrative example for sulfonate ester impurity formation. *Organic Process Research and Development,* Vol. 13, pp. 429-433.

Valerio, L. G. (2009). In silico toxicology for the pharmaceutical sciences. *Toxicology and Applied Pharmacology,* Vol. 241, pp. 356-370.

Valvo, L., Alimenti, R., Alimonti, S., Raimondi, S., Foglietta, F. & Campana, F. (1997). Development and validation of a liquid chromatographic method for the determination of related substances in verapamil hydrochloride. *Journal of Pharmaceutical and Biomedical Analysis,* Vol. 15, pp. 989-996.

Vijayan, M., Deecaraman, M. & Pudupalayam, K. T. (2007). In vitro genotoxicity of piperacillin impurity-A. *African Journal of Biotechnology,* Vol. 6, pp. 2074-2077.

Wade, D. R., Airy, S. C. & Sinsheimer J. E. (1978). Mutagenecity of aliphatic epoxides. *Mutation Research,* Vol. 58, pp. 217-223.

Yasueda, S., Higashiyama, M., Shirasaki, Y., Inada, K. & Ohtori, A. (2004). An HPLC method to evaluate purity of a steroidal drug, loteprednol etabonate. *Journal of Pharmaceutical and Biomedical Analysis,* Vol. 36, pp. 309-316.

Yu, Y., Huang, T., Yang, B., Liu, X. & Duan, G. (2007). Development of gas chromatography–mass spectrometry with microwave distillation and simultaneous solid-phase microextraction for rapid determination of volatile constituents in ginger. *Journal of Pharmaceutical and Biomedical Analysis*, Vol. 43, pp. 24-31.

18

Measurement Uncertainty in Forensic Toxicology: Its Estimation, Reporting and Interpretation

Rod G. Gullberg
Clearview Statistical Consulting, Snohomish, WA, USA

1. Introduction

All measurements, regardless of their purpose, context or quality, possess uncertainty. No measurement is performed with absolute perfection since all are approximations. Uncertainty, however, does not mean there is anything wrong or inappropriate with the results. Uncertainty is simply a measure of the confidence we have in our best estimate and results from limitations in our technology, our methods, our standards and our limited understanding of the property being measured. [Drosg] Uncertainty is a fundamental property of the natural world in which we live and work. Moreover, no measurement is fully interpretable within a given context until the full process generating the result is understood. The general additive measurement function observed in equation 1 illustrates this basic limitation of all measurements:

$$Y = \mu + \beta + \varepsilon \tag{1}$$

where: Y = the measurement result
μ = the true value of the measurand
β = measurement error due to bias
ε = random measurement error
Our measurement is an imperfect representation of the measurand due to bias and random error components. Bias may be corrected for when reliably determined with traceable controls. Random error, on the other hand, cannot be corrected for but can be minimized to an acceptable level. Figure 1 illustrates how these two contributors to uncertainty influence measurement results - where we have assumed a normal distribution. Bias is simply the difference between the mean and the reference value while random error, determined by the variance or standard deviation, defines the width of the distribution. Figure 1 also illustrates another important property of measurement - all results are random variables that arise from a specified distribution. As a result they have a fixed mean and variance from which confidence intervals can be determined – an useful metric for defining uncertainty. The fact that uncertainty exists in our measurements, however, should not alarm us. We simply need to understand it, acknowledge it, estimate it in a statistically valid way, report it and ensure that it is fit-for-purpose.

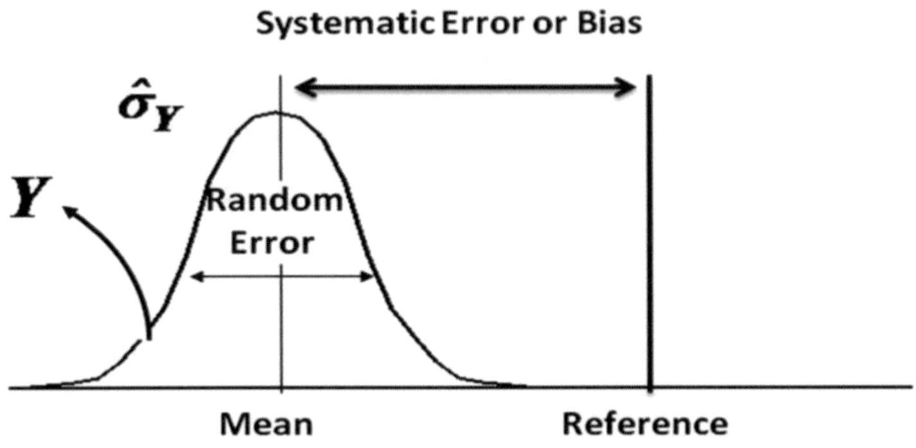

Fig. 1. Measurement results, Y, are random representations from a distribution having a fixed mean and variance. The variance defines the random error while the mean relative to a reference defines their bias

Forensic toxicologists have a conceptual understanding of measurement uncertainty. However, most would probably find it difficult to actually compute a statistically valid estimate of the uncertainty, accounting for all relevant factors, and report it in an intuitive and comprehendible fashion for a jury to understand. For most analytical measurements performed by forensic toxicologists, both quantitative and qualitative, the formalization of measurement uncertainty is not generally considered or provided. This is due, in large part, to the lack of customer demand. The primary customers of forensic toxicologists are the courts and members of the legal community. They do not understand measurement uncertainty and are not aware of its relevance or importance. This, however, is changing. The legal community is becoming more aware of the concept and is now demanding it in several jurisdictions. The uncertainty allows the user to judge the quality and validity of the measurement results for a given application. Several factors have contributed to this renewed interest in measurement uncertainty. One is a recent report from the National Academy of Sciences in 2009. The NAS report states, "All results for every forensic science method should indicate the uncertainty in the measurements that are made,...". (NAS, 2009) The report was largely critical of the forensic sciences arguing the lack of a strong scientific foundation for their claims and practices. Another influencing factor has been the US Supreme Court decision in 1993 of Daubert vs. Merrell Dow Pharmaceuticals. The court required one of four criteria for admissibility to be "...the technique's known or potential rate of error...". (Daubert vs. Merrell Dow, 1993) The ruling requires that uncertainty be considered and accompany the introduction of measurement results in court. Finally, accrediting agencies are now requiring that forensic laboratories perform and report measurement uncertainty as part of their analytical protocol. The ASCLD/LAB-International accreditation program, for example, has adopted the ISO/IEC 17025 program and requires in part that, "...the laboratory estimate the measurement uncertainty for any area of testing or calibration where the customer makes the request or the jurisdiction or statute requires such". (ASCLD/LAB, 2011) These and other factors have now brought attention on this issue to measurement uncertainty. Forensic toxicologists need to address the issue and be prepared to compute, report and explain measurement uncertainty.

Moreover, providing the uncertainty along with measurement results is one important step in ensuring evidence-based inference. (Mnookin, et.al., 2011) We intend to illustrate and explain here several practical ways this can be accomplished.

Very basically, measurement uncertainty is best described by an interval, symmetric about the measurement result and within which we claim that the true value (the measurand) exists with some level of probability. The end points of this interval are called uncertainty or confidence limits. This interval quantifies the precision of the measurement result. Figure 2 illustrates this concept of uncertainty. The classical statistical view would state that the measurand (μ) is a fixed quantity and the measurement result along with the interval limits are random variables. The probability, therefore, relates to the random interval actually encompassing the fixed true value (μ). This involves some subtle distinctions between classical and Bayesian statistics which will not be discussed further here. Suffice it to say, our general approach regarding the estimation of measurement uncertainty will be classical in nature.

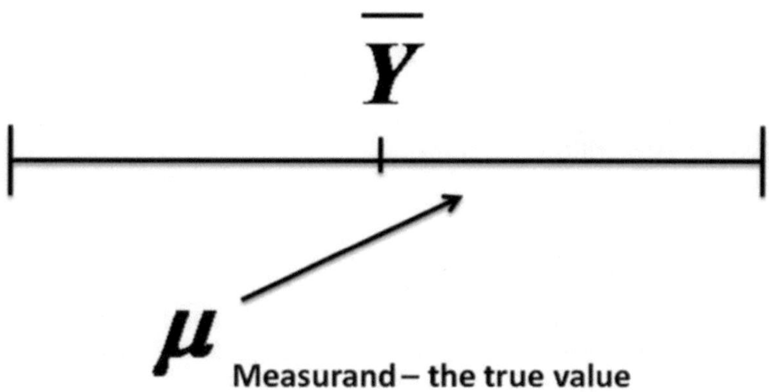

Fig. 2. Measurement uncertainty is best viewed as an interval symmetric about the mean and within which we claim the measureand lies with some stated level of probability

Not all measurement processes are capable of providing a rigorous and statistically valid estimate of uncertainty. This fact is acknowledged by metrologists and by the ISO 17025 document in particular. (IEC/ISO 17025, 2000) For these situations, ISO 17025 requires that the analyst or laboratory at least identify the uncertainty components and make a reasonable effort to express the uncertainty. All of the published guides on measurement uncertainty recognize that every measurement context is different and there are multiple ways for estimation. Accordingly, forensic toxicologists should develop a well reasoned documented approach that can be justified to both the legal and accrediting communities.

Consider the following two separate blood alcohol concentrations measured on samples from two different individuals: **0.086 g/dL, 0.104 g/dL.** Which result presents the stronger inference that the subject's true blood alcohol concentration exceeds 0.080 g/dL? Very simply, we do not know. We have no information regarding the measurement process or the uncertainty for each. Now consider the same two results along with their two standard deviation uncertainty estimates: **0.086 ± 0.005 g/dL, 0.104 ± 0.027 g/dL.** From this we now see that the first results (0.086 ± 0.005 g/dL) provide the stronger evidence that the individual's true blood alcohol concentration exceeds 0.080 g/dL. Figure 3 illustrates this as well. The result of 0.104 g/dL actually has a significant probability that the true value is below 0.080 g/dL. This illustrates the additional value provided by measurement uncertainty, particularly in the cases near critical prohibited limits. Such information would be important for a court to consider.

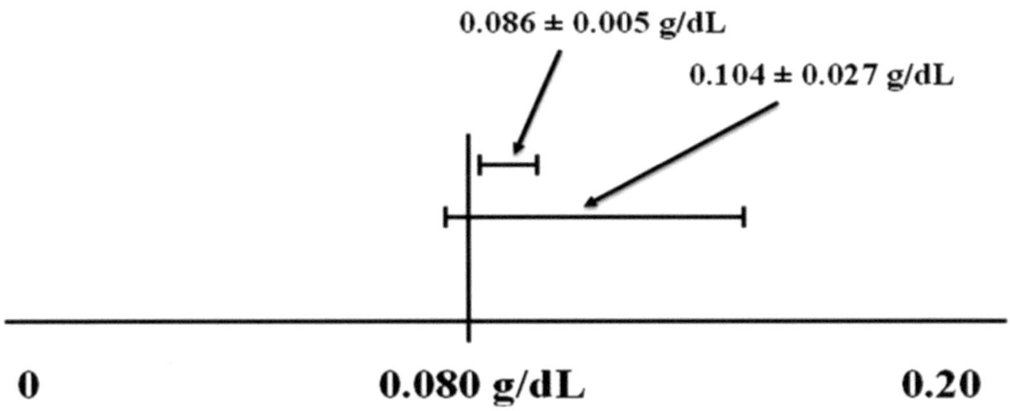

Fig. 3. Including measurement uncertainty adds considerable information when interpreting measurement results near critical concentrations

1.1 The meaning of Fit-for-purpose

Fitness-for-purpose (FFP) is a very important concept in analytical measurements designed to be used in important decision making contexts. FFP is the assurance that a measurement result will be suitable or appropriate for its intended applications. FFP is closely associated with uncertainty and the confidence that is necessary for a measurement result in a particular application. Measurement results in forensic toxicology have significant implications for the rights and property of individuals. Major consequences result from their interpretation in a legal context. For this reason, measurement results generated by forensic toxicologists must have a high level of confidence with minimum uncertainty to ensure their FFP. Determining the FFP in forensic toxicology can be challenging. (Thompson and Fearn, 1996) Toxicologists and customers should both contribute to establishing the appropriate FFP in a forensic context. Forensic toxicologists should continually strive to optimize their process and enhance the quality.

1.2 Published resources

There are a few important resource documents regarding measurement uncertainty that should be read and kept as references by the forensic toxicologist. These represent standards in the field of metrology. They are rigorous and well grounded theoretically. However, this does not mean there is uniform acceptance of these documents. There is a great deal of literature debating their application and interpretation. (Bich and Harris, 2006, Deldossi and Zappa 2009, Kacker,et.al. 2007, Kacker,et.al. 2010, Krouwer, 2003, Kristiansen, 2003) Three references of significant importance are:

1. *Guide to the Expression of Uncertainty in Measurement (GUM):* (ISO, 2008) This is commonly referred to as the *GUM* document and is published by ISO along with several other international standards organizations. The *GUM* provides primarily a

"bottom-up" approach to uncertainty estimation. They generally begin with an assumed measurement model and then proceed to employ the general method of error propagation.

2. EURACHEM/CITAC Guide, *Quantifying Uncertainty in Analytical Measurement:* (EURACHEM/CITAC, 2000) This document is similar to the *GUM* and provides all of the basic terminology and computations. The illustrated examples are more relevant to chemistry and may be more helpful to toxicologists.
3. NIST Technical Note 1297, *Guidelines for Evaluating and Expressing the Uncertainty of NIST Measurement Results:* (NIST, 1994) This document is brief but includes the key concepts and definitions. There are very few illustrated examples.

All of these documents are available on the internet and can be downloaded free of charge. There are also a large number of other documents and guidelines regarding measurement uncertainty available on the internet. As one begins to read this large body of literature it soon becomes apparent that there is no consensus in the analytical sciences on the best approach to estimating measurement uncertainty.

2. The measurement model

The measurement model is a mathematical function where the measurement result (the response variable) is expressed explicitly as a function of several input (predictor) variables. Equation 2 shows the general form:

$$Y = f\left(X_1, X_2, \ldots, X_n\right) \tag{2}$$

where: Y = the measurement result

X_i = the predictor or input variables

The values of X in equation 2 may represent quality control results, bias estimates, traceability components, a total measurement method component, calibrant materials, etc. Moreover, the values of X may themselves be functions of other input variables. The function f may be additive as illustrated in equation 3:

$$Y = X_1 + X_2 + \ldots + X_n \tag{3}$$

For additive models with independent input variables, the uncertainty is found from the root sum square (RSS) of the variance terms for each component as illustrated in equation 4:

$$u_Y = \sqrt{u_{X_1}^2 + u_{X_2}^2 + \ldots + u_{X_n}^2} \tag{4}$$

where: $u_{X_i}^2$ = the variance estimate for the ith variable

The function f may, on the other hand, be multiplicative as in equation 5:

$$Y = X_1 \cdot X_2 \cdot \ldots \cdot X_n \tag{5}$$

For the multiplicative model with independent variables the uncertainty is found by employing the RSS of the coefficients of variation squared as in equation 6:

$$\frac{u_{\overline{Y}}}{\overline{Y}} = \sqrt{CV_{X_1}^2 + CV_{X_2}^2 + \ldots + CV_{X_n}^2} \tag{6}$$

Notice also that equation 6 incorporates the mean $\overline{Y}$ and yields the standard deviation of the mean. This will result when we incorporate the appropriate sample sizes (values of n) for each term within the radical sign of equation 6. The function f may even be a combination of additive and multiplicative terms as in equation 7:

$$Y = \frac{X_1 \cdot X_2}{X_3 + X_4} - X_5 \tag{7}$$

In this case the uncertainty must be estimated by employing the general method of error propagation. The equation for this estimation is derived from the first-order (linear term) of the Taylor series expansion: (Ku, 1966)

$$\frac{u_{\overline{Y}}}{\overline{Y}} = \sqrt{\left[\frac{\partial Y}{\partial X_1}\right]^2 u_{X_1}^2 + \left[\frac{\partial Y}{\partial X_2}\right]^2 u_{X_2}^2 + \ldots + \left[\frac{\partial Y}{\partial X_n}\right]^2 u_{X_n}^2} \tag{8}$$

Equation 8 also assumes that all of the input variables are independent. When this is not the case, a covariance term must be added as seen in equation 9:

$$\frac{u_{\overline{Y}}}{\overline{Y}} = \sqrt{\sum_{i=1}^{n}\left[\frac{\partial Y}{\partial X_i}\right]^2 u_{X_i}^2 + 2\left[\frac{\partial Y}{\partial X_i}\right]\left[\frac{\partial Y}{\partial X_j}\right] Cov\left(X_i, X_j\right)} \tag{9}$$

where:

$$Cov\left(X_i, X_j\right) = r_{\left(X_i, X_j\right)} S_{X_i} S_{X_j}$$

The value of r in equation 9 is the correlation coefficient between the two input variables. For each pair of input variables that are correlated an additional covariance term would need to be added. A simple example of a concentration measurement function that could apply to either blood or breath alcohol measurement is shown in equation 10:

$$C_{Corr} = \frac{C_0 R}{\overline{X}} \tag{10}$$

where: C_{Corr} = the corrected measurement concentration result
C_0 = the raw measurement results (either a mean or a single observation)
R = the traceable reference control value
$\overline{X}$ = the mean results from measuring the control reference standard (R)

Since equation 10 is multiplicative and we assume all three variables are independent we could employ the RSS for the CV's squared according to equation 11. Notice that we have incorporated the values of n, which may vary for each term, where this information is known. This will result in $u_{C_{Corr}}$ representing the standard deviation (or standard error) of the mean. Equation 12 illustrates a more complicated model that may represent the measurement of breath alcohol concentration. Bias in the breath test instrument is adjusted for by measuring controls which have been measured by gas chromatography and which in turn has had its bias accounted for by measuring other traceable controls.

$$\frac{u_{C_{Corr}}}{C_{Corr}} = \sqrt{CV_{C_0}^2 + CV_R^2 + CV_{\overline{X}}^2} = \sqrt{\left[\frac{\frac{u_{C_0}}{\sqrt{n_{C_0}}}}{C_0}\right]^2 + \left[\frac{u_R}{R}\right]^2 + \left[\frac{\frac{u_X}{\sqrt{n_X}}}{\overline{X}}\right]^2} \tag{11}$$

$$\overline{Y}_{Corr} = \frac{\overline{Y}_0 \cdot GC_{Sol} \cdot R}{\overline{X} \cdot K \cdot GC_{Cont}} \tag{12}$$

where: $\overline{Y}_0$ = the mean of the original n measurements

GC_{Sol} = the mean of the simulator solution measurements by gas chromatography

R = the traceable reference value of alcohol in water solutions purchased from a commercial vendor

$\overline{X}$ = the mean of the breath test instrument measuring the simulator solution heated to 34°C

K = 1.23 the ratio of partition coefficients relating to the simulator heated to 34°C

GC_{Cont} = the mean results from measuring the traceable controls on the gas chromatograph

Notice also that equation 12 is simply a set of correction factors that adjust for bias in the gas chromatograph as well as in the breath test instrument:

$$\overline{Y}_{Corr} = \frac{\overline{Y}_0 \cdot GC_{Sol} \cdot R}{\overline{X} \cdot K \cdot GC_{Cont}} = \overline{Y}_0 \cdot \left[\frac{GC_{Sol}}{\overline{X} \cdot K}\right] \cdot \left[\frac{R}{GC_{Cont}}\right] = \overline{Y}_0 \cdot f_{Inst} \cdot f_{GC} \tag{13}$$

where: f_{Inst} = correction factor for the breath test instrument

f_{GC} = correction factor for the gas chromatograph

The uncertainty estimates for R and K will generally be Type B estimates available from certificates of analysis or other documentation. The other four factors will be Type A estimates since they are based on actual experimental results. The uncertainty computation for equation 13 can be determined from employing either the RSS method of equation 6 (since the function is multiplicative) or the error propagation method of equation 8. Both will yield the same estimate. We have illustrated only a few of the many measurement functions that may be relevant for forensic toxicologists. More examples are found in the *EURACHEM/CITAC Guide* as well as other literature sources. (Kristiansen and Peterson, 2004) The important point is to try and develop a model best describing the measurement process which will facilitate selecting the most appropriate uncertainty computation to perform. Where the measurement model is unknown it is common to assume a multiplicative form. The justification for this is the fact that variation generally increases with concentration, a property of a multiplicative model. (Kristiansen, 2001)

3. Traceability

Traceability is defined within the *VIM* document as a "...property of a measurement result whereby the result can be related to a reference through a documented unbroken chain of calibrations, each contributing to the measurement uncertainty". (ISO/VIM, 2008) Figure 3 illustrates this concept of traceability which links a measurement result (breath alcohol) to a national metrological authority with each link propagating its own uncertainty. The magnitude of uncertainty will increase with each additional level of the metrological chain. Since standards are imperfect there is the associated uncertainty that must be included as part of the final combined measurement uncertainty. The ultimate reference is usually a property maintained and defined by some metrological authority such as a National Metrological Institute (NMI). Chemical analytes are generally considered traceable to a method or standard reference material (SRM) such as NIST 1828b. There are other intermediate standards often used between the measurement result and the NMI. These are referred to as Certified Reference Materials (CRM) or simply Reference Materials (RM). (Thompson, 1997) Traceability is important for establishing the property of comparability and to determine and correct for bias. Uncertainty information regarding traceable standards are found on the certificates of analysis (COA).

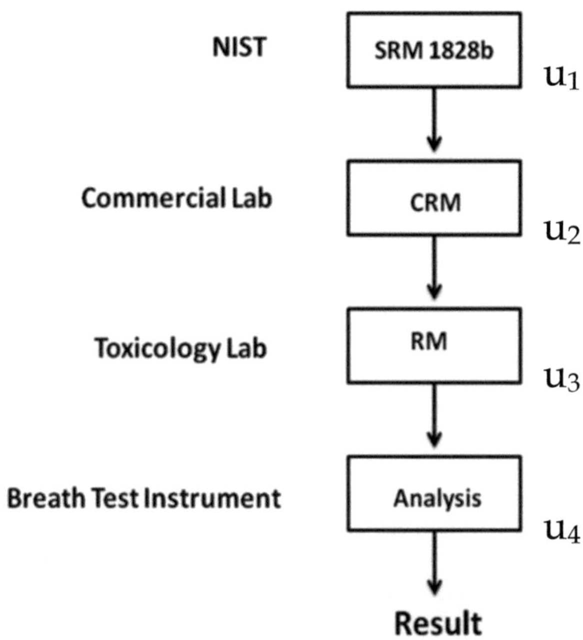

Fig. 4. Illustrating traceability where a measurement result is linked through an unbroken chain of comparisons to the national metrological authority

4. Practical steps for estimating measurement uncertainty

There are several valid approaches to estimating and quantifying measurement uncertainty. For our present purposes, we will present a very general "bottom-up" corresponding to the *GUM* document. Later, we will discuss other approaches as well. We will assume the following eight basic steps for estimating measurement uncertainty that should generally apply for most quantitative measurements in forensic toxicology:

1. Clearly define the property to be measured (the measurand)
2. Identify the measurement function
3. Identify the components contributing to the measurement uncertainty
4. Quantify the standard uncertainty for each component
5. Combine the standard uncertainties for each component and compute the combined uncertainty
6. Compute the expanded uncertainty and the confidence interval
7. Produce the uncertainty budget
8. Report the results

Next, we present these steps in some detail. In addition we will present an example of blood alcohol measurement by gas chromatography and illustrate how each of the steps can be applied. We will assume duplicate blood alcohol results of 0.081 and 0.082 g/dL for this example.

4.1 Clearly define the measurand

It is very important that the customer and the toxicologist have a clear understanding of exactly the property being measured. Interpretation will then be applied to a specific measurand in a specific context where FFP can be appropriately determined. For our example we will assume that the measurand is the venous whole blood alcohol concentration collected from a specific individual at a specific time and location.

4.2 Identify the measurement function

We will assume the following basic model for our measurement of blood alcohol concentration (BAC) by headspace gas chromatography:

$$C_{corr} = \frac{C_0 R}{\overline{X}} \cdot f_{dilutor} \tag{14}$$

where: C_{corr} = the corrected BAC results

C_0 = the mean of the original measurement results

R = the traceable reference control value

$\overline{X}$ = the mean results from measuring the controls

$f_{dilutor}$ = the correction factor for the dilutor

Equation 14 is a basic multiplicative model that includes four components of uncertainty and corrects for analytical bias.

4.3 Identify the components of uncertainty

From equation 14 we see four components that contribute to the combined uncertainty in the corrected BAC. These include: (1) the original duplicate measurement results of the blood alcohol concentration, (2) the reference value (R) representing a traceable unbiased control standard purchased from a commercial laboratory having a certificate of analysis, (3) the mean of the replicate measurements $\left(\overline{X}\right)$ of the traceable control and (4) the correction factor $\left(f_{dilutor}\right)$ for the dilutor used in preparing both the controls and blood samples before analysis. We will assume $f_{dilutor} = 1$.

4.4 Quantify the standard uncertainties for the components

For our example we will assume the values for the four parameters are those shown in Table 1. The uncertainty for the reference value (R) is a Type B uncertainty which comes from the certificate of analysis provided by the vendor preparing the control standard. The uncertainty for the replicate measurements of the control standard is simply the standard deviation determined from n=8 measurements of the control standard. The uncertainty for the dilutor was determined from the certificate of analysis. Since the dilutor is designed to provide 10 ml volume we see a small bias exists. This is not corrected for since the same bias would influence both the control standard measurements as well as the blood samples. For this reason we assume $f_{dilutor} = 1$. The actual value of the $f_{dilutor}$ in table 1 (10.15ml), however, will be used to estimate its uncertainty. The uncertainty associated with the blood alcohol results reported in table 1 (0.00072 g/dL) requires some further explanation. The uncertainty associated with these BAC results represents total method uncertainty. This estimate will be determined from a large number of duplicate BAC results generated within the same laboratory over a long period of time (approximately one year). This would include variation from sample preparation, multiple instruments, multiple calibrations, multiple analysts, multiple uses of the dilutor and time. Figure 5 illustrates an uncertainty function generated from duplicate blood alcohol data analyzed in the forensic laboratory of New Zealand. (Stowell, e.tal., 2008) For illustration purposes, we will assume this model is relevant to our example. Each point in the plot represents the standard deviation associated with a single determination and is generated from the following equation for a pooled estimate:

$$u_B = \sqrt{\frac{\sum_{i=1}^{k} d_i^2}{2k}} \tag{15}$$

where: u_B = the standard deviation for a single measurement of blood alcohol concentration
d_i = the difference between duplicate results for the ith sample
k = the total number of duplicate samples within the bin

Duplicate results are pooled into bins of 0.010 g/dL to generate the uncertainty estimates throughout the concentration range. The result is an estimate of the uncertainty as a function of concentration and reveals the general increase in variation with concentration. Some would advocate the use of a characteristic function rather than an uncertainty function. (Thompson and Coles, 2011) A characteristic function is generated from regressing the variance against the concentration squared. Before estimating our method uncertainty from these functions, we need to determine our corrected BAC result. This is done as follows:

$$C_{corr} = \frac{C_0 R}{\overline{X}} \cdot f_{dilutor} = \frac{(0.0815)(0.100)}{(0.0986)} \cdot 1 = 0.0827\, g / dL \tag{16}$$

We now use this corrected result to estimate our method uncertainty from the model in figure 5. Based on the linear uncertainty function in figure 5 we obtain a method uncertainty of 0.00076 g/dL. Developing the characteristic function for the same data set yields a method uncertainty estimate of 0.00072 g/dL. Therefore, we will use the value of 0.00072 g/dL for example, as we see in table 1.

Parameter	Values	Type	Standard Uncertainty	n
C0	(0.082, 0.081 g/dL)0.0815 g/dL	A	0.00072g/dL	2
R	0.100 g/dL	B	0.0004 g/dL	1
$\overline{X}$	0.0986 g/dL	A	0.0008 g/dL	8
$f_{dilutor}$	10.15 ml	B	0.050 ml	10

Table 1. Estimates, standard uncertainties and the number of measurements for the four parameters assumed to contribute to the combined uncertainty of blood alcohol measurement

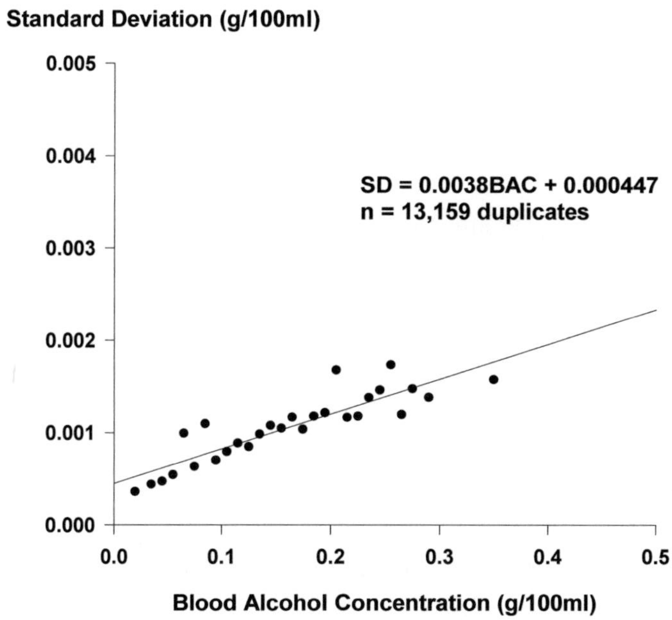

Fig. 5. An uncertainty function plotting pooled standard deviation estimates against their concentration determined from a large number of duplicate blood alcohol results

4.5 Combine the standard uncertainties and compute the combined uncertainty

We first determine our combined uncertainty using the general method of error propagation found in equation 8 assuming independence amongst the predictor variables. Putting our values determined from equation 16 into equation 8 we obtain equation 17. Since our measurement function is multiplicative we also estimate our combined uncertainty using equation 6 and assuming independence we obtain equation 18. Notice that we have included the actual estimate for $f_{dilutor}$ of 10.15 ml. This will ensure the appropriate value is determined for the uncertainty of the dilutor component. For purposes of bias correction in the measurement function of equation 14, however, we assume the value of $f_{dilutor} = 1.0$. From equations 17 and 18 we see that both the RSS method of equation 6 and the error propagation method of equation 8 yield nearly identical results.

$$u_{C_{Corr}} = \sqrt{\left[\frac{R}{\overline{X}}\cdot f_{dilutor}\right]^2 u_{C_0}^2 + \left[\frac{C_0}{\overline{X}}\cdot f_{dilutor}\right]^2 u_R^2 + \left[-\frac{C_0 R}{\overline{X}^2}\right]^2 u_{\overline{X}}^2 + \left[\frac{C_0 R}{\overline{X}}\right]^2 u_{f_{dilutor}}^2}$$

$$u_{C_{Corr}} = \sqrt{\left[\frac{0.100}{0.0986}\cdot 1\right]^2\left[\frac{0.00072}{2}\right]^2 + \left[\frac{0.0815}{0.0986}\cdot 1\right]^2\left[\frac{0.0004}{1}\right]^2 + \left[-\frac{(0.0815)(0.100)}{(0.0986)^2}\cdot 1\right]^2\left[\frac{0.0008}{8}\right]^2 + \left[\frac{(0.0815)(0.100)}{0.0986}\right]^2\left[\frac{0.050}{10}\right]^2} \quad (17)$$

$$u_{C_{Corr}} = 0.00065\, g/dL$$

$$\frac{u_{\overline{Y}}}{\overline{Y}} = \sqrt{\left[\frac{\frac{u_{C_0}}{\sqrt{n}}}{C_0}\right]^2 + \left[\frac{\frac{u_R}{\sqrt{n}}}{R}\right]^2 + \left[\frac{\frac{u_{\overline{X}}}{\sqrt{n}}}{\overline{X}}\right]^2 + \left[\frac{\frac{u_{f_{dilutor}}}{\sqrt{n}}}{f_{dilutor}}\right]^2}$$

$$\frac{u_{\overline{Y}}}{0.0827} = \sqrt{\left[\frac{\frac{0.00072}{\sqrt{2}}}{0.0815}\right]^2 + \left[\frac{\frac{0.0004}{\sqrt{1}}}{0.100}\right]^2 + \left[\frac{\frac{0.0008}{\sqrt{8}}}{0.0986}\right]^2 + \left[\frac{\frac{0.050}{\sqrt{10}}}{10.15}\right]^2} \quad (18)$$

$$u_{\overline{Y}} = 0.0827(0.0081) = 0.00067\, g/dL$$

4.6 Compute the expanded uncertainty and uncertainty interval

The expanded uncertainty is denoted by the value U and is determined from: $U = ku_C$ where k = a coverage factor and u_C = the combined uncertainty. The expanded uncertainty is then used to generate an uncertainty interval as

$$\overline{Y} \pm ku_c \;\Rightarrow\; \overline{Y} \pm U \quad (19)$$

where: $\overline{Y}$ = the unbiased mean measurement result, k = the coverage factor and U = the expanded uncertainty. Notice that u_C is actually the standard deviation of the mean. This results from the fact that we included the appropriate sample sizes, where available, for each term in equations 17 and 18. Sample size also determines degrees of freedom and whether the normal distribution can be assumed or if the t-distribution should be employed. Sample size should be determined as part of the measurement design to ensure sufficient quality control and statistical power. Coverage factors of k=2 or k=3 are common and represent approximately 95% and 99% uncertainty intervals respectively. Selecting k=2 or 3 assumes large degrees of freedom (sample size ≥ 30). Sample sizes less than 30 should employ the Students t distribution. From table 1 we see that none of the sample sizes exceed ten. However, we could argue that the method uncertainty associated with the duplicate blood alcohol results (0.00072 g/dL), determined from the data in figure 5, was generated from over 11,000 duplicate blood alcohol results. This should clearly justify the use of k=2 or 3 for approximate estimates of the 95% and 99% expanded uncertainty intervals. For our present example, however, we will assume we have the limited number of observations noted in table 1 and illustrate the calculation of what is called the "effective degrees of freedom", which may be necessary in some forensic contexts. For this purpose we employ the Welch-Satterthwaite equation which assumes the estimation of the effective degrees of freedom for a probability distribution formed from several independent normal distributions as in equation 20. (Ballico, 2000, Kirkup and Frenkel, 2006)

$$\nu_{eff} = \frac{u_C^4}{\sum_{i=1}^{k} \frac{u_i^4}{\nu_i}} \tag{20}$$

where: ν_{eff} = the effective degrees of freedom

u_C^4 = the combined uncertainty

u_i^4 = the uncertainty associated with the ith component

k = the number of components contributing to the combined uncertainty

The uncertainty terms $\left(u_i^4\right)$ can be determined either from the coefficients of variation (CV) or from partial derivatives determined from the measurement function in equation 14. If the CV estimates are used we do not incorporate the sample size n for each term. We will determine the CV estimates for our example. We first compute the combined uncertainty again as in equation 21.

$$\frac{u_C}{C_{Corr}} = \sqrt{\left[\frac{u_{C_0}}{C_0}\right]^2 + \left[\frac{u_R}{R}\right]^2 + \left[\frac{u_{\overline{\overline{X}}}}{\overline{\overline{X}}}\right]^2 + \left[\frac{u_{f_{dilutor}}}{f_{dilutor}}\right]^2}$$

$$\frac{u_C}{0.0827} = \sqrt{\left[\frac{0.00072}{0.0815}\right]^2 + \left[\frac{0.0004}{0.100}\right]^2 + \left[\frac{0.0008}{0.0986}\right]^2 + \left[\frac{0.050}{10.15}\right]^2} = 0.0011\, g/dL \tag{21}$$

Next, we incorporate these results into equation 20 as follows:

$$\nu_{eff} = \frac{u_C^4}{\sum_{i=1}^{k} \frac{u_i^4}{\nu_i}} = \frac{\left[\frac{0.0011}{0.0827}\right]^4}{\frac{\left[\frac{0.00072}{0.0815}\right]^4}{1} + \frac{\left[\frac{0.0004}{0.100}\right]^4}{\infty} + \frac{\left[\frac{0.0008}{0.0986}\right]^4}{7} + \frac{\left[\frac{0.050}{10.15}\right]^4}{9}} = 4.6 \approx 4$$

From this computation we see that the effective degrees of freedom can be some non-integer value, in which case the value is generally truncated. Notice also that the uncertainty associated with the reference value (R) has an infinite number of degrees of freedom. This is because it is a Type B uncertainty determined from a certificate of analysis where we assume the uncertainty in the uncertainty estimate (0.0004 g/dL) is zero with correspondingly large degrees of freedom. As a result this term disappears from the computation. Each of the other degrees of freedom is determined from n-1. From these results we would estimate our value from the t-distribution to be: $t_{0.975,4} = 2.776$ for estimating a 95% uncertainty interval. Using these results along with our combined uncertainty determined from equation 18 we would obtain a 95% uncertainty interval of: $\overline{Y} \pm k u_C \Rightarrow 0.0827 \pm 2.776(0.00067) \Rightarrow 0.0827 \pm 0.0019 \Rightarrow 0.0808\ to\ 0.0846\, g/dL$.

We now have an interval within which we would expect a large fraction (approximately 95%) of the expected values of the measurand to exist. If we were to assume k=2 to generate an approximate 95% uncertainty interval we would obtain: $0.0827 \pm 2(0.00067) \Rightarrow 0.0827 \pm 0.0013 \Rightarrow 0.0814 \ to \ 0.0840 \, g / dL$. We see that this interval is slightly narrower than that employing the effective degrees of freedom estimate. Choosing the appropriate coverage factor will be a decision made within each forensic laboratory. A 99% interval (k=3) will provide a higher degree of confidence that may be important in forensic applications. This is particularly true where results are near prohibited legal limits. Whatever decision is made, the value for k should be clearly identified in the program policy or SOP manuals and strictly adhered to in practice. In this example we have assumed our expanded interval to be an "uncertainty interval" rather than a "confidence interval". The *GUM* document prefers the term "uncertainty interval" or "level of confidence". (ISO/GUM, 2008) Others, however, interpret U as representing a confidence interval which has a specific definition in the classical statistical sense.

4.7 Produce the uncertainty budget

Table 2 illustrates one form of an uncertainty budget for our example. The uncertainty budget lists the components contributing to the combined uncertainty along with the percent of their contribution to the total. The percent contributions were determined from the terms under the radical sign in equation 18. This is very useful for identifying which components are the major contributors and which may be reasonably ignored. The *GUM* document states that any contributions less than one-third of the largest contributor can be safely ignored. (ISO/GUM, 2008) Based on this we see that the analytical and dilutor components could be safely ignored in this example. However, from a forensic perspective it may be better to include all components considered, providing full disclosure. We see that the total method contributes the largest component at 59%. This is expected because of all of the contributing sub-components involved: analysts, calibrations, time, dilutions, etc. This analysis does not include, however, the venous blood sampling performed by the phlebotomist who typically performs only one venipuncture. Moreover, many laboratories do not even consider sampling as a component of their combined uncertainty. They simply consider their uncertainty estimates corresponding to the sample "as received in the laboratory". Jones, for example, has considered sampling as a source of uncertainty in some of his published work. (Jones, 1989)

Source	Type	Distribution	Standard Uncertainty	Percent[1]
Traceability	B	Normal	0.0004 g/dL	24%
Analyical	A	Normal	0.0008 g/dL	13%
Dilutor	B	Normal	0.050 ml	4%
Total Method	A	Normal	0.00072 g/dL	59%
Combined Uncertainty			0.00067 g/dL	
Expanded Uncertainty (k=2.776)			0.0019 g/dL	
95% confidence interval			0.0808 to 0. 0846 g/dL	

[1]Percent of contribution to total combined uncertainty

Table 2. Uncertainty budget for the illustrated example

4.8 Report the results

One of the most important, yet often overlooked, elements of determining measurement uncertainty is reporting the results. A great deal of thought should be given to this aspect of measurement. The end-user should be consulted to determine exactly what is needed for their application. There should be sufficient information so the results and their associated uncertainty are fully interpretable and unequivocal for a specific application without reference to additional documentation. This will necessitate some textual explanation in addition to the numerical results. One possibility for our blood alcohol example above is:

The duplicate whole blood alcohol results were 0.082 and 0.081 g/dL with a corrected mean result of 0.0827 g/dL. An expanded combined uncertainty of 0.0019 g/dL assuming a coverage factor of k=2.776 with an effective degrees-of-freedom of 4 and a normal distribution was generated from four principle components contributing to the uncertainty. An approximate 95% confidence interval for the true mean blood alcohol concentration is 0.0808 to 0.0846 g/dL.

In addition to the statement, a figure similar to that of figure 3 could be provided which might assist the court in placing the results in some geometric perspective. The format for reporting the results should be considered flexible. As time goes on there will no doubt be the need for revision to ensure clarity in communication and interpretation.

4.9 Assumptions of this approach

There were a number of assumptions employed in estimating the uncertainty illustrated above. The customer should appreciate these assumptions to allow for full and clear interpretation. Very generally, the assumptions are:

1. The blood alcohol measurement results are normally distributed
2. All standard uncertainties are valid estimates
3. The method uncertainty is probably over estimated due to some "double counting"
4. The method of confidence interval estimation will be robust
5. With a fixed mean (μ), 95% of the intervals will bracket μ
6. The confidence interval expresses the uncertainty due to sampling variability only
7. This entire approach to estimating the uncertainty is uncertain.
8. We have assumed that all uncertainty components are independent

We would not advocate that these assumptions be listed as part of the reported results. Rather, they should be available if requested by the end-user and toxicologists should be prepared to discuss them.

5. Breath alcohol measurement example

Our next example illustrates the uncertainty estimation for a breath alcohol measurement. We will assume the following measurement function which was presented earlier as equation 12:

$$\overline{Y}_{Corr} = \frac{\overline{Y}_0 \cdot GC_{Sol} \cdot R}{\overline{X} \cdot K \cdot GC_{Cont}} \quad (22)$$

where: $\overline{Y}_0$ = the mean of the original n measurements

GC_{Sol} = the mean of the simulator solution measurements by gas chromatography

R = the traceable reference value

$\overline{X} =$ mean of the breath test instrument measuring the simulator solution heated to 34°C

$K =$ 1.23 the ratio of partition coefficients

$GC_{Cont} =$ the mean results from measuring the traceable controls on the gas chromatograph

For this example we assume that simulator solutions are prepared and tested by gas chromatography within the toxicology laboratory. Commercially purchased standards (CRM) are used as calibrators and controls on the gas chromatograph. Certificates of analysis are used as Type B uncertainties to establish the traceability. For this example we will assume the following data are available for the six components of equation 22: Duplicate BrAC results: 0.081 and 0.085 g/210L, $\overline{Y}_0 =$ 0.0830 g/210L, GC_{Sol} : mean = 0.0985 g/dL u = 0.0007 g/dL n=15, $R =$ 0.100 g/dL u = 0.0003 g/dL, $\overline{X}$: mean = 0.0795 g/210L u = 0.0012 g/210L n=10, $K =$ 1.23 u = 0.012 and GC_{Cont} : mean = 0.1015 g/dL u = 0.0006 g/dL n=28. We begin by computing the corrected mean BrAC results according to:

$$\overline{Y}_{Corr} = \frac{(0.0830\,g/210L)(0.0985\,g/dL)(0.100\,g/dL)}{(0.0795\,g/210L)(1.23)(0.1015\,g/dL)} = 0.0824\,g/210L$$

The estimate for the uncertainty in $\overline{Y}_0$ will come from an uncertainty function seen in figure 6 and developed from a large number of duplicate breath alcohol tests using equation 15. The total method uncertainty for our example determined from the linear model in figure 6 and using the corrected mean BrAC of 0.0824 g/210L is 0.0031 g/210L. Since our model in equation 22 is multiplicative we employ the RSS for the CV values and assume independence amongst all components. The combined uncertainty estimate is seen in equation 23. Next we estimate the 95% uncertainty interval and obtain:

$$\overline{Y} \pm k u_C \Rightarrow \overline{Y} \pm U \Rightarrow 0.0824 \pm 2(0.00239) \Rightarrow 0.0824 \pm 0.0048$$
$$0.0776 \text{ to } 0.0872\,g/210L$$

Since the n for estimating the uncertainty function in figure 6 was very large, we assume an infinite degrees of freedom and use k=2 for estimating an approximate 95% confidence interval. Table 3 shows the uncertainty budget for this analysis. From the uncertainty budget we see that the total method accounted for the majority of the combined uncertainty (84%). This is not surprising since the breath sampling component, contained within the total method uncertainty function of figure 6, has significant variation. The budget also shows that the reference traceability, the GC measurement of the controls and the GC measurement of the simulator solution all provide 1% or less to the combined uncertainty. They could reasonably be ignored in this example. We now report our results as follows:

The duplicate breath alcohol results were 0.081 and 0.085 g/210L with a corrected mean result of 0.0824 g/210L. An expanded combined uncertainty of 0.0048g/210L assuming a coverage factor of k=2 with an infinite number of degrees-of-freedom and a normal distribution was generated from six principle components contributing to the uncertainty. An approximate 95% confidence interval for the true mean breath alcohol concentration is 0.0776 to 0.0872 g/210L.

$$\frac{u_{\overline{Y}}}{\overline{Y}} = \sqrt{CV_{\overline{Y}_0}^2 + CV_{GC_{Sol}}^2 + CV_R^2 + CV_{\overline{X}}^2 + CV_K^2 + CV_{GC_{Cont}}^2}$$

$$\frac{u_{\overline{Y}}}{\overline{Y}_{Corr}} = \sqrt{\left[\frac{\frac{u_{\overline{Y}_0}}{\sqrt{n}}}{\overline{Y}_0}\right]^2 + \left[\frac{\frac{u_{GC_{Sol}}}{\sqrt{n}}}{GC_{Sol}}\right]^2 + \left[\frac{\frac{u_R}{\sqrt{n}}}{R}\right]^2 + \left[\frac{\frac{u_{\overline{X}}}{\sqrt{n}}}{\overline{X}}\right]^2 + \left[\frac{\frac{u_K}{\sqrt{n}}}{K}\right]^2 + \left[\frac{\frac{u_{GC_{Cont}}}{\sqrt{n}}}{GC_{Cont}}\right]^2} \tag{23}$$

$$\frac{u_{\overline{Y}}}{0.0824} = \sqrt{\left[\frac{\frac{0.0031}{\sqrt{2}}}{0.0824}\right]^2 + \left[\frac{\frac{0.0007}{\sqrt{15}}}{0.0985}\right]^2 + \left[\frac{\frac{0.0003}{\sqrt{1}}}{0.100}\right]^2 + \left[\frac{\frac{0.0012}{\sqrt{10}}}{0.0795}\right]^2 + \left[\frac{\frac{0.012}{\sqrt{1}}}{1.23}\right]^2 + \left[\frac{\frac{0.0006}{\sqrt{28}}}{0.1015}\right]^2}$$

$$u_{\overline{Y}} = 0.0824(0.0290) = 0.00239\, g / 210L$$

The approximate 95% uncertainty interval estimated for this example shows that the lower limit falls below the critical legal driving level of 0.080 g/210L. We may be interested in knowing the probability that the true population mean BrAC is above 0.080 g/210L. This can be estimated by first considering our confidence interval in the following form:

$$P\left[\overline{Y} - Z_{(1-\alpha/2)}\, S_{\overline{Y}} \le \mu \le \overline{Y} + Z_{(1-\alpha/2)}\, S_{\overline{Y}}\right] = \pi \tag{24}$$

Since we are interested in determining the probability that μ exceeds the lower limit we rewrite equation 24 as follows:

$$P\left[\overline{Y} - Z_{(1-\alpha/2)}\, S_{\overline{Y}} \le \mu \le \infty\right] = \pi \tag{25}$$

We set the lower limit expressed in equation 25 equal to 0.080 g/210L and solve for $Z_{(1-\alpha/2)}$:

$$\overline{Y} - Z_{(1-\alpha/2)}\, S_{\overline{Y}} = 0.080 \Rightarrow 0.0824 - Z_{(1-\alpha/2)}\,(0.00239) = 0.080 \Rightarrow Z_{(1-\alpha/2)} = 1.0$$

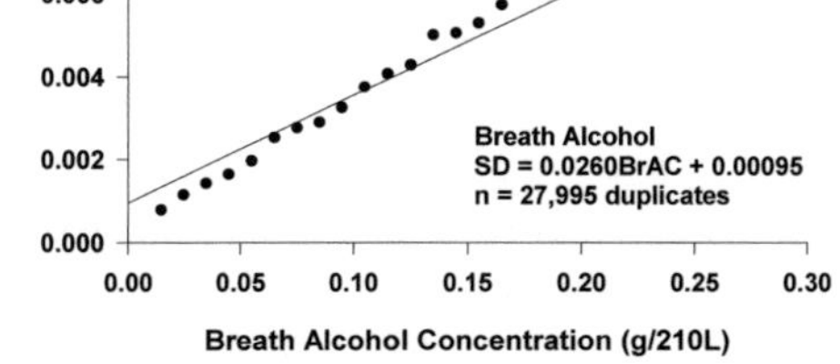

Fig. 6. An uncertainty function plotting pooled standard deviation estimates against their concentration determined from a large number of duplicate breath alcohol results

Source	Type	Distribution	Standard Uncertainty	Percent[1]
Total Method	A	Normal	0.0031 g/210L	84%
GC Solution	A	Normal	0.0007 g/dL	0.5%
Reference	B	Normal	0.0003 g/dL	1%
Breath Instrument	A	Normal	0.0012 g/210L	3%
Simulator Part. Coef	B	Normal	0.012	11%
GC Controls	A	Normal	0.0006 g/210L	0.5%
Combined Uncertainty			0.00239 g/210L	
Expanded Uncertainty (k=2)			0.0048 g/210L	
95% confidence interval			0.0776 to 0. 0872 g/210L	

[1] Percent of contribution to total combined uncertainty

Table 3. Uncertainty budget for the illustrated breath alcohol example

Next, we rearrange our probability statement, introduce the value for $Z_{(1-\alpha/2)}$, and refer to the standard normal tables:

$$P\left[\overline{Y} - Z_{1-\alpha/2}\, S_{\overline{Y}} \le \mu\right] = P\left[\frac{\overline{Y} - \mu}{S_{\overline{Y}}} \le Z_{1-\alpha/2}\right] = P\left[Z \le Z_{1-\alpha/2}\right] = P\left[Z \le 1.0\right] = 0.8413$$

There is a probability of 0.8413 that the individual's true mean BrAC exceeds 0.080 g/100ml. This may or may not rise to the level of proof beyond a reasonable doubt, depending on the opinion of the court. This example illustrated the use of simulator control standards produced within a local toxicology laboratory including their associated uncertainties. Some jurisdictions, however, choose to purchase simulator control standards rather than prepare their own. If that were the case in this example, we could have eliminated the GC solutions and GC controls from our uncertainty estimates. The simulator partition coefficient would have remained while the reference value would have been obtained from the certificate of analysis from the manufacturer and considered a Type B uncertainty. Therefore, rather than having to include the GC solution and GC control components separately in the combined uncertainty estimate, they should already be included within the manufacturer's estimate of combined uncertainty, depending, of course, on how the solution standards were prepared and tested.

6. Dealing with measurement bias

Our principle objective here will be to illustrate several ways for treating uncorrected bias. Bias or systematic error is common in all measurements. Some consider different types of bias such as: (1) method bias, (2) laboratory bias and (3) run bias. (O'Donnell and Hibbert, 2005) Not all, however, would agree with the need for classifications of bias. (Kadis, 2007, O'Donnell and Hibbert, 2007) Regardless of its classification or source, all forms of bias should ideally be determined and corrected for employing traceable control standards. As this is done, the uncertainty of that correction must be included as one of the components in the combined uncertainty. Occasionally, the analyst may determine that the bias is small and insignificant and not correct for it. There are ways to handle uncorrected bias as well by adding an additional component to the combined uncertainty. We will consider some examples here. Estimations for bias can come from internal quality control, proficiency test data, collaborative studies or method validation data. (Kane, 1997)

6.1 Preparing an alcohol in water control solution

We will assume in this example that we desire to prepare an ethanol in water solution to be used as a control standard. We want to prepare this solution to have a concentration of approximately 0.10 g/dL. Our measurement function will be as follows: (Philipp et.al., 2010)

$$C = \frac{m_{Etoh} PD}{m_{Solution}} \tag{26}$$

where: C = the concentration of ethanol in water
m_{Etoh} = the mass measurement of ethanol
P = the purity of the ethanol
D = the density of the ethanol
$m_{Solution}$ = the mass measurement of the combined solution of ethanol and water
Preparing a control standard gravimetrically has advantages. (Gates, et.al., 2009) There is better traceability for the mass measurements and no concern regarding the uncertainty in volume measurements. We will assume the purity (P) to be 0.995 with a Type B standard uncertainty of 0.002 determined from the certificate of analysis. We further assume that the density (D) of the solution is 0.997 g/ml (OIML, King and Lawn, 1999) with a Type B standard uncertainty of 0.00054 g/ml (King and Lawn, 1999), determined from the certificate of analysis from the manufacturer of a density meter. For both the purity and the density we will assume the uniform distribution in order to estimate their standard uncertainties. The values for the density are obtained from published tables for ethanol/water solutions. The density of the solution will be a function of the mass fraction of ethanol. The higher the mass fraction of ethanol the closer the density will be to 0.789 g/ml - the density of pure ethanol. The lower the mass fraction of ethanol the closer the density will be to 1.00 g/ml - the density of water. Since the density of the solution depends on the mass fraction of ethanol and we have selected a density of 0.997 g/ml (corresponding to a mass fraction of approximately 0.101%) and we desire a total solution mass of 1800 g, we need to have the mass of ethanol equal to 1.82 g. We will need to weigh 1.82 g of ethanol and place it into solution with water and add water until we have a total mass of 1800g. We will assume that the total solution mass is weighed on a scale that has had replicate measurements (n=30) of a 2 Kg traceable check weight (Type B uncertainty of 0.016 Kg) with a mean result of 1,940 g and a standard uncertainty of 30 g. This will be used to estimate the standard uncertainty in the measurement of $m_{Solution}$. We now recognize that there is a bias in the weighing of the total solution. The measured mass of the solution is low by 3.0%. This will affect the mass of the ethanol necessary to maintain the density of 0.997 and mass fraction of 0.101%. As a result the mass of the ethanol will need to be 1.87 g. The mass of ethanol was weighed on a different scale that also has a set of replicate measurements (n=23) of a 2.0 g traceable check weight (Type B standard uncertainty of 0.014g) with a mean result of 2.08 g and a standard uncertainty of 0.02g. This scale has a bias of +4.0%. We now incorporate our assumed measurement information into equation 26:

$$C = \frac{m_{Etoh} PD}{m_{Solution} \cdot \frac{R_{2Kg}}{\overline{X}}} = \frac{(1.87g)(0.995)(0.997g/ml)}{(1800g)\left(\frac{2000g}{1940g}\right)} = 0.00100g/ml = 0.1000g/dL \quad (27)$$

where: $\frac{R_{2Kg}}{\overline{X}}$ = the correction factor for the bias in the scale used to weigh the total solution

Notice that we only correct for the bias in the scale used to weigh the total solution but not for the scale used to weigh the ethanol. The question now is how to deal with the +4.0% bias in the one scale. We begin by estimating the combined uncertainty ignoring the bias (assuming it is zero) and assuming independence of all variables. Since equation 27 is a multiplicative model we employ the RSS of the CV's squared as in equation 28. Notice that the standard uncertainty in the solution mass measurement comes from the repeatability measurements of the 2.0 Kg traceable check standards. There is no separate uncertainty estimate for the single measurement of the total solution of 1800 g. Employing the Welch-Sattherwaite equation to compute the effective degrees of freedom for our example we obtain:

$$v_{eff} = \frac{\left[\frac{0.00210}{0.1000}\right]^4}{\frac{\left[\frac{.02}{2.08}\right]^4}{22} + \frac{\left[\frac{.002}{0.995}\right]^4}{\infty} + \frac{\left[\frac{0.00054}{0.997}\right]^4}{\infty} + \frac{\left[\frac{30}{1800}\right]^4}{29} + \frac{\left[\frac{16}{2000}\right]^4}{\infty}} = 63.8 \approx 63$$

$$\frac{u_C}{C} = \sqrt{CV^2_{m_{Etoh}} + CV^2_P + CV^2_D + CV^2_{m_{Sol}} + CV^2_{R_{2Kg}}}$$

$$\frac{u_C}{C} = \sqrt{\left[\frac{\frac{u_{m_{Etoh}}}{\sqrt{n}}}{m_{Etoh}}\right]^2 + \left[\frac{\frac{u_P}{\sqrt{n}}}{P}\right]^2 + \left[\frac{\frac{u_D}{\sqrt{n}}}{D}\right]^2 + \left[\frac{\frac{u_{m_{Sol}}}{\sqrt{n}}}{m_{Sol}}\right]^2 + \left[\frac{\frac{u_{R_{2Kg}}}{\sqrt{n}}}{R_{2Kg}}\right]^2} \quad (28)$$

$$\frac{u_{\overline{Y}}}{0.1000} = \sqrt{\left[\frac{\frac{0.02}{\sqrt{23}}}{2.08}\right]^2 + \left[\frac{\frac{0.002}{\sqrt{3}}}{0.995}\right]^2 + \left[\frac{\frac{0.00054}{\sqrt{3}}}{0.997}\right]^2 + \left[\frac{\frac{30}{\sqrt{30}}}{1800}\right]^2 + \left[\frac{\frac{16}{\sqrt{1}}}{2000}\right]^2}$$

$$u_{\overline{Y}} = 0.1000(0.0089) = 0.00089g/dL$$

The 95% confidence interval for our estimated concentration would be:

$$\overline{Y} \pm t_{0.975,63} u_c \Rightarrow 0.1000 \pm 2.00(0.00089) \Rightarrow 0.1000 \pm 0.00178 \Rightarrow 0.0982 \text{ to } 0.1018$$

The next option for dealing with the bias in the mass measurement of the ethanol is to correct for it. This is always the recommended practice and consistent with the *GUM* document. Correcting the ethanol mass for the +4.0% bias yields a result of 1.80 g. Placing this corrected value into equation 27 yields a corrected concentration of 0.000962 g/ml or 0.0962 g/dL. Now we must account for the uncertainty in the 2.0g reference check weight by including its Type B uncertainty in equation 28 where we add the additional term:

$\left[\frac{\frac{u_{R_{2g}}}{\sqrt{1}}}{R_{2g}}\right]^2 = \left[\frac{\frac{0.014}{\sqrt{1}}}{2.00}\right]^2$ and, when including the corrected concentration, we obtain: $u_C = 0.0986(0.0113) = 0.00111\, g/dL$. The uncertainty budget is shown in table 4 both when ignoring the bias and when including the bias correction. From table 4 we see that including the additional balance bias, the combined uncertainty increased by 25% and contributed 38% to the combined uncertainty. The bias, in this example, is clearly significant and as a result should be corrected for. Before illustrating our next approach to handling uncorrected bias, we will evaluate the bias in our example to determine its significance. To do so we employ the following t-test:

$$t = \frac{C - R}{\sqrt{u_C^2 + u_R^2}} = \frac{2.08 - 2.00}{\sqrt{\left[\frac{\frac{0.02}{\sqrt{23}}}{2.08}\right]^2 + \left[\frac{\frac{0.014}{\sqrt{1}}}{2.00}\right]^2}} = 10.9 \quad (29)$$

The critical value for a two-tailed test with α=0.05 and effective degrees of freedom of 51 from the t-distribution is $t_{0.975,51} = 2.01$. The results from equation 29 show the bias to be largely significant and should be corrected for. There are times when measurement bias is known to exist but is not corrected for. The analyst may believe the bias to be small and insignificant or it may be too complex to correct for. There are several methods that have been proposed for including the uncertainty due to uncorrected bias. (Maroto,et.al., 2002, Petersen, et.al., 2001) All of these effectively increase the expanded uncertainty by some amount to account for the uncorrected bias. Moreover, including an uncertainty component

			Percent[1]	
Source	**Type**	**Standard Uncertainty**	**Ignoring Bias**	**Correcting Bias**
Mass of Ethanol	A	0.02 g	5%	3%
Purity of Ethanol	B	0.002	1%	1%
Density of Solution	B	0.00054 g/ml	1%	1%
Mass of Solution	A	30 g	12%	7%
2.0 Kg Reference	B	16 g	81%	50%
2.0 g Reference	B	0.014 g		38%
Combined Uncertainty			0.00089 g/dL	0.00111 g/dL

[1] Percent of contribution to total combined uncertainty

Table 4. Uncertainty budget for the preparation of the control ethanol solution resulting from a corrected bias is always less than the uncertainty component resulting from uncorrected bias. (Synek, 2005, Linsinger, 2008) One approach is to include the bias within the radical sign and estimate the expanded uncertainty (U) as follows:

$$U = kC\sqrt{CV_{m_{Etoh}}^2 + CV_P^2 + CV_D^2 + CV_{m_{Sol}}^2 + CV_{R_{2Kg}}^2 + bias^2} \tag{30}$$

Since all of the other terms within the radical sign are dimensionless relative variances, we must transform the bias into dimensionless relative units. Doing this with our example and assuming k=2 we obtain:

$$U = 2(0.1000)\sqrt{\left[\frac{\frac{0.02}{\sqrt{23}}}{2.08}\right]^2 + \left[\frac{\frac{0.002}{\sqrt{3}}}{0.995}\right]^2 + \left[\frac{\frac{0.00054}{\sqrt{3}}}{0.997}\right]^2 + \left[\frac{\frac{30}{\sqrt{30}}}{1800}\right]^2 + \left[\frac{\frac{16}{\sqrt{1}}}{2000}\right]^2 + \left[\frac{\frac{0.08}{\sqrt{23}}}{2.00}\right]^2}$$

$$U = 2(0.1000)(0.0122) = 0.0024\, g / dL$$

The combined uncertainty with this approach is 0.00122 g/dL compared to 0.00111 g/dL when correcting for the bias and 0.00089 g/dL when ignoring the bias. Another approach is to incorporate the coverage factor k into the radical sign but without effecting the bias term as follows:

$$U = C\sqrt{k^2\left[CV_{m_{Etoh}}^2 + CV_P^2 + CV_D^2 + CV_{m_{Sol}}^2 + CV_{R_{2Kg}}^2\right] + bias^2} \tag{31}$$

With this approach the combined uncertainty remains the same but the expanded uncertainty becomes 0.00196 g/dL. As expected, this is slightly less than the expanded uncertainty determined from equation 30 which was 0.0024 g/dL. A third approach is basically the same as correcting for the bias and is expressed as:

$$Y \pm U + bias \quad \Rightarrow \quad \bar{y} - (U + bias) \le Y \le \bar{y} + (U - bias) \tag{32}$$

For our example, the bias in the mass of the ethanol was +0.08g. The corrected mass of the ethanol should be 1.79 g rather than the 1.87 g value measured. Using the correct value of 1.79 g, the corrected concentration of the ethanol should be 0.0957 g/dL. This indicates that we have a bias in the estimated concentration of +0.0043 g/dL. Using this value for our bias and assuming an approximate 95% confidence interval, equation 32 becomes:

$$0.1000 - (2(0.00089) + 0.0043) \le Y \le 0.1000 + (2(0.00089) - 0.0043)$$
$$0.0939 \le Y \le 0.0975\, g / dL$$

Notice that this interval is not symmetric around our estimated, yet biased, concentration of 0.1000 g/dL. Instead, it has accounted for the +0.0043 g/dL bias and adjusted for this.

The next proposal for handling uncorrected bias is to simply add the absolute value of the bias to the expanded uncertainty as: $\bar{Y} \pm U + |bias|$. For our example this would result in:

$$\bar{Y}-(U+|bias|) \le Y \le \bar{Y}+(U+|bias|) \Rightarrow \quad 0.1000-0.00608 \le Y \le 0.1000+0.00608$$
$$0.0939 \le Y \le 0.1061\, g\,/\,dL$$

This clearly would yield the largest uncertainty interval compared to the preceding methods and is probably larger than necessary. The final method we will consider yields an expanded uncertainty interval that is also asymmetric about the measurement result. (Phillips, et.al., 1997) This method computes the confidence interval based on the expanded uncertainty (U) estimated as follows:

$$\bar{Y}-U_{-} \le Y \le \bar{Y}+U_{+}$$

$$where: \qquad U_{+}=\begin{cases} ku_c - bias & if\ ku_c - bias > 0 \\ 0 & if\ ku_c - bias \le 0 \end{cases} \tag{33}$$

$$and \quad U_{-}=\begin{cases} ku_c + bias & if\ ku_c + bias > 0 \\ 0 & if\ ku_c + bias \le 0 \end{cases}$$

Using this approach for our example would yield:

$$0.1000-[2(0.00089)+0.0043] \le Y \le 0.1000+0 \Rightarrow \quad 0.0939 \le Y \le 0.1000\,.$$

The asymmetry with this method has accounted for the positive bias and yields the same lower limit as the two preceding methods above. This results from the fact that our estimate is biased high by +0.0043 g/dL and was not corrected for. This last approach has more desirable statistical properties compared to the previous methods and has the advantage of avoiding negative expanded uncertainty limits (where the lower limit is below zero) which could occur at low concentrations. (Phillips, et.al., 1997)

6.2 Estimating bias by recovery

Another approach to estimating and handling bias is with recovery analysis. (Thompson, et.al., 1999) Recovery is the ratio, expressed as a percent, of the measurement result to the reference or true measurand value described by:

$$\%R = \left[\frac{C_0}{C_{Ref}}\right]100 \tag{34}$$

where: %R = percent recovery
C_0 = the measured value
C_{Ref} = the true value of the measurand
Percent recovery is a metric more commonly applied in analytical contexts involving complex matrices with several steps of extraction, sample preparation and analysis of a specified sub-sample. The requirements of this complex procedure for extraction and analysis often results in a loss of the analyte prior to its actual quantitative determination. Hence, we have the concept of %Recovery. The accuracy of the analytical method is determined by its ability to quantify (recover) the full amount of the analyte in the original

matrix. Simply spiking alcohol in a blood sample and measuring it is not a typical application of percent recovery. The recovery is often determined during the method validation phase where a known blank matrix is spiked with a known mass of the relevant analyte. This is often referred to as a "reference recovery" or a "method recovery". (Barwick and Ellison, 1999) When recovery estimates are applied to correct subsequent samples, it is very important that the concentrations and matrix are appropriately similar and that the same full analytical protocol is followed. Measurements of recovery from several spiked samples may be performed with the mean and standard deviation of the percent estimates determined, providing uncertainty estimates for the percent recovery in future measurements. The fractional recovery can be employed as a correction factor in the measurement equation as follows:

$$C_{Corr} = \frac{C_0}{\overline{R}} \tag{35}$$

where: C_{Corr} = the corrected analytical result
C_0 = the original measurement
$\overline{R}$ = the mean fractional recovery

Assume that we are interested in determining the percent recovery of a specific drug for a particular analytical method. Assume that we have two vials of a subject's blood, each containing 1.0 ml and each containing some unknown concentration of the drug of interest. To one tube we add 0.1ml of a known analyte standard having a concentration of 20mg/dL. We have now added a concentration of: $\frac{20mg}{dL}\left[\frac{0.1ml}{0.1ml+1.0ml}\right] = 1.82\frac{mg}{dL}$. To the other tube we simply add 0.1 ml of water. We now measure the concentration of the analyte in each tube in replicate (at least twice) and determine the means to be: Tube with added analyte: 10.8 mg/dL Tube with added water: 9.3 mg/dL. We now compute the percent recovery according to:

$$\%\text{Recovery} = \left[\frac{\text{Measured Difference}}{\text{Concentration Added}}\right]\cdot 100 = \left[\frac{10.8mg/dL - 9.3mg/dL}{1.82mg/dL}\right]\cdot 100 = 82.4\% \tag{36}$$

Assume that we have done this recovery experiment during method validation using blood specimens spiked with the analyte and obtained a mean % recovery of $\overline{R} = 84\%$ with a standard uncertainty of 6% determined from 45 spiked samples. Assume further that we now have a suspect's blood sample and we wish to provide an unbiased estimate of the analyte's concentration using this recovery data. We determine the suspect's sample results to be C_0 = 15.4mg/dL with a standard uncertainty of 0.92mg/dL determined from n=56 measurements of past quality control data. We further assume there are no other significant sources of bias, other than that estimated by the %Recovery. First we could determine whether the mean recovery of 84% was significantly different from 1.0 or not with the following t-test:

$$t = \frac{\left|\overline{R}-1\right|}{u_{\overline{R}}} = \frac{\left|0.84-1\right|}{0.06/\sqrt{45}} = -17.9 \tag{37}$$

The p-value for t = 17.9 with df=44 is <0.00001. We conclude that the mean recovery is very significantly different from 1.0. The recovery estimate should be used to correct the analytical results. Using our mean recovery to correct our analytical results yields: $C_{Corr} = \frac{C_0}{\bar{\bar{R}}} = \frac{15.4}{0.84} = 18.3 mg/dL$. The combined uncertainty in our corrected estimate can now be determined from the RSS method using the CV's squared since we have a multiplicative model and we assume independence according to:

$$\frac{u_C}{C_{Corr}} = \sqrt{CV_{C_0}^2 + CV_{\bar{R}}^2} \Rightarrow \frac{u_C}{18.3} = \sqrt{\left[\frac{\frac{0.92}{\sqrt{56}}}{18.3}\right]^2 + \left[\frac{\frac{0.06}{\sqrt{45}}}{0.84}\right]^2} \Rightarrow u_C = (18.3)(0.0126) = 0.231 mg/dL$$

This results in a relative combined uncertainty of approximately 1.3%. Moreover, the analytical component contributed 45% while the recovery component contributed 65% to the combined uncertainty. The same analysis can be done when spiking blank specimens with a known concentration of the analyte. If we added the same 0.1ml of 20mg/dL concentration to 1.0ml of blank specimen, and quantified the specimen with our analytical method and obtained 1.65 mg/dL, this would become the numerator in equation 36 and we would obtain a recovery estimate of:

$$\% \text{Recovery} = \left[\frac{\textit{Measured Concentration}}{\textit{Concentration Added}}\right] \cdot 100 = \left[\frac{1.65 mg/dL}{1.82 mg/dL}\right] \cdot 100 = 90.7\% \quad .$$

Both methods of spiking blank samples or spiking samples already containing the analyte are used in recovery studies. Moreover, it is important to remember with recovery studies the assumption that no other bias exists. We have briefly considered several ways that have been proposed to handle uncorrected bias. Ideally, bias should always be corrected for - even when statistically insignificant. When the bias is not corrected for, the combined uncertainty statement should include some additional component, thus increasing its magnitude, accounting for the uncorrected bias. Moreover, the customer should be made aware, either in the uncertainty statement or otherwise, when uncorrected bias exists and how it has been accounted for.

7. Uncertainty in post-mortem drug analysis

This example summarizes work recently published where methadone was measured in post-mortem cases. (Linnet, et.al., 2008) One sample of blood was taken from each femoral vein in 27 post-mortem autopsies. LC-MS/MS was the analytical method used to quantify both methadone and its main metabolite, 2-ethyl-1,5-dimethyl-3,3-diphenylpyrrolinium (EDDP). For our present example we will focus only on the quantitative measurement of methadone. While the study did not explicitly present a measurement function, the following would be a reasonable approximation:

$$C_{Corr} = \frac{C_0 \cdot C_{Cal}}{\bar{C}_A} = \frac{C_0 \cdot \frac{m_{Meth} P}{V}}{\bar{C}_A} \tag{38}$$

where: C_{Corr} = the corrected measurement of methadone
C_0 = the original quantitative measurement result of the methadone by LC-MS/MS
C_{Cal} = the reference calibration and/or control value
$\overline{C}_A$ = the mean quantitative measurement of the reference value
m_{Meth} = mass of the reference methadone added to the calibration/control solution
P = the purity of the methadone
V = the volume of the calibration/control methadone solution
The study also presented the following uncertainty estimates, expressed as %CV's, for each of the components in equation 38: $u_{\overline{C}_A} = 3.65\%$ $u_P = 0.29\%$ $u_{m_{Meth}} = 0.53\%$ $u_V = 0.05\%$.

The uncertainty in the purity was determined from employing the uniform distribution and the manufacturer's certificate of analysis stating the purity was 99.99% ± 0.5%. The uncertainty in the original measurements (C_0) was determined from the duplicate sampling, one from each femoral vein. The standard uncertainty for a single determination was determined from each of these results according to:

$$u_M = \sqrt{\frac{\sum_{i=1}^{N}(rd)_i^2}{2N}} = \sqrt{\frac{\sum_{i=1}^{N} d_i^2}{2N}} \tag{39}$$

Equation 39, expressing the computation in two equivalent forms, was designed to estimate the total method (u_M) component of uncertainty. A major part of this was due to the sampling technique from each of the femoral veins. This component was termed pre-analytical (PA). Once the computations were determined from equation 39, the pre-analytical component was determined according to:

$$CV_M^2 = CV_{PA}^2 + CV_A^2 \tag{40}$$

Finally, the combined uncertainty was determined according to:

$$CV_T^2 = CV_{PA}^2 + CV_A^2 + CV_{Cal}^2 = CV_{PA}^2 + CV_A^2 + CV_{m_{Meth}}^2 + CV_P^2 + CV_V^2 \tag{41}$$

Incorporating the uncertainty estimates outlined in Table 1 of the study we obtain:
$CV_T = \sqrt{18.95\%^2 + 3.65\%^2 + 0.53\%^2 + 0.29\%^2 + 0.05\%^2} = 19.3\%$. With this estimate we, and the authors of the study, have assumed independence of the components and a multiplicative measurement model. The uncertainty budget for this example is shown in Table 5, from which we see that the pre-analytical or sampling component contributes by far the most to the combined uncertainty. This is not unexpected since it represents the sampling component. Sampling, when included as a component in the combined uncertainty estimate, is typically the largest contributor. The study reported that amongst the 27 cases, the concentration of methadone ranged from 0.005 to 2.29 mg/kg with a median value of 0.472 mg/kg. The median was appropriately reported, rather than the mean, because the distribution of results was positively skewed. Therefore, we would be interested in this case in computing a 95% confidence interval for the median. The most common approaches to estimating confidence intervals for a median do not involve uncertainty estimates. This results from the fact that the median is a quantile, specifically, the 50th percentile. One method for estimating the approximate 95% confidence interval for the median presented in

this study is to compute estimates of r and s as in equation 42. (Altman, et.al., 2000) For our sample size of n=27 and rounding the estimates to the nearest integer we obtain the results seen in equation 43. This would indicate that the 8th and 20th ordered observations would provide an approximate 95% confidence interval for the population median. The exact level of confidence for this example based on the binomial distribution would be 98.1%. (Altman, et.al., 2000)

Source	**Type**	**%CV**	**Percent[1]**
Pre-Analytical	A	18.95%	96%
Analytical	A	3.65%	3.9%
Mass of Methadone	A	0.53%	0.08%
Purity	B	0.29%	0.02%
Volume	B	0.05%	0%
Combined Uncertainty		19.3%	100%

[1]Percent of contribution to total combined uncertainty

Table 5. Uncertainty budget for the post-mortem measurement of methadone in femoral blood

$$r = \frac{n}{2} - \left[Z_{1-\alpha/2} \cdot \frac{\sqrt{n}}{2} \right] \qquad s = 1 + \frac{n}{2} + \left[Z_{1-\alpha/2} \cdot \frac{\sqrt{n}}{2} \right] \tag{42}$$

$$r = \frac{27}{2} - \left[1.96 \cdot \frac{\sqrt{27}}{2} \right] = 8.4 \approx 8 \qquad s = 1 + \frac{27}{2} + \left[1.96 \cdot \frac{\sqrt{27}}{2} \right] = 19.6 \approx 20 \tag{43}$$

8. Uncertainty in a blood alcohol analysis

The unique aspect of this example will be the addition of the uncertainty due to calibration. We will assume that duplicate blood alcohol results of 0.104 and 0.107 g/dL were obtained from the same headspace gas chromatograph. The following is our assumed measurement function:

$$C_{corr} = \frac{C_0 R}{\overline{X}_{Cont}} \cdot f_{dilutor} \cdot f_{Calib} \tag{44}$$

where: C_{corr} = the corrected BAC results

C_0 = the mean of the original measurement results

R = the traceable reference control value

$\overline{X}_{Cont}$ = the mean results from measuring the controls

$f_{dilutor}$ = the correction factor for the dilutor

f_{Calib} = the correction factor for the calibration

We have added an additional correction factor (f_{Calib}) in equation 44 which we also set equal to one and also include its uncertainty component. We will assume that the instrument was calibrated with a linear five point calibration curve generated by the use of five traceable control standards. The calibration curve was generated by linear least squares yielding the following function:

$$Y = a + bX \tag{45}$$

where: Y = instrument response, X = known control concentration values and a and b are model parameters. The objective in developing a calibration curve is to estimate the true value of a future unknown concentration (X) given some instrument response (Y). Therefore, we find the inverse of equation 45:

$$X = \frac{Y - a}{b}. \tag{46}$$

For our purposes, we are interested in determining the uncertainty in X found in equation 46. The parameters a and b, however, are correlated. We can eliminate the parameter a by solving for a according to $a = \overline{Y} - b\overline{X}$ and then substituting this into equation 46 according to:

$$X_0 = \frac{Y_0 - \left(\overline{Y} - b\overline{X}\right)}{b} \quad \Rightarrow \quad X_0 = \frac{Y_0 - \overline{Y}}{b} + \overline{X} \tag{47}$$

where: X_0 = a future single estimate of concentration
Y_0 = a future single instrument response
$\overline{Y}$ = the mean of the instrument responses during calibration
$\overline{X}$ = the mean of the control samples used during calibration
From equation 47 we see that X_0 is a function of only three random variables: Y_0, $\overline{Y}$, and b. Solving for the uncertainty in X_0 by the method of error propagation we obtain:

$$u_{X_0} = \frac{S_{Y|X}}{b}\sqrt{\frac{1}{m} + \frac{1}{n} + \frac{\left(Y_0 - \overline{Y}\right)^2}{b^2 \sum_{i=1}^{n}\left(X_i - \overline{X}\right)^2}} \tag{48}$$

where: $S_{Y|X}$ = standard error from regression of Y on X in developing the calibration curve
b = the slope of the calibration curve
m = the number of measurements used to estimate X_0
n = the number of measurements used to generate the calibration curve
We will assume specific values for the terms in equation 48 and solve for the uncertainty according to:

$$u_{X_0} = \frac{(0.005)}{(1.02)}\sqrt{\frac{1}{2} + \frac{1}{5} + \frac{(0.1055 - 0.1516)^2}{(1.02)^2\,(0.046)}} = 0.0042$$

Now, for our example we will assume the variables for equation 44 found in Table 6. For purposes of determining the uncertainties in each of the correction factors we assume $f_{Dilutor}$ to be 10.65 and f_{Calib} to be 0.1058 g/dL. However, for estimating the corrected blood alcohol concentration in equation 44 we assume each to be 1.0. Next, we can estimate our corrected blood alcohol concentration according to:

$$C_{corr} = \frac{C_0 R}{\overline{X}} \cdot f_{dilutr} \cdot f_{Calib} = \frac{(0.1055)(0.100)}{(0.1025)} \cdot 1 \cdot 1 = 0.1029\, g / dL$$

We now combine the standard uncertainty components to determine the combined uncertainty according to equation 49. Estimating an approximate 95% uncertainty interval would yield:

$$0.1029 \pm 2(0.0020) \Rightarrow 0.1029 \pm 0.0040 \Rightarrow 0.0989 \text{ to } 0.1069\, g / dL.$$

The percent contribution from each component to the combined uncertainty in this example is: C_0 10%, R 2%, $\overline{X}_{Cont}$ 1% , $f_{Dilutor}$ 1% and f_{Calib} 86%. From this we see that the calibration uncertainty contributed by far the most to the combined uncertainty. This may have resulted from the values assumed for this example and may not reflect most forensic programs. Each laboratory would need to determine this for their particular context. It should also be noted that equation 48 includes the uncertainty only of the least squares estimates and not that of the reference standards used as calibrants. These could be added as separate components. There are other methods to account for the uncertainty in calibration as well. For example, the maximum vertical deviation between the line of identify and the least squares regression line can be divided by the square root of three, assuming the uniform distribution, and

Variable	Estimate	Uncertainty	n
C_0	0.1055	0.0009	2
R	0.100	0.0003	1
$\overline{X}_{Cont}$	0.1025	0.0008	16
$f_{Dilutor}$	10.65	0.05	10
f_{Calib}	0.1058	0.0042	5

Table 6. The values of specific variables assumed for our blood alcohol measurement model

$$\frac{u_{\overline{C}_{Corr}}}{\overline{C}_{Corr}} = \sqrt{\left[\frac{\frac{u_{C_0}}{\sqrt{n}}}{C_0}\right]^2 + \left[\frac{\frac{u_R}{\sqrt{n}}}{R}\right]^2 + \left[\frac{\frac{u_{\overline{X}}}{\sqrt{n}}}{\overline{X}}\right]^2 + \left[\frac{\frac{u_{f_{dilutor}}}{\sqrt{n}}}{f_{dilutor}}\right]^2 + \left[\frac{\frac{u_{f_{Calib}}}{\sqrt{n}}}{f_{Calib}}\right]^2}$$

$$\frac{u_{\overline{C}}}{0.1029} = \sqrt{\left[\frac{\frac{0.0009}{\sqrt{2}}}{0.1029}\right]^2 + \left[\frac{\frac{0.0003}{\sqrt{1}}}{0.100}\right]^2 + \left[\frac{\frac{0.0008}{\sqrt{16}}}{0.1025}\right]^2 + \left[\frac{\frac{0.050}{\sqrt{10}}}{10.65}\right]^2 + \left[\frac{\frac{0.0042}{\sqrt{5}}}{0.1058}\right]^2} \quad (49)$$

$$u_{\overline{Y}} = 0.1029(0.0192) = 0.0020\, g / dL$$

divided by the concentration value of X at that point. This is often termed a "lack of linearity" component.

The preceding examples presented here have been illustrative only. There was no intention that the uncertainty estimates assumed were the only ones to be considered or even represented any specific laboratory program. They were presented simply to illustrate the computations involved. Indeed, there are surely other components to be considered. (Sklerov and Couper, 2011) These must be identified by the forensic toxicologist considering their particular laboratory, protocol, instruments, customers and the required fitness-for-purpose.

9. Different methods for estimating uncertainty

We have illustrated above several examples for estimating the combined uncertainty in contexts relevant to forensic toxicology. These examples have presented the standard bottom-up approach recommended largely by the *GUM* document. There are, however, several other approaches to dealing with uncertainty that have been proposed in the forensic toxicology and metrological literature. Wallace, for example, has proposed a number of different methods for estimating measurement uncertainty. (Wallace, 2010)

9.1 Use of proficiency test data

One method advocated by Wallace is the use of proficiency test data. (Wallace, 2010) Proficiency testing basically consists of an organizing laboratory which, employing well established and traceable methods, prepares and tests the concentrations of several samples. These samples are then sent blindly to participating laboratories with instructions on how the measurements are to be performed, recorded and then returned to the organizing laboratory. The samples are to be treated by the participating laboratories as routine case samples and tested according to their routine protocols. The organizing laboratory summarizes the data reporting means, standard deviations and various plots, including, for example, Z-scores. The standard deviations at various mean concentrations can be used to generate uncertainty functions. Clearly, these estimates will exhibit rather large variation due to the different laboratories, instruments, protocols, analysts, time, etc. These estimates, conditioned on the appropriate concentration, can be used as the total method component in the combined uncertainty estimate. Consider an example where we have duplicate blood alcohol results obtained in the toxicology laboratory of 0.118 and 0.116 g/dL. The laboratory participated in a proficiency study which yielded the uncertainty function observed in figure 7. This figure was actually generated from data available from Collaborative Testing Services [CTS]. For this example we will assume the following measurement function:

$$C_{Corr} = \frac{C_0 R}{\overline{X}} \tag{50}$$

where: C_{Corr} = the corrected measurement result

C_0 = the mean of the original duplicate measurements

R = the reference value for the controls

$\overline{X}$ = the mean result for measuring the reference controls

The mean of our assumed duplicate results is 0.1170 g/dL. The reference value is R=0.100 g/dL with a Type B standard uncertainty of 0.0003 g/dL. The mean measurement of the controls were $\overline{X} = 0.1024\,g/dL$ with n=34 measurements and a standard uncertainty of 0.0009 g/dL. Computing our corrected estimate from equation 56 we obtain 0.1143 g/dL. Using this value to estimate our method uncertainty from the equation found in figure 8 we obtain: $u_M = 0.0369(0.1143)+0.00129 = 0.0055\,g/dL$. Assuming independence and the multiplicative model of equation 50, we now estimate our combined uncertainty as seen in equation 51. The approximate 95% confidence interval (k=2) for the true mean blood alcohol concentration in this example would be:

$$\overline{Y} \pm 2u_{\overline{Y}} \Rightarrow 0.1143 \pm 2(0.0039) \Rightarrow 0.1065\ to\ 0.1221\,g/dL\,.$$

The risk in using proficiency data in this manner is that the actual uncertainty associated with a particular laboratory may be overestimated. Another limitation to keep in mind is that the proficiency data may not have been generated with the same analytical protocol employed within a particular laboratory. Proficiency data, however, does have a large source of variation, which may be acceptable within the forensic context. The uncertainty budget for these results is found in Table 7. The method uncertainty determined from the proficiency test data in this example, contributed by far the most to the combined uncertainty while the reference and analytical components could effectively be ignored.

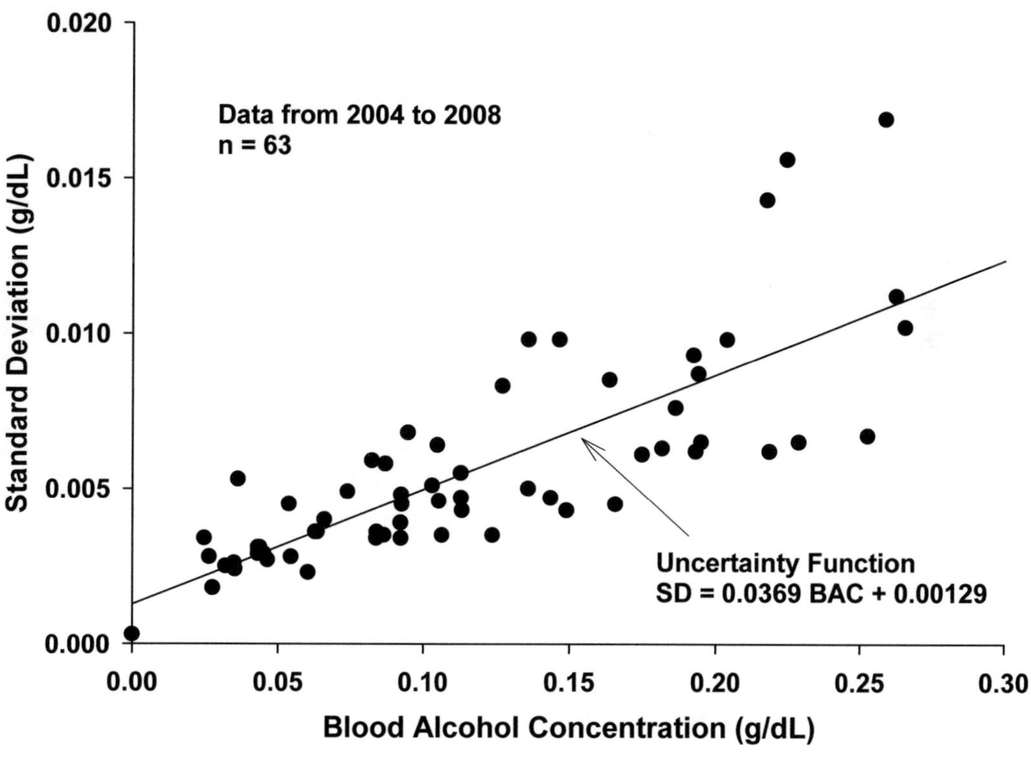

Fig. 7. Plot of the standard deviation against concentration and determination of an uncertainty function from CTS proficiency test blood alcohol data

$$\frac{u_C}{C} = \sqrt{CV_{C_0}^2 + CV_R^2 + CV_{\overline{X}}^2} \quad = \frac{u_C}{C} = \sqrt{\left[\frac{\frac{u_{C_0}}{\sqrt{n}}}{C_0}\right]^2 + \left[\frac{\frac{u_R}{\sqrt{n}}}{R}\right]^2 + \left[\frac{\frac{u_{\overline{X}}}{\sqrt{n}}}{\overline{X}}\right]^2} \tag{51}$$

$$\frac{u_{\overline{Y}}}{0.1143} = \sqrt{\left[\frac{\frac{0.0055}{\sqrt{2}}}{0.1143}\right]^2 + \left[\frac{\frac{0.0003}{\sqrt{1}}}{0.100}\right]^2 + \left[\frac{\frac{0.0009}{\sqrt{34}}}{0.1024}\right]^2} \Rightarrow u_{\overline{Y}} = 0.1143(0.0342) = 0.0039\, g/dL$$

Source	Type	%CV	Percent[1]
Method (Proficiency)	A	5%	99%
Reference	B	0.3%	0.8%
Analytical	A	0.9%	0.2%
Total			100%

[1] Percent of contribution to total combined uncertainty

Table 7. Uncertainty budget resulting from the use of proficiency test data as the estimate for method uncertainty

9.2 Using the guard band approach

Employing a guard band is another approach to accounting for measurement uncertainty. (EURACHEM/CITAC, 2000) Use of the guard band is a tool for determining compliance within specified limits. It establishes a decision rule, particularly relevant where there are critical or prohibited analytical limits which may define, for example, binary outcomes such as pass/fail, guilty/not guilty, etc. These can be important in drunk-driving prosecution where alcohol results (either blood or breath) are introduced to establish whether the subject exceeded the legal limit. Consider the example where an individual provided duplicate breath alcohol results of 0.092 and 0.098 g/210L. A traceable commercially purchased simulator control standard having a reference value of 0.0824 g/210L and a Type B combined uncertainty of 0.0008 g/210L was measured by the breath test instrument. The mean of n=46 measurements with this control was 0.0856 g/210L with a standard uncertainty of 0.0010 g/d10L. We wish to determine an upper limit to the guard band, above which we will be 99% confident that the individual's true mean breath alcohol concentration exceeds 0.080 g/210L. This can be visualized in figure 8 where we see that the upper limit of the guard band is the value 0.080 + ku_C. We must first find the combined uncertainty (u_C) and then the appropriate value of k. The value of k will actually be from the t-distribution in this example and will need to correspond to a 98% confidence interval. The degrees of freedom will be determined from the Welch-Satterthwaite equation. We begin by identifying our measurement function as follows:

$$C_{Corr} = \frac{C_0 R}{\overline{X}} \tag{52}$$

where: C_{Corr} = the corrected breath alcohol concentration
R = the traceable control reference value
$\overline{X}$ = the mean of replicate (n=18) measurements of the reference control standard

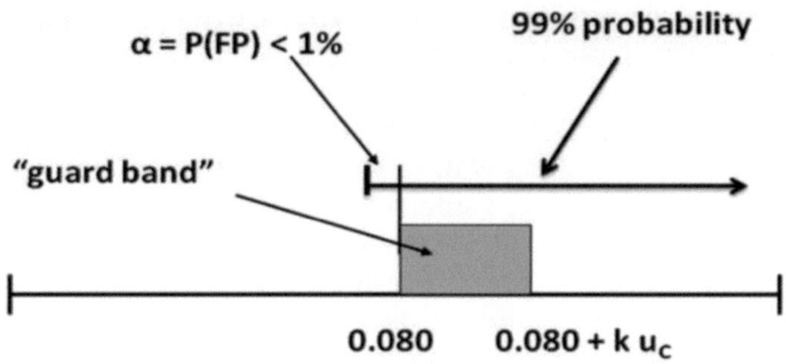

Fig. 8. Illustrating the construction and use of a "guard band" to determine compliance with a specified limit

The corrected mean breath alcohol results in our example is found from equation 52 to be: $C_{Corr} = \frac{(0.0950)(0.0824)}{(0.0856)} = 0.0914\,g/210L$. We will assume that our method uncertainty is determined from the uncertainty function found in figure 6 which results in: $u = 0.0260(0.0914) + 0.00095 = 0.0033\,g/210L$. Given that our measurement function in equation 52 is multiplicative, we now find our combined uncertainty, assuming independence, as in equation 51:

$$\frac{u_{\overline{Y}}}{0.0914} = \sqrt{\left[\frac{\frac{0.0033}{\sqrt{2}}}{0.0914}\right]^2 + \left[\frac{\frac{0.0008}{\sqrt{1}}}{0.0824}\right]^2 + \left[\frac{\frac{0.0010}{\sqrt{46}}}{0.0856}\right]^2} \Rightarrow u_{\overline{Y}} = 0.0914(0.0274) = 0.0025\,g/210L .$$

We now find the relative combined uncertainty by removing the values of n according to:

$$\frac{u_{\overline{Y}}}{0.0914} = \sqrt{\left[\frac{0.0033}{0.0914}\right]^2 + \left[\frac{0.0008}{0.0824}\right]^2 + \left[\frac{0.0010}{0.0856}\right]^2} \Rightarrow u_{\overline{Y}} = 0.0914(0.0391) = 0.0036\,g/210L .$$

Now we determine our effective degrees of freedom using the Welch-Satterthwaite equation as follows:

$$\nu_{eff} = \frac{\left[\frac{0.0036}{0.0914}\right]^4}{\frac{\left[\frac{.0033}{0.0914}\right]^4}{\infty} + \frac{\left[\frac{.0008}{0.0824}\right]^4}{\infty} + \frac{\left[\frac{0.0010}{0.0856}\right]^4}{45}} = 5814.8 \approx \infty$$

Notice that in the Welch-Satterthwaite equation we have changed our degrees of freedom for the total method component to infinity. This is because the standard uncertainty estimate

(0.0033 g/210L) from figure 6 is based on much more than one degree of freedom (n>27,000). The degrees of freedom for the reference standard in the Welch-Satterthwaite equation is set to infinity because it is a Type B uncertainty without information on the degrees of freedom provided. Since we have essentially an infinite number of effective degrees of freedom we select our k (or t) value of 1.96. We can now compute the upper limit for our guard band: 0.080 + 2.33(0.0025) = 0.0858 g/210L. Since the subject's corrected mean breath alcohol concentration exceeds the upper guard band limit of 0.0858 g/210L we conclude there is 99% confidence that the individual's true mean breath alcohol concentration exceeds 0.080 g/210L. Values exceeding 0.080 + ku_c could be considered within the "rejection zone". For a measurement in this region, the probability of a "false rejection" is less than α, the probability of the false-positive error. (Desimoni and Brunetti, 2007) One must also keep in mind that for guard band estimates at different concentrations, the combined uncertainty estimates need to incorporate the method uncertainty appropriate to that concentration. The guard band approach could also be generated based on a large set of historical data and then employed for a period of time. The estimates could be updated annually, for example, to ensure the system remains in statistical control. The assumptions with this approach is that the individuals continue to be tested on the same instrumentation and protocols used to generate the guard band limits and that the system remains in statistical control. The United Kingdom is one jurisdiction that employs a guard band approach. (Walls and Brownlee, 1985) A value of 6mg/dL is subtracted from the mean of duplicate blood alcohol results below 100 mg/dL and 6% is deducted from results over 100 mg/dL. The results of this deduction must exceed their legal limit of 80 mg/dL for prosecution. Denmark employs a similar approach where they deduct 0.1 g/Kg to compute their level for prosecution. (Kristiansen and Petersen, 2004) Similarly, Sweden employs the guard band approach to uncertainty estimation by requiring that the lower 99.9% confidence interval limit for mean results must exceed their legal limit. (Jones and Schuberth, 1989) Guard band calculations could also be incorporated into computerized breath test instruments for immediate determination of critical limits for purposes of prosecution.

9.3 Uncertainty estimation from total allowable error

There is considerable debate regarding the best method for estimating measurement uncertainty and whether it is even necessary. Many argue that measurement uncertainty is unnecessary because it may be misunderstood by the customer or confuse the interpretation. Since bias is only determined with regard to a reference standard, many analytes do not have standards available while others have several. As a result, it is argued that bias may not be validly determined in the first place. Some that argue against the use of measurement uncertainty would advocate the use of total allowable error (TE_a). (Westgard, 2010) Total allowable error is determined from the following linear model:

$$TE_a = |bias| + k\,u_C \quad . \tag{53}$$

The total allowable error combines both bias and random components and estimates the upper limit. In some cases this may over estimate the actual capability of the analytical method or laboratory performance. Moreover, the method of total allowable error does not correct for bias - it simply includes the maximum level allowable. If we were to allow a maximum bias of 4% and the relative combined uncertainty for the method was 2% and we selected a coverage factor of k=2, we would obtain: $TE_a = |4\%| + 2(2\%) = 8\%$. This would provide an upper limit estimate for the customer who could be assured, with a high degree of probability, that the total error would not exceed this limit. One might report the final results in this context as: *The whole blood alcohol results were 0.094 and 0.096 g/dL having a mean of 0.0950 g/dL which did not have an associated total allowable error of more than 8% with approximately 95% probability.* One context appropriate for the application of the total error method is where a single control is measured as part of an analytical run. If the control exceeded the total allowable error, one would not know whether it was due to bias or random sources. However, the result would be caught and the system corrected before resuming routine measurements. One of the criticisms of the method of total allowable error method is that it allows bias to exist without correcting for it. (Dybkaer, 1999, Dybkaer, 1999) Admittedly, the total error method provides a very conservative estimate, a maximum actually, for interpreting measurement uncertainty.

9.4 Monte Carlo methods

Monte Carlo methods are simulation techniques that are more computationally intensive. With faster computers available, these methods are becoming more popular. Monte Carlo methods require assumptions regarding the measurement function along with the distributional form and parameters for each of the input components, being themselves random variables. Random data are then simulated from each of the component distributions, placed into the measurement function, followed by the computation of the measurand. This is done a large number of times, generating a distribution of response values. From these results, the distribution, the expected value and the standard uncertainty of the response variable can be determined. As a result we do not need to assume some distributional form for the response variable and we have a direct, empirically determined estimate of uncertainty. Monte Carlo methods also avoid two limitations of the GUM method - the required linear relationship between the response variable and the components and the justified application of the central limit theorem. (Fernandez, et.al., 2009) Consider the following example of a breath alcohol measurement function where we have six input variables: $\overline{Y}_{Corr} = \dfrac{\overline{Y}_0 \cdot GC_{Sol} \cdot R}{\overline{X} \cdot K \cdot GC_{Cont}}$ and where we assume the following distributions for each of the six input variables: $\overline{Y}_0 \sim N\left(0.1250, 0.0047^2\right)$ the mean of the original n measurements, $GC_{Sol} \sim N\left(0.1025, 0.0008^2\right)$ the mean of the simulator solution measurements by gas chromatography, $R \sim N\left(0.100, 0.0003^2\right)$ the traceable reference value, $\overline{X} \sim N\left(0.0825, 0.0012^2\right)$ the mean of the breath test instrument measuring the simulator solution, $K \sim Unif(1.21, 1.25)$ the ratio of partition coefficients in the simulator heated to 34^0C and $GC_{Cont} \sim N\left(0.0980, 0.0008^2\right)$ the results from measuring the traceable controls on the gas chromatograph. We employ a routine written in R that simulates random results from each of these distributions and computes the response variable $\left(\overline{Y}_{Corr}\right)$. This is done 10,000 times. The resulting distribution for the response variable is seen in figure 9. The expected value for the response variable is 0.1287 g/210L with an empirical 95% confidence interval of 0.1215 to 0.1360g/210L, determined from the distribution of results in figure 9. The sampling/method component was also correctly identified as having the largest contribution to total uncertainty of 85%.

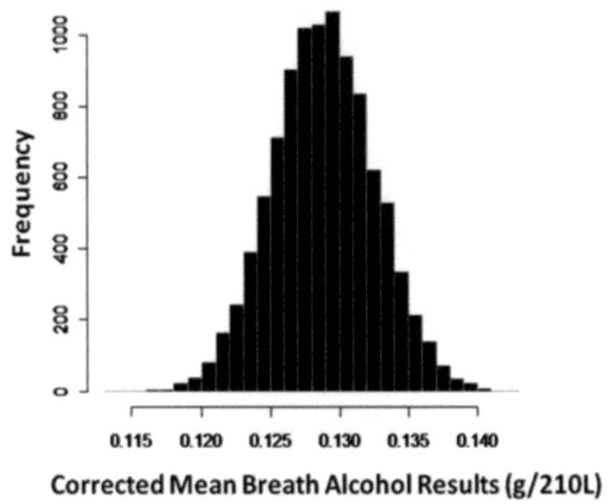

Fig. 9. A distribution of 10,000 Monte Carlo simulated measurement results

10. Uncertainty in qualitative analysis

Several measurements performed in forensic toxicology are qualitative in nature. These measurements typically take the form of a binary response (i.e., pass/fail, yes/no, over/under, present/absent, etc.). They are classification in nature where materials are assigned to discrete groups based on measurement results. Diagnostic tests are one important example of qualitative analyses. Their qualitative results are important indicators of whether some specified threshold has been exceeded or not and are important for the determination of further confirmatory analyses. In some cases the measurement system will respond simply with binary results (green light/red light). At other times the measurement system is quantitative on a continuous scale which can be dichotomized. For example, a pre-arrest breath test instrument employing a fuel cell might measure the breath alcohol on a continuous concentration scale but is interpreted as being greater than or equal to 0.080 g/210L or less than 0.080 g/210L. In either case, the response is considered binary and thus qualitative. The uncertainty associated with qualitative analyses has received much less attention than that of quantitative analysis. The uncertainty in qualitative analyses is basically probabilistic in nature - that is, we are interested in the probability of being correct in our decision. We are concerned primarily with the probability of false positive and false negative results. While there are a number of statistical methods for estimating the uncertainty associated with qualitative or diagnostic test results, there is no consensus as to which is to be preferred. (EURACHEM/CITAC, 2003, Pulido, et.al., 2003, Ellison, et.al., 1998) Some methods involve the simple determination of false-positive (FP) and false-negative (FN) fractions which in turn assess the probability of making a wrong decision. (Pepe, 2003) Other qualitative and quantitative methods employ Baye's Theorem which is argued by many as a superior approach to estimating and interpreting measurement uncertainty. (Gleser, 1998, Weise and Woger, 1992, Kacker and Jones, 2003, Phillips, et.al., 1998). Space does not permit further discussion of these important and useful methods.

11. Discussion

Several examples have been presented here for estimating measurement uncertainty in the context of forensic toxicology. By no means do these examples imply that all possible uncertainty components have been considered. These examples were intended primarily to illustrate the general approach and computations involved. Moreover, while an example may have assumed a blood alcohol context, it could just as well have been applied in the context of breath or drug analysis. While the general approach will be relevant to most methods in forensic toxicology, each laboratory will need to identify and quantify its uncertainty components unique to its protocols and instrumentation. The examples and discussion presented here have also assumed independence among the input or predictor variables. This is certainly not always a valid assumption. In some measurement contexts there will be significant correlation between input variables which must be accounted for. (GUM, EURACHEM/CITAC, Ellison, 2005) While these concepts may be new to some practicing toxicologists, the concept of measurement uncertainty should not raise concerns for the forensic sciences. The emphasis should be on their ability to quantify confidence of measurement results. They should be presented in a manner that emphasizes and demonstrates their fitness-for-purpose. Modern technology should enhance and simplify these computations as well. Spreadsheet programs can be developed which require only the entry of specific values followed by the generation of all uncertainty results. Moreover, such computations can even be incorporated into the software of aalytical instruments. Such technology, when validated, should greatly simplify the process.

Several factors are responsible for the emphasis today on reporting measurement results along with their uncertainty. These include legal, economic, liability, accrediting and technological considerations. As professional toxicologists concerned with providing measurement results of the highest possible quality, we must be prepared to make this extra effort of providing the relevant uncertainty. Since there is no consensus regarding the best approach for computing uncertainty at this time, toxicologists should be familiar with the several approaches suggested here and then select and validate the one which best suits their analytical, procedural and legal context. The literature is rich with material regarding measurement uncertainty and should be carefully reviewed by toxicologists. (Drosg, 2007, Williams, 2008, Fernandez, 2011 Ekberg,et.al., 2011) This effort wll enhance the quality and interpretability of our measurement results and help establish a foundation of "evidence based forensics". The unavoidable fact of measurement uncertainty results in the risk of making incorrect decisions. While ignoring the uncertainty increases this risk, providing the uncertainty reduces and quantifies the risk for the decision maker. This fact alone should motivate the legal community to request and forensic toxicologists to rigorously estimate and provide such estimates.

12. References

Altman, D.G., Machin, D., Bryant, T.N. and Gardner, M.J. (2000). *Statistics with confidence*, (2nd edition), British Medical Journal, London, ISBN 0-7279-1375-1

ASCLD/LAB. (2011) ASCLD/LAB Policy on Measurement Uncertainty, August 2011, Available from: http://www.ascld-lab.org/documents/AL-PD-3051.pdf,

Ballico, M. (2000). Limitations of the Welch-Satterthwaite Approximation for Measurement Uncertainty Calculations. *Metrologia*, Vol.37, pp. 61-64.

Barwick, V.J. & Ellison, S.L.R. (1999). Measurement Uncertainty: Approaches to the Evaluation of Uncertainties Associated with Recovery. *Analyst*, Vol.124, pp. 981-990.

Bich, W., Cox, M. and Harris, P. (2006). Evolution of the 'Guide to the Expression of Uncertainty in Measurement'. *Metrologia*, Vol.43, pp. S161-S166.

Daubert vs. Merrell Dow Pharmaceuticals, Inc., 509 U.S. 579 (1993).

Deldossi, L. and Zappa, D. (2009). ISO 5725 and GUM: Comparison and Comments. *Accred Qual Assur*, Vol.14, pp. 159-166.

Desimoni, E. & Brunetti, B. (2010). About Acceptance and Rejection Zones as Defined in the EURACHEM/CITAC Guide (2007) 'Use of Uncertainty Information in Compliance Assessment'. *Accred Qual Assur*, Vol.15, pp. 45-47.

Drosg, M. (2007). *Dealing with Uncertainties: A Guide to Error Analysis*, Springer, New York.

Dybkaer, R. (1999). Setting Quality Specifications for the Future with Newer Approaches to Defining Uncertainty in Laboratory Medicine. *Scand J Clin Lab Invest*, Vol.59, pp. 579-584.

Dybkaer, R. (1999). From Total Allowable Error via Metrological Traceability to Uncertainty of Measurement of the Unbiased Result, *Accred Qual Assur*, Vol.4, pp. 401-405.

Ekberg, C., Englund, S. & Liljenzin, J.O. (2011). Uncertainty Analysis of Correlated Stability Constants. *Accred Qual Assur*, Vol.16, pp. 185-189.

Ellison, S.L.R., Gregory, S. & Hardcastle, W.A. (1998). Quantifying uncertainty in qualitative analysis. *Analyst*, Vol.123, pp. 1155-1161.

Ellison, L. (2005). Including Correlation Effects in an Improved Spreadsheet Calculation of Combined Standard Uncertainties. *Accred Qual Assur*, Vol.10, pp. 338-343.

EURACHEM/CITAC Guide. (2000). *Quantifying Uncertainty in Analytical Measurement*, 2nd Ed., May 2011, Available from: http://www.measurementuncertainty.org/mu/QUAM2000-1.pdf

EURACHEM/CITAC Guide. (2003). *The Expression of Uncertainty in Qualitative Testing*, May 2011, Available from: http://www.nmschembio.org.uk/dm_documents/LGCVAM2003048_cOjjl.pdf

EURACHEM/CITAC Guide. (2007). *Use of uncertainty in compliance assessment*. Eds. Williams, A. and Ellison, S.L.R., April 2011, Available from: http://www.citac.cc/EURACHEM-CITAC%20Guide%20 %20Use%20of%20uncertainty%20information%20%20in%20compliance%20assessment%20-%202007.pdf

Fernandez, M. (2011). On the use of the 'Uncertainty Budget' to Detect Dominant Terms in the Evaluation of Measurement Uncertainty. *Accred Qual Assur*, Vol.16, pp. 83-88.

Fernandez, M., Calderon, J. & Diez, P. (2009). Implementation in MATLAB of the Adaptive Monte Carlo Method for the Evaluation of Measurment Uncertainties. *Accred Qual Assur*, Vol.14, pp. 95-106.

Gates, K., Chang, N., Dilek, I., Jian, H., Pogue, S. & Sreenivasan, U. (2009). The Uncertainty of Reference Standards - A Guide to Understanding Factors Impacting Uncertainty, Uncertainty Calculations, and Vendor Certifications. *Journal of Analytical Toxicology*, Vol.33, pp. 532-539.

Gleser, L.J. (1998). Assessing Uncertainty in Measurement. *Statistical Science*, Vol.13 No.3, pp. 277-290.

International Organization for Standardization (2008). *International Vocabulary of Basic and General Terms in Metrology (VIM)*, 3rd ed., ISO, Geneva. May 2011, Available from:
http://www.bipm.org/utils/common/documents/jcgm/JCGM_200_2008_pdf

International Organization for Standardization (ISO). (2008). *Guide to the Expression of Uncertainty in Measurement*, ISO, Geneva, 2008. June 2011, Available at:
http://www.bipm.org/utils/common/documents/jcgm/JCGM_100_2008_E.pdf

International Organization of Legal Metrology (OIML), *International Alcoholometric Tables*, Paris, available online at: http://www.oiml.org/publications/R/R022-e75.pdf

ISO/IEC 17025. (2000). General requirements for the competence of testing and calibration laboratories. London: British Standards Institution, pp. 1-26.

Jones, A.W. (1989). Differences Between Capillary and Venous Blood-alcohol Concentrations as a Function of Time After Drinking, with Emphasis on Sampling Variations in Left vs Right Arm. *Clin. Chem.*, Vol.35 No.3, pp. 400-404.

Jones, A.W. & Schuberth, J. (1989). Computer-aided Headspace Gas Chromatography Applied to Blood-alcohol Analysis: Importance of Online Process Control. *Journal of Forensic Sciences*, Vol.34 No.5, pp. 1116-1127.

Kacker, R. & Jones, A. (2003). "On Use of Bayesian Statistics to Make the *Guide to the Expression of Uncertainty in Measurement* Consistent. *Metrologia*, Vol.40, pp. 235-248.

Kacker, R., Sommer, K. & Kessel, R. (2007). Evolution of Modern Approaches to Express Uncertainty in Measurement. *Metrologia*, Vol.44, pp. 513-529.

Kacker, R., Kessel, R. & Sommer K. (2010). Assessing Differences Between Results Determined According to the Guide to the Expression of Uncertainty in Measurement. *Journal of Research of the National Institute of Standards and Technology*, Vol.115 No.6, pp. 453-459.

Kadis, R. (2007). Do We Really Need to Account for Run Bias when Producing Analytical Results with Stated Uncertainty? Comment on 'Treatment of Bias in Estimating Measurement Uncertainty' by G.E. O'Donnell and D.B. Hibbert, *Analyst*, Vol.132, pp. 1272-1274.

Kane, J.S. (1997). Analytical Bias: The Neglected Component of Measurement Uncertainty. *Analyst*, Vol.122, pp. 1283-1288.

King, B. & Lawn, R. (1999). International Interlaboratory Study of Forensic Ethanol Standards. *Analyst*, Vol. 124, pp. 1123-1130.

Kirkup, L. & Frenkel, B. (2006). *An introduction to uncertainty in measurement.* Cambridge University Press, Cambridge, UK.

Kristiansen, J. (2001). Description of a Generally Applicable Model for the Evaluation of Uncertainty of Measurement in Clinical Chemistry. *Clin Chem Lab Med,* Vol.39 No.10, pp. 920-931.

Kristiansen, J. (2003). The Guide to Expression of Uncertainty in Measurement Approach to Estimating Uncertainty: An Appraisal. *Clinical Chemistry,* Vol.49 No.11, pp. 1822-1829.

Kristiansen, J. & Petersen, H.W. (2004). An Uncertainty Budget for the Measurement of Ethanol in Blood by Headspace Gas Chromatography. *J of Analytical Toxicology,* Vol.28, pp. 456-463.

Krouwer, J. (2003). Critique of the Guide to the Expression of Uncertainty in Measurement Method of Estimating and Reporting Uncertainty in Diagnostic Assays. *Clinical Chemistry,* Vol.49 No.11, pp. 1818-1821.

Ku, H.H. (1966). Notes on the Use of Propagation of Error Formulas. *J. Res. Natl. Bureau Standards -C, Eng. Instrum.* 70C (4), pp. 916-921.

Linnet, K., Johansen, S.S., Buchard, A., Munkholm, J. & Morling, N. (2008). Dominance of Pre-analytical Over Analytical Variation for Measurement of Methadone and its Main Metabolite in Postmortem Femoral Blood. *Forensic Science International,* Vol. 179, pp. 78-82.

Marato, A., Boque, R., Riu, J. & Rius, F.X. (2002). Should Non-significant Bias be Included in the Uncertainty Budget? *Accred Qual Assur,* Vol.7, pp. 90-94.

Mnookin, J.L., Cole, S.A., Dror, I.E., Fisher, B.A.J., Houck, M.M., Inman, K., Kaye, D.H., Koehler, J.J., Langenburg, G., Risinger, D.M., Rudin, N., Siegel, J. & Stoney, D.A. (2011). The Need for a Research Culture in the Forensic Sciences. *UCLA Law Review,* Vol.58, pp. 725-779.

National Academy of Science. (2009). *Strengthening Forensic Science in the United States: A Path Forward,* National Research Council, The National Academies Press, Washington, D.C.

O'Donnell, G.E. & Hibbert, D.B. (2005). Treatment of Bias in Estimating Measurement Uncertainty. *Analyst,* Vol.130, pp. 721-729.

O'Donnell, G.E. & Hibbert, D.B. (2007). Reply to 'Do We Really Need to Account for Run Bias When Producing Analytical Results with Stated Uncertainty? Comment on 'Treatment of Bias in Estimating Measurement Uncertainty'. *Analyst,* Vol.132, pp. 1275-1277.

Pepe, M.S. (2003). *The statistical evaluation of medical tests for classification and prediction.* Oxford University Press, Oxford.

Petersen, P.H., Stockl, D., Westgard, J.O., Sandberg, S., Linnet, K. & Thienpont, L. (2001). Models for Combining Random and Systematic Errors. Assumptions and Consequences for Different Models. *Clin Chem Lab Med,* Vol.39 No.7, pp. 589-595.

Philipp, R., Hanebeck, O., Hein, S., Bremser, W., Win, T. & Nehls, I. (2010). Ethanol/Water Solutions as Certified Reference Materials for Breath Alcohol Analyzer Calibration. *Accred Qual Assur,* Vol.15, pp. 141-146.

Phillips, S.D., Eberhardt, K.R. and Parry, B. (1997). Guidelines for Expressing the Uncertainty of Measurement Results Containing Uncorrected Bias. *J of Research of the National Institute of Standards and Technology*, Vol.102 No.5, pp. 577-585.

Phillips, S.D., Estler, W.T., Levenson, M.S. and Eberhardt, K.R., (1998), "Calculation of Measurement Uncertainty Using Prior Information", *J. of Research of the National Institute of Standards and Technology*, Vol.103 No.6, pp. 625-632.

Pulido, A., Ruisanchez, I., Boque, R. & Rius, F.X. (2003). Uncertainty of Results in Routine Qualitative Analysis. *Trends in Analytical Chemistry*, Vol.22 Nol.10, pp. 647-654.

Rocke, D.M. & Lorenzato, S. (1995). A Two-Component Model for Measurement Error in Analytical Chemistry. *Technometrics*, Vol.37 No.2, pp. 176-184.

Sklerov, J.H. & Couper, F.J. (2011). Calculation and Verification of blood Ethanol Measurement Uncertainty for Headspace Gas Chromatography. *J Anal Toxicol*, Vol.35, pp. 402-410.

Stowell, A.R., Gainsford, A.R. & Gullberg, R.G. (2008). New Zealand's Breath and Blood Alcohol Testing Programs: Further Data Analysis and Forensic Implications. *Forensic Science International*, Vol.178, pp. 83-92.

Synek, V. (2005). Attempts to Include Uncorrected Bias in the Measurement Uncertainty. *Talanta*, Vol.65, pp.829-837

Taylor, B.N. & Kuyatt, C.E. (1994). NIST Technical Note 1297, *Guidelines for Evaluating and Expressing the Uncertainty of NIST Measurement Results*, Physics Laboratory, Gaithersburg, MD: National Institute of Standards and Technology. March 2011, Available from: http://physics.nist.gov/Document/tn1297.pdf

Thompson, M. & Fearn, T. (1996). What Exactly is Fitness For Purpose in Analytical Measurement. *Analyst*, Vol.121, pp. 275-278.

Thompson, M. (1997). Comparability and Traceability in Analytical Measurements and Reference Materials. *Analyst*, Vol.122, pp. 1201-1205.

Thompson, M. (1998). Do we really need detection limits? *Analyst*, Vol.123, pp. 405-407.

Thompson, M., Ellison, S.L.R., Fajgelj, A., Willetts, P. & Wood, R. (1999). Harmonized Guidelines for the Use of Recovery Information in Analytical Measurement. *Pure and Applied Chemistry*, Vol.71 No.2, pp. 337-348.

Thompson, M. & Coles, B.J. (2011). Use of the 'Characteristic Function' for Modeling Repeatability Precision. *Accred Qual Assur*, Vol.16, pp. 13-19.

Wallace, J. (2010). Proficiency Testing as a Basis for Estimating Uncertainty of Measurement: Application to Forensic Alcohol and Toxicology Quantitations. *J Forensic Sci*, Vol. 55, pp. 767-773.

Wallace, J. (2010). Ten Methods for Calculating the Uncertainty of Measurement. *Science and Justice*, Vol.50 No.4, pp. 182-186.

Walls, H.J. & A.R. Brownlie. (1985). *Drink, Drugs and Driving.* 2nd ed., Sweet and Maxwell, London, p. 108.

Weise, K. & Woger, W. (1992). A Bayesian Theory of Measurement Uncertainty, *Meas Sci Technol*, Vol.3, pp. 1-11.

Westgard, J.O. (2010). Managing Quality vs. Measuring Uncertainty in the Medical Laboratory. *Clin Chem Lab Med*, Vol.48 No.1, pp. 31-40.

Williams, A. (2008). Principles of the EURACHEM/CITAC Guide 'Use of Uncertainty Information in Compliance Assessment'. *Accred Qual Assur*, Vol.13, pp. 633-638.

19

Toxicokinetics and Organ-Specific Toxicity

P.D. Ward
Johnson & Johnson,
Pharmaceutical Research and Development, L.L.C.,
USA

1. Introduction

Toxicokinetics (TK) refers to the kinetics of absorption, distribution, metabolism, and elimination (ADME) processes where both first and zero order kinetics are expected and these processes can vary over a wide range of doses. The goal of TK and pharmacokinetic studies are similar, which is to define the ADME properties of a drug candidate (Dixit & Ward, 2007). Therefore, the wide range of studies to define these ADME properties (e.g., in vitro and in vivo metabolism, animal mass balance, and distribution studies) performed in the pharmacokinetic evaluation of the drug candidate can also serve to help guide the toxicokinetic evaluation of the same drug candidate with the knowledge that first and zero order kinetics might be expected in the ADME processes at the higher doses of this drug candidate in the safety studies.

Now it is widely accepted that toxic effects can be better extrapolated from animals to humans when these comparisons are based on TK instead of dose alone. For example, the safety margin that is based on the ratio of the animal exposure at no observed adverse effect level (NOAEL) to human exposure at the efficacious dose is a key predictor of human safety risk. To calculate this safety margin, the animal and human exposure is determined by analyzing drug and metabolites concentrations in plasma, which is the most practical and widely accepted way of assessing this risk (Dixit & Ward, 2007). However, most safety issues are not observed in the plasma but in the organs and/or tissues. Therefore, is sampling plasma a good measure of the safety margin for the risk assessment of safety?

Sampling plasma and extrapolating this exposure to organs or tissues assumes that 1) concentration of drug in plasma is in equilibrium with concentrations in tissues, 2) changes in plasma drug concentrations reflect changes in tissue drug concentrations over time, and 3) distribution of drug and its metabolites is not affected by polarized cells (e.g., drug transporters and enzymes) that protect a lot of these tissues. Drug transport into tissues may not be a passive process and may depend on drug transporters (Ward, 2008), thus these assumptions may result in an inaccurate assessment of target organ exposure to drug and metabolites. Even without a drug candidate being a substrate for a drug transporter, lysosomal trapping of weak bases (e.g., liver and lung) or accumulation in membranes (e.g., muscle) can occur that can give rise to preferential distribution of the drug and its metabolites (MacIntyre & Cutler, 1988). Therefore, plasma is sometimes not a good surrogate for tissue levels of drug and its metabolites, especially for the assessment of risk for some types of organ-specific toxicity.

The following case examples will illustrate how focusing on drug and metabolites in these tissues (where toxicity is observed) instead of plasma increases understanding of the nature of the toxicity and in some cases allows the efficient identification of a backup drug that has markedly less potential to cause that specific organ toxicity under investigation. These case examples are categorized by the different organs where toxicity was investigated and are generated from the author's personal experience in the pharmaceutical industry.

2. Case example: Toxicokinetics and testicular toxicity

This case example (described below) will highlight 1) preferential distribution of parent and metabolites to tissue, 2) a predominant metabolite that is different in the tissue versus plasma, and 3) accumulation of parent and metabolite that occurs in tissue and not in plasma. Furthermore, the case example will highlight that focusing on tissue burden of the drug and its metabolites (and not plasma concentrations) may actually ensure that a backup does not produce the same toxicity.

2.1 Testicular toxicity in rat

In a 13-week rat safety study, testicular atrophy was observed in rats at all doses tested (10, 50, and 250 mg/kg/day); however, these findings were not observed in the 2-week study. At the dose of 250 mg/kg/day, testicular atrophy was observed in approximately 50% of all rats. At doses of 10 and 50 mg/kg/day, these findings were observed in only 10% of rats but responsibility of Drug A for this toxicity could not be discounted (i.e., unequivocal). Therefore, no NOAEL could be assigned in this study, which markedly complicated the further development of this drug candidate.

2.2 Role of toxicokinetics in rat testicular toxicity

From the rat quantitative whole body autoradiography (QWBA) study, preferential distribution of Drug A-derived radioactivity to the testes was observed; furthermore, this radioactivity was retained in the testes markedly longer compared to other tissues (Figure 1). Since distribution of radioactivity included both parent and its metabolites and the dose in the rat QWBA study was based on the lowest dose of the rat safety study (i.e., 10 mg/kg/day), a cold study was initiated where rats were dosed with a single oral dose of Drug A at 50 mg/kg (similar to the mid dose in the rat safety study). After this single oral dose, the plasma, testes, and epididymes of the rats were collected at different time points and analyzed for Drug A and its two known metabolites (M1 and M2). Interestingly, the predominant metabolite in plasma (i.e., M2) was not the predominant metabolite in testes. M1 preferentially distributed to the testes from plasma; whereas, M2 had limited distribution to this tissue (Table 1 and 2). Furthermore, the T_{max} of M1 was 48 hours in testes suggesting a large accumulation potential of this metabolite in testes compared to plasma. Indeed after a follow-up study for six months of repeated daily oral dosing, M1 accumulated approximately five-fold in the testes; whereas, the parent did not accumulate (Figure 2). Furthermore, parent and M1 did not accumulate in the plasma during the 6-month rat safety study (data not shown).

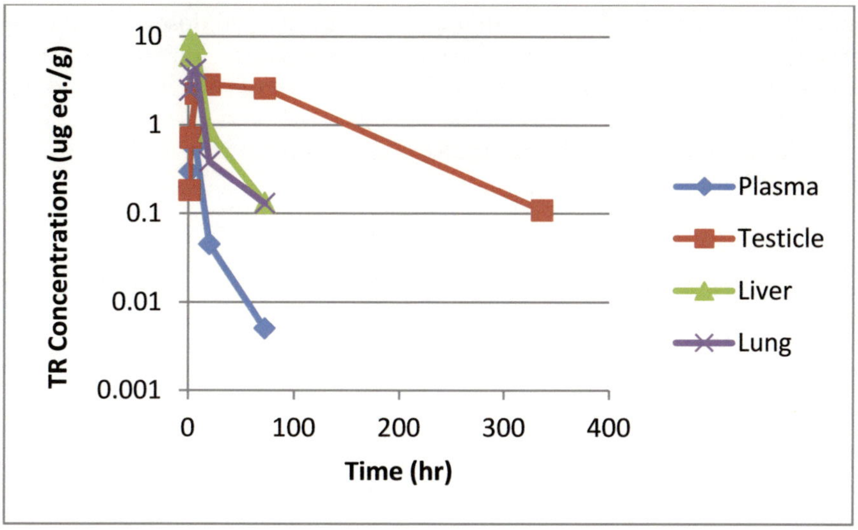

Fig. 1. Total Radioactivity (TR) Concentrations versus Time Profile of Drug A-derived Radioactivity in Rat Plasma, Testicle, Liver, and Lung.
Long Evans rats were dosed with a single oral dose of 10 mg/kg [^{14}C]-labeled Drug A. At different times after this dose, rats were sacrificed via exsanguination (cardiac puncture) under isoflurane anesthesia and blood (approximately 2 to 10 mL) was collected into tubes containing K_2EDTA immediately prior to collection of carcasses for QWBA. Samples were maintained on wet ice and refrigerated until aliquoted and centrifuged to obtain plasma. Immediately after blood collection the animals were prepared for QWBA. The carcasses were immediately frozen in a hexane/dry ice bath for approximately 8 minutes. Each carcass was drained, blotted dry, placed into an appropriately labelled bag, and placed on dry ice or stored at approximately -70°C for at least 2 hours. Each carcass was then stored at approximately -20°C. The frozen carcasses were embedded in chilled carboxymethylcellulose and frozen into blocks. Embedded carcasses were stored at approximately -20°C in preparation for autoradiographic analysis.

		Half Life (hr)	T_{max} (hr)	C_{max} (ng/mL or g)	AUC_{last} (ng*hr/mL or g)	AUC_{inf} (ng*hr/mL or g)
Plasma	M1	4	4	29	401	410
Plasma	M2	6	4	1033	11983	12025
Plasma	Parent	5	4	3712	43454	43491
Testes	M1	46	48	1182	156763	158157
Testes	M2	7	4	76	412	947
Testes	Parent	54	8	9061	684074	692652
Epididymes	M1	9	8	1441	25949	26064
Epididymes	M2	7	4	231	1215	2908
Epididymes	Parent	51	8	6676	115682	116647

Table 1. Toxicokinetic Profile of Drug A and its Metabolites in Rat Plasma, Testes, and Epididymes.

Fed Sprague Dawley rats (n=27) were administered a single oral dose of 50 mg/kg Drug A. Testes, epididymes, and plasma were collected at 1, 4, 8, 24, 48, 72, 96, 168, and 336 hours post dose from three rats at each time point. Bioanalysis of plasma, testes, and epididymes for Drug A (Parent) and its metabolites M1 and M2 was performed. Toxicokinetic parameters were determined on plasma, testes, and epididymes.

		C_{max}	AUC_{last}	AUC_{inf}
Testes	M1	40	391	386
Testes	M2	0.07	0.03	0.08
Testes	Parent	2	16	16
Epididymes	M1	49	65	64
Epididymes	M2	0.22	0.10	0.24
Epididymes	Parent	2	3	3

Table 2. Tissue to Plasma Ratios of Drug A and its metabolites in Rat Plasma, Testes, and Epididymes.

See description of Table 1 for experimental details. After toxicokinetic parameters were determined on testes, epididymes, and plasma, tissue to plasma ratios were calculated.

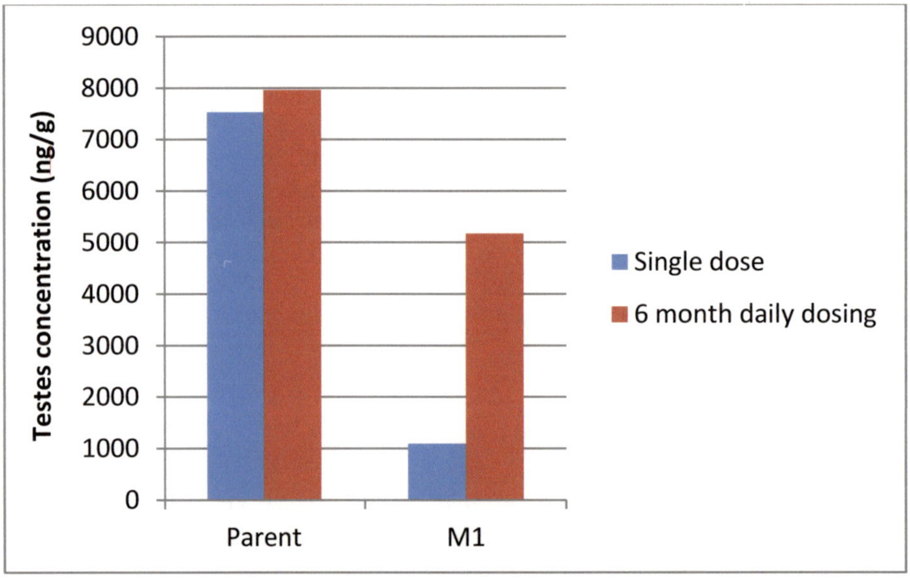

Fig. 2. Distribution of Drug A and its Metabolite, M1, in the Rat Testes after 6 Months of Repeated Daily Dosing (50 mg/kg/day) Compared to a Single Oral Dose (50 mg/kg)

Fed Sprague Dawley rats (n=4) were administered a single oral dose or repeated daily oral doses of 50 mg/kg/day Drug A for 6 months. Testes were collected at 24 hours post dose. Bioanalysis of testes for Drug A (Parent) and M1 was performed. Concentrations of Drug A and M1 after 6 months of repeated daily oral dosing (50 mg/kg/day) were compared to a single oral dose (50 mg/kg) at 24 hours post dose (see description of Table 1 for experimental details of the single oral dose study).

2.3 Identification of a backup molecule with limited potential for testicular toxicity

In order to identify a backup to this molecule (e.g., Drug A), screening potential backups in terms of their toxicity potential to rat testicular atrophy was not practical because of the time required for the toxicity to be observed (i.e., more than 2 weeks). Therefore, another method of screening potential backups needed to be initiated.

To aid the identification of this backup, the rat QWBA study of a prior drug candidate for this target (referred to as Drug B) was assessed where Drug B did not induce testes toxicity in rat during long-term safety studies. Interestingly, Drug B-derived radioactivity was approximately equivalent in blood and testes (Table 3), suggesting that the reduced burden of this tissue may have markedly lowered the susceptibility for this toxicity compared to the structurally similar molecule, Drug A. This markedly lowered distribution to the testes was also mirrored in the volume of distribution calculated after an single intravenous administration of Drug A and B, where the volume of distribution was markedly lower for Drug B compared to Drug A in every animal species tested (e.g., rat, dog, and monkey). Therefore to select future backups of Drug A into development, the volume of distribution was calculated from similar studies with administration of potential backup drug candidates via the intravenous route. These studies led to the identification of a potential drug candidate with similar distribution properties of Drug B (i.e, lower volume of distribution in every animal species tested after a single intravenous dose compared to Drug A). This potential backup to Drug A (referred to as Drug C) was then assessed in a rat QWBA study. In this study, Drug C-derived radioactivity was approximately equivalent in blood and testes (Table 4). From these encouraging results, Drug C was advanced into further development where no testicular toxicity has been observed in long-term rat safety studies. These results support the hypothesis that reduced tissue burden of the drug and its metabolites may actually predict that a backup does not produce the same toxicity.

Time (hr)	0.5	2	4	8	12	24	48	72	120
Blood	21.0	17.0	15.5	8.22	3.09	0.153	ND	ND	ND
Testis	2.84	7.54	15.4	9.98	5.26	0.346	0.135	BLQ	BLQ

Table 3. Tissue Concentrations (μg equivalents/g) of Drug B-derived Radioactivity in Rat Plasma and Testis.

Long Evans rats were dosed with single oral dose of 30 mg/kg [^{14}C]-labeled Drug B. See description of Figure 1 for experimental details.

Time (hr)	1	4	8	24	72	168	336
Blood	4530	1280	310	58.3	BLQ	ND	ND
Testis	2240	989	456	105	BLQ	BLQ	BLQ

Table 4. Tissue Concentrations (μg equivalents/g) of Drug C-derived Radioactivity in Rat Plasma and Testis.

Long Evans rats were dosed with a single oral dose of 10 mg/kg [^{14}C]-labeled Drug C. See description of Figure 1 for experimental details.

2.4 Conclusion

Knowledge of tissue toxicokinetics will increase the understanding about the potential mechanism of an organ-specific toxicity and can potentially assist in identifying a backup drug candidate that has a markedly lower potential for this organ-specific toxicity.

3. Case example: Toxicokinetics and liver toxicity

This case example (described below) will highlight an investigation into liver toxicity where the mechanism of the liver toxicity was questioned. This drug candidate induced a strong pharmacological response; therefore, an investigation was launched to investigate whether the liver toxicity induced by this drug was a result of its strong pharmacology or an off target effect (i.e., independent of its targeted receptor pharmacology) from one of the metabolites of the drug.

3.1 Liver toxicity in dog

In a dog toleration study at the lowest dose tested (10 mg/kg), slight, acute central-lobular and portal inflammation with individual hepatocyte necrosis was observed. Therefore, no NOAEL could be assigned in this study which markedly complicated the further development of this drug candidate.

3.2 Role of toxicokinetics in dog liver toxicity

Even though this drug candidate was known to elicit a strong pharmacological response that could be capable of inducing the adverse effect observed in the dog toleration study, the potential of this drug candidate to form an acyl glucuronide (M2) in liver was evident and thus this metabolite may also be the cause of these adverse effects (Kenny et al., 2005). Furthermore, the potential preferential distribution of this drug candidate to the liver may also predispose its adverse effects. Therefore to investigate these hypotheses, the plasma and liver (also kidney and fat for comparison) were analyzed for drug candidate and its metabolites in the dog after 14 days of repeated daily oral doses of the drug candidate (i.e., parent).

After toxicokinetic evaluation of the tissues and plasma, the concentrations of parent in liver were consistently lower than plasma at 2, 6, and 24 hours postdose, suggesting no preferential distribution of the drug to the liver (Table 5). Furthermore, the acyl glucuronide metabolite (M2) along with other metabolites (M1, M3, and M4) were only observed in the plasma and not in the liver (Table 6), suggesting that these metabolites were not the cause of the observed liver toxicity. These results suggested that the observed liver toxicity in dog was caused by the strong pharmacological response of the drug candidate and probably not caused by an off target effect of M2 (or any other metabolites observed in plasma). Furthermore, the lack of preferential distribution of parent to the liver indicated that the toxicokinetic analysis of plasma exposure was correct in evaluating the risk for observed liver toxicity in the potential further development of this drug candidate.

3.3 Conclusion

Toxicokinetic evaluation of tissue (where toxicity is observed) and plasma for drug and its metabolites will allow further mechanistic understanding of the cause of the observed tissue toxicity and will aid in the choice of the most relevant matrix for sampling in order for the correct evaluation of risk in further development of the drug candidate.

Day	Time (hr)	Concentration (μg/mL or g)							
		Plasma	Plasma + Acid	Liver	Liver + Acid	Kidney	Kidney + Acid	Fat	
Day 1	2	292	373	130	168	209	180	59	Mean
		35	114	17	24	46	68	11	SD
	6	286	284	131	96	181	123	65	Mean
		112	92	35	12	102	57	4	SD
	24	54	48	46	28	68	34	61	Mean
		44	37	24	16	37	25	5	SD
Day 14	2	295	381	226	140	245	90	73	Mean
		141	208	100	27	160	38	12	SD
	6	293	275	284	128	187	94	71	Mean
		89	110	72	29	27	35	5	SD
	24	39	37	41	29	52	36	72	Mean
		54	53	40	24	61	43	3	SD

Table 5. Concentration-Time Profile of Parent in Dog Plasma, Liver, Kidney, and Fat.

Fed Beagle dogs (n=18) were administered a single oral dose or repeated daily oral doses for 14 days of 10 mg/kg drug. Liver, kidney, fat, and plasma were collected at 2, 6, and 24 hours post dose from three dogs at each time point with and without formic acid (formic acid was added to potentially increase the stability of the acyl glucuronide metabolite). Bioanalysis of liver, kidney, fat, and plasma for drug candidate was performed.

		Plasma		Plasma + Acid		Liver		Liver + Acid	
Metabolite	Type	Day 1	Day 14	Day 1	Day 14	Day 1	Day 14	Day 1	Day 14
Parent	-	116,860,326	123,174,663	122,389,879	122,716,072	27,431,252	36,110,995	28,993,390	29,924,921
M1	Oxidation + Sulfation	ND	ND	ND	ND	ND	ND	ND	ND
M2	Glucuronidation	5,299,597	3,790,520	3,552,836	2,817,400	ND	ND	ND	ND
M3	Oxidation	ND	ND	ND	ND	ND	ND	ND	ND
M4	Oxidation	453,680	1,035,337	553,582	1,045,264	ND	ND	ND	ND

ND = not detected

Table 6. Peak Area Counts Versus Time Profile of Parent and its Metabolites in Dog Plasma, Liver, Kidney, and Fat.

Fed Beagle dogs (n=18) were administered a single oral dose or repeated daily oral doses for 14 days of 10 mg/kg drug. Liver, kidney, fat, and plasma were collected at 24 hours post dose from three dogs at each time point with and without formic acid (formic acid was added to potentially increase the stability of the acyl glucuronide metabolite). Bioanalysis of liver, kidney, fat, and plasma for drug (Parent) and it metabolites (M1, M2, M3, and M4) was performed. Peak areas were integrated for both parent and metabolites in each matrix. Data from kidney and fat are not shown.

4. Case example: Toxicokinetics and central nervous system (CNS) toxicity

This case example (described below) will highlight an investigation into CNS toxicity where the lead drug candidate displayed CNS toxicity in the monkey and a backup molecule needed to be identified. This example highlights utilization of the efflux transporter, P-glycoprotein (Pgp), to limit the tissue distribution of the backup drug candidate to the CNS in order to limit CNS toxicity potential.

4.1 CNS toxicity in monkey

In a Cynomolgus monkey toleration study at the 100 mg/kg/day dose (repeat daily oral dosing), test article-related clinical signs observed in the male monkey were characterized by vomiting, ptosis, decreased activity, prostration, tremors, convulsion and ataxia. A slight safety margin was identified (approximately 7-fold); however, this margin was not large enough to confidently advance this drug candidate into longer GLP safety studies in monkey.

4.2 Role of toxicokinetics in monkey CNS toxicity

Unfortunately, the brains of these monkeys were not sampled after the monkey toleration study. However, plasma and brain exposures in the mouse were known for this drug candidate. Mice express similar membrane proteins (e.g., Pgp and BCRP) in their blood brain barrier compared to Cynomolgus monkeys (Ito et al., 2011); therefore, we hypothesized that brain penetration of this drug candidate in mouse may approximate the respective brain penetration in monkey.

The brain to plasma ratio of this drug candidate was large (i.e., 22) in mouse; furthermore, drug was retained in the mouse brain compared to plasma (Figure 3). These results suggested that the drug candidate was preferentially distributed to the brain with a large accumulation potential. This large accumulation potential suggested that the safety margin (established in the monkey toleration study) might decrease with the increased duration of the safety studies, further compromising the developability of this lead candidate.

4.3 Identification of a backup molecule with limited potential for CNS toxicity

In order to identify a backup molecule with limited potential for the observed CNS toxicity of the lead drug candidate, screening potential backup molecules for CNS toxicity in monkey would be resource intensive. Furthermore from an animal usage and management perspective, reduction of potential primate mortality was optimal. Since toxicological screening for a potential backup was unfavorable, reduction in the distribution of a backup to the CNS was a possible solution. Marked structural alterations of the physiochemical properties for this chemical series to alter CNS distribution were not possible since these alterations markedly reduced potency for the pharmacological receptor. Interestingly, some of these molecules (in the same chemical series) were identified as substrates for Pgp. In the MDR1-MDCK cell model, the efflux ratio of the Pgp substrates was between 2 and 3. Since Pgp is known to reduce CNS distribution through efflux of drug candidate from the apical membrane of the endothelial cells in the blood brain barrier into the blood (Cordon-Cardo et al., 1989), the effect of Pgp on the CNS distribution of these potential backup molecules was determined in the mouse (as discussed previously, monkeys were not a practical model for this exploration). CNS concentrations were approximately 10-fold less for one of these backup drug candidates compared to the lead drug candidate (Figure 4). Therefore, this backup drug candidate was advanced into clinical trials and CNS toxicity was never observed in monkey and human.

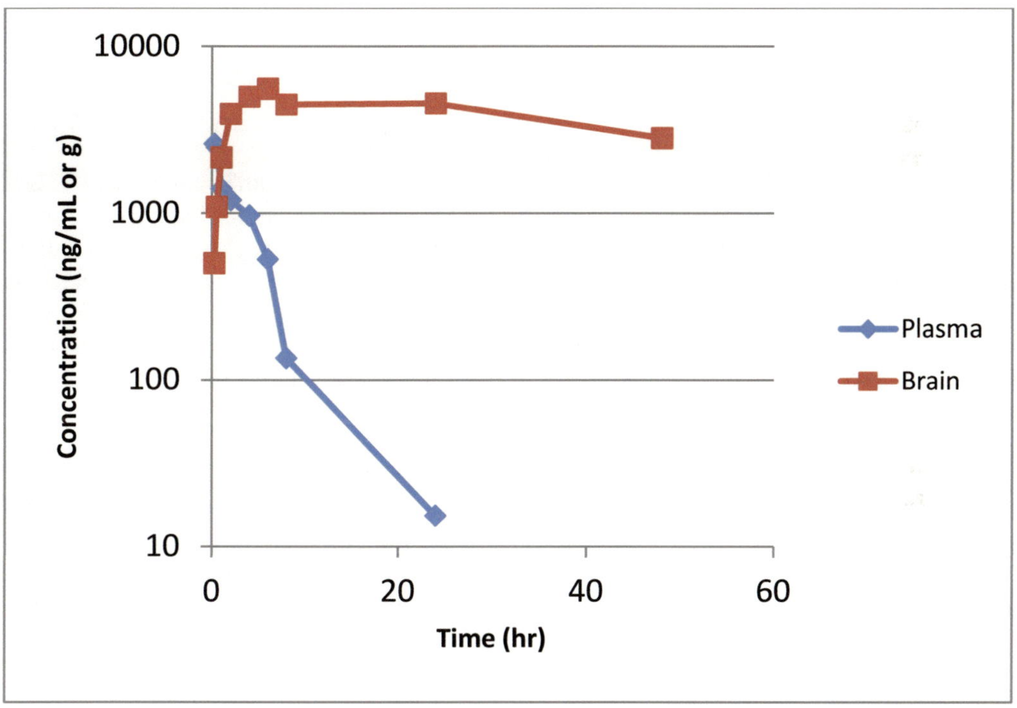

Fig. 3. Concentration-Time Profile of Lead Drug Candidate in Mouse Brain and Plasma after a Single Oral Dose (20 mg/kg)
Fasted CD1 mice (n=27) were administered a single oral dose (20 mg/kg) of the lead drug candidate. Brains and plasma were collected at 0.25, 0.5, 1, 2, 4, 6, 8, 24, and 48 hours post dose from three mice at each time point. Bioanalysis of brain and plasma of the lead drug candidate was performed.

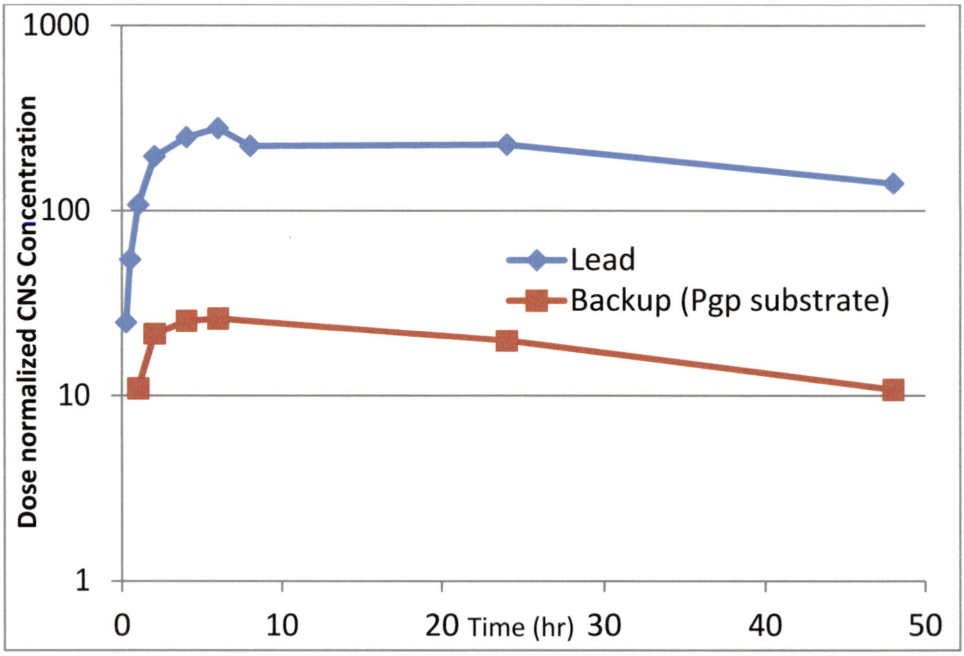

Fig. 4. Dose Normalized CNS Concentration-Time Profile of Drug Candidate in Mouse Brain and Plasma after a Single Oral Dose (20 mg/kg for lead and 5 mg/kg for backup)
Fasted CD1 mice (n=54) were administered a single oral dose of 20 mg/kg of the lead or 5 mg/kg of the backup drug candidate. For the lead drug candidate, brains were collected at 0.25, 0.5, 1, 2, 4, 6, 8, 24, and 48 hours post dose from three mice at each time point. For the backup drug candidate, brains were collected at 0.5, 1, 4, 6, 24, and 48 hours post dose from three mice at each time point. Bioanalysis of brains for the lead and backup drug candidate was performed.

4.4 Conclusion

Development of a backup drug candidate that is a substrate for efflux transporters which limit its distribution to the CNS (e.g., Pgp) can reduce the potential for this backup to cause CNS toxicity where the prior lead drug candidate demonstrated this toxicity in animal safety studies.

5. Future use of safety margins in tissues

In the future, more thorough risk assessment of safety will include safety margins from exposure of drug and its metabolites in the tissues (in addition to plasma) where organ specific toxicity is observed. The challenge in this endeavor is the assessment of drug exposure in human tissues since these tissues cannot be easily sampled from most human volunteers. Therefore, creative sampling methods must be applied. For example, noninvasive in vivo measurements such as sampling excreta (urine, feces, bile, and semen) will be useful. Furthermore, in vitro systems such as the hepatocyte sandwich-culture model (Chandra & Brouwer, 2004), and humanized mice (Jiang et al., 2011), combined with physiologically based pharmacokinetic (PBPK) modelling (Kusuhara & Sugiyama, 2010) can also replace the need for direct sampling of human tissues.

5.1 Sampling excreta to estimate drug and metabolites in tissues

The concept of sampling excreta to estimate drug and metabolites in human tissues is still evolving. The importance of understanding absolute abundance of metabolites from sampling excreta was highlighted by the need to understand the importance of metabolites in safety testing or MIST (Baillie et al., 2002; Smith & Obach, 2005). Smith and Obach concluded that the risk assessment of metabolites would seem more prudent if it was based on absolute mass and not proportion of drug-related material (Smith & Obach, 2005); therefore, sampling excreta and analyzing total amount of metabolite excreted would be more useful than sampling plasma (especially at higher dose of the drug). The recommendation for sampling excreta was based on determining the entire body burden of the metabolites for this MIST guidance and less about sampling excreta to estimate drug and metabolites in tissues.

In animals, the concept of sampling excreta to estimate drug and metabolites in tissues has been applied in a limited fashion. For example in beef steers treated with gentamicin, a small residue remains bound to the kidney cortex tissue for many months (this residue is unacceptable at the time of slaughter). Interestingly, plasma levels of gentamicin declined rapidly to no detectable levels within 3 days after intramuscular administration of gentamicin, while measurable amounts in urine persisted for 75 days before the concentration of gentamicin declined to levels too low to quantitate by the available liquid chromatography tandem mass spectrometry (LC/MS/MS) technique (Chiesa et al., 2006). An estimated correlation between an extrapolation of urine gentamicin concentration to the corresponding kidney tissue sample suggested a urine to kidney tissue relationship of 1:100. A test system sufficiently sensitive to a urine gentamicin concentration of 1 ng/mL correlated with the estimated 100 ng/g gentamicin limit applied to the fresh kidney of the recently slaughtered bovine (Chiesa et al., 2006). This example highlights the utility of measuring excreta (e.g., urine) to better estimate concentrations of drug in tissue (e.g., kidney).

The challenge of excreta being a surrogate model to assess concentrations of drug and metabolites in human tissues is the limited understanding of how concentrations of drug and metabolites in the excreta will relate to the concentrations in the respective tissue. This challenge can be minimized by establishing a relationship between the concentration of drug and metabolites for excreta and tissues in animals (as illustrated by the above example with gentamicin in beef steers). In addition, translating that relationship from animal to human with in silico tools (e.g., PBPK modelling) and in vitro and in vivo human models (e.g., primary in vitro human cell models and humanized mice) will increase the confidence in including safety margins from exposure of drug and its metabolites in the tissues (in addition to plasma) where organ specific toxicity is observed. Below is a case example where the utility of semen as a surrogate model to assess the concentrations of drug and metabolites in dog testes was investigated.

5.1.1 Case example: Utility of semen as a potential matrix to estimate drug and metabolites in testes

In this case example, the potential of semen was evaluated as a matrix to determine the concentration of Drug A (same drug candidate described in the section for Toxicokinetics and Testicular Toxicity) and its metabolite (M1) in dog testes (for potential extrapolation to human). For this study, dogs were given a single oral dose of Drug A and then at different time points dogs were ejaculated to collect semen and their testes were sampled. The toxicokinetic profile of M1 in semen and testes was similar (Table 7). Furthermore, the exposure of parent in testes also approximated the exposure of parent in semen where the exposure of Drug A in semen was approximately 2.5-fold higher than the exposure in testes (Table 7). These results suggest that semen approximated the exposure of Drug A and M1 in testes. Therefore, excreta may be a possible surrogate matrix to estimate tissue concentrations of drug candidate and its metabolites; however, supplementary systems like primary in vitro human cell models and humanized mice, combined with PBPK modelling, will be needed to extrapolate these results to human.

		Half Life (hr)	T_{max} (hr)	C_{max} (ng/mL or g)	AUC_{last} (ng*hr/mL or g)	AUC_{inf} (ng*hr/mL or g)
Testes	M1	13	7	2890	80787	81831
Testes	M2	3	1	28	87	108
Testes	Parent	18	7	12000	232701	233251
Semen	M1	16	7	3680	75766	75867
Semen	M2	ND	ND	ND	ND	ND
Semen	Parent	5	4	42700	593334	593391

Table 7. Toxicokinetic Profile of Drug A and its Metabolites in Dog Testes and Semen.

Before dosing, Beagle dogs (n=9) were trained for ejaculation 2 times/week. Dogs were administered a single oral dose of 15 mg/kg Drug A. Testes (n = 1/time point) were collected at 1, 4, 7, 24, 48, 72, 96, 168, and 336 hours post dose from dogs at each time point. Semen was also collected in the period between dosing and sacrifice. Bioanalysis of semen and testes for Drug A and its metabolites, M1 and M2, was performed. Toxicokinetic parameters were then determined.

5.2 Utility of PBPK to estimate drug and metabolites in tissues

PBPK models aid in the understanding of the disposition of chemicals in the body in different animal species, including humans. In toxicological research, PBPK modelling was initiated approximately 30 years or so, and mainly from an environmental toxicology perspective. For example, PBPK models were developed for polychlorinated biphenyls, methylene chloride, and other persistent lipophilic compounds starting in the mid 1980s (Andersen, 1995). In the past, the utilization of PBPK models in safety assessment departments within the pharmaceutical industry was not common, although the utilization of PBPK models is gaining momentum.

The utility of PBPK models is to extrapolate from one environment to another; for example, PBPK models extrapolate from high to low dose, different routes of administration, interspecies, and different durations of exposure. All of these extrapolations are potentially needed to bridge knowledge of drug and metabolites concentrations in the tissues of safety assessment species (e.g., rat, dog, and monkey) to human tissues (Thompson et al., 2007).

For the best extrapolation, the mechanism of interaction leading to toxicity would be known; for example, a known biological process that is disturbed by a known entity, parent, and/or metabolite (Andersen, 1995). However in many cases, this mechanism is not known and PBPK models can assist in possibly identifying these mechanisms. Especially when modelling efforts address the appropriate questions, the systematic discovery of these mechanisms is possible. The key is to develop models with appropriate measures of tissue concentrations in animals and possibly excreta concentrations in animals and humans. To strengthen this extrapolation, in vitro systems, such as primary in vitro human cell models (e.g., hepatocyte sandwich-cultured cell model and proximal tubule cell monolayers), and humanized mice, will also provide vital parameters (e.g., pharmacokinetics rate constants) for the PBPK modelling in order to extrapolate tissues concentrations from animal to human. In 2001, a consensus building workshop sponsored by the Society of Toxicology concluded that the human in vitro systems, through quantitative measurements and PBPK modelling, can play an important role in dose-response assessment (MacGregor et al., 2001). Therefore in the near future, the combination of these technologies may allow researchers the ability to estimate drug and metabolites concentrations in human tissues.

5.3 Utility of supplementary human models to estimate drug and metabolites in tissues

The primary challenge in calculating safety margins in tissues where organ-specific toxicity is observed is the access to human tissue samples for the measurement of drug and its metabolites. One method to address this challenge is to simulate the distribution of drug and its metabolites in a human in vitro model. For example, development of valid and reliable techniques to quantify biliary excretion of drugs in healthy human volunteers is difficult. Measurements of drug concentrations in bile can only be obtained from patients diagnosed with diseases of the gallbladder and biliary tract who require medical procedures that allow this measurement (Ghibellini et al., 2006). However, there is a promising, recent technique to estimate bile in healthy human volunteers with an oroenteric catheter to aspirate duodenal secretions, and gamma scintigraphy to determine gallbladder contraction. This technique allowed the comparison of the biliary clearance of three compounds estimated with sandwich-cultured human hepatocytes (a human in vitro model). The rank order of biliary clearance predicted from in vitro corresponded well with the in vivo biliary clearance values in mL/min/kg for Tc-99m mebrofenin (7.44 vs 16.1), Tc-99m sestamibi (1.20 vs 5.51), and Tc-99m piperacillin (0.028 vs 0.032) (Ghibellini et al., 2007). Since sandwich-cultured human hepatocytes need to uptake drug across their sinusoidal membrane in order to excrete the drug across their canalicular membrane for the in vitro measurement of biliary excretion, this verification of a good prediction of this human in vitro model from the clinical study suggests that the intracellular concentration within these sandwich-cultured human hepatocytes can also estimate concentrations of drug in the human hepatocyte in vivo. Therefore, in vitro models have the potential to supplement costly and difficult sampling in healthy human volunteers to estimate drug and metabolite concentrations in tissues and excreta. However, significantly more research is needed to realize this potential in existing models and to expand the amount of models for in vitro human tissue models.

Another possible human model to estimate drug and metabolites in organs and/or tissues is mice with humanized organs and/or tissues. To create this model, a severe combined immunodeficient (SCID) mouse line is injected with human cells from the human tissue into the respective mouse tissue. For example, injection of cryopreserved human hepatocytes through a small, left flank incision into the inferior splenic pole in a SCID mouse created a mouse with humanized liver that was replaced by more than 80% of human hepatocytes (Okumura et al., 2007). In this chimeric mice model, cefmetazole (CMZ) excretions in urine and feces were 81.0 and 5.9% of the dose, respectively; however, excretions in urine and feces in control SCID mice were 23.7 and 59.4% of the dose, respectively (Okumura et al., 2007). Because CMZ is mainly excreted in urine in humans, the excretory profile in chimeric mice was demonstrated to be similar to humans. Interestingly in the chimeric mice, the hepatic mRNA expression of human drug transporters (e.g., MDR1, BSEP, MRP2, BCRP, OCT1, and OATP1B1/1B3) were detectable; whereas, the hepatic mRNA expression of mouse drug transporters in the chimeric mice was significantly lower than in the control SCID mice (Okumura et al., 2007). In conclusion, chimeric mice exhibited a humanized profile of drug excretion, suggesting that this chimeric mouse line would be a useful animal model to predict human ADME. Most studies have focused on humanized liver models; however, the potential for humanization of other organs and/or tissues in the mouse is evident in the near future. These new potential models will markedly improve the ability to estimate drug and metabolite concentrations in human organs and/or tissues.

6. Conclusion

For the determination of a safety margin, drug and metabolites concentrations are sampled in plasma, which is the most practical and widely accepted way of assessing this risk. However, most safety issues are not observed in the plasma but in the organs and/or tissues. Assumptions about concentrations of drug and metabolites in tissues from extrapolation with plasma may result in an inaccurate assessment of target organ exposure to drug and metabolites. Therefore, plasma is sometimes not a good surrogate for tissue levels of drug and its metabolites, especially for the assessment of risk for some types of organ-specific toxicity.

Knowledge of toxicokinetics of an organ-specific toxicity can potentially assist in identifying a backup drug candidate that has a markedly lower potential for this organ-specific toxicity. Therefore, a hypothetical plan may be generated where focusing on tissue burden of the drug and its metabolites may actually ensure that a backup does not produce the same toxicity. For example, identifying a backup drug candidate with limited tissue distribution to the tissue where organ-specific toxicity was observed (e.g., testicular toxicity) markedly reduced the potential of these backups to cause these toxicities; furthermore, development of a backup drug candidate that is a substrate for efflux transporters which limit its distribution to the CNS (e.g., Pgp) can reduce the potential for this backup to cause CNS toxicity.

In the future, innovative models such as 1) noninvasive in vivo measurements such as sampling excreta (e.g., urine, feces, bile, and semen), 2) in vitro systems, such as primary in vitro human cell models (hepatocyte sandwich-cultured model), 3) humanized mice, and 4) PBPK models, will provide more insight into the concentration of drug and metabolites in human organs and/or tissues. Therefore, these innovations will provide a more thorough risk assessment of safety which will include safety margins from exposure of drug and its metabolites in the tissues (in addition to plasma) where organ specific toxicity is observed.

7. Acknowledgment

I would like to thank 1) Rita Geerts, Wenying Jian, Rick Edom, and David La for their contribution towards the rat testicular toxicity section; 2) Gregory Reich and Freddy Schoetens for their contribution towards the dog liver toxicity section; 3) David La for his contribution towards the monkey CNS toxicity section; and 4) Rob Thurmond, David Evans, Sandra Snook, Jan de Jong, and David La for reviewing this chapter.

8. References

Andersen, M.E. (1995). Development of physiologically based pharmacokinetic and physiologically based pharmacodynamic models for applications in toxicology and risk assessment. *Toxicol Lett,* Vol.79, No.1-3, pp. 35-44, ISSN 0378-4274

Baillie, T.A., Cayen, M.N., Fouda, H., Gerson, R.J., Green, J.D., Grossman, S.J., Klunk, L.J., LeBlanc, B., Perkins, D.G., & Shipley, L.A. (2002). Drug metabolites in safety testing. *Toxicol Appl Pharmacol,* Vol.182, No.3, pp. 188-196, ISSN 0041-008X

Chandra, P., & Brouwer, K.L. (2004). The complexities of hepatic drug transport: current knowledge and emerging concepts. *Pharm Res,* Vol.21, No.5, pp. 719-735, ISSN 0724-8741

Chiesa, O.A., von Bredow, J., Heller, D., Nochetto, C., Smith, M., Moulton, K., & Thomas, M. (2006). Use of tissue-fluid correlations to estimate gentamicin residues in kidney tissue of Holstein steers. *J Vet Pharmacol Ther,* Vol.29, No.2, pp. 99-106, ISSN 0140-7783

Cordon-Cardo, C., O'Brien, J.P., Casals, D., Rittman-Grauer, L., Biedler, J.L., Melamed, M.R., & Bertino, J.R. (1989). Multidrug-resistance gene (P-glycoprotein) is expressed by endothelial cells at blood-brain barrier sites. *Proc Natl Acad Sci U S A,* Vol.86, No.2, pp. 695-698, ISSN 0027-8424

Dixit, R., & Ward, P.D. (2007). Use of Classical Pharmacokinetic Evaluations in Drug Development and Safety Assessment, In: *Toxicokinetics and Risk Assessment,* Lipscomb, J.C., & Ohanian, E.V. (Ed.), pp. 95-122, Informa Healthcare USA Inc., ISBN 978-0-8493-3722-2, New York, NY

Ghibellini, G., Leslie, E.M., & Brouwer, K.L. (2006). Methods to evaluate biliary excretion of drugs in humans: an updated review. *Mol Pharm,* Vol.3, No.3, pp. 198-211, ISSN 1543-8384

Ghibellini, G., Vasist, L.S., Leslie, E.M., Heizer, W.D., Kowalsky, R.J., Calvo, B.F., & Brouwer, K.L. (2007). In vitro-in vivo correlation of hepatobiliary drug clearance in humans. *Clin Pharmacol Ther,* Vol.81, No.3, pp. 406-413, ISSN 0009-9236

Ito, K., Uchida, Y., Ohtsuki, S., Aizawa, S., Kawakami, H., Katsukura, Y., Kamiie, J., & Terasaki, T. (2011). Quantitative membrane protein expression at the blood-brain barrier of adult and younger cynomolgus monkeys. *J Pharm Sci,* Vol.100, No.9, pp. 3939-3950, ISSN 1520-6017

Jiang, X.L., Gonzalez, F.J., & Yu, A.M. (2011). Drug-metabolizing enzyme, transporter, and nuclear receptor genetically modified mouse models. *Drug Metab Rev,* Vol.43, No.1, pp. 27-40, ISSN 1097-9883

Kenny, J.R., Maggs, J.L., Tettey, J.N., Harrell, A.W., Parker, S.G., Clarke, S.E., & Park, B.K. (2005). Formation and protein binding of the acyl glucuronide of a leukotriene B4 antagonist (SB-209247): relation to species differences in hepatotoxicity. *Drug Metab Dispos,* Vol.33, No.2, pp. 271-281, ISSN 0090-9556

Kusuhara, H., & Sugiyama, Y. (2010). Pharmacokinetic modeling of the hepatobiliary transport mediated by cooperation of uptake and efflux transporters. *Drug Metab Rev,* Vol.42, No.3, pp. 539-550, ISSN 1097-9883

MacGregor, J.T., Collins, J.M., Sugiyama, Y., Tyson, C.A., Dean, J., Smith, L., Andersen, M., Curren, R.D., Houston, J.B., Kadlubar, F.F., Kedderis, G.L., Krishnan, K., Li, A.P., Parchment, R.E., Thummel, K., Tomaszewski, J.E., Ulrich, R., Vickers, A.E., & Wrighton, S.A. (2001). In vitro human tissue models in risk assessment: report of a consensus-building workshop. *Toxicol Sci,* Vol.59, No.1, pp. 17-36, ISSN 1096-6080

MacIntyre, A.C., & Cutler, D.J. (1988). The potential role of lysosomes in tissue distribution of weak bases. *Biopharm Drug Dispos,* Vol.9, No.6, pp. 513-526, ISSN 0142-2782

Okumura, H., Katoh, M., Sawada, T., Nakajima, M., Soeno, Y., Yabuuchi, H., Ikeda, T., Tateno, C., Yoshizato, K., & Yokoi, T. (2007). Humanization of excretory pathway in chimeric mice with humanized liver. *Toxicol Sci,* Vol.97, No.2, pp. 533-538, ISSN 1096-6080

Smith, D.A., & Obach, R.S. (2005). Seeing through the mist: abundance versus percentage. Commentary on metabolites in safety testing. *Drug Metab Dispos,* Vol.33, No.10, pp. 1409-1417, ISSN 0090-9556

Thompson, C., Sonawane, B., Nong, A., & Krishnan, K. (2007). Considerations for Applying Physiologically Based Pharmacokinetic Models in Risk Assessment, In: *Toxicokinetics and Risk Assessment,* Lipscomb, J.C., & Ohanian, E.V. (Ed.), pp. 123-140, Informa Healthcare USA Inc., ISBN 978-0-8493-3722-2, New York, NY

Ward, P. (2008). Importance of drug transporters in pharmacokinetics and drug safety. *Toxicol Mech Methods,* Vol.18, No.1, pp. 1-10, ISSN 1537-6524

20

Environmental Toxicants Induced Male Reproductive Disorders: Identification and Mechanism of Action

Kuladip Jana and Parimal C. Sen
Division of Molecular Medicine,
Bose Institute, Kolkata,
India

"Several observations on poor trends in Male Reproductive Health have been reported during the last Decades. These difficult trends include the increasing prevalence of Testicular Cancer, Low and possibly declining Semen Quality, high and possibly rising frequencies of Cryptorchidism (Undescended Testis) and malformation of the Penis (Hypospadias) as well as a increasing demand for Assisted Reproduction".

1. Introduction

The phrase 'endocrine disruption' has seemingly become inextricably linked with terms like 'environmental oestrogens' and 'falling sperm counts'. While these connections aid understanding about these issues, they represent a simplified view of the field of endocrine disruption. There is currently no strong data to suggest that environmental endocrine disrupters (EDCs) are responsible for the observed disintegration in human male reproductive health, but there are secular trends to suggest that it is declining. There is, however, very good evidence that lifestyle factors (e.g. smoking, alcohol consumption and/or use of cosmetics) can have an impact on fertility (Sharpe & Franks 2002; Sharpe & Irvine, 2004). Similarly, the notion that all EDCs act by mimicking oestrogen (environmental oestrogens) is too simplistic. The current literature illustrates that EDCs can act as oestrogens, anti-oestrogens, anti-androgens, steroidogenic enzyme inhibitors and can also act via interaction with the thyroid hormones and their receptors, or within the brain and the hypothalamo–pituitary axis, as well as the immune system (Fisher, 2004; Jana et al., 2006; 2010a). Reports of declining sperm counts over the past 50 years and other disturbing trends alerted scientists to the possibility that exposure to chemicals in the environment may damage male reproductive health (Carlsen et al., 1992). Testicular cancer, the most common malignancy in men 15-44 years of age, has increased markedly in incidence in this century in virtually all countries studied. The incidence of hypospadias, a developmental malformation of the male urethra, appears to be increasing worldwide. Cryptorchidism (undescended testicle), another developmental defect, may have increased in some human populations and appears to be increasing in wildlife (Toppari et al., 1996; Fisher, 2004, Sharpe, 2010). The causes of these trends have not been identified and relevant toxicological data about male reproductive effects of environmental toxicants are limited. Recent research efforts have focused on the possibility that exposures to hormonally active compounds, particularly during childhood and *in utero,* are to blame, at least in part, for changes in semen quality, increasing rates of testicular cancer, and malformations of the male urogenital tract (Sharpe, 2010). The ability to investigate environmental determinants of these indicators of male reproductive health is currently limited by available methodologies and data.

1.1 The male reproductive system: Environmental influence

Global changes in semen quality are suggested to be produced by the enhanced exposure to environmental chemicals contained in pesticides, food sources, cosmetics, plastics, electronics, and other synthetic materials (Carlsen et al., 1992). The biological basis for this hypothesis is the action of certain chemical compounds, both naturally occurring and anthropogenic (man-made), on endogenous hormone receptors and hormone-dependent pathways. These chemicals are termed hormonally active agents, environmental estrogens, hormone mimics, and endocrine disrupters/disruptors (US. EPA, 1998a; 1998b; National Research Council [NRC], 1989). A wide range of mechanisms of action are described for endocrine disrupters, including agonists of the estrogen receptor (ER) genistein, diethylstilbestrol (DES; Roy et al., 1997), and bisphenol A (BPA; Kuiper et al., 1998); androgen receptor (AR) antagonists such as vinclozolin (Wong et al., 1995), linuron, procymidone (Gray et al., 1999), phthalates (Foster et al., 2001), and *p,p'*-dichlorodiphenyl dichloroethylene (*p,p'*-DDE; Kelce et al., 1995) and aryl hydrocarbon receptor (AhR) agonists, which include dioxins (Toyoshiba et al., 2004), polychlorinated biphenyls (PCB), polycyclic aromatic hydrocarbons (PAH), and polychlorinated dibenzofurans (PCDF; Peterson et al., 1993). Exposure to endocrine-disrupting chemicals may occur through environmental routes (air, soil, water, food) or via occupational exposures (**Figure 1**) (Sharpe & Irvine, 2004).

1.2 The testis: Male reproductive organ

The testis is both an endocrine gland and a reproductive organ, responsible for the production of hormones and male gametes and an important target for endocrine disruption. The testis consists of two types of tissues: seminiferous tubules, supported by Sertoli cells, and the interstitial compartment, comprised of Leydig cells (Fisher, 2004; Akingbemi, 2005). Testicular functions (spermatogenesis steroidogenesis) are regulated by the hypothalamic-pituitary-testicular (HPT) axis which involves the pituitary gonadotropins luteinizing hormone (LH) and follicle-stimulating hormone (FSH; Jana et al., 2006). Testicular functions are proposed to be regulated by a number of hormones and growth factors in addition to FSH, LH, and androgens, including insulin-like growth factor, oxytocin, and transforming growth factor-α and estrogens (Pryor et al., 2000).

1.2.1 Spermatogenesis

Spermatogenesis is the formation of the male gamete or spermatozoa. Spermatogenesis is dependent on the integrity of the architecture of the seminiferous tubules and Sertoli cells and endocrine regulation and is regulated by testosterone and FSH. In response to LH, Leydig cells produce androgens, including testosterone, which along with FSH bind to their respective Sertoli cell receptors to regulate spermatogenesis. Spermatogenesis requires unique associations between Sertoli cells and developing male germ cells such that the seminiferous tubules are lined by Sertoli cells and joined by tight junctions forming the

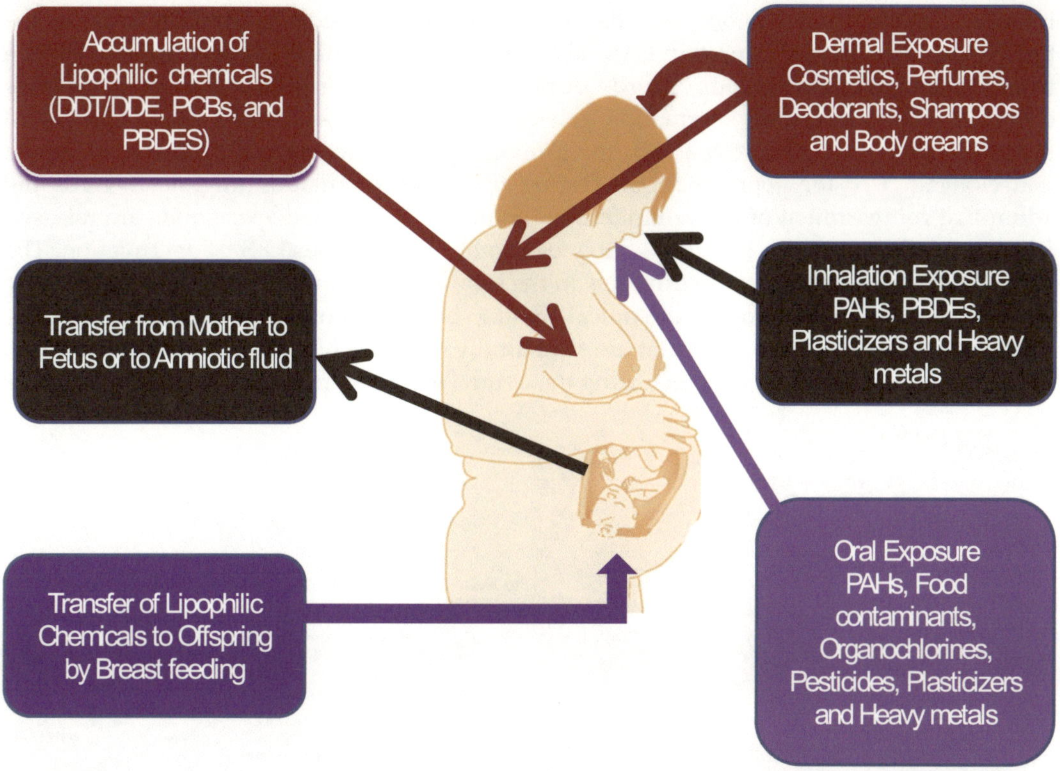

Fig. 1. Routes of human exposure to some common environmental chemicals. DDE= 1, 1-dichloro-2, 2-bis (p- chlorophenyl) ethylene; DDT= dichlorodiphenyltrichloroethane; PAHs= polycyclic aromatic hydrocarbons; PCBs= polychlorinated biphenyls. (Modified from Sharpe & Irvine, BMJ, 2004).

blood–testis barrier (BTB; Walker & Cheng, 2005). There are three major phases of spermatogenesis: (1) spermatogonial phase, (2) spermatocyte phase, and (3) spermatid phase (**Figure 2**). In the first phase the diploid spermatogonia undergo mitosis and create stem cells and diploid primary spermatocytes. During the second phase the primary spermatocytes undergo two rounds of meiosis, producing haploid spermatids. Finally, the spermatids begin a differentiation phase, sometimes referred to as spermiogenesis, during which the immature gametes develop into mature spermatozoa (O'Donnell et al., 2001). Spermatids continue their differentiation (spermiogenesis) while physically associated with the Sertoli cells. Spermiogenesis includes polarization of the spermatid, formation of the acrosome cap and flagellum, condensation, elongation of the nucleus, and cytoplasmic re-modelling to produce the characteristic appearance of the mature spermatozoa. Spermatozoa are morphologically mature but immotile and are then released into the lumen of the seminiferous tubules (spermiation). At this stage these immotile testicular spermatozoa are not yet capable of fertilization (O'Donnell et al., 2001). The BTB between Sertoli cells comprises a co-existing tight junction (TJ), desmosome, gap junction and a testis-specific adherens junction (AJ) called the basal ectoplasmic specialization (ES). The basal ES is typified by the presence of actin filament bundles 'sandwiched' between the plasma membrane and the cisternae of endoplasmic reticulum in two neighbouring Sertoli cells.

However, recent studies show that the unique structural aspects of the BTB, such as the presence of focal adhesion protein FAK, also render the testis highly susceptible to damage from environmental toxicants. Third, during spermiogenesis when round spermatids differentiate into elongated spermatids, genetic material in the spermatid head condense to form the tightly packed nucleus with the formation of an acrosome above the head region and elongation of the spermatid tail. During this time, spermatids migrate towards the adluminal compartment of the seminiferous tubule until elongated spermatids are released into the tubule lumen via the disassembly of another ES, the apical ES, at spermiation. The apical ES anchors developing spermatids in the seminiferous epithelium until they are fully developed. Thus, disruption of the apical ES (e.g. by environmental toxicants) causes the premature release of spermatids that are structurally defective (e.g. lack of acrosome and/or tail) and which are incapable of fertilizing the ovum (Wong & Cheng, 2011).

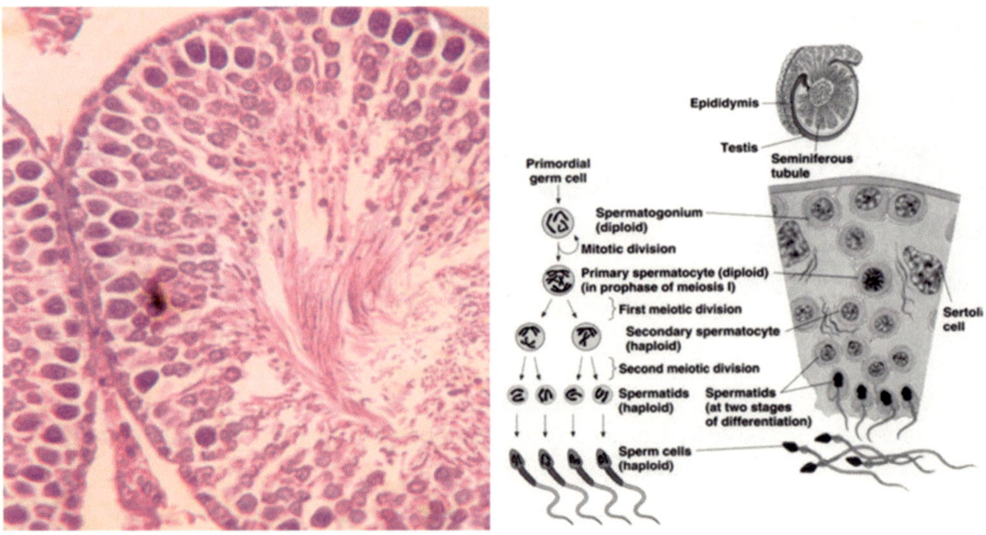

Fig. 2. The process of normal mammalian spermatogenesis with three major phases: (1) spermatogonial phase, (2) spermatocyte phase, and (3) spermatid phase.

1.2.2 Sperm maturation

The immotile spermatozoa are transported from the lumen of the seminiferous tubules by peristaltic contractions of adjacent myoid cells. The spermatozoa are suspended in a fluid secreted by Sertoli cells and migrate through a series of ductules within the testis (rete testis), passing through the efferent ductules and eventually entering the epididymis. The efferent ductules concentrate the spermatozoa by reabsorbing fluid (O'Donnell et al., 2001). There is evidence from transgenic mice that this fluid resorption is regulated by estrogen (Hess et al., 1997). The segments of the epididymis, caput, corpus, and cauda secrete proteins, and endocytose secreted proteins from the epididymal lumen to contribute to the maturation of the spermatozoa (O'Donnell et al., 2001). It is within the epididymis that the spermatozoa gain motility machinery. However, these spermatozoa remain immotile as they are pushed through the rest of the reproductive tissues via peristaltic contractions. It is during this final passage that seminal fluid is produced by the seminal vesicles, which contributes about 70% to the semen, and the prostate gland, which contributes another 10–

30%. Seminal fluid is comprised of proteins, enzymes, fructose, mucus, vitamin-C, flavins, phosphorylcholine, and prostaglandins (Purvis et al., 1986). Decreases in seminal fluid volume may therefore indicate diminished seminal vesicle or prostate functions.

1.3 The role of androgens in male reproductive tract development

Male reproductive tract development is a dynamic process requiring the interaction of many factors and hormones. One of the major factors essential for the development of the male internal and external male reproductive tract are the androgens, testosterone and dihydrotestosterone (DHT) (Phillips & Tanphaichitr, 2008). Androgens are produced by the testes during fetal and neonatal development and are essential for the maintenance of the Wolffian duct that differentiates into the epididymis, vas deferens and the seminal vesicles. The masculinization of these reproductive structures is mediated by testosterone. The masculinization of the external genitalia and prostate is largely mediated by DHT which is a more potent metabolite of testosterone and is produced by the action of the enzyme 5α-reductase. The central role of androgens in driving these developmental processes illustrates why chemicals that can interfere with the synthesis or action of androgens can have deleterious consequences for the developing male genital tract. Administration of the anti-androgen, flutamide (an androgen receptor antagonist), during male reproductive tract development resulted in abnormalities in the formation of the external genitalia - hypospadias and cryptorchidism; internally, agenesis of the epididymis, vas deferens and prostate (Mylchreest et al., 2000). Within the testis, degeneration of the seminiferous epithelium and Leydig cell hyperplasia were common (although this may be a consequence of the cryptorchidism rather than an anti-androgenic effect). The male pups also displayed retained thoracic nipples and a reduced anogenital distance (feminised) which are both indicative of reduced androgen action in fetal life (Mylchreest et al., 2000). In summary, both testosterone- and DHT-mediated male reproductive tract development is impaired by flutamide when administered over the period of reproductive tract differentiation.

1.4 Problems with male reproductive health

1.4.1 Semen quality

Reports suggesting that sperm counts have declined in certain areas of industrialized countries throughout the world have contributed to concern about a possible worldwide decline in human semen quality (Swan et al., 1997). A meta-analysis by Carlsen et al.,(1992) reported a worldwide decline in sperm counts over the preceding 50 years, concluding that mean sperm concentrations had decreased by almost 50% from 1940 to 1990. Numerous researchers have attempted to determine whether this apparent decline is real or due to unrecognized biases in data collection and analysis. Confounding Variables may account for the observed findings. Potential confounders include increasing donor age, duration of abstinence, frequency of ejaculation, and even the season of sample collection, all of which influence sperm variables. Other suggested confounders include smoking, chemicals and radiation exposures, stress, ethnicity, and a variety of physical conditions including varicocele, infection, and genital abnormalities such as hypospadias and cryptorchidism. Theories explaining the apparent geographic disparities in sperm counts are currently only speculative, and include environmental, socioeconomic, racial, and methodologic differences (Swan et al., 1997). Fisch et al., (1996) reported yearly fluctuations in mean sperm counts and birth rates (Fisch et al., 1997), suggesting that this may be a more important variable than previously considered.

1.4.2 Testicular cancer

Testicular cancer is often quoted as the commonest cancer of young men. The secular trends across Europe and the United States show that it is increasing in incidence in Caucasian men (SEER 2003). There is widespread geographical variation and the incidence of testicular cancer can vary up to 10-fold between countries. In Denmark in 1980, the age standardised incidence rate per 100 000 population was 7.8% whereas in Lithuania it was 0.9%, although in all countries where registry data has been analysed there was an annual increase of 2.3–3.4% (Adami et al., 1994). The increase in testicular cancer has been linked to a birth cohort effect, suggesting that factors affecting in utero development may be important (Bergstrom et al., 1996). Testicular germ cell cancer arises from cells which have similar characteristics to fetal germ-cells; these pre-malignant cells are termed carcinoma-in situ (CIS) cells (Rajpert-De Meyts et al., 2003). How these cells persist during development and what causes them to proliferate after puberty is not well understood, although it is thought that the factors that promote normal germ cell division may also be important in promoting CIS proliferation. Abnormal intrauterine hormone levels i.e. decreased androgen and/or increased oestrogen levels are believed to be important in the occurrence of testicular cancer (Sharpe & Skakkebaek 1993). Similarly, decreased androgen and/or increased oestrogen levels have also been implicated in the occurrence of cryptorchidism, hypospadias and low sperm counts (Sharpe & Skakkebaek 1993). Although genetics almost certainly plays a major role in the etiology of the disease, other etiologies, including environmental factors, need to be elucidated to explain why, for example, major differences in testicular cancer rates exist among the relatively genetically homogenous Scandinavian countries. Increases in testicular cancer rates are not recent phenomena. A doubling in incidence was documented in Denmark within 25 years after the initiation of cancer registration in 1943 (Ekbom & Akre, 1998). Mortality data from Great Britain show an increase in mortality due to testicular cancer beginning in the 1920s (Davies, 1981). These mortality data raise an important distinction: if environmental risk factors play a role in testicular cancer incidence, relevant exposures must therefore have existed since the turn of the century. This would make it less likely that organochlorines such as DDT and other endocrine-disrupting chemicals are possible etiologic agents. Research is ongoing to explore new genetic markers for early detection of carcinoma *in situ* cells in semen, as well as to define the role of hormonal assays (e.g., inhibin-B) as screening tools for testicular cancer and carcinoma *in situ*.

1.4.3 Congenital abnormalities (Cryptorchidism and hypospadias)

Cryptorchidism and hypospadias are abnormalities normally detected at birth (congenital abnormalities). Cryptorchidism occurs when the testis does not descend into the scrotal sac; this is generally unilateral but can be bilateral. Hypospadias is a developmental abnormality of the penis in which the urethral opening is not located at the tip of the glans penis but can occur anywhere along the shaft. Determining whether there is a real increase in hypospadias and/or cryptorchidism is confounded by changes in diagnostic criteria and recording practices which make the registry data unreliable (Toppari et al., 1996). Despite this, cryptorchidism is the most common congenital abnormality of the newborn (2–4% incidence) and trends for hypospadias suggest a progressive increase; based on registry data, hypospadias is the second most common (0.3–0.7% at birth) congenital malformation (Sharpe, 2003). Prospective studies are underway, which employ standardised diagnostic criteria, to collect robust data about the current incidence of cryptorchidism and hypospadias. This will allow the monitoring of future trends and allow international comparisons on the incidences of these disorders. However, two male genital birth defects, hypospadias and cryptorchidism, both apparently representing mild degrees of feminization, have become important in the ongoing debate regarding the significance of endocrine disruptors or other environmental influences on male development (Sharpe & Skakkebaek, 1993). Several researchers have reported increases in each of these defects in the past three decades. To evaluate the hypothesis of common etiologies, pre- and peri-natal determinants of hypospadias, cryptorchidism, testicular cancer, and infertility are under investigation. Abnormal sex hormone exposure during critical periods of development has been postulated as a likely shared pathologic mechanism (Toppari et al., 1996).

1.4.4 There is a link between these male reproductive health issues

The strongest evidence suggesting a link between these male reproductive tract disorders, aside from the (largely imperfect) data which suggests they are all increasing in incidence, is the fact that epidemiologically the occurrence of one disorder is a risk factor for the occurrence of another (Skakkebaek et al., 2001, Sharpe, 2003). This has led to the proposal that low sperm counts, hypospadias, cryptorchidism and testicular germ cell cancer are interrelated disorders comprising a 'testicular dysgenesis syndrome' (TDS; Skakkebaek et al., 2001, Sharpe, 2003, 2010; **Figure 3**). The disorders that comprise TDS all have their roots in fetal development, suggesting that a possible causal link lies in abnormal hormone synthesis or action during reproductive tract development. From the historical literature, it is well known that the administration of diethylstilboestrol (DES; a potent synthetic oestrogen) to pregnant humans and rodents causes reproductive tract abnormalities in the offspring (Stillman, 1982). In male rodents, neonatal administration of DES induces a reduction in the number of Sertoli cells (the major somatic cell type which supports spermatogenesis) (Sharpe et al., 2003). There is also data suggesting DES administration to humans induces an increase in the incidence of cryptorchidism, although it is less certain whether hypospadias and testicular cancer show any significant increase (Stillman, 1982). DES only induces male reproductive tract abnormalities after administration at very high doses, which are probably not relevant to environmental considerations. However, what is of more concern is that, when administered at high doses, DES and other potent oestrogens are capable of reducing androgen levels and expression of the androgen receptor protein relative to control rats (McKinnell et al., 2001, Rivas et al., 2002). This raises the important question of whether some of the genital tract abnormalities that arise from in utero administration of potent oestrogens are caused by lowered androgen levels and/or action.

1.5 Anti-androgenic compounds in the environment

There are a number of commonly used environmental chemicals that have been identified as having anti-androgenic properties. These chemicals have been administered to pregnant rodents during the period of reproductive tract development. When the male pups were examined, they displayed many of the abnormalities associated with flutamide administration. Some chemicals (vinclozolin, procymidone, linuron, p,p'DDE (1,1,1-dichloro-2,2-bis(p-chlorophenyl)ethane) act as androgen receptor antagonists, others (phthalate esters) reduce androgen synthesis, but it is likely that other modes of action are also involved in the toxicity induced by these compounds (Gray et al.,2001). The following sections provide information on a few well-characterised examples of anti-androgenic compounds (i.e. vinclozolin, linuron, p,p' DDE and phthalates etc.) and common environmental toxins reported to be involved in male reproductive toxicity.

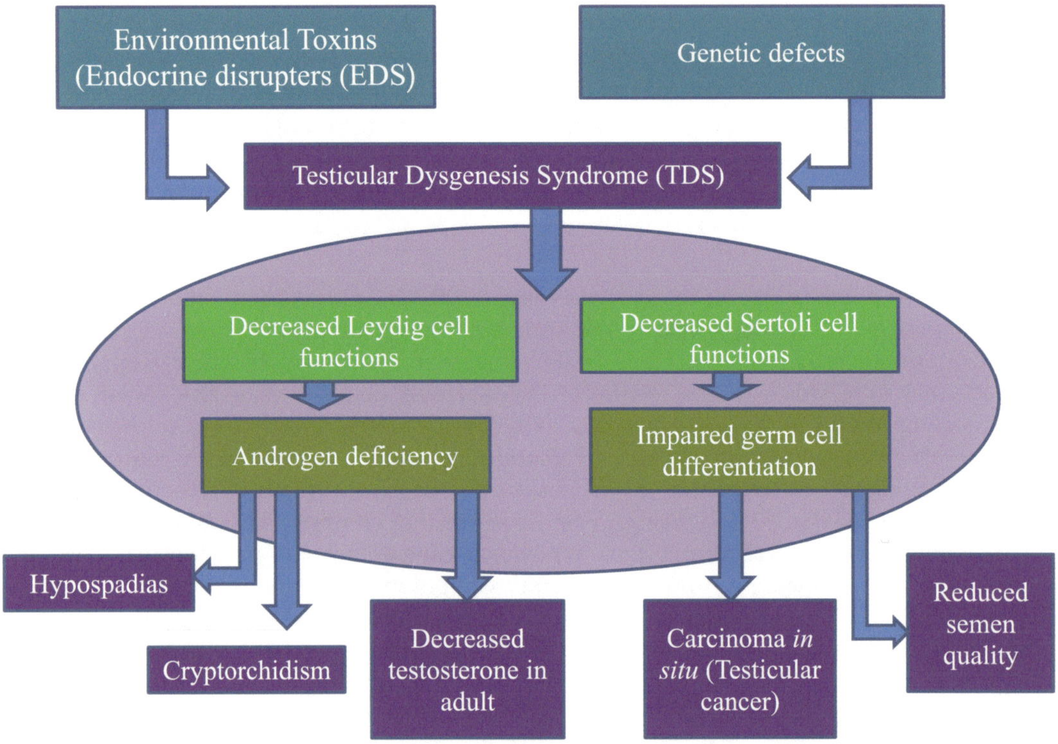

Fig. 3. Testicular dysgenesis syndrome. Both genetic and environmental factors affect testicular development and functions. Damage of the testicular cells (Leydig cells and Sertoli cells), disrupts androgen production from Leydig cells and secretion of paracrine factors from sertoli cells, leading to birth defects (hypospadias, cryptorchidism) and impaired germ cell differentiation, apparent later as reduced semen quality or in the worst cases as carcinoma *in situ* (CIS) of the testis and consequent testicular cancer. (Modified from Skakkeback et al. Human Reproduction, 2001).

1.5.1 Polychlorinated Biphenyls (PCB)

PCB make up a group of synthetic organic chemicals containing about 200 individual compounds. Some PCB bind to ERs and consequently PCB may exert their toxic effects through estrogenic activity (McKinney & Waller, 1998). Alternatively, some PCB may produce reproductive toxicity through the production of free radicals. Rats exposed to mixtures of PCB demonstrated decreased superoxide dismutase and catalase activity in the testes following exposure (Peltola et al., 1994). PCB congeners have different mechanisms of action and therefore different effects on biological systems. Longitudinal studies of children with in utero or lactational exposure to PCB and other environmental chemicals are essential to assess the long-term effects of endocrine disruption. Prenatal and lactational exposure to PCB may exert adverse effects on male reproduction during subsequent adulthood. A well-studied population exposed to PCB/PCDF-contaminated rice oil (Yu-Cheng exposure;

Taiwan 1978–79) was followed to determine effects on male reproductive health. Median serum PCB levels measured in Yu-Cheng mothers was 26.8 ng/ml: a relatively high PCB exposure that would be expected to affect fetal development. Sexual development and semen quality were evaluated in Yu-Cheng sons, aged 16 yr and older. Seminal volume and sperm concentration were not different between exposed and control boys. However, proportions of sperm with normal morphology and motility were reduced in exposed boys (Guo et al., 2000). The effects of PCB exposure on semen quality in men from the general population appear to affect differentiation of spermatids (spermiogenesis) and post-testicular development (sperm maturation), which would manifest as decreased sperm morphology and motility, respectively. Further studies of PCB exposure—both individual congeners and PCB mixtures—and sperm parameters are required.

1.5.2 DDT and *p,p* '-DDE

The persistent pesticide, DDT, is broken down in the environment, and one of its metabolites is p,p'-DDE, which has been shown to act as an androgen receptor antagonist both in vivo and in vitro (Kelce et al., 1995). Studies in which p,p'-DDE was administered to rats during development (gestational day (GD)14–18; 100 mg/kg/day) affected androgen-dependent aspects of male development such that it reduced anogenital distance, caused nipple retention and, depending on the rat strain, induced hypospadias (You et al., 1998). Another DDT derivative, methoxychlor and its metabolites, have been shown to interact with both oestrogen receptors and the androgen receptor (AR). The methoxychlor metabolite, 1,1-Trichloro-2,2-bis (4 hydroxyphenyl) ethane, is an oestrogen receptor (ER)- α agonist, an ER-β antagonist and an androgen receptor (AR) antagonist (Gray et al., 2001). This illustrates that these chemicals may act by more than one mechanism to induce effects on the exposed population. Moreover, several population studies conducted to examine the effects of DDT and metabolite exposure on male reproductive health support the hypothesis that DDT exposure is related to reduced semen quality. Significantly higher seminal concentrations of *p,p'*-DDE were also reported in infertile patients compared to a fertile control group in India. Seminal fluid levels of fructose, γ-glutamyl transpeptidase, and acid phosphatase were positively correlated with *p,p'*-DDE concentrations in infertile men. The high concentration of fructose, a marker for seminal vesicle function and an important energy source for sperm, may indicate non-utilization of fructose by sperm. DDT exposure may be associated with abnormal metabolism in sperm, including decreased fuel utilization, in infertile men (Pant et al., 2004). Mexican men living in the areas where DDT was used for malaria control, but without occupational exposure to DDT, exhibited serum levels of *p,p'*-DDE approximately 350-fold greater than Canadian men exposed to background environmental levels. *p,p'*-DDE concentrations in the Mexican men were correlated with increases in SHBG concentration and negatively correlated with testosterone levels. Both semen volume and total sperm number were inversely correlated to *p,p'*-DDE levels. Thus, androgen levels and semen quality are adversely affected by high *p,p'*-DDE body burden (Ayotte et al., 2001). The studies examining DDT exposure and semen quality report consistent effects on sperm motility and sperm morphology, similar to the PCB studies. The increased SHBG concentrations associated with serum *p,p'*-DDE described by Ayotte et al.,(2001) provides a possible mechanism for observed reductions in plasma testosterone and sperm number. By inducing SHBG synthesis, *p,p'*-DDE may exert its antiandrogenic effects by reducing the amount of bioavailable testosterone, thereby impairing spermatogenesis.

Further, more extensive correlation studies on the serum levels of DDT and metabolites in mothers of infertile men are required. These studies would provide insight into the effects of in utero exposure to DDT on semen quality of adult males.

1.5.3 Dioxins

Tetrachlodibenzo-*p*-dioxin (TCDD) is a carcinogen, demonstrated to target the endocrine system in experimental animals. Humans are exposed to dioxins through pulp and paper industry emissions, use of contaminated herbicides (now reduced in industrialized countries), and waste incineration emissions. Dioxins are lipophilic, slowly metabolized, and thus are not easily eliminated leading to bioaccumulation. Secondary dioxin exposures include dietary uptake via contaminated breast milk, meat, fish, and other dairy. Dioxins along with polycyclic aromatic hydrocarbons (PAH) and polyhalogenated biphenyls bind to the aryl hydrocarbon receptor (AhR). AhR ligands induce cell proliferation, differentiation, and apoptosis, although the mechanisms of these stimulations are not fully understood. It is known that human sperm possess AhR and may therefore be directly susceptible to dioxin (Khorram et al., 2004). A range of endocrine effects are reported in experimental animals following dioxin exposure. These include disruption of the HPT axis feedback mechanisms leading to alterations in serum levels of testosterone, dihydrotestosterone (DHT), E2, and LH, as well as modifications of the metabolism processes/events of estrogens and androgens (Birnbaum & Tuomisto, 2000). There are few published studies reporting human exposure to dioxins. Agent Orange, which contains TCDD as its contaminant, was used during the Vietnam War and exposure was documented in veterans of Operation Ranch Hand (the unit responsible for aerial herbicide spraying in Vietnam from 1962 to 1971; (Stone, 2007). Detectable TCDD levels in serum and seminal plasma were evident in U.S. veterans two to three decades following their Vietnam military service. Reproductive parameters including serum testosterone, FSH, LH, and testicular abnormalities were not associated with serum TCDD levels in the exposed men. It may be possible that the effects of dioxin on reproductive parameters were no longer evident at the time of the study, several decades after the use of Agent Orange. As semen quality can only be evaluated by follow-up study, the acute effects of exposure to Agent Orange on male reproductive health are unknown. Another study of 101 men from the general population in Belgium assessed TCDD exposure and semen quality. TCDD exposure was measured as dioxin-like activity in serum. Increases in serum dioxin-like activity were associated with decreased seminal volume resulting in elevated sperm concentrations. Total testosterone levels were significantly reduced in men with high serum dioxin-like activity. However, there was no significant association with LH, inhibin B, FSH, total sperm numbers, or sperm morphology (Dhooge et al., 2006). There are few epidemiological studies evaluating reproductive outcomes and particularly semen quality following TCDD and dioxin exposure. However, it is more relevant to consider the effects of dioxin at environmental concentrations on male reproductive health. A possible mechanism for infertility may be mediated by dioxin interacting with AhR on human sperm with implications for capacitation, acrosome reaction, sperm–egg binding, and fertilization. More studies are required to examine the effects of dioxin on semen quality.

1.5.4 Phthalates esters

Phthalate esters are abundant industrial chemicals used in the production of plastics and are present in many personal care products including cosmetics. Phthalates are a family of compounds and only a few induce male reproductive tract abnormalities. Gray et al., (2000) compared the ability of six phthalate esters (diethylhexyl phthalate, DEHP; benzylbutyl phthalate, BBP; diisononyl phthalate, DINP; dimethyl phthalate, DMP; diethyl phthalate, DEP; dioctyl terephthalate, DOTP; all administered at 750 mg/kg body weight from GD14 to postnatal day (PND) 3) to induce malformations of the reproductive tract. This study assessed changes in many androgenic endpoints and found that only DEHP, BBP and to a lesser degree DINP induced alterations in all aspects of androgen-regulated male reproductive endpoints. Exposure to diethyl hexyl and dibutyl phthalates is associated with adverse effects on sperm motility (Fredricsson et al., 1993). Animal studies consistently demonstrated that phthalate esters are male reproductive toxicants (Park et al., 2002), with exposure associated with testicular atrophy, spermatogenetic cell loss, and damage to the Sertoli cell population. Phthalate monoesters target Sertoli cell functions in supporting the spermatogenesis process. This may be due to the effect of phthalates in reducing the ability of Sertoli cells to respond to FSH (Hauser et al., 2005). Initial reports on the effects of phthalates on male reproductive tract development focussed on the gross changes such as reduced anogenital distance, hypospadias, malformed epididymis and, in later studies, nipple retention (Mylchreest et al., 2000). Only a few studies give a more detailed account of the histological changes observed in the testis after in utero phthalate exposure and demonstrate that the fetal testis is directly affected by phthalates during fetal and neonatal testis differentiation (Parks et al., 2000; Fisher et al., 2003). Some of these alterations are permanent and affect the function of the testis in adult life and are similar to the histological changes which are now being shown in patients with testicur dysgenesis syndrome (TDS; Skakkebaek et al., 2003). The production of testosterone is critical for the normal masculinization of the male reproductive tract, as already discussed. It has been shown that DBP and DEHP are both capable of inhibiting the production of testosterone by the fetal testis (Parks et al., 2000; Fisher et al., 2003). Testosterone synthesis by the fetal testis is first detectable by GD15, reaches a peak at around GD18/19, and remains high until birth. However, phthalate treatment induces a 60–85% reduction in testosterone synthesis during this critical developmental window, reducing testosterone levels to a similar level to those found in females (Parks et al., 2000). This reduction in testosterone is a factor in the occurrence of hypospadias and cryptorchidism observed after phthalate treatment. This is not to suggest that phthalate exposure causes TDS in humans, merely that the administration of very high doses of DBP to pregnant rats induces a TDS-like syndrome in the male offspring that shows many analogous features to human TDS. It is plausible, given how highly conserved the pathways of fetal development are, that phthalate administration may disrupt some common mechanistic pathways which if altered in humans could be helpful in determining the pathogenesis of human TDS. In both the human syndrome and the rodent model, abnormal testicular development or dysgenesis is evident by the abnormal organisation of these tissues. In humans, histological evidence of testicular dysgenesis (immature seminiferous tubules with undifferentiated Sertoli cells, microcalcifications and Sertoli cell only (SCO) tubules, Leydig cell hyperplasia, morphologically distorted tubules and the presence of carcinoma *in situ* (CIS) cells) have been found in biopsies of the contralateral testes of testicular germ cell cancer patients and in biopsies from patients with infertility, hypospadias and cryptorchidism (Skakkebaek et al., 2003). These studies support the hypothesis that all of these disorders (low sperm counts, cryptorchidism, hypospadias and testicular cancer) are associated with TDS. The in utero administration of DBP to rodents during the sensitive period of tissue morphogenesis permanently alters the testis and produces foci of testicular dysgenesis (immature seminiferous tubules with undifferentiated Sertoli cells, SCO tubules, Leydig cell hyperplasia, morphologically distorted tubules and the presence of abnormal germ cells) which persist in the adult animal (Fisher et al., 2003). The downstream consequences of altered Sertoli cell (and subsequently Leydig cell) function may be a key cause of many of the observed changes in both human TDS and the rat TDS-like model due to the central role of this cell type in driving testis morphogenesis in both rodents and humans. Several population studies evaluated phthalate ester exposure and semen quality. A randomized controlled study of men with unexplained infertility reported a negative correlation between seminal plasma phthalate ester concentration and sperm morphology (Rozati et al., 2002). Environmental phthalate levels measured by urinary metabolite, were reported to be associated with increased DNA damage in sperm (Duty et al., 2003). The studies measuring phthalate levels and semen quality seem to suggest an effect on sperm morphology and motility, rather than on total sperm numbers. Hauser et al.,(2005) suggest a mechanism by which PCB exposure may extend the bioavailability of phthalate metabolites, which in turn adversely affect semen quality. As human exposure consists of phthalate mixtures, along with xenobiotics, studies designed to test or measure single phthalate esters fail to appropriately characterize risks associated with these chemicals.

1.5.5 Phytoestrogens

Phytoestrogens are nonsteroidal plant-derived compounds with potent estrogenic activity. There are four main groups of phytoestrogens: isoflavonoids, flavonoids, coumestans, and lignans. Phytoestrogens exert their action via multiple mechanisms. Phytoestrogens interact with both ERα and ERβ, thereby inducing weak estrogenic and antiestrogenic actions (Kuiper et al., 1998). Coumestrol and genistein, two phytoestrogens, exhibit a higher affinity for ERß than for ERα (Whitten & Naftolin, 1998). Some phytoestrogens exert an inhibitory action on steroidogenic enzymes (Strauss et al., 1998). For example, isoflavonoids and lignans inhibit 5α-reductase activity, thereby reducing the conversion of testosterone to the active form DHT. A number of phytoestrogens, including lignans, isoflavonoids daidzein and equol, enterolactone, and genistein, were found to induce SHBG production in the liver (Adlercreutz et al., 1987). There are few studies measuring the effects of phytoestrogens on semen parameters in men. The effects of short-term phytoestrogen supplementation on semen quality and endocrine function were examined in a group of young, healthy males. Subjects received 500 mg supplements containing 40 mg of phytoestrogens isoflavones genistein, daidzein, and glycitein daily for 2 months and donated semen and blood for 2 months before and 4 months after supplementation (Mitchell et al., 2001). Testicular volume was not influenced by phytoestrogen supplementation; nor did serum E2, testosterone, FSH, or LH differ between the supplement-taking group and the control group who did not take supplements. Finally, phytoestrogen supplementation did not produce changes in seminal volume, sperm concentration, sperm count, and sperm motility (Mitchell et al., 2001). A case report described therapeutic phytoestrogen supplementation (80 mg/day for 6 months) to an oligospermic man, which did sufficiently improve semen parameters such that intrauterine insemination was performed and the couple was able to conceive (Casini et al., 2006). To date, evidence linking dietary consumption of phytoestrogens and reduced semen quality is insufficient and requires further study.

1.5.6 Pesticides, fungicides and herbicides

The U.S Environmental Protection Agency (EPA) defines a pesticide as "any substance or mixture of substances intended for preventing, destroying, repelling, or lessening the damage of any pest," which may include plants, weeds, animals, insects, and fungus. Many epidemiological studies use the generic term *pesticides* to refer to a broad range of structurally unrelated compounds with different mechanisms of action, biological targets, and target pests. Epidemiological studies that evaluate the effects of these chemicals on male reproductive parameters often lack direct, quantitative measures of exposure. A study of participants from The Study for Future Families evaluated semen quality and pesticide exposures in male partners of pregnant women attending prenatal clinics in Missouri and Minnesota (Swan et al., 2003) Urinary levels of metabolites from the pesticides alachlor, diazinon, atrazine, and metolochlor were detected more often in men from Missouri, representative of the pesticides used in the agricultural practices of this state. Pesticide metabolites of chlorpyrifos/chlorpyrifos methyl (3,5,6-trichloropyridinol) and methyl parathion (4-nitrophenol) were detected more frequently in men from Minnesota. For the Missouri group, there was an association between low semen quality and urinary levels of chlorpyrifos and parathion metabolites. Further, increased levels of herbicides alachlor and metoachlor were associated with decreased sperm morphology and concentration. In contrast, there was no association between levels of any of these pesticides and their metabolites and semen parameters within the Minnesota group (Swan et al., 2003). A follow-up study focused on the men from Missouri, using a nested case-control design (cases: men with low semen parameters; controls: men with normal parameters). Urinary levels of metabolites of eight currently used pesticides were measured and correlated with semen quality. Men with elevated metabolite levels of alachlor and atrazine (herbicides) and diazinon (2-isopropoxy-4-methyl-pyrimidinol insecticide) were significantly more likely to have poor semen quality than controls (Swan, 2006). This study provide evidence that environmental exposures differ between regions, even within the same country. Different agricultural practices will create regional variation in the amounts and types of pesticides used, leading to differences in biological effects. A study in male infertility patients in Massachusetts measured urinary metabolites of carbaryl/naphthalene and chlorpyrifos. Sperm concentration, motility, and, to a lesser extent, morphology were reduced in men with elevated exposure to carbaryl/naphthalene (as measured by urinary levels of the metabolite 1-naphthol) and to chlorpyrifos (as measured by urinary levels of the metabolite 3,5,6-trichloro-2-pyridinol [TCPY]) (Meeker et al., 2004). The mechanism of action of carbaryl may be related to the production of reactive oxygen species (ROS) rather than endocrine disruption. Carbaryl produced lipid peroxidation at low concentrations, which in turn induced the sperm plasma membrane to lose its fluidity and integrity, thereby impairing sperm motility (Meeker et al., 2004). Generally, the studies reviewed here demonstrated a relationship between pesticide exposure and reduced semen quality. However, toxicology studies using animal models are essential to understand the biological mechanisms underlying the adverse reproductive affects caused by pesticide exposure in the male.

1.5.6.1 Vinclozolin

Vinclozolin is a dicarboximide fungicide that has two active metabolites, M1 and M2, which have anti-androgenic properties. In vivo and in vitro experiments demonstrate that these compounds act as potent androgen receptor antagonists, and administration to pregnant rats results in abnormalities of androgen-regulated sexual differentiation similar to those induced by flutamide, e.g. reduced anogenital distance, nipple retention, hypospadias, undescended testes and small or absent accessory glands (Gray et al., 2001). Studies have tried to define the 'sensitive window' for exposure to vinclozolin, and have determined that administration to pregnant rats during gestational day (GD) 14–19 induced reproductive tract malformations, with treatment over GD16–17 causing the most severe malformations (Wolf et al., 2000). This illustrates that the whole period of male reproductive tract differentiation is sensitive to the effects of anti-androgens.

1.5.6.2 Linuron

Linuron is a urea-based herbicide which acts as a weak androgen receptor antagonist in vitro and in vivo, and disrupts androgen-dependent male reproductive tract development after gestational exposure (Gray et al., 2001). When administered to pregnant rats (GD 14–18; 100 mg/ kg/day) the male pups displayed a reduced anogenital distance and retention of areolas (Gray et al., 1999). Linuron failed to induce either hypospadias or undescended testes, suggesting that linuron affects testosterone-but not DHT-mediated development, though how this occurs is not known (McIntyre et al., 2002).

1.5.7 Tobacco smoke

It is beyond the scope of this review to provide a detailed review of the literature on cigarette smoking and semen quality. However, PAH (polycyclic aromatic hydrocarbons), the major carcinogenic components of cigarette smoke (Vine, 1996), were found to activate aryl hydrocarbon receptor (AhR), suggesting that tobacco smoke may represent a chemical mixture with endocrine disrupting activity. There is extensive evidence demonstrating that exposure to tobacco smoke is associated with reduced semen quality (Vine, 1996). An inverse dose-dependent relationship between smoking and semen volume, total sperm count, and percent motile sperm was reported following a large cross-sectional study of 2542 healthy Danish men. Sperm concentration was 19% lower in heavy smokers compared to non-smokers. Serum LH and testosterone were positively correlated with smoking (Ramlau-Hansen et al., 2007). The incidence of bilateral cryptorchidism in a sample of cryptorchid Danish boys was increased in children of smoking mothers. Testicular biopsies from boys exposed in utero/neonatal to tobacco smoke demonstrated a decreased number of spermatogonia and gonocytes per tubule cross section (Thorup et al., 2006). Similarly, a large cross-sectional European study of 889 Danish men, 221 men from Norway, 313 Lithuanian men, and 190 men from Estonia reported reductions of sperm concentrations by 20% in sons exposed to prenatal tobacco smoke (Jensen et al., 2004), while a separate study described an inverse dose-dependent association between sperm concentration and prenatal tobacco exposure, measured in adult sons of 522 Danish women (Jensen et al., 2005). The association between impaired semen quality and smoking is fairly well established (Vine, 1996). Although epidemiological studies of male reproductive function were designed to avoid the confounding effects of smoking, by limiting samples to non-smokers or segmenting samples according to smoking status, the interaction effects of tobacco smoke, alcohol, and other lifestyle factors are often not considered. An important study by Robbins et al.,(1997) did investigate the interactions of caffeine, alcohol, and cigarette smoking on sperm aneuploidy, determining that incidence of sperm abnormalities decreased after controlling for age and other lifestyle factors.

1.5.8 Medications and male reproductive toxicity

There are a variety of prescription medications that can lead to male infertility, often temporary but sometimes permanent. Arthritis medication, depression drugs, high blood pressure medication, drugs for digestive problems as well as antibiotics and cancer drugs are just a few of the medications that can lead to interferences with sperm production, sexual function and ejaculation (Nudell et al., 2002). Here is a look at some of the common medications and drugs that can cause a man to experience fertility problems.

1.5.8.1 Antihypertensive

Although most men who are treated for hypertension are older, the recent focus on the importance of blood pressure control has led to greater numbers of younger patients on antihypertensives. Many of these medications are commonly associated with erectile dysfunction but most do not directly affect fertility. One exception is spironolactone, which acts as an anti-androgen and has been associated with impaired semen quality. Calcium channel blockers (e.g. nifedipine) have been reported to cause reversible functional defects in sperm, impairing their ability to fertilize eggs without affecting sperm production or standard semen analysis parameters; however, not all investigators report these types of effects. Diuretics can affect function by decreasing penile blood flow, and beta-blockers may affect libido and erectile function (Benoff et al., 1994).

1.5.8.2 Hormones

Diethylstilbestrol (DES) was given to pregnant women in the 1950s, and reports of epididymal cysts and cryptorchidism (undescended testes) in males with prenatal DES exposure have raised concerns about fertility; however, follow-up studies on adult men with prenatal DES exposure have revealed no adverse effects on fertility (Wilcox et al., 1995). Exogenous androgens are well known to induce hypogonadotropic hypogonadism. This may be induced directly by testosterone supplementation or by use of synthetic anabolic steroids, leading to azoospermia. This hypogonadism is usually reversible but may take 3 to 6 months, and some patients do not recover pituitary function. It is important to remember that testosterone replacement therapy in younger men may lead to infertility. Dehydroepiandrosterone (DHEA) is a natural steroid prohormone precursor of androsterone, testosterone, and estrogen. DHEA is commonly taken and easily available over the counter. Antiandrogens and estrogens can adversely affect fertility by altering the HPG axis or decreasing libido or erectile function, while progesterones act by decreasing libido or erectile function (Nudell et al., 2002).

1.5.8.3 Antiandrogens

Finasteride and dutasteride are antiandrogens that act by inhibiting 5-alpha-reductase. Finasteride has also been used to treat male-pattern baldness. These drugs increase the risk of low ejaculate volumes and libido, as well as cause erectile and ejaculatory dysfunction; however, men taking low doses of finasteride for hair loss have shown no changes in semen parameters (Overstreet et al., 1999).

1.5.8.4 Antibiotics

Many antibiotics have been reported to exert adverse effects on male fertility; however, there are few human data on the majority of these medications. High doses of nitrofurantoin have been reported to cause early maturation arrest at the primary spermatocyte stage but the more common short-term low-dose therapy is not likely detrimental. While in vitro data on erythromycin, tetracycline, and gentamycin suggest the potential for adverse effects on fertility, documentation of an in vivo effect in humans is lacking (Hargreaves et al., 1998). Sulfasalazine, used in the treatment of ulcerative colitis, is well known to cause defects in human sperm concentration and motility. Aminoglycosides, type of antibiotics is generally used for serious bacterial infections, like TB, and are administered under medical supervision. Aminoglycosides can negatively impact sperm production while neomycin has been shown to reduce both sperm count and motility. Macrolides, in addition to being used to treat chlamydia and Legionnaires disease, macrolides are similar to penicillin and can be used in place of it in people with a penicillin allergy. Macrolides research has mainly focused on animals, where it has been found that the antibiotic can decrease sperm motility as well as kill off sperm. It is believed that the antibiotic produces similar results in humans (Schlegel et al., 1991).

1.5.8.5 Psychotherapeutic agents

Many psychotherapeutic agents affect male fertility by suppressing the HPG axis and decreasing erectile function and libido. Indeed, one of the most significant side effects of the antidepressants is elevation of serum prolactin, leading to significant but reversible suppression of spermatogenesis (Nudell et al., 2002). Psychotherapeutic agents include antipsychotics, tricyclic and selective serotonin reuptake inhibitor (SSRI) or selective norepinephrine reuptake inhibitor (SNRI) antidepressants, monoamine oxidase inhibitors (MAOIs), phenothiazines, and lithium. There are now large numbers of patients taking SSRI or SNRI medications, many of which have significant fertility effects.

1.5.8.6 Anticancer drugs

Doxorubicin hydrochloride, Goserelin acetate, methotrexate, or fluorouracil all are the drugs used to treat various types of cancer. However, these drugs have significant side effects on sexual behaviour, altered fertility and sperm count (Nudell et al., 2002).

1.5.8.6.1 Chemotherapeutic agents

Chemotherapy for the treatment of cancer can have devastating effects on male fertility through the impairment of spermatogenesis; indeed, alkylating agents, antimetabolites, and the vinca alkaloids are all gonadotoxins. The alkylating agent, cyclophosphamide alters male fertility; treatment with 1-2 mg/kg for more than 4 months increases the incidence of azospermia and oligospermia in adult male patients (Qureshi et al., 1972). In patients with testicular cancer, the cumulative dose of cisplatin determines whether spermatogenesis is impaired irreversibly. Most patients will become azoospermic, with the majority recovering spermatogenesis within 4 years. The majority of Hodgkin's disease or leukemia patients become azoospermic after chemotherapy; this may or may not lead to permanent sterility. After treatment with mitoxantrone, vincristine, vinblastine, and prednisone combination therapy plus abdominal radiotherapy for Hodgkin's disease, sperm counts and motility were restored to pre-treatment levels in most patients (Magelseen et al., 2006).

1.5.8.7 Miscellaneous medications

Cimetidine has been reported to have antiandrogenic effects that induce gynecomastia and decreases in sperm count. Immune modulators are commonly used but, unfortunately, clear human data regarding male fertility for interferon or the immunosuppressant mycophenolate mofetil are lacking. Although cyclosporine has been found to induce impaired fertility in rats, there are no human data available (Nudell et al., 2002). Epilepsy has been associated with decreased testosterone levels and increased estrogen levels leading to reductions in libido and to erectile dysfunction. Medications used to treat epilepsy (eg, valproate, oxcarbazepine, and carbamazepine) may worsen hormonal abnormalities and have been associated with some sperm morphologic defects (Isojarvi et al., 2004).

1.5.9 Recreational and illicit substances and male reproductive toxicity

Heavy marijuana use has been associated with gynecomastia, decreased serum testosterone levels, decreased sperm concentration, and pyospermia (white cells in the semen indicating possible infection) (Close et al., 1990). Patients experience variable sensitivity to marijuana, and it may take 2 to 3 months for symptoms to improve.

Oligospermia (abnormally low sperm concentration in the ejaculate) and defects in sperm morphology and motility have been reported in users of cocaine. Opiates have also been shown to decrease libido and erectile function through induction of hypogonadotropic hypogonadism. This also is important to note when prescribing opioids for pain. Chronic opioid use whether, oral or intrathecal, may lead to sexual dysfunction (Bracken et al., 1990). Cumulative evidence suggests that cigarette smoking may have a deleterious effect on male fertility by reducing sperm production, motility, and morphology. Cigarette smoking may also lead to development of pyospermia, decreased sperm penetration, and hormonal alterations (Nudell et al., 2002; Close et al., 1990). Long-term abuse of alcohol has detrimental effects in the HPG axis. Alcoholics exhibit significant decreases in semen volume, sperm count, motility, and number of morphologically normal sperm. They also show signs of pyospermia. Alcohol in excess can thus exert profound deleterious effects on all aspects of the male reproductive system. However, there is no evidence that moderate alcohol intake impairs male fertility (Nudell et al., 2002; Close et al., 1990).

The examples of few chemicals which are reported to disrupt the sex hormones and/or damage the male in animal studies are summarized below (Woodruff et al., 2008).

Common environmental Toxicants	Common uses and routes of exposure	The effects on male reproductive system
Heavy Metals (Mainly cadmium, Lead and arsenic)	Population exposed to cadmium and lead via contaminations found in drinking water and food, while occupational exposure takes place during mining or manufacturing of batteries and pigments or industrial activities such as smelting and refining metals and municipal waste incineration.	a. Testicular toxicity b. Low sperm count and motility and density. c. Reduce male fertility d. Foetal toxicity and malformation of male organs.
Volatile organic compounds (Toluene, benzene and xylene)	Mostly occupational exposure in industrial workers.	a. Testicular toxicity b. Low sperm count and motility and density. c. Reduce male fertility
Phthalates DBP = di(n)butylphthalate DiBP =di(iso)butylphthalate	Phthalates are a group of chemicals used to impart flexibility to plastic polyvinyl chloride (PVC) products as	a. Testicular toxicity b. Reduce anogenital distance, hypospadias and

Common environmental Toxicants	Common uses and routes of exposure	The effects on male reproductive system
BBP = benzyl butyl phthalate DEHP = di(2-ethylhexyl)phthalate DPP = dipentyl phthalate DINP = diisononyl phthalate DCHP = dicyclohexyl phthalate	well as in other applications, including pharmaceuticals, and pesticides. There is widespread human exposure with reported uses in building materials, household furnishings, clothing, cosmetics, dentures, medical tubing and bags, toys, modelling clay, cars, lubricants, waxes and cleaning materials. Exposure may arise via the air, through absorption when used on the skin, and through the diet.	undescended of testes in immature male. c. Reduce male fertility d. Foetal toxicity and malformation of male organs.
Paraben	Paraben is the name given to a group of chemicals used as preservatives in cosmetics and body care products, including deodorants, creams and lotions. They are able to penetrate the skin	a. Hormone mimicking activities b. Reduce synthesis of testosterone
Triclosan	Triclosan is an anti-bacterial and anti-fungal chemical widely used in personal care products such as some soaps, toothpaste etc. Triclosan has also been added to plastic products such as kitchen chopping boards.	a. Hormone mimicking activities b. Reduce synthesis of testosterone
Triclocarban	Triclocarban (TCC or 3,4,4'-trichlorocarbanilide) is also used as an anti- bacterial in personal care products such as soaps.	a. It has sex hormone disrupting properties.
BPA (Bisphenol A)	BPA is the building block of polycarbonate plastic used in baby bottles, CDs, motor cycle windshields etc. It is also used for the production of epoxy resins used in the coating of the food packaging.	a. Oestrogenic activities b. Altered male reproductive organs and induce early puberty c. Anti androgenic activity.
Penta-BDE (Penta-brominated diphenyl ether)	There are actually 3 commercial PBDE products, which predominantly contain deca, octa and penta-BDEs, and are therefore called by these names. PBDEs are used as flame retardants to prevent fire taking hold quickly. Penta-BDE is used in polyurethane foam, for example, in mattresses and car and aeroplane seats. Apart from exposure via dust it is possible to transfer from hand to mouth.	a. Altered male reproductive organs c. Anti androgenic properties.

Common environmental Toxicants	Common uses and routes of exposure	The effects on male reproductive system
PCBs	PCBs are used in a variety of applications, including electrical applications, dielectric fluids for transformers and capacitors, hydraulic and heat transfer systems, lubricants, gasket sealers, paints, fluorescent lights, plasticizers, adhesives, carbonless copying paper, flame retardants, and brake linings. Human exposure also arises due to contamination of the food chain.	a. Hormone mimicking activities b. Anti androgenic properties.
Dioxins	Dioxins are a group of chemicals which are not intentionally produced, but are emitted during incomplete or relatively low temperature combustion. They can come from industrial or domestic sources, wherever a chlorine source is present. Such sources include, for example, domestic bonfires with PVC plastic, incinerators, certain chemical and metal factories (particularly aluminium recovery sites), paper pulp production using chlorine, and coal burning in power stations and in fire-places in the home. Exposure can arise from inhalation, but mainly comes from contamination of food.	a. Sex hormone disruptor b. Testicular dysfunctions c. Low sperm count d. Sperm abnormalities
Diesel fuel Exhaust	As diesel is used as a fuel in many cars and lorries, diesel exhaust is widespread.	a. Disrupts androgen action b. Prenatal exposure in animals leads to endocrine disruption after birth and suppresses testicular function in male rats.
Tobacco smoke (Polycyclic aromatic hydrocarbons (PAH)	It includes active or passive smoking	a. Blocks androgen synthesis b. Testicular dysfunctions c. Low sperm count d. Sperm abnormalities
Alkylphenols Nonylphenol Octylphenol	Nonylphenol is the breakdown product of the surface active agent, nonylphenol ethoxylate. Many uses including in domestic cleaning and industrial and institutional cleaning, and in textiles and leather processing. Octyl phenol is used in the production	a. Hormone mimicking activities b. Reduce synthesis of testosterone c. Reduce testicular size d. reduce male fertility and sperm number and quality.

Common environmental Toxicants	Common uses and routes of exposure	The effects on male reproductive system
	of phenol/ formaldehyde resins (Bakelite) and in the production of octylphenol ethoxylates, and used in the formulation of printing inks and in tyre manufacture	
DDT (break-down product DDE).	DDT is an insecticide which was used extensively on crops, but is now only used in a few countries against the malaria-bearing mosquito. DDT and DDE last in the soil for a very long time, potentially for hundreds of years. Unfortunately, due to this persistence, it is still found in some produce, such as vegetables, fish and liver. DDE is also found as a persistent contaminant in our bodies. The DDT breakdown product or metabolite, p,p'-DDE, is able to block testosterone.	a. Hormone mimicking activities b. Reduce synthesis of testosterone
Linuron Diuron	Linuron and diuron are herbicide used to control weeds on hard surfaces such as roads, railway tracks and in crops and forestry. It has been detected in tap water and as a residue in vagetables such as carrots, parsnips and spinach.	a. Anti-androgenic properties
Vinclozolin Procymidone Iprodione Prochloroz Fenarimol	These are all fungicide used on fruits and vegetables.	a. Blocks testosterone action b. Reduce testosterone synthesis c. Anti-androgenic properties d. Feminize male offspring.
Fenarimol Fenitrothion Chlorpyrifos-methyl	These are all insecticides are used, for example, on apples, plums, barries, peas, sweet corn and cereals. Those have been found as a contaminant of fruit, such as oranges and grapes etc.	a. Blocks testosterone action b. Reduce testosterone synthesis c. Anti-androgenic properties
Ketoconazole	Ketoconazole is as an anti-fungal product in pharmaceuticals to treat fungal infections of the skin.	a. Blocks testosterone action b. Reduce testosterone synthesis
Pyrethroid pesticides Permethrin Beta-cyfluthrin Cypermethrin	Some pyrethroid pesticides such as Permethrin beta-cyfluthrin, cypermethrin, are still in use, with for example, the latter found as a residue in apples, beans, melons and oranges	a. Blocks testosterone action b. Reduce testosterone synthesis c. Anti-androgenic properties

Common environmental Toxicants	Common uses and routes of exposure	The effects on male reproductive system
Certain sun-screens 4-MBC 3-BC	A few ultraviolet (UV) filters have been found as contaminants in waste water treatment plants and rivers.	a. Estrogenic activity b. Anti-androgenic activity c. Interfere male sexual activity d. delay male puberty e. reduce reproductive organ weights in male offspring.
Heat, Ionizing radiation, Non-ionizing radiation, microwaves, electromagnetic fields	Mostly occupational exposures in home or industry as well as the mobile phone users.	a. Testicular toxicity b. Low sperm count and motility and density. c. Reduce male fertility d. Azospermia
Chemotherapeutic drugs (Cisplatin, cyclophosphamide, procarbazine, and doxirubicine, and vincristine etc.)	Anticancer treatment.	a. Testicular dysfunctions b. Low sperm count and motility and density. c. Infertility d. Azospermia and oligospermia.

2. Identifying hazards

A discrepancy exists between the number of chemicals in commerce (approximately 84,000) and the number that have been evaluated in model species for reproductive toxicity potential (4,000) (U.S. EPA 1998a and 1998b). It is not feasible to allocate additional resources to test the 80,000 or so untested chemicals through traditional testing protocols, particularly given that about 2,000 new chemicals are introduced into commerce each year (U.S. EPA 1998). Instead, new, more rapid methods are needed to screen large numbers of chemicals and to identify those that are potential reproductive hazards. In the near term, top priorities will be to develop the most promising alternative models and to test their ability to appropriately classify the toxicity of sets of known toxicants and non-toxicants.

2.1 High-throughput assays

High-throughput assays evaluate the effect of a test substance on a single biologic process using an automated manner that allows thousands or tens of thousands of compounds to be tested in a short time at a reasonable cost. Robotics and genetic engineering make it possible to produce large quantities of receptors or genetically engineered cells for use in these assays. Knowledge about mechanisms of toxicity is often central to the strategy of high-throughput assays. For example, cells are being developed that are bioengineered to express human hormone receptors for estrogens and androgens. These cells can be used for high-throughput chemical screening for steroid hormone receptor affinity or the potential to act as endocrine disruptors. Both isoforms of recombinant human estrogen receptor and human androgen receptor are commercially available for this purpose. Based on the same principles, other batteries of high-throughput assays are available to screen for activity against various receptors and cytochrome P-450 enzyme isoforms (Lawson et al., 2003). The availability and application of these assays will undoubtedly expand as we understand more about the relevance of each protein in toxicologic processes.

2.2 Structure-activity prediction

Methods for predicting activity from structure continue to be developed and refined. Computer programs use available empirical information about the toxicity of existing compounds and their chemical characteristics to predict whether a new compound will have similar toxicity. These programs have not performed well in the area of reproductive and developmental toxicity, probably because reproductive processes are complex and effects may be elicited through multiple modes and mechanisms. As science progresses and we learn more about mechanisms of toxicity at the molecular level, however, structure-activity computer programs will become more exact and predictive. The best examples are the programs that are being developed and refined for estrogen receptor binding (Tong et al., 1997).

2.3 Integration of human studies and tests of model species

Though 4,000 chemicals have been tested in model species, few chemicals have been adequately evaluated for reproductive effects in humans and contain a partial list of known human developmental and adult toxicants. Because the interpretation of studies of model species is often not straightforward and because field studies are labor and resource intensive, a systematic approach is needed to select and prioritize chemicals for epidemiologic studies. Moorman et al., (2000) recently proposed a process for selecting chemicals for human field studies. In this process, information gained from model species testing conducted by the National Toxicology Program (NTP) was reviewed for significant adverse reproductive effects and potency of the toxicants. The evaluative process then combined this information with human exposure information available in public databases to arrive at a list of high-priority candidates for studies in humans.

2.4 New biomarkers for humans and model species

In 1977, men exposed to dibromochloropropane (DBCP), a pesticide that is now banned in the United States, were found to be azoospermic and oligospermic (Whorton et al., 1977). Currently, a variety of biomarkers are used to assess the potential adverse reproductive effects due to toxic chemical exposures. Bioindicators of sperm production and quality (semen volume, sperm concentration, sperm motility, sperm morphology) are routinely evaluated in ejaculated semen samples in men and in suspensions of epididymal sperm from test species (epididymal sperm reserves, sperm motility, and sperm morphology) (Moline et al., 2000; U.S. EPA 1998a). During the past decade, computer-assisted methods developed to improve and automate the evaluation of sperm motion and morphology have been added to the battery of routine sperm measures, and guidance for their use and interpretation has been made available through a number of workshops (ILSI 1999; Seed et al.,1996). Furthermore, baseline data on the relationship between various semen or epididymal sperm measures and fertility have emerged from a number of large studies designed to address this question (Zinaman et al.,2000). Thus, these measures are widely accepted biomarkers of adverse reproductive effects that are suitable for application in both human and model species studies. Serum hormone measures can also be determined in humans and test species. Inhibin B has been proposed as an indicator of testicular function and a possible surrogate for sperm measures (Anderson and Sharpe 2000). The recognition that sperm functional tests are also desirable has led to development of various new tests that have only recently been applied to toxicology. Biomarkers of the genetic integrity of sperm are designed to identify risks for paternally mediated developmental effects. Sperm proteins are being tested as biomarkers of fertility to detect specific deficits in sperm function (as opposed to decreased sperm output). Although details of such tests are beyond the scope of this review, **Table 1.** provides a list of new tests and references regarding methodology and examples of use. Further research is needed to make these tests more practical and more cost effective and to determine their ultimate utility for hazard identification and elucidation of modes and mechanisms of toxicant action.

Target	Bioassay	Function assessed
Sperm fertilizing ability	SP-22 protein Sperm antigens Ubiquitin	Sperm function Acrosome reaction
Sperm maturity	Cytoplasmic droplets Heat shock protein A2	Sperm morphology
Sperm DNA	CMA3 staining COMET DNA adducts TUNEL SCSA	Chromatin damage DNA damage
Sperm chromosomes	FISH	Aneuploidy, Brakage Translocation
Sperm count surrogate	Inhibin-B	Endocrine feedback of spermatogenesis.

Abbreviations: CMA3 staining, Chromomycin A3 staining; COMET, Single-cell gel electrophoresis assay; FISH, Fluorescence in situ hybridization; SCSA, Sperm chromatin structure assay; TUNEL, Terminal deoxynucleotidyl transferase-mediated dUTP-biotin end-labeling (Lawson et al., 2003)

Table 1. The Biomarkers for the assessment of male reproductive toxicity by Chemical agents (Lawson et al., 2003).

2.5 Estimating occupational exposure

Establishing that a significant number of workers or members of the general population are or will be exposed to a potential reproductive toxicant is central to priority setting. NIOSH's National Occupational Hazard Survey and National Occupational Exposure Survey conducted in 1972-1974 and 1981-1983, respectively, has been used extensively to identify substances of common exposure (NIOSH 1978, 1988). These surveys are the only comprehensive assessments of general industry where the number of workers potentially exposed to chemical agents has been estimated. However, these databases are outdated and of limited use because they indicate only potential exposure. NIOSH is currently planning a new hazard surveillance activity that will target industry sectors on a rolling basis, beginning with the health care sector. Public health researchers will continue to require updated exposure surveys to keep up with the changing workplace exposures and monitor new exposures that may be potential reproductive toxicants. New technologies such as geographic information systems (GIS) allow mapping of industries and specific chemical exposures. Use of GIS to identify geographic areas with high volume of use of suspect chemicals might be an effective method of identifying populations with greater potential occupational and environmental exposures. Biomonitoring is a valuable tool for estimating occupational exposure. The National Report on Human Exposure to Environmental Chemicals is a new and ongoing assessment of the U.S. population's exposure to environmental chemicals. The first edition of the report presents levels of 27 environmental chemicals, including metals (e.g., lead, mercury, and uranium), cotinine (a marker of tobacco smoke exposure), organophosphate pesticide metabolites, and phthalate metabolites. This is a significant step forward in assessing the potential human toxicity of a class of chemicals known to be reproductive and developmental toxicants in rodents. Improved methods for analysis of exposure, especially of age and time effects, are likely to impact the characterization of occupational exposure in these studies (Richardson and Wing 1998). Current research approaches usually consider the action of single, unique toxicants on outcomes of interest, creating yet another challenge to drafting a reproductive hazards agenda. The more common human exposure scenario is to mixtures of toxicants at low concentrations, episodically and over the long term. Attention to cumulative exposure over years of a working lifetime and total aggregate exposure to toxicants from multiple exposure sources, as well as classical considerations of exposure routes, must also be addressed. Methodologic approaches must enlarge and mature to consider the effects and modulation of effects mediated by both exposure to mixtures of toxicants and the complexities of exposure mode at low dose and over prolonged duration.

2.6 Mechanistic research

Understanding mechanisms of action of toxicants is important for a number of reasons, including *a*) supporting the biologic plausibility of an observed association between chemical exposure and adverse outcome; *b*) uncovering common pathways of actions of different agents; *c*) extrapolating across species for risk assessment; *d*) improving the predictability of human morbidity from responses of model species; and *e*) predicting responses to mixed exposures (Lawson et al., 2003). Mechanistic studies are not new in toxicology; however, new tools in genomics, proteomics, and bioinformatics present unprecedented opportunities to advance our understanding of toxicant action at a molecular level. Genomic information and the ability to screen most or all of the genome of an increasing number of organisms for changes in gene expression are revolutionizing the way in which biologic effects data are gathered. It is now possible to determine the effects of a toxicant exposure on gene expression of most of the genome of mice and rats. This will allow us to generate testable hypotheses about the mechanism of action of toxicants. It will also open up the possibility of identifying markers of exposure or effect specific to a particular insult that can be used in field studies. As with any new technology, a number of problems will need to be overcome for the promise of genomics to be realized. The first will be to manage the large volume of information produced by gene expression experiments. Gene chips may contain thousands or tens of thousands of sequences. Experience shows that any perturbation in a biologic system leads to numerous changes in gene expression. An entire field of bioinformatics is being developed to help collect, organize, and manage the data to identify changes related temporally, by dose, or by metabolic pathway. The second challenge will be to separate those changes in gene expression pivotal to the toxic response from those that are more generalized responses to any stimulus. The third challenge will be to quantitatively relate changes in expression of critical genes with toxicity, which is manifested at a more complex level of biologic organization (i.e., the cell, organ, or organism). Real comfort in this genomic approach will come only with experience and the development of a large database.

2.7 Gene-environment interactions

Reproductive toxicants can affect human populations over the total life span, including the *in utero* and perinatal periods, childhood, puberty, and adulthood. Thus, extending research efforts to address stage-specific sensitivity is recommended. Another emerging approach allows the identification of populations at potentially increased risk from toxicant exposure by characterizing genetic polymorphisms of metabolizing enzymes in exposed cohorts. Such methods may identify vulnerable subpopulations on the basis of inherent (genetic) differences in their ability to metabolize a toxicant.

2.8 Identifying genes that increase sensitivity to reproductive toxicants

Genetic factors that elevate risk for disease can be grouped into two categories: those for which having a particular allele conveys a high risk for the disease regardless of other (e.g., environmental) influences and those associated with only small increases in risk of the disease. The latter, termed susceptibility genes are being identified at an increasing rate. The interaction of these alleles with environmental agents or other susceptibility alleles ultimately determines whether the disease will be manifested. Much work has been done to understand the role of these genes for reproductive toxicity.

2.9 Potential information from genetics to advance epidemiologic studies

If epidemiologic studies could identify genetic-toxicant interactions by comparing the prevalence of a particular genetic marker (polymorphism) or a group of markers in affected and unaffected populations, this information could be used to target environmental, behavioral, or medical interventions (Khoury 1997). Ultimately, validation of genetic testing to link a particular genotype with exposure to a specific chemical to the increased prevalence of a particular reproductive disorder would require epidemiologic confirmation (Khoury & Dorman 1998).

2.10 Communication

An essential component of future reproductive studies will be improved communication. Because of the complex mechanisms involved in reproductive research, collaboration across scientific disciplines must be conducted. In addition, notification of research results and recommendations must be communicated to workers and the affected public in a manner that is timely, accessible, and easily understood. A primary goal of reproductive research is to reduce the high percentages of adverse outcomes such as infertility, pregnancy loss, and congenital malformations. Although certain limitations exist that are unique to reproductive research, many advances in technology and methodologies have been recently developed that will aid researchers in their efforts to *a*) understand mechanisms by which toxicants exert their effects, *b*) identify populations at risk, and *c*) evaluate reproductive and developmental hazards to improve public health.

3. Methods of assessing male reproductive capacity

The determination of sperm concentration, morphology, and motility remains the primary clinical assay for male infertility (WHO, 1999). The WHO guidelines on semen quality provide reference semen parameters as follows: sperm concentration >20 million/ml, 50% motility, and at least 50% normal morphology (WHO, 1999). *Oligospermia* is the term for semen with <20 million/ml sperm in ejaculate, and *asthenospermia* for semen with sperm <50% motility or <25% rapid progressive motility, *teratospermia* for reduced percent sperm with normal morphology, and *azoospermia* for the absence of sperm in the ejaculate (Braude & Rowell, 2003). It is unknown whether endocrine disrupter exposure represents a subset of the environmental risk factors for male infertility, as there are few studies that examine exposure and human semen quality. Moreover, toxicants can affect the male reproductive system at one of several sites or at multiple sites. These sites include the testes, the accessory sex glands, and the central nervous system, including the neuroendocrine system.

3.1 The contribution of experimental models

The usefulness of experimental animal models is usually perceived as limited to hazard identification using the test protocols specified by regulatory agencies. However, animal models can also provide valuable support to reproductive risk assessment on many other fronts. If the focus is on human exposure, animal studies can be designed to confirm reproductive toxicity when initial observations in exposed humans are suggestive of an adverse effect. Furthermore, such observations can be extended across a wide range of exposures in animals, using any route of exposure and any specified dose versus time scenario. For example, when human exposure is likely to be acute or intermittent, animal models are ideal for defining critical exposure windows based on developmental stage or for revealing the pathogenesis of an effect at various times after exposure through recovery. This is particularly important with respect to male reproductive effects because alterations in semen quality or fertility may not become evident until sometime after the exposure, particularly if an early stage of spermatogenesis is targeted. A rodent model is most commonly used for the study of reproductive and developmental toxicity (Claudio et al., 1999). To use toxicology data derived from animal studies to advantage in risk assessment, it is critical to identify and understand species-specific differences in physiology and metabolism that may affect the response to the toxicant in question. Rodent models have, for example, been used to determine the relationship between sperm end points and function (fertility) (Chapin et al., 1997). Determining that a substance is toxic to the male reproductive system is only the first step: The next step is to examine its mechanisms of toxicity. Mechanistic information allows for predictions about the potential toxicity of individual compounds or complex mixtures in humans, for better understanding of the windows of vulnerability in the development of the male reproductive system, and for developments of possible preventive or curative measures. Acute short-term exposure models combined with serial exposure models give a complete picture of the range of effects (Claudio et al., 1999). Exposing animals over a long period of time allows for the detection of transgenerational effects from chemicals, such as male-mediated developmental effects. If developmental effects appear, researchers can go back and administer a dose during that critical period of development to refine knowledge about how such problems occur. Early developmental end points measurable in animal research include anogenital distance at birth, testis position, genital malformations, secondary sex characteristics, and serum hormone levels. Acute short-term exposures, on the other hand, can be useful for identifying critical windows of exposure. Acute exposures followed over time can help identify the pathogenesis of a lesion, isolate the cell type that is susceptible to damage (germ cells, spermatocytes, or spermatid), and determine genetic effects, including the repair capability of affected genes. Serial sacrifice studies are best used for identifying the earliest detectable pathologic changes in target organs, cells, or processes. Multigeneration studies, in particular continuous breeding studies, yield the most thorough assessment of the many complex processes that result in reproductive and developmental toxicity.

3.2 Epidemiologic approaches

Epidemiologic methods for assessing the impact of hazardous substances on male reproductive health include *a*) questionnaires to determine reproductive history and sexual function, *b*) reproductive hormone profiles, and *c*) semen analysis. The choice of appropriate methodologies to study the effects of reproductive toxicants is predicated on the investigators' understanding of several factors: the nature of the exposed population; the source, the levels, and the known routes of exposure; the organ systems in which a toxicant exerts its actions; the hypothesized mechanisms of a toxicant's actions; and the techniques available to assess the effects of toxicants in the relevant organ systems (Wyrobeck et al., 1997). **Table 2** outlines the methods currently available for assessing the principal targets of male reproductive toxicants in humans--the testes, the accessory sex glands, the neuroendocrine system, and sexual function. Researchers and clinicians interested in male reproductive health and fertility are using increasingly sophisticated methods adapted from the fields of assisted reproductive technology and reproductive toxicology, including assays of sperm function, genetic integrity, and biomarkers of DNA damage. For population-based studies involving occupational groups or communities with environmental exposures, issues related to the cost, validity, precision, and utility of these methods must be carefully considered.

The testis, the site of sperm cell production and the target organ for genetic damage, is most often studied. To establish the extent of toxicity to the testis, researchers can measure the size of the testis, obtain a semen sample, or take a testicular biopsy. Standard semen analyses (including semen volume, sperm concentration, total sperm count, motility, and morphology) have been the primary research tools for studying the effects of toxicants on the male reproductive system. Epidemiologic studies have successfully utilized semen quality as a marker of fertility (Fisch et al., 1997). The uncertainties associated with traditional semen measures have led to the recent development of assays of sperm function and genetic integrity; these assays may prove more sensitive and more specific reflections of toxicant-induced effects (e.g., aneuploidy or reduced sperm motility) in individuals (Martin et al., 1997). However, The accessory sex glands, which include the epididymis, prostate, and seminal vesicle, may also be targets of toxicants (Schrader, 1997). Ethylene dibromide is one substance that affects the accessory sex glands after occupational exposure. Alterations in sperm viability, as measured by eosin stain exclusion or by hypo-osmotic swelling or alterations in sperm motility variables, suggest a problem with the accessory sex glands. Biochemical analysis of seminal plasma provides insights into glandular function by

Sl. No.	Methods of Assessment:
1.	Testosterone (T) , Prolactin, LH, FSH, and Inhibin-B concentrations.
2.	Semen volume and pH.
3.	Sperm density/Sperm count.
4.	Sperm morphology and morphometry
5.	Sperm motility (% of motile and velocity), Sperm viability (Vital stain and Hyper Osmotic Swelling (HOS)).
6.	Sperm function assays (Acrosome reaction, Hemizona assay of sperm binding and sperm penetration assay).
7.	Sperm genetic analysis (Sperm chromatin stability assay, Comet assay. Assessment of chromosomal aneuploidy and Nuclear microdeletions).
8.	Marker chemicals from accessory glands (Epididymis is represented by glyceryl-phosphorylcholine, Seminal vesicles by fructose, and the Prostate gland by zinc).
9.	Nocturnal penile measurements.
10.	Personal reproductive history (Pubertal development, Paternity (Pregnancy timing and outcomes), Sexual functions (Erection, Ejaculation, Orgasm and Libido)).

Table 2. Assessment of Male Reproductive Capacity in Humans (Moline et al., 2000).

evaluating marker chemicals secreted by each respective gland (Schrader, 1997). For example, the epididymis is represented by glycerylphosphorylcholine, the seminal vesicles by fructose, and the prostate gland by zinc. Measures of semen pH and volume provide additional general information on the nature of seminal plasma, reflecting post testicular effects. A toxicant or its metabolite may act directly on accessory sex glands to alter the quantity or quality of their secretions. Alternatively, the toxicant may enter the seminal plasma and affect the sperm or may be carried to the site of fertilization by the sperm and affect the ova or conceptus. The presence of toxicants or their metabolites in seminal plasma can be analyzed using atomic absorption spectrophotometry or gas chromotography/mass spectrometry. Impact on the neuroendocrine system is another mechanism whereby toxicants can disturb the male reproductive system. To establish the extent of endocrine dysfunction, hormone levels can be measured in blood and urine. The profile recommended by NIOSH to evaluate endocrine dysfunction associated with reproductive toxicity consists of assessing serum concentrations of follicle-stimulating hormone (FSH), luteinizing hormone (LH), testosterone, and prolactin (Schrader, 1997). Because of the pulsatile secretion of LH, testosterone, and to a much lesser extent FSH, and the variability in the evaluation of reproductive hormones, it is recommended that three blood samples be drawn at set intervals in the early morning and the results pooled or averaged for clinical assessment. In epidemiologic field studies, however, multiple blood samples are impractical and may decrease participation rates. Alternatively, LH and FSH can be measured in urine, providing indices of gonadotropin levels that are relatively unaffected by pulsatile secretion. However, if an exposure can affect hepatic metabolism of sex steroid hormones (Apostoli et al., 1996), urinary measures of excreted testosterone metabolite (androsterone) or estradiol metabolite (estrone-3-glucuronide) are not recommended. Moreover, future assessment of reproductive hormones may extend to inhibin, activin, and follistatin, polypeptides that are secreted primarily by the gonads and that act on the pituitary to increase (activin) or decrease (inhibin and follistatin) FSH synthesis and secretion. Within the gonads, these peptides regulate steroid hormone synthesis and may also directly affect spermatogenesis. Ongoing studies are investigating the utility of serum inhibin-B level as an important marker of Sertoli cell function and *in utero* developmental toxicity (Jensen et al., 1997). Other indicators of central nervous system toxicity are reported alterations in sexual function, including libido, erection, and ejaculation. There is not much literature on occupational exposures causing sexual dysfunction in men (Schrader, 1997); however, there are suggestions that lead, carbon disulfide, stilbene, and cadmium can affect sexual function. These outcomes are difficult to measure because of the absence of objective measures and because sexual dysfunction can be attributed to and affected by psychologic or physiologic factors (Schrader, 1997).

3.3 Biomarkers of genetic damage

Biomarkers of chromosomal and genetic damage are increasingly used in the search to understand abnormal reproductive health outcomes, in part because of the possibility that there may be identifiable genetic polymorphisms which make an individual more susceptible to the adverse reproductive effects from exogenous substances. These assays provide promising and sensitive approaches for investigating germinal and potentially heritable effects of exposures to agents and for confirming epidemiologic observations on smaller numbers of individuals. Efficient technology for examining chromosomal abnormalities in sperm has only been developed recently. Chromosomal abnormalities are primarily of two types: numerical and structural. Both kinds can be attributed in some cases to paternal factors. Karyotype studies have shown that although oocytes demonstrate a higher frequency of numerical chromosomal abnormalities, human sperm demonstrate a higher frequency of structural abnormalities with less frequent numerical abnormalities (Moosani et al., 1995). In assessing sperm exposure to toxicants, it is therefore imperative to assess DNA structural integrity and not just chromosomal count. Aneuploidy is a chromosomal abnormality that causes pregnancy loss, perinatal death, congenital defects, and mental retardation. Aneuploidy, a disorder of chromosome count, is observed in approximately 1 in 300 newborns. It is speculated that of all species, humans experience the highest frequency of aneuploidy at conception, with estimates ranging from 20 to 50% (Moosani et al., 1995). Spontaneous abortions occur in at least 10-15% of all clinically recognized pregnancies. Of these, 35% contain chromosomal aneuploidy. Despite such a high frequency, there is little information about what causes this abnormality in humans. Paternal origins of aneuploidy and other genetic abnormalities can be analyzed by studying chromosome complements in human sperm. Two types of analyses provide data on chromosomal abnormalities in human sperm: sperm karyotype analysis and fluorescence *in situ* hybridization (FISH) (Moosani et al., 1995). Each technique has advantages and disadvantages. Sperm karyotyping is performed after sperm have fused with hamster oocytes. It provides precise information on numerical and gross structural abnormalities of all chromosomes from a given spermatozoon. However, only a limited number of sperm can be evaluated in each assay, and only those sperm that fertilize the oocytes are analyzable. Furthermore, this assay is technically difficult, labor intensive, expensive, and requires the use of animals. Also, it is better suited for clinical than for field studies because it must be performed on fresh semen. FISH, on the other hand, relies on the use of chromosome-specific probes to detect extra chromosomes (aneuploidy) or chromosome breaks or rearrangements in sperm. It is performed directly on sperm cells, eliminating the need for the use of animals. Although information is gained only for several chromosomes at a time, slides can be reprobed to increase the number of chromosomes evaluated. Furthermore, FISH can be conducted on archived sperm (either frozen or dried on slides), making it ideal for use in field studies. However, because the incidence of sperm aneuploidy is low, many cells (up to 10,000 per semen sample) must be evaluated, which requires significant scoring times. In comparison to karyotype analysis, however, FISH is relatively inexpensive and technically simpler, and data are obtained on all sperm, not just the ones that are capable of fertilization. These two techniques complement each other, with FISH providing information on large numbers of cells and karyotyping providing more precise and detailed information (Robbins et al., 1997).

3.4 Develop biomarkers of exposures and male reproductive health for research and clinical use

Resources must be invested in developing more advanced biomarkers of exposure to reproductive toxicants and of male reproductive health outcomes. Advanced biomarkers would allow for the development of toxicant-specific tests (e.g., polycyclic aromatic hydrocarbon-DNA adducts) and the detection of subclinical changes that might have significant health implications but which now go unnoticed by current measures. New biomarkers of semen quality are advantageous in that they can both describe male reproductive capacity and indicate toxic effects independent of the female partner's reproductive health. New tests could more accurately measure sperm function, fertilization potential, and the transmission of an intact male genome. Genetic testing may provide valuable tools for researchers and clinicians. For example, the sperm chromatin stability assay and FISH are used to assess genetic structure after exposure to a potential toxicant. Recently, single nucleotide polymorphisms have been used in the assessment of gene-environment interactions.

4. Mechanism of male reproductive toxicity

The disruption of spermatogenesis may be represented by four mechanisms, including (1) epigenetic changes to the genome, (2) apoptosis of germ cells, (3) dysregulation of androgenic signaling, and (4) disruption of Sertoli and other spermatogenesis support (Phillips & Tanphaichitr, 2008) (**Figure 4**). The first mechanism is relatively novel and was only demonstrated in vitro by one group thus far. Rats exposed in vitro to anti-androgenic pesticides vinclozolin or methoxychlor demonstrated heritable changes in methylation status of genomic DNA. These epigenetic effects included impaired male fertility and were evident in the F3 and F4 generations (Anway et al., 2005). Reduced sperm number or altered sperm morphology may be indicative of problems during spermatogenesis and spermiogenesis and may be produced by the direct loss of developing spermatocytes. Adult rats exposed *in utero* to flutamide, an antiandrogen, exhibit hypo-spermatogenesis associated with increased apoptosis of adult germ cells (Maire et al., 2005). Anti-androgenic exposure is associated with elevation of pro-apoptotic molecules, including Fas-L (Maire et al., 2005), caspase-3 and caspase-6, Bax, Bak, and Bid, and a decrease in anti-apoptotic molecules Bcl2 and Bclw (Bozec et al., 2004) in rat models. Di(2-ethylhexyl) phthalate (DEHP) exposure in rats induces testicular apoptosis via a mechanism involving ERK1/2-induced up-regulation of PPAR (peroxisome proliferators-activated receptor) -γ, RXR

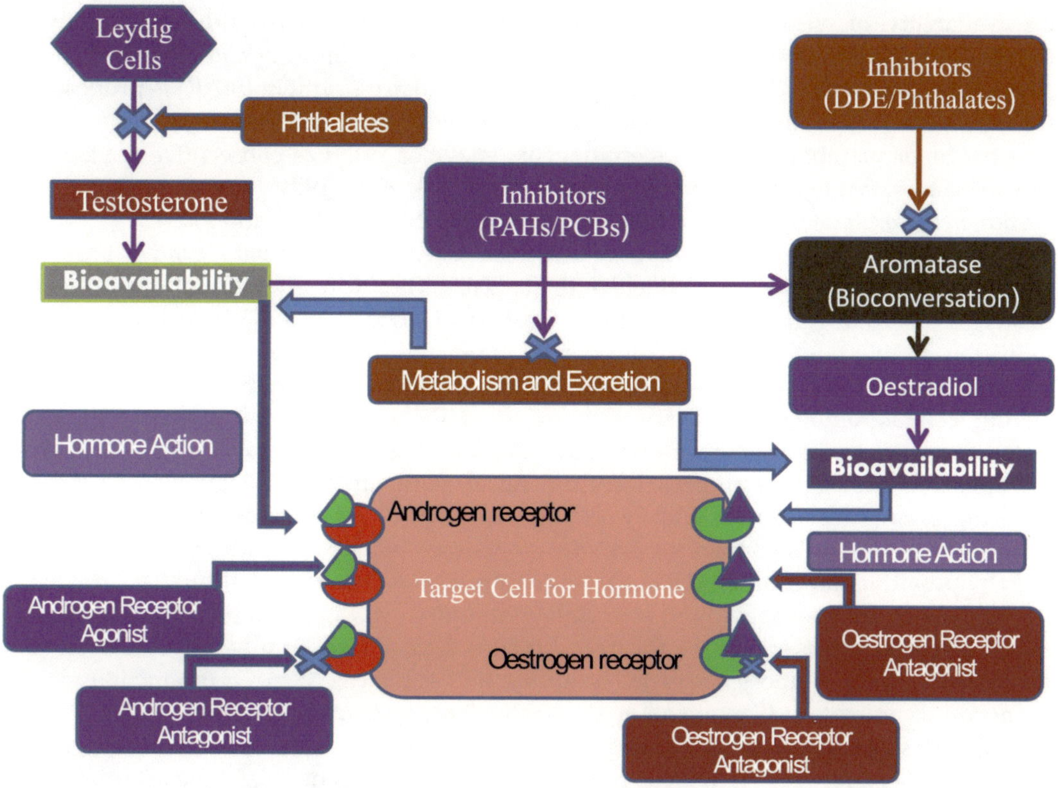

Fig. 4. Possible Pathways of endocrine disruption by environmental chemicals. DDE= 1, 1-dichloro-2, 2-bis (p-chlorophenyl) ethylene; DDT= dichlorodiphenyltrichloroethane; PAHs= polycyclic aromatic hydrocarbons; PCBs= polychlorinated biphenyls. (Modified from Sharpe & Irvine, BMJ, 2004).

(retinoid X receptor)-α and p21, and down-regulation of pRB, cyclin D, CDK2, cyclin E, and CDK4 (Ryu et al., 2007). Neonatal estrogen treatment (DES, ethinyl estradiol [EE]) increased apoptosis at all stages of spermatogenesis in the rat (Atanassova et al., 1999). Thus, apoptosis is a likely mechanism for some mechanisms of endocrine disruption in the testis (Jana et al., 2010b). Testicular androgenic signalling may be impaired via several mechanisms, including decreased Leydig cell population, impaired Leydig cell steroidogenesis, and dysregulation of the HPT axis. Abnormal development and maturation of the Leydig cell population reduces the steroidogenic potential of the testis. *In utero* exposure to phthalate esters is associated with morphological abnormalities of the male reproductive tract, including decreased anogenital distance, cryptorchidism, hypospadias, diminished Leydig cell population, and decreased testicular testosterone (Mylchreest et al., 2000; Fisher et al., 2003). Phthalate esters such as DEHP are proposed to exert antiandrogenic and estrogenic mechanisms of action and disrupt hormone synthesis via an AhR pathway (Ge et al., 2007). Low-dose BPA exposure in utero reduced the size of the epididymis and decreased anogenital distance and increased prostate size (Gupta, 2000) in adult mice. Leydig cell maturation and development include expression of genes related to endocrine signaling (LH receptors, AR) and steroidogenesis. Steroidogenesis is dependent on availability of cholesterol to the cytochrome P-450 cholesterol side chain cleavage (P450scc) enzyme complex within the mitochondria, the rate-limiting and regulated step in steroidogenesis (Miller, 1988). Steroidogenic acute regulatory protein (StAR) is proposed as the candidate protein for the acute regulation of steroidogenesis. StAR transports cholesterol into the inner membrane, where steroidogenic enzymes catalyze consecutive reactions to convert cholesterol to testosterone in Leydig cells (Clark et al., 1994, Jana et al., 2008; 2010a; 2010b). *In utero* exposure to exogenous estrogens (EE, DES, genistein, and BPA) downregulate expression of a number of testicular genes including *Cyp17, Cyp11a,* and *StAR* expression in the rat and mouse (Fielden et al., 2002). The expression of a number of genes related to steroidogenesis (*Scarb1, Star, Cyp11a1, HSD3b1,* and *CYP17a1*) was altered following in utero exposure to di(*n*-butyl) phthalate (Barlow et al., 2003). Testicular androgen signalling may also be impaired through suppression of normal HPT regulation of Leydig cell steroidogenesis. Disruption of the HPT axis, thereby reducing testicular testosterone levels, was demonstrated in the rat following exposure to a range of endocrine disrupters. Exposure to estrogens DES and EE also impaired HPT signalling in the rat, reducing plasma testosterone and increasing plasma FSH (Atanassova et al., 1999). Both Leydig and Sertoli cells contain the enzyme aromatase and convert androgens to estrogens, thereby providing an intratesticular source of estrogens (O'Donnell et al., 2001). Atrazine, a herbicide with antiandrogenic and estrogenic properties, was found to produce a number of adverse reproductive effects in the rat. Atrazine has a low affinity for androgen and estrogen receptors, reduces androgen synthesis, and enhances estrogen production via the induction of aromatase (Sanderson et al., 2000). Thus, testicular physiology is sensitive to perturbations of androgenic and estrogenic signalling, such that xenobiotic exposures might result in reduced fertility. Sertoli cell number is directly representative of the spermatogenic potential of the testis. Ablation of the Sertoli cell population, or loss of Sertoli cell function, is therefore another mechanism by which endocrine disrupters may impair spermatogenesis. Exposure to prenatal DES or EE reduced adult population of Sertoli cells in rats (Atanassova et al., 1999) and supports the hypothesis that *in utero* exposure to estrogens contributes to impaired spermatogenesis in the adult. It is also noteworthy that human spermatogenesis is much less efficient than in rodents, such that small decreases in the population of Sertoli cells would be expected to have large effects on male fertility in human. Estrogenic disruption of the testis is perhaps the most well characterized example of endocrine disruption of spermatogenesis; however, it is also worthy to note that estrogens play important roles in development of hormone responsive tissue, including Leydig cells and development and differentiation of the fetal male reproductive tract (Tsai-Morris et al., 1986). ERs, both alpha and beta (ERα and ERß), are found throughout the male reproductive tract and represent a transcriptional mechanism by which endocrine disrupters may alter gene expression. In rodents, ERα is expressed by all developmental stages of Leydig cells (fetal, neonatal/pubertal/adult), seminiferous tubules, efferent ductules, and epididymis but not Sertoli cells. ERß is expressed in all stages of rodent Leydig and Sertoli cell development and in efferent ductules and epididymis (O'Donnell et al., 2001). The existence of plasma membrane ERs along with the different tissue distribution, C-terminal ligand-binding domain and N-terminal transactivation domain of ERα and ERß provide possible explanations for the differential effects of so-called weak estrogens like BPA (Wozniak et al., 2005). These are but a few of the mechanisms by which endocrine disrupters might impair spermatogenesis. Other mechanisms include dysregulation of bioavailable androgens via increased synthesis of sex hormone binding globulin (SHBG) and other plasma binding proteins (Haffner, 1996) and disruption of testicular androgen signaling by AhR ligands, PAH and nicotine, contained in tobacco smoke (Kizu et al., 2003) and many others. Further that, increasing evidence suggests an induction of oxidative stress in the testis represents another common response after exposure to environmental toxicants (Jana et al., 2010a & 2010b). Increase in oxidative stress can be seen in ≤80% of clinically proven infertile men, and exposure to environmental toxicants is a major factor contributing to such an increase (Tremellen, 2008). Environmental toxicants that have been shown to induce oxidative stress in the testis are highly heterogeneous, with different chemical structures, and include cadmium (Liu et al., 2009), bisphenol A (Kabuto et al., 2004) and 2,3,7,8-tetrachlorodibenzo-p-dioxin (Dhanabalan & Mathur, 2009).

Interestingly, these environmental toxicants commonly increase oxidative stress by down regulating the production of antioxidant enzymes such as superoxide dismutase, catalase and glutathione peroxidase. In turn, excessive amounts of reactive oxygen species (ROS) are produced. ROS damage the lipids, proteins, carbohydrates and DNA in cells (Jana et al., 2010a & 2010b; **Figure 5**). Importantly, these observations were confirmed in studies illustrating that co-administration of antioxidants such as vitamin E with environmental toxicants could alleviate the pathophysiological effects (e.g. reduction in sperm count) of toxicants in the testis (Latchoumycandane & Mathur, 2002). These findings demonstrate that oxidative stress induced by environmental toxicants is one of the major contributing factors to male infertility. In fact, oxidative stress has long been linked to male infertility; although most studies have focused on its roles in causing abnormalities in germ cells and apoptosis (Sikka, 2001; Turner and Lysiak, 2008). Recent studies have shown that environmental toxicant-induced oxidative stress can cause male infertility by disrupting the cell junctions and adhesion between Sertoli–Sertoli cells and/or Sertoli–germ cells via the phosphatidylinositol 3-kinase (PI3K)/c-Src/focal adhesion kinase (FAK) signaling pathway (Wong & Cheng, 2011). Oxidative stress is known to increase epithelial and endothelial permeability by disrupting tight junctions (TJ) and adherens junctions (AJ) between cells (Sandoval and Witt, 2008). Activation of the PI3K/c-Src signalling pathway in response to oxidative stress induced by environmental toxicants could be a common mechanism by which the toxicants trigger damage to the testis. Early evidence shows that the toxic effects of 2,3,7,8-tetrachlorodibenzo-p-dioxin in the testis are caused by an induction in c-Src kinase activity. Furthermore, significant increase in the c-Src level has also been detected in the testis after cadmium exposure in rodents, indicating that c-Src is activated in response to multiple environmental toxicants (Wong et al., 2004; Wong & Cheng, 2011) **(Figure 6).**

The MAPK pathways have emerged as a common signaling platform for multiple environmental toxicants (**Figure 6**). Three MAPKs (extracellular-signal-regulated kinase (ERK), c-Jun N-terminal kinase (JNK) and p38) have been shown to be activated in the testis after exposure to environmental toxicants. MAPKs are involved in regulating normal reproductive functions in the testis, which include spermatogenesis (e.g. cell-cycle progression, meiosis, BTB dynamics, cell adhesion dynamics and spermiogenesis), steroidogenesis, sperm hyperactivation and acrosome reaction (Almog & Naor 2010). As a result, unregulated activation of MAPKs by environmental toxicants imposes an array of pathophysiological effects on Sertoli cells, germ cells and Leydig cells in the testis. These include an increase in DNA damage and apoptosis, disruption of cell junctions and steroidogenesis (Li et al., 2009; Wong & Cheng, 2011). MAPKs are activated by oxidative stress induced by environmental toxicants in cells and tissues. For example, blocking oxidative stress by free-radical scavengers (e.g. N-acetyl cysteine), reverses cadmium-induced MAPK activation (Chen, et al., 2008). This phenomenon is partly regulated by the inhibition of Ser/Thr protein phosphatases 2A (PP2A) and 5 (PP5) by oxidative stress, which results in an increase in phosphorylation of MAPK (Chen, et al., 2008). In addition, activation of ERK can lead to phosphorylation of c-Src, FAK and paxillin under oxidative stress, implying that MAPKs might be one of the upstream targets to activate these non-receptor tyrosine kinases (Li et al., 2009) **(Figure 6).** Activation of MAPKs by environmental toxicants also upregulates the expression of proinflammatory cytokines such as nuclear factor kB (NFkB), and tumor necrosis factor-α (TNFα) in macrophages and monocytes (Lecureur et al., 2005), which can diffuse from microvessels in the interstitial space and disrupt the BTB because they are known to perturb the Sertoli cell TJ-permeability barrier (Li et al., 2009). Similarly, cadmium and pollutants from motorcycle exhausts (e.g. polycyclic aromatic hydrocarbons) increase the expression of transforming growth factor-β (TGF-β) and interleukin-6 (IL-6) in the testis, respectively (Lui et al., 2009). TNFα, TGF-β and IL-1α are known to disrupt Sertoli–Sertoli and Sertoli–germ cell junctions via downregulation (Li et al., 2006) and/or redistribution of junctional proteins (Wong & Cheng, 2005) such as occludin, ZO-1 and N-cadherin in the seminiferous epithelium. Consequently, the loss of integral membrane proteins at the cell–cell interface causes disruption of the BTB and adhesion of germ cells in the seminiferous epithelium, which lead to the premature release of germ cells from the epithelium and hence infertility (Li et al., 2006; Li et al., 2009; Wong & Cheng, 2011). Furthermore, proinflammatory cytokines (e.g. IL-6 and TNFα) activate leukocytes to produce ROS, which amplifies the deleterious effects of environmental toxicant-induced oxidative stress (Tremellen, 2008). The male reproductive system has emerged as one of the major targets of environmental toxicants. Although acute exposure to toxicants contributes to apoptosis and the necrosis of testicular cells, chronic and sub-lethal exposure is prevailing in the general public (Hauser & Sokol 2008). Due to the unusually long half-lives of some of these toxicants in the mammalian body (e.g. cadmium has a mean half-life of >15 years), chronic and low-level exposure to humans could cause long-term unwanted health effects. The disruptive effects of environmental toxicants on cell junctions mediated by non-receptor tyrosine kinases (e.g. c-Src and FAK) and cytokines through oxidative stress because such damage is often observed in low-level exposure before apoptosis occurs (Li et al., 2006; Li et al., 2009). Significantly, these signalling pathways converge to utilize polarity proteins to regulate intercellular junctions. Polarity proteins (which are known to control cell adhesion in the testis) thus emerge as novel targets for therapeutic intervention to limit environmental toxicant-induced infertility. Although it is equally important to study the epigenetic (e.g. vinclozolin) and endocrine-disruptive (e.g. BPA, dioxin, cadmium) effects of environmental toxicants, it is increasingly clear that these toxicants are imposing an immediate deleterious effect in the testis via disruption of cell junctions between testicular cells due to increase in oxidative stress. In addition, endocrine-disrupting toxicants that affect estrogen levels might cause a disturbed balance of ROS and oxidative stress because estrogen is an important free-radical scavenger in humans, besides being essential for spermatogenesis (Carreau and Hess, 2010).

Recent studies have emphasized the importance of assessing the effects of a mixture of environmental toxicants on male reproductive function because humans are exposed to an array of chemicals that might antagonize or agonize each other (Hauser & Sokol 2008).

Although this type of study is inherently difficult to undertake, it is crucial for a full understanding of the impact of environmental toxicants on the reproductive system. However, much work is needed to understand the precise molecular events and mechanism(s) regulated by environmental toxicants to target c-Src, FAK, MAPK and polarity proteins in the testis. Only then can we identify specific phosphorylation targets or isoforms so that small-molecule agonists and/or antagonists can be designed to limit systemic toxicity in vivo.

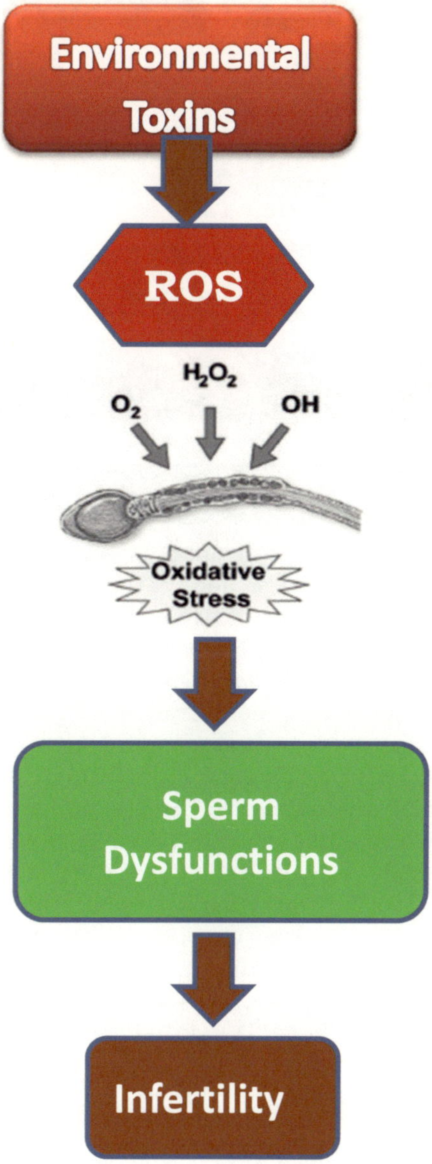

Fig. 5. Primary pathologies of male reproductive system in connection with environmental toxins, oxidative stress and infertility.

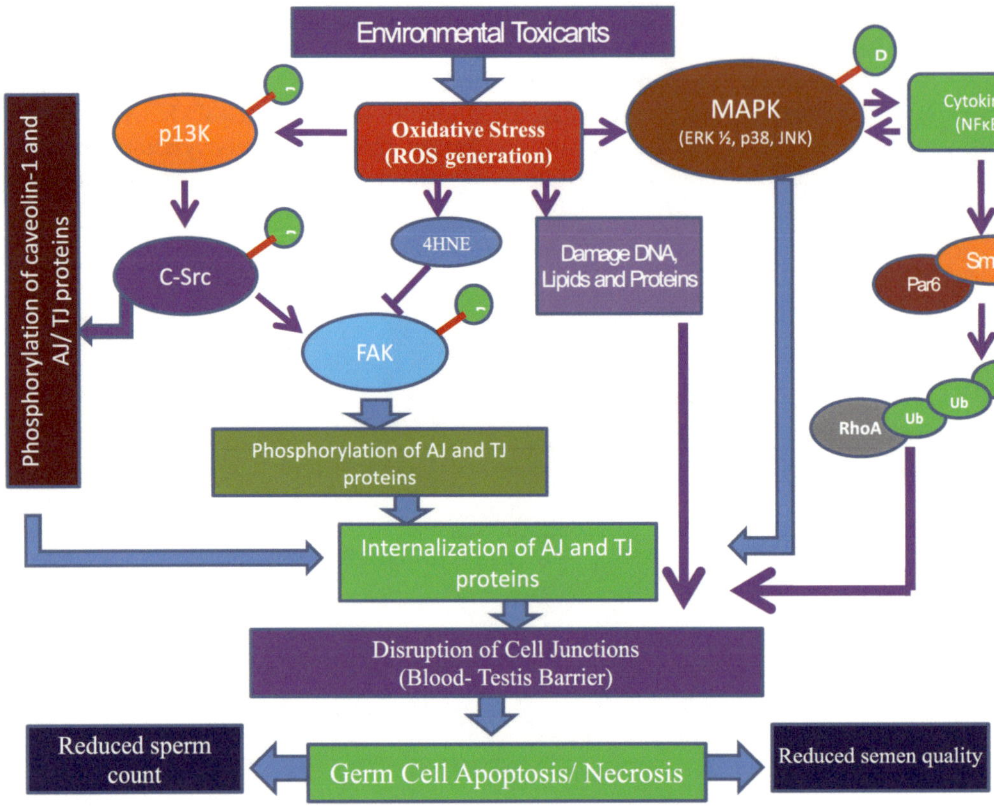

Fig. 6. Molecular signalling pathways of testicular toxicity by environmental toxicants through the induction of oxidative stress. Oxidative stress induced by environmental toxicants activates the PI3K/ C-src/FAK pathway, which subsequently controls the phosphorylation of TJ and/or AJ proteins. This leads to the internalization of TJ and AJ proteins at the cell–cell interface. In addition, environmental toxicants induce the production of cytokines which are also regulated by the activation of MAPK through oxidative stress. Cytokines stimulate the production of reactive oxygen species (ROS) from leukocytes to further increase oxidative stress. Cytokines and the activation of MAPK together result in endocytic vesicle- mediated internalization of TJ and AJ proteins. Polarity proteins such as Par6 are also involved in mediating the action of cytokines to recruit the E3 ubiquitin ligase Smurf1 for the poly ubiquitination and degradation of RhoA, which is important for the disruption of cell junctions. This illustrates that crosstalk exists between the PI3K/C-Src/FAK and cytokines/ MAPK pathways via polarity proteins as their common downstream signalling mediators. The disruption of cell junctions ultimately leads to the germ cell apoptosis and necrosis and as a result sperm count and quality of semen are reduced. (Modified from Wong & Cheng, Trends in Pharmacological Sciences, 2011).

5. Conclusions

In view of the fact that the preliminary concerns arose about environmental chemicals or toxins and declining sperm counts, there has been an explosion of research in this area. The initial 'environmental oestrogen' hypothesis has been superseded by a more refined definition of EDCs. It is now accepted that there are a plethora of ways in which the environmental chemicals can potentially act on the endocrine as well as male reproductive systems. Though supportive data must need to determine whether human male reproductive health is declining or not. However; the hypothesis of a 'testicular dysgenesis syndrome' is an important advancement and may aid our understanding of the underlying aetiology of these disorders. Within the reproductive tract, the male is exquisitely vulnerable to the effects of anti-androgens during development due the dependence on the synthesis and action of androgens for the masculinization of the male reproductive tract. The ability of phthalates to suppress androgen synthesis during development and to induce testicular dysgenesis together with cryptorchidism and hypospadias has close parallels with human TDS. However, the crucial question regarding whether the level of environmental chemicals is sufficient to impact on human male reproductive health remains unanswered, although advances will be made from studying the effects of multi-component EDC mixtures in both in vitro and in vivo test systems. Moreover, it has been observed that in wildlife, there is a increasing rates of testicular cancer, to the debate regarding trends in sperm counts, there has been increasing concern that hazardous substances in the environment adversely affect male reproductive health. The ultimate benefits of this chapter that should serve as a framework for future studies to improve our knowledge in this area. By better defining the problems, learning about the mechanisms responsible for adverse effects, and developing panels of relevant biomarkers, we will make progress toward preventing future adverse effects on male reproductive health.

6. Acknowledgment

The authors acknowledge the financial support provided by the Bose Institute, Kolkata.

7. References

[1] Adami H.O., Bergstrom R., Mohner M., Zatonski W., Storm H., Ekbom A., Tretli S., Teppo L., Ziegler H. & Rahu M. 1994. Testicular cancer in nine northern European countries. *International Journal of Cancer, Vol* 59, pp. 33–*38.*

[2] Adlercreutz, H., Höckerstedt, K., Bannwart, C., Bloigu, S., Hämäläinen, E., & Fotsis, T. and Ollus, A. 1987. Effect of dietary components, including lignans and phytoestrogens, on enterohepatic circulation and liver metabolism of estrogens and on sex hormone binding globulin (SHBG). *Journal of Steroid Biochemistry,* Vol 27, pp.1135–1144.

[3] Almog, T. & Naor, Z. 2010. The role of mitogen activated protein kinase (MAPK) in sperm functions. *Molecular Cellular Endocrinology,* Vol 314, pp.239–243.

[4] Akingbemi, B.T. 2005. Estrogen regulation of testicular function. *Reproductive Biology and Endocrinology,* Vol 3: pp. 51.

[5] Anderson RA., & Sharpe RM. 2000. Regulation of inhibin production in the human male and its clinical applications. *International Journal of Andrology,* Vol. 23, pp.136–144.

[6] Anway, M.D., Cupp, A.S., Uzumcu, M. & Skinner, M.K. 2005. Epigenetic transgenerational actions of endocrine disruptors and male fertility. *Science* , Vol. 308, pp. 1466–1469.

[7] Apostoli, P., Romeo, L., Peroni, E., Ferioli, A., Ferrari, S., Pasini, F., & Aprili, F.1996. Steroid hormone sulphation in lead workers. *British Journal of Industrial Medicine,* Vol. 46, pp.204-208.

[8] Atanassova, N., McKinnell, C., Walker, M., Turner, K. J., Fisher, J. S., Morley, M., Millar, M. R., Groome, N. P. & Sharpe, R. M. 1999. Permanent effects of neonatal estrogen exposure in rats on reproductive hormone levels, Sertoli cell number, and the efficiency of spermatogenesis in adulthood. *Endocrinology* , Vol.140, pp. 5364–5373.

[9] Ayotte, P., Giroux, S., Dewailly, E., Hernandez Avila, M., Farias, R., Danis, P. & Villanueva Diaz, C. 2001. DDT spraying for malaria control and reproductive function in Mexican men. *Epidemiology.* Vol. 12 pp. 366–367.

[10] Barlow, N. J., Phillips, S. L., Wallace, D. G., Sar, M., Gaido, K. W. & Foster, P. M. 2003. Quantitative changes in gene expression in fetal rat testes following exposure to di(n-butyl) phthalate. *Toxicological Sciences*, Vol.73, pp. 431–441.

[11] Bergstrom R., Adami H.O., Mohner M., Zatonski W., Storm H., Ekbom A., Tretli S., Teppo L., Akre O. & Hakulinen T. 1996. Increase in testicular cancer incidence in six European countries: a birth cohort phenomenon. *Journal of the National Cancer Institute*, Vol. 88, *pp. 727–733.*

[12] Benoff, S., Cooper, G.W., & Hurley I, et al. 1994. The effect of calcium ion channel blockers on sperm fertilization potential. *Fertility and Sterility.* Vol. 62, pp. 606–617.

[13] Birnbaum, L. S. & Tuomisto, J. 2000. Non-carcinogenic effects of TCDD in animals. *Food Additives and Contaminants*, Vol.17, pp. 275–288.

[14] Bracken, M.B., Eskenazi, B., Sachse, K., McSharry, J.E., Hellenbrand, K., & Leo-Summers, L. 1990. Association of cocaine use with sperm concentration, motility, and morphology. *Fertility and Sterility.* Vol. 53, pp. 315–322.

[15] Bozec, A., Chuzel, F., Chater, S., Paulin, C., Bars, R., Benahmed, M. &Mauduit, C. 2004. The mitochondrial-dependent pathway is chronically affected in testicular germ cell death in adult rats exposed in utero to anti-androgens. *Journal of Endocrinology*, Vol.183, pp. 79–90.

[16] Braude, P. & Rowell, P. 2003. Assisted conception. II—In vitro fertilisation and intracytoplasmic sperm injection. *British Medical Journal*, Vol. 327, pp. 852–855.

[17] Carlsen, E., Giwercman, A., Keiding, N. & Skakkebaek. N.E. 1992. Evidence for decreasing quality of semen during past 50 years. *British Medical Journal Vol.* 305, *pp. 609–613.*

[18] Carreau, S. & Hess, R.A. 2010. Oestrogens and spermatogenesis, *Philos. Trans. R. Soc. Lond. B: Biol. Sci.* Vol. 365, pp.1517–1535.

[19] Casini, M. L., Gerli, S. & Unfer, V. 2006. An infertile couple suffering from oligospermia by partial sperm maturation arrest: can phytoestrogens play a therapeutic role? A case report study. *Gynecological Endocrinology*, Vol.22, pp. 399–401.

[20] Chapin, R.E., Sloane, R.A., & Haseman, J.K. 1997. The relationships among reproductive endpoints in Swiss mice, using the reproductive assessment by continuous breeding database. *Fundamental Applied Toxicology*, Vol. 38, pp.129-142.

[21] Chen, L. et al., 2008. Cadmium activates the mitogen-activated protein kinase (MAPK) pathway via induction of reactive oxygen species and inhibition of protein phosphatases 2A and 5. *Free Radical Biology and Medicine* Vol.45, pp. 1035–1044.

[22] Clark, B. J., Wells, J., King, S.R. & Stocco, D. M. 1994. The purification, cloning, and expression of a novel luteinizing hormone-induced mitochondrial protein in MA-10 mouse Leydig tumor cells. Characterization of the steroidogenic acute regulatory protein (StAR). *Journal of Biological Chemistry*, Vol. 269, pp.28314–28322.

[23] Claudio, L., Bearer, C.F., & Wallinga, D. 1999. Assessment of the U.S. Environmental Protection Agency methods for identification of hazards to developing organisms. Part I: the reproduction and fertility testing guidelines. *American Journal of Industrial Medicine*, Vol. 35, pp.543-553.

[24] Close, C.E., Roberts, P.L., & Berger, R.E. 1990. Cigarettes, alcohol and marijuana are related to pyospermia in infertile men. *Journal of Urology*. Vol. 144, pp. 900–903.
[25] Davies, J.M. 1981. Testicular cancer in England and Wales; some epidemiological aspects. *Lancet* Vol. 1(8226), pp.928-932.
[26] Dhanabalan, S. & Mathur, P.P. 2009. Low dose of 2,3,7,8 tetrachlorodibenzo-p-dioxin induces testicular oxidative stress in adult rats under the influence of corticosterone, *Experimental Toxicology and Pathology*, Vol.61, pp. 415–423.
[27] Dhooge, W., van Larebeke, N., Koppen, G., Nelen, V., Schoeters, G., Vlietinck, R., Kaufman, J.-M. & Comhaire, F. 2006. Serum dioxin-like activity is associated with reproductive parameters in young men from the general Flemish population. *Environ. Health Perspect.* , 114: 1670–1676.
[28] Ekbom, A., & Akre, O. 1998. Increasing incidence of testicular cancer--birth cohort effects. *Acta Pathologica, Microbiologica et Immunologica Scandinavica* Vol.106, pp.225-231.
[29] Evans, B. A., Griffiths, K. and Morton, M. S. 1995. Inhibition of 5 alpha-reductase in genital skin fibroblasts and prostate tissue by dietary lignans and isoflavonoids. *Journal of Endocrinology*, Vol.147, pp. 295–302.
[30] Fielden, M. R., Halgren, R. G., Fong, C. J., Staub, C., Johnson, L., Chou, K. & Zacharewski, T. R. 2002. Gestational and lactational exposure of male mice to diethylstilbestrol causes long-term effects on the testis, sperm fertilizing ability in vitro, and testicular gene expression. *Endocrinology* , Vol.143, pp. 3044–3059.
[31] Fisch H., Andrews, H., Hendricks, J., Goluboff, E.T., Olson, J.H., & Olsson, C.A. 1997. The relationship of sperm counts to birth rates: a population based study. *Urology*, Vol. 157, pp.840-844.
[32] Fisch, H., Goluboff, E.T., Olson, J.H., Feldshuh, J., Broder, S.J., & Barad, D.H. 1996. Semen analyses in 1,283 men from the United States over a 25-year period: no decline in quality. *Fertility and Sterility*, Vol.65, pp.1009-1014.
[33] Fisher, J.S. 2004. Environmental anti-androgens and male reproductive health: focus on phthalates and testicular dysgenesis syndrome. *Reproduction* Vol. 127, pp. 305-315.
[34] Fisher, J. S., Macpherson, S., Marchetti, N. & Sharpe, R. M. 2003. Human 'testicular dysgenesis syndrome': A possible model using in-utero exposure of the rat to dibutyl phthalate. *Human Reproduction*, Vol.18, pp. 1383–1394.
[35] Foster, P. M., Mylchreest, E., Gaido, K. W. & Sar, M. 2001. Effects of phthalate esters on the developing reproductive tract of male rats. *Human Reproduction Update* , Vol. 7, pp. 231–235.
[36] Fredricsson, B., Moller, L., Pousette, A. & Westerholm, R. 1993. Human sperm motility is affected by plasticizers and diesel particle extracts. *Pharmacology & Toxicology* , Vol. 72, pp. 128–133.
[37] Gray, L.E., Ostby, J., Furr, J., Wolf, C.J., Lambright, C., Parks, L., Veeramachaneni, D.N., Wilson, V., Price, M., Hotchkiss, A., Orlando, E. & Guillette, L. 2001. *Effects of Environmental Antiandrogens on Reproductive Development in Experimental Animals.* Human Reproduction Update, Vol. 7, pp. 248–264.
[38] Gray, L.E., Ostby, J., Price, M., Veeramachaneni, D.N., & Parks, L. 2000. Parinatal exposure to the pathalates DEHP, BBP and DIVD, but not DEP, BMP or DOTP alters sexual differentiation of the male rats. *Toxicological Sciences,* Vol. 58, pp. 350-365.
[39] Gray, L.E., Wolf, C., Lambright, C., Mann, P., Price, M., Cooper, R. L. & Ostby, J. 1999. Administration of potentially antiandrogenic pesticides (procymidone, linuron, iprodione, chlozolinate, *p, p'*-DDE, and ketoconazole) and toxic substances (dibutyl-

and diethylhexyl phthalate, PCB 169, and ethane dimethane sulphonate) during sexual differentiation produces diverse profiles of reproductive malformations in the male rat. *Toxicology and Industrial Health*, Vol.15, pp. 94–118.

[40] Ge, R. S., Chen, G. R., Tanrikut, C. & Hardy, M. P. 2007. Phthalate ester toxicity in Leydig cells: Developmental timing and dosage considerations. *Reproductive Toxicology* , Vol.23, pp. 366–373.

[41] Guo, Y. L., Hsu, P. C., Hsu, C. C. & Lambert, G. H. 2000. Semen quality after prenatal exposure to polychlorinated biphenyls and dibenzofurans. *Lancet* , Vol.356, pp. 1240–1241.

[42] Gupta, C. 2000. Reproductive malformation of the male offspring following maternal exposure to estrogenic chemicals. *Proc. Soc. Exp. Biol. Med.* , Vol. 224, pp. 61–68.

[43] Haffner, S. M. 1996. Sex hormone-binding protein, hyper-insulinaemia, insulin resistance and noninsulindependent diabetes. *Hormone Research,* Vol.45, pp. 233–237.

[44] Hargreaves, C.A., Rogers, S., Hills, F., Rahman, F., Howell, R.J. & Homa, S.T. 1998. Effects of co-trimoxazole, erythromycin, amoxycillin, tetracycline and chloroquine on sperm function in vitro. *Human Reproduction,* vol. 13, pp. 1878–1886.

[45] Hauser, R. & Sokol, R., 2008. Science linking environmental contaminant exposures with fertility and reproductive health impacts in the adult male, *Fertilily and Sterility,* Vol. 89: pp. e59–e65.

[46] Hauser, R., Williams, P., Altshul, L. & Calafat, A. M. 2005. Evidence of interaction between polychlorinated biphenyls and phthalates in relation to human sperm motility. *Environmental Health Perspectives,* Vol.113, pp. 425–430.

[47] Hess, R. A., Bunick, D., Lee, K. H., Bahr, J., Taylor, J. A., Korach, K. S., & Lubahn, D. B. 1997. A role for oestrogens in the male repro- ductive system. *Nature.* Vol.390, pp. 509–512.

[48] Isojarvi, J.I., Lofgren, E., & Juntunen K.S., et al. 2004. Effect of epilepsy and antiepileptic drugs on male reproductive health. *Neurology.* Vol. 62, pp. 247–253.

[49] ILSI. 1999. An Evaluation and Interpretation of Reproductive Endpoints for Human Health Risk Assessment (Daston G, Kimmel C, eds), *International Life Sciences Institute Press,* Washington, DC.

[50] Jana, K., Jana, S., & Samanta, P.K. 2006. Effects of chronic exposure to sodium arsenite on hypothalamo-pituitary-testicular activities in adult rats: possible an estrogenic mode of action. *Reproductive Biology Endocrinology,* Vol. 4: pp.9-22.

[51] Jana, K., Samanta, P.K., & De, D.K. 2010a. Nicotine diminishes testicular gametogenesis, steroidogenesis and steroidogenic acute regulatory protein expression in adult albino rats: possible influence on pituitary gonadotropins and alteration of testicular antioxidant status. *Toxicological Sciences,* vol.116, pp. 647-59.

[52] Jana, K., Yin, X., Schiffer, R.B., Chen, J-J., Pandey, A.K., Stocco, D.M., Grammas, P., & Wang, X. 2008. Chrysin, a natural flavonoid enhances steroidogenesis and steroidogenic acute regulatory protein gene expression in mouse Leydig cells. *Journal of Endocrinology,* vol.197, pp. 315-323.

[53] Jana, K., Jana, N., De, D.K., & Guha, S.K. 2010b. Eathanol induces mouse spermatogenic cell apoptosis in vivo through overexpression of Fas/Fas-L, p53, and caspase-3 along with cytochrome-c translocation and glutathione depletion. *Molecular Reproduction & Development,* vol. 77, pp. 820-833.

[54] Jensen, M. S., Mabeck, L. M., Toft, G., Thulstrup, A. M. & Bonde, J.P. 2005. Lower sperm counts following prenatal tobacco exposure. *Human Reproduction,* vol. 20, pp. 2559–8566.

[55] Kabuto, H. et al., 2004. Exposure to bisphenol A during embryonic/fetal life and infancy increases oxidative injury and causes underdevelopment of the brain and testis in mice, *Life Sciences*, Vol. 74, pp. 2931–2940.
[56] Kelce, W. R., Stone, C. R., Laws, S. C., Gray, L. E., Kemppainen, J. A. & Wilson, E. M. 1995. Persistent DDT metabolite p, p'-DDE is a potent androgen receptor antagonist. *Nature*, vol. 375, pp. 581–585.
[57] Khorram, O., Garthwaite, M., Jones, J. & Golos, T. 2004. Expression of aryl hydrocarbon receptor (AHR) and aryl hydrocarbon receptor nuclear translocator (ARNT) mRNA expression in human spermatozoa. *Med. Sci. Monit.*, vol. 10, pp. 135–138.
[58] Khoury, M.J., & Dorman, J.S. 1998. The human genome epidemiology network. *American Journal of Epidemiology*, vol.148, pp.1–3.
[59] Khoury, M.J. 1997. Genetic epidemiology and the future of disease prevention and public health. Epidemiologic Reviews, Vol. 19, pp.175–180.
[60] Kizu, R., Okamura, K., Toriba, A., Kakishima, H., Mizokami, A., Burnstein, K. L. & Hayakawa, K. 2003. A role of aryl hydrocarbon receptor in the antiandrogenic effects of polycyclic aromatic hydrocarbons in LNCaP human prostate carcinoma cells. *Archies of Toxicology*, vol. 77, pp. 335–343.
[61] Kuiper, G. G., Lemmen, J. G., Carlsson, B., Corton, J. C., Safe, S. H., van der Saag, P. T., van der Burg, B., & Gustafsson, J. A. 1998. Interaction of estrogenic chemicals and phytoestrogens with estrogen receptor beta. *Endocrinology* vol. 139, pp. 4252–4263.
[62] Latchoumycandane, C. & Mathur, P.P. 2002. Effects of vitamin E on reactive oxygen species-mediated 2,3,7,8-tetrachlorodi-benzo-p-dioxin toxicity in rat testis, *Journal of Applied Toxicology*, vol. 22, pp. 345–351.
[63] Lawson, C.C., Schnorr, T.M., Daston, G.P., Grajewski, B., Marcus, M., & McDiarmid, M. et al., 2003. An Occupational Reproductive Research Agenda for the Third Millennium. *Environmental Health Perspectives*, vol.111, pp. 584-592.
[64] Lecureur, V. et al., 2005. ERK-dependent induction of TNFalpha expression by the environmental contaminant benzo(a)pyrene in primary human macrophages, *FEBS Letters*, vol. 579, pp. 1904–1910.
[65] Li, M.W.M. et al., 2006. Tumor necrosis factor {alpha} reversibly disrupts the blood-testis barrier and impairs Sertoli-germ cell adhesion in the seminiferous epithelium of adult rat testes, *Journal of Endocrinology*, vol.190, pp. 313–329.
[66] Li, M.W.M., Murk, D.D., & Cheng, C.Y. 2009. Mitogen-activated protein kinases in male reproductive function. *Trends in Molecular Medicine*, vol. 15, pp. 159-168.
[67] Liu, J. et al., 2009. Role of oxidative stress in cadmium toxicity and carcinogenesis, *Toxicology and Applied Pharmacology*, vol. 238, pp. 209–214.
[68] Maire, M., Florin, A., Kaszas, K., Regnier, D., Contard, P., Tabone, E., Mauduit, C., Bars, R. & Benahmed, M. 2005. Alteration of transforming growth factor-beta signaling system expression in adult rat germ cells with a chronic apoptotic cell death process after fetal androgen disruption. *Endocrinology*, Vol. 146, pp. 5135–5143.
[69] Magelssen, H., Brydoy, M. & Fossa, S.D. 2006. The effects of cancer and cancer treatments on male reproductive function. *Nat Clin Pract Urol.* Vol. 3, pp. 312–322.
[70] Martin, R.H., Ernst, S., Rademaker, A., Barclay, L., Ko, E., & Summers, N. 1997. Chromosomal abnormalities in sperm from testicular cancer patients before and after chemotherapy. *Human Genetics*, vol. 99, pp.214-218.
[71] McIntyre, B.S., Barlow, N.J. & Foster, P.M. 2002. Male rats exposed to linuron *in utero* exhibit permanent changes in anogenital distance, nipple retention, and epididymal malformations that result in subsequent testicular atrophy. *Toxicological Sciences*, vol. 65, pp. 62–70.

[72] McKinnell, C., Atanassova, N., Williams, K., Fisher, J.S., Walker, M., Turner, K.J., Saunders, T.K. & Sharpe, R.M. 2001. Suppression of androgen action and the induction of gross abnormalities of the reproductive tract in male rats treated neonatally with diethylstilbestrol. *Journal of Andrology*, vol. 22, pp. 323–*338*.

[73] McKinney, J.D. & Waller, C.L. 1998. Molecular determinants of hormone mimicry: Halogenated aromatic hydrocarbon environmental agents. *Journal of Toxicology and Environmental Health B*, Vol.1, pp. 27–58.

[74] Meeker, J.D., Ryan, L., Barr, D.B., Herrick, R.F., Bennett, D.H., Bravo, R. & Hauser, R. 2004. The relationship of urinary metabolites of carbaryl/naphthalene and chlorpyrifos with human semen quality. *Environmental Health Perspectives* , vol. 112, pp. 1665–1670.

[75] Miller, W.L. 1988. Molecular biology of steroid hormone synthesis. *Endocrine Reviews* , vol. 9, pp. 295–318.

[76] Mitchell, J.H., Cawood, E., Kinniburgh, D., Provan, A., Collins, A. R. & Irvine, D. S. 2001. Effect of a phytoestrogen food supplement on reproductive health in normal males. *Clinical Science (Lond.)*, vol. 100, pp. 613–618.

[77] Moline, J.M., Golden, A., Bar-Chama, N., Smith, E., Rauch, M.E., & Chapin RE, et al., 2000. Exposure to hazardous substances and male reproductive health: a research framework. *Environmental Health Perspectives*, vol. 108, pp.803–813.

[78] Moorman, W.J., Ahlers, H.W., Chapin, R.E., Daston, G.P., Foster, P.M.D., & Kavlock, R.J., et al., 2000. Prioritization of NTP reproductive toxicants for field studies. *Reproductive Toxicology*, vol. 14, pp. 293–301.

[79] Moosani, N., Pattinson, H.A., Carter, M.D., Cox, D.M., Rademaker, A.W., & Martin, R.H. 1995. Chromosomal analysis of sperm from men with idiopathic infertility using sperm karyotyping and fluorescence in situ hybridization. *Fertility and Sterility*, vol. 64, pp. 811-817.

[80] Mylchreest, E., Wallace, D. G., Cattley, R. C. & Foster, P. M. 2000. Dose-dependent alterations in androgen-regulated male reproductive development in rats exposed to di(*n*-butyl). *Toxicological Sciences*, vol. 55, pp. 143–151.

[81] NIOSH. 1978. *National Occupational Hazards Survey*. Vol III. Survey Analysis and Supplemental Tables. DHHS (NIOSH) Publication no. 78-114, National Institute for Occupational Safety and Health, Cincinnati, OH.

[82] NIOSH. 1988. *National Occupational Exposure Survey Analysis of Management Interview Responses*. DHHS (NIOSH) Publ no. 89-103, National Institute for Occupational Safety and Health, Cincinnati, OH.

[83] O'Donnell, L., Robertson, K. M., Jones, M. E. & Simpson, E. R. 2001. Estrogen and spermatogenesis. *Endocrinine Reviews*, vol. 22, pp. 289–318.

[84] Overstreet, J.W., Fuh, V.L., & Gould, J. et al. 1999. Chronic treatment with finasteride daily does not affect spermatogenesis or semen production in young men. *Journal of Urology*, vol. 162, pp.1295–1300.

[85] Nudell, D.M., Monoski, M.M. & Lipshultz, L.I. 2002. Common medications and drugs: how they affect male fertility. *Urol Clin North Am.* Vol. 29, pp. 965–973.

[86] Pant, N., Mathur, N., Banerjee, A.K., Srivastava, S. P. & Saxena, D.K. 2004. Correlation of chlorinated pesticides concentration in semen with seminal vesicle and prostatic markers. *Reproductive Toxicology*, vol. 19, pp. 209–214.

[87] Park, J.D., Habeebu, S.S. & Klaassen, C.D. 2002. Testicular toxicity of di-(2-ethylhexyl)phthalate in young Sprague-Dawley rats. *Toxicology* , vol. 171, pp. 105–115.

[88] Parks, L.G., Ostby, J.S., Lambright, C.R., Abbott, B.D., Klinefelter, G.R., Barlow, N.J. & Gray, L.E. Jr. 2000. The plasticizer diethylhexyl phthalate induces malformations by decreasing fetal testosterone synthesis during sexual differentiation in the male rat. *Toxicological Sciences*, vol. 58, pp. 339–349.

[89] Peltola, V., Mantyla, E., Huhtaniemi, I. & Ahotupa, M. 1994. Lipid peroxidation and antioxidant enzyme activities in the rat testis after cigarette smoke inhalation or administration of polychlorinated biphenyls or polychlorinated naphthalenes. *Journal of Andrology* , vol. 15, pp. 353–361.

[90] Peterson, R.E., Theobald, H.M. & Kimmel, G.L. 1993. Developmental and reproductive toxicity of dioxins and related compounds: Cross-species comparisons. *Critical Reviews in Toxicology* , vol. 23, pp. 283–335.

[91] Phillips, K.P. & Tanphaichitr N. 2008. Human exposure to endocrine disrupters and semen quality, *Journal of Toxicology and Environmental Health Part B*. vol. 11, pp. 188-220

[92] Pryor, J.L., Hughes, C., Foster, W., Hales, B.F., & Robaire, B. 2000. Critical windows of exposure for children's health: The reproduc- tive system in ani mals and humans. *Environmental Health Perspectives*, vol. 108, pp. 491–503.

[93] Purvis, K., Magnus, O., Morkas, L., Abyholm, T., & Rui, H. 1986. Ejaculate composition after masturbation and coitus in the human male. *International Journal of Andrology*, vol. 9, pp. 401–406.

[94] Qureshi, M.S., Pennington, J.H., Goldsmith, H.J., & Cox, P.E. 1972. Cyclophosphamide therapy and sterility. *Lancet*, vol. 16, pp. 1290-1291.

[95] Rajpert-De Meyts, E., Bartkova, J., Samson, M., Hoei-Hansen, C.E., Frydelund-Larsen, L., Bartek, J. & Skakkebaek, N.E. 2003. The emerging phenotype of the testicular carcinoma in situ germ cell. *Acta Pathologica, Microbiologica et Immunologica Scandinavica*, vol. 111, pp. 267–*278*.

[96] Ramlau-Hansen, C.H., Thulstrup, A. ., Aggerholm, A.S., Jensen, M.S., Toft, G. & Bonde, J. P. 2007. Is smoking a risk factor for decreased semen quality? A cross-sectional analysis. *Human Reproduction, vol.* 22, pp. 188–196.

[97] Richardson, D.B., & Wing, S. 1998. Methods for investigating age differences in the effects of prolonged exposures. *American Journal of Industrial Medicine*, vol. 33, pp.123–130.

[98] Rivas, A., Fisher, J.S., McKinnell, C., Atanassova, N. & Sharpe, R.M. 2002. Induction of reproductive tract developmental abnormalities in the male rat by lowering androgen production or action in combination with a low dose of diethylstilbestrol: evidence for importance of the androgen–estrogen balance. *Endocrinology*, vol. 143, pp. 4797–*4808*.

[99] Robbins, W.A., Vine, M.F., Truong, K.Y. & Everson, R.B. 1997. Use of FISH (fluorescence in situ hybridization) to assess effects of smoking, caffeine, and alcohol on aneuploidy load in sperm of healthy men. *Environmental Molecular Mutagenesis*, vol. 30, pp. 175–183.

[100] Roy, D., Palangat, M., Chen, C.W., Thomas, R.D., Colerangle, J., Atkinson, A., and Yan, Z.J. 1997. Biochemical and molecular changes at the cellular level in response to exposure to environmental estrogen-like chemicals. *Journal of Toxicology and Environmental Health*, vol. 50, pp.1–29.

[101] Rozati, R., Reddy, P.P., Reddanna, P. & Mujtaba, R. 2002. Role of environmental estrogens in the deterioration of male factor fertility. *Fertility and Sterility*, vol. 78, pp. 1187–1194.

[102] Ryu, J.Y., Whang, J., Park, H., Im, J. Y., Kim, J., Ahn, M. Y., Lee, J., Kim, H. S., Lee, B. M., Yoo, S.D., Kwack, S. J., Oh, J. H., Park, K. L., Han, S. Y. & Kim, S.H. 2007. Di(2-ethylhexyl) phthalate induces apoptosis through peroxisome proliferators-activated receptor-gamma and ERK 1/2 activation in testis of Sprague-Dawley rats. *Journal of Toxicology and Environmental Health part A*, vol. 70, pp. 1296–1303.

[103] Sanderson, J.T., Seinen, W., Giesy, J.P. & van den Berg, M. 2000. 2-Chloro-*s*-triazine herbicides induce aromatase (CYP19) activity in H295R human adrenocortical carcinoma cells: A novel mechanism for estrogenicity?. *Toxicological Sciences*, vol. 54: pp. 121–127.

[104] Sandoval, K.E. & Witt, K.A. 2008. Blood-brain barrier tight junction permeability and ischemic stroke. *Neurobiology of Disease*, vol. 32, pp. 200–219.

[105] Schrader SM. 1997. Male reproductive toxicity. In: *Handbook of Human Toxicology* (Massaro EJ, ed). pp. 962-980, CRC Press, Boca Raton, FL.

[106] Schlegel, P.N., Chang, T.S. & Marshall, F.F. 1991. Antibiotics: potential hazards to male fertility. *Fertility and Sterility*, vol. 55, pp. 235–242.

[107] Seed, J., Chapin, R.E., Clegg, E.D., Dostal, L.A., Foote, R.H., & Hurtt, M.E., et al., 1996. Methods for assessing sperm motility, morphology, and counts in the rat, rabbit, and dog: a consensus report. *Reproductive Toxicology*, vol. 10, pp. 237–244.

[108] Sharpe, R.M., & Irvine, D.S. 2004. How strong is the evidence of a link between environmental chemicals and adverse effects on human reproductive health. *BMJ*,. vol. 328, pp. 447-451.

[109] Sharpe RM & Franks S. 2002. Environment, lifestyle and infertility - an inter-generational issue. *Nature Cell Biology 4,* (Suppl) S33–S40.

[110] Sharpe, R.M. 2003. The 'oestrogen hypothesis' - where do we stand now? *International Journal of Andrology*, vol. 26, pp. 2–15.

[111] Sharpe, R.M. 2010. Environmental/lifestyle effects on spermatogenesis. *Phil. Trans. R. Soc. B.*, vol. 365, pp. 1697- 1712.

[112] Sharpe, R.M., & Skakkebaek, N.E. 1993. Are oestrogens involved in falling sperm counts and disorders of the male reproductive tract? *Lancet*, vol. 29, pp. 1392-1395.

[113] Sikka, S.C. 2001. Relative impact of oxidative stress on male reproductive function, *Current Medicinal Chemistry*, vol. 8, pp. 851–862.

[114] Skakkebaek, N.E., Holm, M., Hoei-Hansen, C., Jorgensen, N. & Rajpert-De Meyts, E. 2003. Association between testicular dysgenesis syndrome (TDS) and testicular neoplasia: evidence from 20 adult patients with signs of maldevelopment of the testis. *Acta Pathologica, Microbiologica et Immunologica Scandinavica*, vol. 111, pp. 1–9.

[115] Skakkebaek, N.E., Rajpert-De Meyts, E. & Main, K.M. 2001. Testicular dysgenesis syndrome: an increasingly common developmental disorder with environmental aspects. *Human Reproduction*, vol. 16, pp. 972–978.

[116] Stillman, R.J. 1982. *In utero* exposure to diethylstilbestrol: adverse effects on the reproductive tract and reproductive performance and male and female offspring. *American Journal of Obstetrics and Gynecology*, vol. 142, pp. 905–921.

[117] Stone, R. 2007. Epidemiology. Agent Orange's bitter harvest. *Science*, vol. 315, pp. 176–179.

[118] Strauss, L., Santti, R., Saarinen, N., Streng, T., Joshi, S. & Makela, S. 1998. Dietary phytoestrogens and their role in hormonally dependent disease. *Toxicology Letters*, vol. 102–103, pp. 349–354.

[119] Swan, S.H., Elkin, E.P., & Fenster, L. 1997. Have sperm densities declined? A reanalysis of global trend data. *Environmental Health Perspectives*, vol. 105, pp. 1228-1232.

[120] Swan, S.H. 2006. Semen quality in fertile US men in relation to geographical area and pesticide exposure. *International Journal of Andrology* , vol. 29, pp. 62–68.

[121] Swan, S.H., Kruse, R.L., Liu, F., Barr, D.B., Drobnis, E.Z., Redmon, J.B., Wang, C., Brazil, C., Overstreet, J.W. & Study for Future Families Research Group. 2003. Semen quality in relation to biomarkers of pesticide exposure. *Environmental Health Perspective,* vol. 111, pp. 1478–1484.

[122] Tong, W., Perkins, R., Sterlitz, R., Collantes, E.R., Keenan, S., & Welsh, W.J., et al.,1997. Quantitative structure-activity relationships (QSARs) for estrogen binding to the estrogen receptor: predictions across species. *Environmental Health Perspectives,* vol. 105, pp. 1116–1124.

[123] Toppari, J., Larsen, J.C., Christiansen, P., Giwercman, A., Grandjean, P., Guillett, L.J. Jr., et al., 1996. Male reproductive health and environmental xenoestrogens. *Environmental Health Perspectives,* vol. 104 (Suppl 4), pp. 741–803.

[124] Tremellen, K. 2008. Oxidative stress and male infertility – a clinical perspective, *Human Reproduction Update*, vol. 14, pp. 243–258.

[125] Tsai-Morris, C.H., Knox, G., Luna, S. & Dufau, M.L. 1986. Acquisition of estradiol-mediated regulatory mechanism of steroidogenesis in cultured fetal rat Leydig cells. *Journal of Biological Chemistry*, vol. 261, pp. 3471–3474.

[126] Toyoshiba, H., Yamanaka, T., Sone, H., Parham, F. M., Walker, N. J., Martinez, J. & Portier, C.J. 2004. Gene interaction network suggests dioxin induces a significant linkage between aryl hydrocarbon receptor and retinoic acid receptor beta. *Environmental Health Perspectives* , vol. 112, pp. 1217–1224.

[127] Turner, T.T. & Lysiak, J.J. 2008. Oxidative stress: a common factor in testicular dysfunction, *Journal of Androl* , vol. 29, pp. 488–498.

[128] U.S. EPA. 1998a. Health Effect Test Guidelines. Reproduction and Fertility Effects. OPPTS 870.3800, U.S. Environmental Protection Agency, Washington DC.

[129] U.S. EPA. 1998b. Endocrine Disruptor Screening and Testing Advisory Committee (EDSTAC); Final Report. U.S. EPA, Washington, DC.

[130] Vine, M.F. 1996. Smoking and male reproduction: A review. *International Journal of Andrology*, vol. 19, pp. 323–337.

[131] Walker, W.H., & Cheng, J. 2005. FSH and testosterone signaling in Sertoli cells. *Reproduction*, vol. 130, pp.15–28.

[132] Whelan EA, Grajewski B, Wild DK, Schnorr TM, & Alderfer R. 1996. Evaluation of reproductive function among men occupationally exposed to a stilbene derivative. II. Perceived libido and potency. *American Journal of Industrial Medicine*, vol. 29, pp.59–65.

[133] Whitten, P.L. & Naftolin, F. 1998. Reproductive actions of phytoestrogens. *Bail. Clin. Endocrinol. Metab.* , vol. 12, pp. 667–690.

[134] Wilcox, A.J., Baird, D.D., Weinberg, C.R., Hornsby, P.P. & Herbst, A.L. 1995. Fertility in men exposed prenatally to diethylstilbestrol. *New England Journal of Meicine.* Vol. 332, pp. 1411–1416.

[135] Whorton, D., Krauss, R.M., Marshall, S., & Milby, T.H. 1977. Infertility in male pesticide workers. *Lancet*, vol. 2, pp. 1259–1261.

[136] Wolf, C.J., LeBlanc, G.A., Ostby, J.S. & Gray, L.E. Jr. 2000. Characterization of the period of sensitivity of fetal male sexual development to vinclozolin. *Toxicological Sciences*, vol. 55, pp.152–161.

[137] Wong C.H. & Cheng, C.Y. 2005. Mitogen-activated protein kinases, adherens junction dynamics, and spermatogenesis: A review of recent data. *Developmental Biology*, vol. 286, pp. 1-15.

[138] Wong, C.H., Murk, D.D., Lui, W.Y., & Cheng, C.Y. 2004. Regulation of blood-testis barrier dynamics: an in vivo study. Journal of Cell Sciences, vol. 117, pp. 783-798.

[139] Wong, E.W.P. & Cheng, C.Y. 2011. Impacts of environmental toxicants on male reproductive dysfunction. *Trends in Pharmacological Sciences*, vol. 32, pp. 290-299.

[140] Wong, C., Kelce, W.R., Sar, M. & Wilson, E.M. 1995. Androgen receptor antagonist versus agonist activities of the fungicide vinclozolin relative to hydroxyflutamide. *Journal of Biological Chemistry*, vol. 270, pp. 19998–20003.

[141] Woodruff, T.J., Carlson, A., Schwartz, J.M., & Giudice, L.C. 2008. Proceedings of the sumit on environmental challenges to reproductive health and fertility: executive summary. *Fertility and Sterility*, vol. 89, pp. 281-300.

[142] World Health Organization (WHO). 1999. WHO laboratory manual for the examination of human sperm and semen-cervical mucus interaction, *4th ed, Cambridge University Press*, Cambridge, NY.

[143] Wozniak, A.L., Bulayeva, N.N. & Watson, C.S. 2005. Xenoestrogens at picomolar to nanomolar concentrations trigger membrane estrogen receptor-α-mediated Ca++ fluxes and prolactin release in GH3/B6 pituitary tumor cells. *Environmental Health Perspectives,* vol. 113, pp. 431–439.

[144] Wyrobeck, A.J., Schrader, S.M., Perreault, S.D., Fenster, L., Huszar, G., Katz, D.F., Osorio, A.M., Sublet, V., & Evenson, D. 1997. Assessment of reproductive disorders and birth defects in communities near hazardous chemical sites. III: Guidelines for field studies of male reproductive disorders. *Reproductive Toxicology*, vol. 11, pp. 243-259.

[145] You, L., Casanova, M., Archibeque-Engle, S., Sar, M., Fan, L.Q. & Heck, H.A. 1998. Impaired male sexual development in perinatal Sprague-Dawley and Long-Evans hooded rats exposed *in utero* and lactationally to p,p' *-DDE. Toxicological Sciences,* vol. 45, pp.162–173.

[146] Zinaman, M.J., Brown, C.C., Selevan, S.G., & Clegg, E.D. 2000. Semen quality and human fertility: a prospective study with healthy couples. *Journal of Andrology*, vol. 21, pp. 145–153.